ENDOSCOPIC TECHNIQUES IN GASTROENTEROLOGY

Dr. Ahmed Mohamed Helmy

ALLIED
HEALTH
PRESS

Endoscopic Techniques in Gastroenterology

Author: **Dr. Ahmed Mohamed Helmy**

Allied Health Press
4164 Lakeshore Road
Burlington ON L7L 1A4
Canada
www.alliedhealthpress.com
Email: orders@arclereducation.com

ISBN: 978-1-77956-833-5

Allied Health Press publishes wide variety of books and eBooks. For more information about Allied Health Press and its products, visit our website at www.alliedhealthpress.com

ABOUT THE AUTHOR

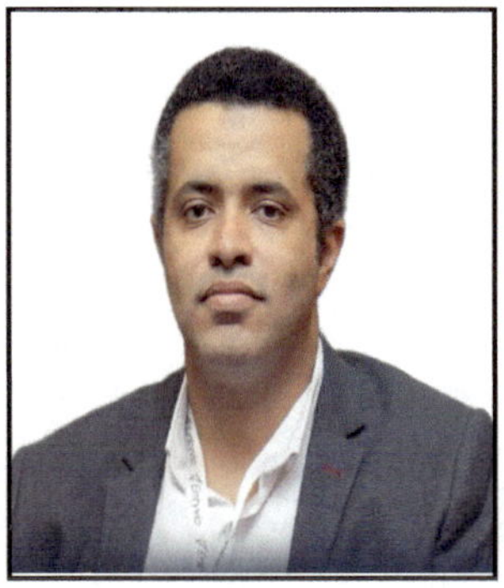

Dr. Ahmed Helmy is a physician with over 15 years of extensive experience in internal medicine, gastroenterology, hepatology, and gastrointestinal (GI) endoscopy. His clinical acumen is rooted in a solid academic foundation and years of dedicated practice in both hospital and academic settings.He began his medical career at Raghi GIT and Hepatology Hospital, Assiut University, where he completed a rigorous residency program. Building on that, he earned a master's degree in gastroenterology, hepatology, and infectious diseases from the same esteemed institution. To further refine his technical skills, Dr. Helmy pursued advanced training and received a GI endoscopy diploma from Ain Shams University, one of Egypt's leading medical universities.

Dr. Helmy currently serves as a consultant of gastroenterology and endoscopy at Assiut P.Staff Hospital, where he specializes in the diagnosis, treatment, and procedural management of a broad spectrum of gastrointestinal conditions. His clinical focus includes chronic liver disease, inflammatory bowel disease, gastrointestinal bleeding, and advanced endoscopic techniques.

In addition to his clinical role, Dr. Helmy is a recognized leader in gastroenterology research. His scholarly interests center around improving diagnostic accuracy and therapeutic strategies in hepatogastroenterology. He has contributed to academic forums, with particular emphasis on liver disease epidemiology, novel endoscopic technologies, and the intersection of infectious diseases with GI disorders. His work has informed evidence-based practices and has been instrumental in shaping regional treatment protocols. Dr. Helmy remains committed to advancing the field through a combination of patient-centered care, academic collaboration, and continuous research innovation.

Brief Table of Contents

1. Introduction to Endoscopy 1
2. Instrumentation and Equipment 35
3. Patient Preparation and Sedation 65
4. Upper Gastrointestinal Endoscopy (Esophagogastr-oduodenoscopy – EGD) 95
5. Colonoscopy 127
6. Sigmoidoscopy and Proctoscopy 157
7. Endoscopic Retrograde Cholangiopancreatography (ERCP) 187
8. Endoscopic Ultrasound (EUS) 217
9. Capsule Endoscopy 249
10. Enteroscopy Techniques 281
11. Therapeutic Endoscopy 311
12. Advanced Imaging in Endoscopy 341
13. Pediatric Endoscopy 375
14. Complications of Endoscopy 407
15. Endoscopy in Inflammatory Bowel Disease (IBD) 441

Index 473

Detailed Table of Contents

List of Figures *xv*
Preface *xxiii*

CHAPTER 1

Introduction to Endoscopy 1

Introduction of Endoscopy **1**
1.1. Historical Background **5**
1.1.1. Early Developments in Endoscopic Techniques 6
1.1.2. Key Figures in the Evolution of Endoscopy 7
1.1.3. Milestones in Technology and Instrumentation 8
1.2. Types of Endoscopic Procedures **9**
1.2.1. Gastrointestinal Endoscopy 10
1.2.2. Bronchoscopy 11
1.2.3. Urological Endoscopy 12
1.3. Indications for Endoscopy **13**
1.3.1. Diagnostic Purposes 13
1.3.2. Therapeutic Interventions 14
1.3.3. Screening for Diseases 15
1.4. Preparation for Endoscopy **16**
1.4.1. Patient Assessment and Medical History 17
1.4.2. Pre-Procedure Instructions 18
1.4.3. Importance of Informed Consent 18
1.5. Risks and Complications **19**
1.5.1. Common Risks Associated with Endoscopy 20
1.5.2. Potential Complications During the Procedure 21
1.5.3. Post-Procedure Care and Monitoring 22
1.6. Advances in Endoscopic Technology **23**
1.6.1. Innovations in Imaging Techniques 24
1.6.2. Development of Minimally Invasive Tools 25
1.6.3. Future Trends in Endoscopic Research 25
Summary **27**
References **30**

CHAPTER 2

Instrumentation and Equipment 35

Introduction **35**
2.1. Types of Instrumentation **38**
2.1.1. Analytical Instrumentation 39
2.1.2. Measurement Instrumentation 40
2.1.3. Control Instrumentation 41
2.2. Common Equipment in Laboratories **42**
2.2.1. Spectrophotometers 42
2.2.2. Chromatographs 43
2.2.3. Microscopes 44
2.3. Instrumentation in Medical Applications **45**
2.3.1. Diagnostic Equipment 46
2.3.2. Monitoring Devices 47
2.3.3. Therapeutic Instruments 48
2.4. Industrial Instrumentation **48**
2.4.1. Process Control Systems 49
2.4.2. Quality Assurance Tools 50

2.4.3. Safety Instrumentation 51
2.5. Advances in Instrumentation Technology **52**
2.5.1. Automation and Robotics 53
2.5.2. Digital vs. Analog Instrumentation 54
2.5.3. Integration of Artificial Intelligence (AI) in Instrumentation 54
2.6. Maintenance and Calibration of Equipment **55**
2.6.1. Importance of Regular Maintenance 56
2.6.2. Calibration Procedures 57
2.6.3. Troubleshooting Common Issues 58
Summary **59**
References **62**

CHAPTER 3

Patient Preparation and Sedation **65**

Introduction **65**
3.1. Understanding Patient Preparation **68**
3.1.1. The Role of Patient History in Preparation 69
3.1.2. Physical Assessments Before Sedation 70
3.1.3. Psychological Considerations for Patients 71
3.2. Types of Sedation **72**
3.2.1. Minimal Sedation and Its Applications 73
3.2.2. Moderate Sedation and Its Benefits 74
3.2.3. Deep Sedation and Its Risks 75
3.3. Pre-Sedation Protocols **76**
3.3.1. Fasting Guidelines Before Sedation 76
3.3.2. Medication Review and Adjustments 77
3.3.3. Informed Consent Process 78
3.4. Monitoring During Sedation **78**
3.4.1. Vital Signs and Their Significance 79
3.4.2. Use of Monitoring Equipment 80
3.4.3. Role of Healthcare Professionals in Monitoring 81
3.5. Post-Sedation Care **82**
3.5.1. Recovery Room Protocols 83
3.5.2. Assessing Patient Readiness for Discharge 84
3.5.3. Instructions for Post-Procedure Care 84
3.6. Complications and Risks **85**
3.6.1. Common Complications Associated with Sedation 86
3.6.2. Risk Factors That Increase Complications 87
3.6.3. Strategies for Minimizing Risks 87
Summary **89**
References **92**

CHAPTER 4

Upper Gastrointestinal Endoscopy (Esophagogastr-oduodenoscopy – EGD) **95**

Introduction **95**
4.1. Indications for Esophagogastroduodenoscopy (EGD) **99**
4.1.1. Evaluation of Gastrointestinal Symptoms 100
4.1.2. Diagnosis of Esophageal Disorders 101
4.1.3. Assessment of Gastric and Duodenal Conditions 102
4.2. Preparation for Esophagogastroduodenoscopy (EGD) **103**
4.2.1. Pre-procedure Instructions for Patients 104
4.2.2. Dietary Restrictions Before the Procedure 105
4.2.3. Medications and Anesthesia Considerations 105
4.3. The Esophagogastroduodenoscopy (EGD) Procedure **106**
4.3.1. Description of the Equipment Used 107
4.3.2. Step-by-Step Process of the Procedure 108
4.3.3. Duration and Setting of the Procedure 109
4.4. Risks and Complications **109**
4.4.1. Common Risks Associated with Esophagogastroduodenoscopy (EGD) 110
4.4.2. Rare but Serious Complications 111
4.4.3. Management of Complications if They Occur 111
4.5. Post-Procedure Care **112**
4.5.1. Recovery Process and Monitoring 113
4.5.2. Dietary Recommendations After Esophagogastroduodenoscopy (EGD) 114
4.5.3. Follow-Up Appointments and Results Discussion 115

4.6. Advances in Esophagogastroduodenoscopy (EGD) Technology 116
4.6.1. Innovations in Endoscopic Equipment 117
4.6.2. Development of Minimally Invasive Techniques 117
4.6.3. Future Trends in Gastrointestinal Endoscopy 118
Summary 120
References 123

CHAPTER 5

Colonoscopy 127

Introduction 127
5.1. Purpose of Colonoscopy 130
5.1.1. Screening for Colorectal Cancer (CRC) 131
5.1.2. Diagnosing Gastrointestinal Disorders 132
5.1.3. Monitoring Inflammatory Bowel Diseases (IBD) 133
5.2. The Colonoscopy Procedure 133
5.2.1. Preparation for the Procedure 134
5.2.2. The Actual Procedure Process 135
5.2.3. Post-Procedure Care and Recovery 136
5.3. Risks and Complications 137
5.3.1. Common Risks Associated with Colonoscopy 138
5.3.2. Rare But Serious Compli cations 139
5.3.3. Factors That Increase Risk 140
5.4. Benefits of Colonoscopy 140
5.4.1. Early Detection of Cancer 141
5.4.2. Prevention of Colorectal Cancer (CRC) 142
5.4.3. Improved Management of Gastrointestinal Conditions 143
5.5. Patient Experience 144
5.5.1. Emotional and Psychological Aspects 145
5.5.2. Patient Testimonials and Perspectives 145
5.5.3. Addressing Common Fears and Misconceptions 146
5.6. Alternatives to Colonoscopy 147
5.6.1. Other Screening Methods 148
5.6.2. Pros and Cons of Alternatives 149
5.6.3. Recommendations for Different Patient Needs 149
Summary 151
References 154

CHAPTER 6

Sigmoidoscopy and Proctoscopy 157

Introduction 157
6.1. Historical Background 160
6.1.1. Development of Sigmoidoscopy and Proctoscopy Techniques 161
6.1.2. Key Figures in the Advancement of These Procedures 162
6.1.3. Evolution of Medical Instruments Used 163
6.2. Indications for Procedures 163
6.2.1. Diagnostic Purposes for Gastrointestinal Disorders 164
6.2.2. Screening for Colorectal Cancer 165
6.2.3. Evaluation of Inflammatory Bowel Diseases (IBD) 166
6.3. Procedure Overview 167
6.3.1. Preparation Required for Patients 168
6.3.2. Step-by-Step Process of Sigmoidoscopy 168
6.3.3. Step-by-Step Process of Proctoscopy 169
6.4. Risks and Complications 170
6.4.1. Common Risks Associated with Both Procedures 171
6.4.2. Potential Complications During and After the Procedures 172
6.4.3. Strategies for Minimizing Risks 172
6.5. Patient Experience 173
6.5.1. What Patients Can Expect During the Procedures 174
6.5.2. Pain Management and Sedation Options 175
6.5.3. Post-Procedure Care and Recovery 176
6.6. Comparison of Sigmoidoscopy and Proctoscopy 177
6.6.1. Differences in Scope and Reach of Each Procedure 177
6.6.2. Advantages and Disadvantages of Each Method 178
6.6.3. Situational Appropriateness for Each Procedure 179

Summary 181

References 184

CHAPTER 7

Endoscopic Retrograde Cholangiopancreatography (ERCP) 187

Introduction 187

7.1. Indications for Endoscopic Retrograde Cholangiopancreatography (ERCP) 191

7.1.1. Diagnosis of Biliary Tract Disorders 192

7.1.2. Management of Pancreatic Diseases 193

7.1.3. Treatment of Bile Duct Obstructions 194

7.2. Procedure of Endoscopic Retrograde Cholangiopancreatography (ERCP) 195

7.2.1. Pre-Procedural Preparations 195

7.2.2. Step-by-Step Process of the Procedure 196

7.2.3. Post-Procedural Care and Monitoring 197

7.3. Risks and Complications 198

7.3.1. Common Complications Associated with Endoscopic Retrograde Cholangiopancreatography (ERCP) 199

7.3.2. Risk Factors That Increase Complications 199

7.3.3. Strategies for Minimizing Risks 200

7.4. Diagnostic Applications 201

7.4.1. Use of Endoscopic Retrograde Cholangiopancreatography (ERCP) in Diagnosing Cholangitis 202

7.4.2. Role of Endoscopic Retrograde Cholangiopancreatography (ERCP) in Identifying Pancreatic Tumors 203

7.4.3. Evaluation of Biliary Stones Through Endoscopic Retrograde Cholangiopancreatography (ERCP) 203

7.5. Therapeutic Applications 204

7.5.1. Endoscopic Removal of Bile Duct Stones 205

7.5.2. Stenting Procedures for Bile Duct Obstructions 206

7.5.3. Management of Strictures in the Biliary System 207

7.6. Advances in Endoscopic Retrograde Cholangiopancreatography (ERCP) Technology 207

7.6.1. Innovations in Endoscopic Equipment 208

7.6.2. Development of Imaging Techniques 209

7.6.3. Future Trends in Endoscopic Retrograde Cholangiopancreatography (ERCP) Procedures 210

Summary 211

References 214

CHAPTER 8

Endoscopic Ultrasound (EUS) 217

Introduction 217

8.1. Mechanism of Action 221

8.1.1. Description of the Endoscopic Ultrasound (EUS) Procedure 222

8.1.2. Types of Ultrasound Waves Used 223

8.1.3. Role of Endoscopes in Endoscopic Ultrasound (EUS) 223

8.2. Indications for Endoscopic Ultrasound (EUS) 224

8.2.1. Diagnosis of Gastrointestinal Disorders 225

8.2.2. Evaluation of Pancreatic Conditions 226

8.2.3. Staging of Cancers 227

8.3. Advantages of Endoscopic Ultrasound (EUS) 227

8.3.1. Minimally Invasive Nature 228

8.3.2. High-Resolution Imaging Capabilities 229

8.3.3. Ability to Perform Fine-Needle Aspiration (FNA) 230

8.4. Limitations of Endoscopic Ultrasound (EUS) 231

8.4.1. Technical Challenges and Limitations 232

8.4.2. Patient-Related Factors Affecting Outcomes 233

8.4.3. Comparison with Other Imaging Modalities 233

8.5. Endoscopic Ultrasound (EUS) in Clinical Practice 234

8.5.1. Role in Gastroenterology 235

8.5.2. Use in Oncology 236

8.5.3. Integration with Other Diagnostic Tools 236

8.6. Future Directions in Endoscopic Ultrasound (EUS) 237

8.6.1. Technological Advancements 238

8.6.2. Potential for New Applications 239

8.6.3. Research and Clinical Trials 240

Summary 242

References 245

CHAPTER 9

Capsule Endoscopy 249

Introduction to Capsule Endoscopy 249

9.1. The Technology Behind Capsule Endoscopy 253

9.1.1. Description of the Capsule Design and Components 254

9.1.2. Mechanism of Action During the Procedure 255

9.1.3. Comparison with Traditional Endoscopic Methods 256

9.2. Indications for Capsule Endoscopy (CE) 257

9.2.1. Diagnosis of Small Bowel Disorders 257

9.2.2. Evaluation of Gastrointestinal Bleeding 258

9.2.3. Assessment of Inflammatory Bowel Diseases (IBD) 259

9.3. Procedure and Patient Experience 260

9.3.1. Preparation Required Before the Procedure 261

9.3.2. Step-by-Step Overview of the Capsule Ingestion Process 262

9.3.3. Post-Procedure Monitoring and Data Retrieval 263

9.4. Advantages of Capsule Endoscopy 263

9.4.1. Non-Invasive Nature of the Procedure 264

9.4.2. Enhanced Visualization of the Small Intestine 265

9.4.3. Increased Patient Comfort and Compliance 266

9.5. Limitations and Challenges 267

9.5.1. Potential for Incomplete Visualization 268

9.5.2. Risk of Capsule Retention in the Gastrointestinal Tract 268

9.5.3. Limitations in Diagnostic Capabilities Compared to Traditional Methods 269

9.6. Future Directions in Capsule Endoscopy 270

9.6.1. Technological Advancements on the Horizon 271

9.6.2. Potential Integration with Artificial Intelligence (AI) 272

9.6.3. Expanding Applications in Gastrointestinal Health 273

Summary 274

References 277

CHAPTER 10

Enteroscopy Techniques 281

Introduction 281

10.1. Historical Background 284

10.1.1. Development of Enteroscopy Techniques 285

10.1.2. Key Milestones in Enteroscopy 285

10.1.3. Evolution of Technology in Enteroscopy 286

10.2. Types of Enteroscopy 287

10.2.1. Push Enteroscopy 288

10.2.2. Balloon-Assisted Enteroscopy 289

10.2.3. Double-Balloon Enteroscopy 290

10.3. Indications for Enteroscopy 291

10.3.1. Diagnosis of Small Bowel Diseases 291

10.3.2. Management of Gastrointestinal Bleeding 292

10.3.3. Evaluation of Suspected Malignancies 293

10.4. Preparation for Enteroscopy 294

10.4.1. Patient Assessment and Selection 295

10.4.2. Pre-procedural Instructions 295

10.4.3. Sedation and Anesthesia Considerations 296

10.5. Enteroscopy Procedure 297

10.5.1. Step-by-Step Overview of the Procedure 298

10.5.2. Role of the Endoscopist 299

10.5.3. Use of Imaging and Tools During Enteroscopy 300

10.6. Complications and Risks 300

10.6.1. Common Complications Associated with Enteroscopy 301

10.6.2. Risk Factors for Adverse Events (AEs) 302

10.6.3. Strategies for Minimizing Risks 302

Summary 304

References 307

CHAPTER 11

Therapeutic Endoscopy 311

Introduction 311

11.1. Historical Background 314

11.1.1. Development of Endoscopic Techniques 314

11.1.2. Milestones in Therapeutic Endoscopy 315

11.1.3. Evolution of Technology in Endoscopy 317

11.2. Types of Therapeutic Endoscopy **318**
11.2.1. Gastrointestinal Endoscopy 318
11.2.2. Bronchoscopic Procedures 319
11.2.3. Urological Endoscopy 320
11.3. Indications for Therapeutic Endoscopy **321**
11.3.1. Diagnosis of Gastrointestinal Disorders 321
11.3.2. Treatment of Malignancies 322
11.3.3. Management of Bleeding and Obstructions 323
11.4. Techniques and Procedures **324**
11.4.1. Endoscopic Mucosal Resection (EMR) 325
11.4.2. Endoscopic Retrograde Cholangiopancreatography (ERCP) 326
11.4.3. Endoscopic Ultrasound (EUS) 326
11.5. Risks and Complications **327**
11.5.1. Common Complications Associated with Procedures 328
11.5.2. Risk Factors Influencing Complications 329
11.5.3. Strategies for Minimizing Risks 330
11.6. Future Directions in Therapeutic Endoscopy **331**
11.6.1. Innovations in Endoscopic Technology 331
11.6.2. Potential for Robotic-Assisted Endoscopy 332
11.6.3. Research Trends and Clinical Trials 333
Summary **335**
References **338**

CHAPTER 12

Advanced Imaging in Endoscopy 341

Introduction **341**
12.1. Historical Background of Endoscopy **345**
12.1.1. Early Techniques and Limitations 346
12.1.2. Development of Fiber-Optic Technology 346
12.1.3. Milestones in Imaging Advancements 347
12.2. Types of Advanced Imaging Techniques **348**
12.2.1. High-Definition Endoscopy 349
12.2.2. Narrow-Band Imaging (NBI) 350
12.2.3. Confocal Laser Endomicroscopy (CLE) 351
12.3. Benefits of Advanced Imaging in Endoscopy **352**
12.3.1. Enhanced Visualization of Tissues 353
12.3.2. Improved Diagnostic Accuracy 354
12.3.3. Reduction in Unnecessary Biopsies 354
12.4. Applications of Advanced Imaging in Various Medical Fields **355**
12.4.1. Gastroenterology 356
12.4.2. Pulmonology 358
12.4.3. Urology 358
12.5. Challenges and Limitations **359**
12.5.1. Cost and Accessibility of Advanced Imaging Technologies 360
12.5.2. Training and Expertise Required for Practitioners 361
12.5.3. Potential for Overdiagnosis and Overtreatment 362
12.6. Future Trends in Endoscopic Imaging **362**
12.6.1. Integration of Artificial Intelligence (AI) 363
12.6.2. Development of Portable Imaging Devices 364
12.6.3. Innovations in Imaging Software and Analysis 365
Summary **367**
References **370**

CHAPTER 13

Pediatric Endoscopy 375

Introduction **375**
13.1. Historical Background **378**
13.1.1. Development of Endoscopic Techniques 379
13.1.2. Milestones in Pediatric Endoscopy 379
13.1.3. Evolution of Equipment and Technology 380
13.2. Types of Pediatric Endoscopy **381**
13.2.1. Gastrointestinal Endoscopy 382
13.2.2. Bronchoscopy 383
13.2.3. Ureteroscopy 384
13.3. Indications for Pediatric Endoscopy **385**
13.3.1. Diagnostic Purposes 385
13.3.2. Therapeutic Interventions 386
13.3.3. Management of Congenital Anomalies 387
13.4. Preparation for Pediatric Endoscopy **388**
13.4.1. Pre-Procedure Assessments 389
13.4.2. Parental Involvement and Education 390
13.4.3. Anesthesia Considerations 390
13.5. Risks and Complications **391**

13.5.1. Common Risks Associated with Procedures 392
13.5.2. Long-term Complications 393
13.5.3. Strategies for Risk Mitigation 394
13.6. Advances in Pediatric Endoscopy 394
13.6.1. Technological Innovations 395
13.6.2. Minimally Invasive Techniques 396
13.6.3. Future Directions in Research 397
Summary 399
References 402

CHAPTER 14

Complications of Endoscopy 407

Introduction 407
14.1. Types of Endoscopic Procedures 411
14.1.1. Gastrointestinal Endoscopy 411
14.1.2. Bronchoscopy 412
14.1.3. Urological Endoscopy 413
14.2. Common Complications 414
14.2.1. Perforation of Organs 415
14.2.2. Infection Risks 416
14.2.3. Bleeding During or After the Procedure 416
14.3. Patient-Related Factors 417
14.3.1. Pre-Existing Medical Conditions 418
14.3.2. Age and Overall Health 419
14.3.3. Medication Interactions 420
14.4. Technical Factors 421
14.4.1. Equipment Malfunction 421
14.4.2. Operator Skill and Experience 422
14.4.3. Procedure Complexity 423
14.5. Prevention Strategies 424
14.5.1. Pre-Procedural Assessments 425
14.5.2. Use of Advanced Technology 426
14.5.3. Training and Certification for Practitioners 427
14.6. Management of Complications 428
14.6.1. Immediate Response Protocols 429
14.6.2. Long-Term Follow-up Care 429
14.6.3. Patient Education and Support 430
Summary 432
References 435

CHAPTER 15

Endoscopy in Inflammatory Bowel Disease (IBD) 441

Introduction 441
15.1. Types of Inflammatory Bowel Disease (IBD) 444
15.1.1. Crohn's Disease 445
15.1.2. Ulcerative Colitis (UC) 445
15.1.3. Indeterminate Colitis (IC) 446
15.2. Role of Endoscopy in Diagnosis 447
15.2.1. Visualizing the Gastrointestinal Tract 448
15.2.2. Biopsy Collection for Histological Analysis 449
15.2.3. Differentiating Between Types of Inflammatory Bowel Diseases (IBD) 450
15.3. Therapeutic Endoscopy Techniques 451
15.3.1. Endoscopic Mucosal Resection (EMR) 452
15.3.2. Balloon Dilatation for Strictures 452
15.3.3. Endoscopic Submucosal Dissection (ESD) 453
15.4. Risks and Complications of Endoscopy 454
15.4.1. Perforation of the Gastrointestinal Tract 455
15.4.2. Infection Risks 456
15.4.3. Bleeding During or After Procedure 456
15.5. Advances in Endoscopic Technology 457
15.5.1. High-Definition Imaging 458
15.5.2. Capsule Endoscopy 459
15.5.3. Artificial Intelligence (AI) in Endoscopic Procedures 460
15.6. Patient Perspectives and Experiences 460
15.6.1. Psychological Impact of Endoscopy 461
15.6.2. Patient Education and Preparation 462
15.6.3. Post-Procedure Care and Follow-Up 463
Summary 465
References 468

Index 473

LIST OF FIGURES

Figure 1.1. Endoscopy
Figure 1.2. Upper endoscopy
Figure 1.3. Endoscopic procedures types
Figure 1.4. The first endoscopic equipment
Figure 1.5. The evolution of endoscopy: From early techniques
Figure 1.6. Evolution of the endoscope: (a) Lichtleiter endoscope (1806), (b) Mikulicz gastroscope (1881), (c) Schindler's gastroscope (1932) and (d) Hirschowitz fiberscope (1957)
Figure 1.7. Minimally invasive robotic surgery systems
Figure 1.8. Current surgical and endoscopic bariatric procedures
Figure 1.9. Upper GI endoscopy procedure
Figure 1.10. Bronchoscopy
Figure 1.11. Endoscopy urology installation
Figure 1.12. Three sources of possible extracellular vesicles (EVs) for diagnostic purposes
Figure 1.13. Prepare for your endoscopy procedure
Figure 1.14. Patient assessment
Figure 1.15. Informed consent
Figure 1.16. Common risks associated with endoscopy
Figure 1.17. Complications during the procedure
Figure 1.18. Post-procedure care and monitoring
Figure 1.19. Advances in endoscopy
Figure 2.1. Instrumentation and equipment
Figure 2.2. Instrumentation
Figure 2.3. Lab Equipment
Figure 2.4. Instrumentation
Figure 2.5. Analytical instrumentation
Figure 2.6. Measurement instrumentation
Figure 2.7. Common equipment in laboratories
Figure 2.8. Spectrophotometers
Figure 2.9. Chromatography
Figure 2.10. Microscopes

Figure 2.11. Medical diagnostic equipment
Figure 2.12. Industrial instrumentation
Figure 2.13. Quality assurance tools
Figure 2.14. Robotic process automation (RPA)
Figure 2.15. The transformative role of artificial intelligence (AI) in biomedical instrumentation
Figure 2.16. Calibration procedure of a control valve
Figure 3.1. Anesthesia patient preparation
Figure 3.2. Patient preparation
Figure 3.3. Enhancing patient comfort with sedation dentistry
Figure 3.4. Understanding patient preparation
Figure 3.5. The importance of patient's medical history
Figure 3.6. Physical exam
Figure 3.7. Providing psychological support
Figure 3.8. Types of sedation
Figure 3.9. Minimal sedation
Figure 3.10. Moderate sedation
Figure 3.11. Pediatric deep sedation
Figure 3.12. Conducting a medication review
Figure 3.13. Monitoring during anesthesia
Figure 3.14. Continuous vital signs monitoring
Figure 3.15. Patient monitoring
Figure 3.16. Post anesthesia care
Figure 3.17. Post-operative care
Figure 4.1. Esophagogastroduodenoscopy (EGD) procedure (Upper endoscopy)
Figure 4.2. Upper gastrointestinal endoscopy
Figure 4.3. Esophagogastroduodenoscopy (EGD) procedure for diagnosis
Figure 4.4. Upper endoscopy procedure
Figure 4.5. Upper GI endoscopy indications types
Figure 4.6. These are the symptoms of gastrointestinal syndrome
Figure 4.7. Esophageal disorders
Figure 4.8. Esophagogastroduodenoscopy (EGD) procedure
Figure 4.9. Pre-procedure instructions
Figure 4.10. Anesthesia medications
Figure 4.11. Esophagogastroduodenoscopy (EGD) procedure
Figure 4.12. Profession medical equipment Aq-100 video endoscopy camera
Figure 4.13. Esophagogastroduodenoscopy (EGD) procedure

Figure 4.14. Medical complications
Figure 4.15. Post-operative care
Figure 4.16. Recovery monitoring
Figure 4.17. Post-surgery diet plan: How to get on the fastest road to recovery
Figure 4.18. Artificial intelligence (AI) in endoscopy
Figure 4.19. Using robotic endoscopic platforms to perform gastric endoscopy
Figure 5.1. Colonoscopy
Figure 5.2. Colon health
Figure 5.3. Colonoscopy: Purpose
Figure 5.4. Colorectal cancer screening options
Figure 5.5. Ultrasound in diagnosing gastrointestinal disorders
Figure 5.6. Colonoscopy procedure.
Figure 5.7. Colonoscopy preparation
Figure 5.8. Preventing colorectal cancer: The vital role of colonoscopy screening
Figure 5.9. Post-operative care
Figure 5.10. Colonoscopy risks and complications
Figure 5.11. Intramural cecal hematoma: A rare complication after colonoscopy
Figure 5.12. Risk factors of colorectal cancer
Figure 5.13. Benefits of a colonoscopy
Figure 5.14. Colorectal cancer
Figure 5.15. Robotic surgery for digestive & gastrointestinal conditions
Figure 5.16. Patient perspectives
Figure 5.17. Colon cancer – Alternatives to colonoscopy
Figure 6.1. Sigmoidoscopy vs. colonoscopy
Figure 6.2. Sigmoidoscopy
Figure 6.3. Flexible sigmoidoscopy
Figure 6.4. Sigmoidoscopy procedure
Figure 6.5. Proctoscopy
Figure 6.6. Evaluation of surgical instruments
Figure 6.7. Colorectal cancer screening options
Figure 6.8. Inflammatory bowel disease (IBD)
Figure 6.9. Sigmoidoscopy and proctoscopy
Figure 6.10. Sigmoidoscopy procedure
Figure 6.11. Proctoscopy
Figure 6.12. Value of patient experience
Figure 6.13. Sigmoidoscopy patient education

Figure 6.14. Sedation and pain management
Figure 6.15. Post-operative care
Figure 6.16. Flexible sigmoidoscopy
Figure 7.1. Endoscopic retrograde cholangiopancreatography (ERCP)
Figure 7.2. Endoscopic retrograde cholangiopancreatography (ERCP)
Figure 7.3. Endoscopic retrograde cholangiopancreatography (ERCP) machine
Figure 7.4. Endoscopic retrograde cholangiopancreatography (ERCP) indications
Figure 7.5. Biliary tract disorders
Figure 7.6. Pancreatic disease
Figure 7.7. Bile duct obstruction
Figure 7.8. Pre-procedure preparation
Figure 7.9. Patient monitoring
Figure 7.10. Prevention and management of endoscopic retrograde cholangiopancreatography (ERCP)-related complications
Figure 7.11. Risk management: How to minimize risk and secure success
Figure 7.12. Understanding cholangitis
Figure 7.13. Pancreatic cancer
Figure 7.14. Bile duct stone removal
Figure 7.15. Stent placement in a patient with common bile duct obstruction
Figure 7.16. Mastering endoscopic retrograde cholangiopancreatography (ERCP) techniques
Figure 8.1. Endoscopic ultrasound (EUS)
Figure 8.2. Endoscopic ultrasound (EUS)
Figure 8.3. Endoscopic ultrasound (EUS)
Figure 8.4. Endoscopic ultrasound (EUS): procedure
Figure 8.5. Role of endoscopes in endoscopic ultrasound (EUS)
Figure 8.6. Indications for endoscopic ultrasound (EUS)
Figure 8.7. Staging of cancers
Figure 8.8. Advantages of endoscopic ultrasound (EUS)
Figure 8.9. High-resolution imaging capabilities of endoscopic ultrasound (EUS)
Figure 8.10. Ability to perform fine-needle aspiration
Figure 8.11. Technical challenges and limitations endoscopic ultrasound (EUS)
Figure 8.12. Comparison with other imaging modalities endoscopic ultrasound (EUS) serves
Figure 8.13. Role in gastroenterology
Figure 8.14. Future directions in the field of endoscopic ultrasound (EUS)
Figure 8.15. Potential for new applications
Figure 8.16. Research and clinical trials

Figure 9.1. Capsule endoscopy
Figure 9.2. Purpose of capsule endoscopy
Figure 9.3. Importance in modern gastrointestinal diagnostics
Figure 9.4. Technology behind capsule endoscopy
Figure 9.5. Description of the capsule design and components
Figure 9.6. Mechanism of action during the procedure capsule endoscopy involves
Figure 9.7. Comparison with traditional endoscopic methods
Figure 9.8. Diagnosis of small bowel disorders
Figure 9.9. Evaluation of gastrointestinal bleeding
Figure 9.10. Assessment of inflammatory bowel diseases (IBD)
Figure 9.11. Step-by-step overview of the capsule ingestion process
Figure 9.12. Post-procedure monitoring and data retrieval
Figure 9.13. Advantages of capsule endoscopy
Figure 9.14. Non-invasive nature of capsule endoscopy in gastrointestinal diagnostics
Figure 9.15. Increased patient comfort Increased patient comfort and compliance and compliance
Figure 9.16. Risk of capsule retention in the gastrointestinal tract
Figure 9.17. Future directions in capsule endoscopy
Figure 9.18. Technological advancements on the horizon
Figure 10.1. Enteroscopy techniques
Figure 10.2. Importance of enteroscopy in gastrointestinal diagnostics
Figure 10.3. Development of enteroscopy techniques
Figure 10.4. Types of enteroscopy
Figure 10.5. Balloon-assisted enteroscopy
Figure 10.6. Double-balloon enteroscopy
Figure 10.7. Diagnosis of small bowel diseases
Figure 10.8. Management of gastrointestinal bleeding
Figure 10.9. Preparation for enteroscopy
Figure 10.10. Patient assessment and selection
Figure 10.11. Pre-procedural instructions
Figure 10.12. Enteroscopy procedure
Figure 10.13. Role of the endoscopist
Figure 10.14. Complications and risks use of with capsule enteroscopy techniques
Figure 10.15. Strategies for minimizing the risks of enteroscopy techniques
Figure 11.1. Therapeutic endoscopy
Figure 11.2. Importance in modern medicine

Figure 11.3. Development of endoscopic techniques
Figure 11.4. Milestones in therapeutic endoscopy
Figure 11.5. Evolution of technology in endoscopy
Figure 11.6. Gastrointestinal endoscopy
Figure 11.7. Urological endoscopy
Figure 11.8. Indications for therapeutic endoscopy
Figure 11.9. Treatment of malignancies
Figure 11.10. Management of bleeding and obstructions
Figure 11.11. Endoscopic mucosal resection (EMR)
Figure 11.12. Endoscopic retrograde cholangiopancreatography (ERCP)
Figure 11.13. Endoscopic ultrasound (EUS)
Figure 11.14. Common complications associated with procedures
Figure 11.15. Risk factors influencing complications
Figure 11.16. Future directions in therapeutic endoscopy
Figure 11.17. Potential for robotic-assisted endoscopy
Figure 11.18. Research trends and clinical trials
Figure 12.1. Advanced imaging in endoscopy
Figure 12.2. Importance of imaging in endoscopic procedures
Figure 12.3. Overview of advancements in imaging technology in endoscopy
Figure 12.4. Development of fiber-optic technology
Figure 12.5. Milestones in imaging advancements
Figure 12.6. High-definition endoscopy
Figure 12.7. Narrow-band imaging (NBI)
Figure 12.8. Confocal laser endomicroscopy (CLE)
Figure 12.9. Enhanced visualization of tissues in endoscopy
Figure 12.10. Reduction in unnecessary biopsies
Figure 12.11. Gastroenterology
Figure 12.12. Pulmonology
Figure 12.13. Cost and accessibility of advanced imaging technologies
Figure 12.14. Potential for overdiagnosis and overtreatment
Figure 12.15. Integration of artificial intelligence (AI)
Figure 12.16. Innovations in imaging software and analysis
Figure 13.1. Pediatric endoscopy
Figure 13.2. Importance in pediatric medicine
Figure 13.3. Milestones in pediatric endoscopy

Figure 13.4. Evolution of equipment and technology
Figure 13.5. Gastrointestinal endoscopy
Figure 13.6. Bronchoscopy is an essential procedure
Figure 13.7. Indications for pediatric endoscopy have garnered increased attention
Figure 13.8. Management of congenital anomalies
Figure 13.9. Pre-procedure assessments
Figure 13.10. Parental involvement role in shaping educational outcomes for children
Figure 13.11. Anesthesia considerations
Figure 13.12. Long-term complications
Figure 13.13. Advances in pediatric endoscopy
Figure 13.14. Technological innovations
Figure 13.15. Future directions in research
Figure 14.1. Complications of endoscopy
Figure 14.2. Endoscopy
Figure 14.3. Overview of potential complications
Figure 14.4. Gastrointestinal endoscopy
Figure 14.5. Bronchoscopy
Figure 14.6. Urological endoscopy
Figure 14.7. Perforation of organs
Figure 14.8. Bleeding during or after the procedure
Figure 14.9. Pre-existing medical conditions
Figure 14.10. Medication interactions
Figure 14.11. Equipment malfunction
Figure 14.12. Prevention strategies
Figure 14.13. Advancement of technology in the field of endoscopy
Figure 14.14. Training and certification for practitioners
Figure 14.15. Management of complications arising from endoscopic
Figure 14.16. Long-term follow-up care
Figure 14.17. Patient education and support
Figure 15.1. Endoscopy in inflammatory bowel disease (IBD)
Figure 15.2. Importance of endoscopy in diagnosis and management
Figure 15.3. Types of inflammatory bowel disease (IBD)
Figure 15.4. Ulcerative colitis (UC) represents a chronic inflammatory bowel disease (IBD)
Figure 15.5. Indeterminate colitis (IC)
Figure 15.6. Role of endoscopy in diagnosis

Figure 15.7. Visualizing the gastrointestinal tract
Figure 15.8. Differentiating between types of inflammatory bowel diseases (IBD)
Figure 15.9. Therapeutic endoscopy techniques
Figure 15.10. Balloon dilatation for strictures
Figure 15.11. Perforation of the gastrointestinal tract
Figure 15.12. Bleeding during or after procedure
Figure 15.13. Advances in endoscopic technology
Figure 15.14. Capsule endoscopy
Figure 15.15. Artificial intelligence (AI) in endoscopic procedures
Figure 15.16. Psychological impact of endoscopy
Figure 15.17. Post-procedure care and follow-up

PREFACE

Endoscopic examination of the gastrointestinal tract has revolutionized clinicians' methods of diagnosis and treatment of gastrointestinal disease. Through direct visualization of mucosal surfaces, endoscopic techniques have developed previously blind techniques into precise, image-guided interventions. Advances in optics, illumination, and digital detectors have improved to provide brighter images of the esophageal, gastric, and intestinal mucosa to visualize inflammation, ulceration, neoplasia, and less apparent lesions. Parallel to these advances in endoscopes, developments in accessory equipment, forceps, snares, and hemostatic devices, have broadened the scope of endoscopy from simple observation to active intervention, reducing the need for open surgery in a large number of cases.

Over the past decades, endoscopic procedures have expanded to encompass high-resolution imaging, ultrasound capability, and capsule-based technology. These methods not only optimize diagnostic yield but also enable minimally invasive treatment to minimize hospital stay, decrease patient discomfort, and lower overall healthcare costs. With continuous research, new methodologies , such as molecular imaging and artificial intelligence–assisted interpretation are going to further enhance diagnostic accuracy. The dynamic evolution of endoscopic practice has made the practitioner keep in mind a steady commitment to technical expertise, patient safety, and evidence-based practice.

This book, *Endoscopic Techniques in Gastroenterology*, brings together authoritative coverage of the entire scope of endoscopic procedures. It contains both basic training in equipment and patient care protocols and in-depth descriptions of specialty techniques. Authors are experts in adult and pediatric gastroenterology, endoscopic surgery, and gastrointestinal pathology. The book integrates procedural information, clinical pearls, and safety considerations designed to support best practice and best outcomes.

- Chapter 1 gives a background in endoscopy and principles, highlighting by tracing the evolution of scopes from stiff tubes to modern-day flexible instruments. The chapter condenses the physics of light transmission and lenses, outlines significant milestones in technology development, and discusses the training pathway for endoscopists.
- Chapter 2 deals with instrumentation and design and function of equipment. It describes the structure of video endoscopes, disposable versus reusable accessories, and quality control in equipment maintenance. Broad guidelines for the selection of scopes and ancillary instruments based on clinical needs are provided.
- Chapter 3 covers patient preparation and sedation practice. Topics include assessment of risk, fasting protocols, bowel preparation procedures for lower GI endoscopy, and

selection of sedation or anesthesia. Monitoring parameters for vital signs and the handling of complications from sedation are emphasized.

- Chapter 4 Upper GI endoscopy or esophagogastroduodenoscopy (EGD) — summarizes indications, technique of procedure, biopsy techniques, and management of frequently acquired findings , such as erosive esophagitis, Barrett's mucosa, and peptic ulcer. Therapeutic interventions like dilatation of stricture and foreign body removal are also covered.
- Chapter 5 discusses the detailed procedures of colonoscopy. It gives an account of the insertion and navigation of the scope in the colon, methods of polypectomy, and protocols of screening for colorectal cancer. Ideal practice for complete examination and reducing patient discomfort is highlighted.
- Chapter 6 addresses proctoscopy and sigmoidoscopy separately from total colonoscopy. The chapter discusses indications for flexible sigmoidoscopy, techniques of rectal biopsy, and the diagnostic role of proctoscopy in the treatment of anorectal disorders , such as hemorrhoids, fissures, and neoplasms.
- Chapter 7 is dedicated to endoscopic retrograde cholangiopancreatography (ERCP). The chapter covers methods of cannulation of the bile and pancreatic ducts, injection of contrast, and therapeutic maneuvers like stone extraction, stenting, and control of postsphincterotomy bleeding.
- Chapter 8 covers endoscopic ultrasound (EUS), an integration of endoscopy and high-frequency ultrasound scanning. It discusses echoendoscope maneuvering, interpretation of images, and fine-needle aspiration methods. Clinical applications in staging gastrointestinal cancer and diagnosing submucosal lesions are presented.
- Chapter 9 presents capsule endoscopy as an ingestible imaging system for noninvasive visualization of the small bowel. The chapter discusses patient selection, preparation protocols, data acquisition, and interpretation of findings in obscure gastrointestinal bleeding and Crohn's disease.
- Chapter 10 addresses enteroscopy modalities for greater access to the small bowel. Double-balloon, single-balloon, and spiral enteroscopy techniques are compared. Procedural step-by-step information on scope progression, lesion visualization, and therapeutic maneuvers is addressed.
- Chapter 11 deals with therapeutic endoscopy , such as hemostasis, resection of mucosa, and closure techniques. Chapter 11 provides step-by-step guidelines for endoscopic clipping, injection therapy, thermal coagulation, and endoscopic mucosal resection (EMR) and endoscopic submucosal dissection (ESD) for excision of early neoplastic lesions.
- Chapter 12 is focused on advanced imaging modalities of endoscopy. The subjects dealt with are chromoendoscopy, narrow-band imaging, confocal laser endomicroscopy, and autofluorescence. The chapter explains how such modalities enhance lesion characterization and enable targeted biopsies.
- Chapter 13 is focused on the special considerations of pediatric endoscopy. The anatomy variations, guidelines for sedation, and instrument sizes are dealt with. Case examples address diagnostic challenges and therapeutic approaches in children with congenital abnormalities, inflammatory bowel disease, and functional GI disorders.

- Chapter 14 addresses potential complications of endoscopy , including bleeding, perforation, infection, and cardiopulmonary complications. The chapter elucidates prevention maneuvers, early recognition signs, and management algorithms for adverse events to ensure patient safety.
- Chapter 15 addresses endoscopy for inflammatory bowel disease (IBD), diagnostic and therapeutic uses. The chapter outlines the measurement of disease activity, mucosal healing, and endoscopic therapies for stricture dilation and fistula in ulcerative colitis and Crohn's disease.

Target readers are gastroenterologists-in-training, experienced endoscopists seeking to update their skills, surgeons with endoscopic experience, and allied health staff responsible for the operation of endoscopy units. The text also serves as a reference for clinical teachers and researchers concerned with the ongoing improvement of gastrointestinal endoscopy.

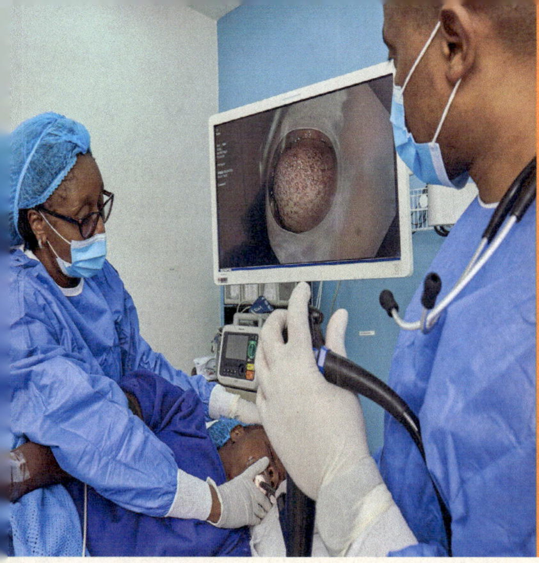

Chapter 1

INTRODUCTION TO ENDOSCOPY

Contents

Introduction of Endoscopy 1
1.1. Historical Background 5
1.2. Types of Endoscopic Procedures 9
1.3. Indications for Endoscopy 13
1.4. Preparation for Endoscopy 16
1.5. Risks and Complications 19
1.6. Advances in Endoscopic Technology 23
Summary 27
References 30

Introduction of Endoscopy

Endoscopy is a medical practice that involves the use of certain devices, known as endoscopes, in examining the inside of the organs and body cavities. The procedure is usually minimally invasive and primarily used to enable doctors to diagnose and treat many conditions in the gastrointestinal system, lungs, and other systems. By applying an endoscope, most of the time with a light source and camera attached, medical professionals are able to obtain real-time video and pictures of the infected area. The application of endoscopy in medicine has significantly enhanced the accuracy of diagnosis, allowing for the identification of diseases , such as ulcers, cancer, and inflammatory diseases. Its non-invasiveness, to accompany the applicability of performing therapeutic interventions in the same session, indicates endoscopy's growing importance in modern medicine. The evolving landscape in endoscopic technology has incorporated numerous advancements that increase its efficacy and safety. One such advancement is the integration of artificial intelligence (AI) in endoscopy, which has begun transforming traditional methods by improving adenoma and early cancer detection rates. Recent studies indicate that integration of AI in colonoscopy has the ability to dramatically increase the adenoma detection rate (ADR) above high-definition colonoscopy by itself, resulting in enhanced patient outcomes (Aziz et al., 2022). Moreover, newer imaging modalities , such as chromoendoscopy and magnified endoscopy enable better visualization of subtle pathologies. The integration of AI with such advanced imaging modalities is not only at the cusp of simplifying endoscopic procedures but also at the cusp of reducing the likelihood of missing significant lesions, ultimately enhancing the quality of care provided to patients. Beyond technology innovation, the term 'endoscopy' also encompasses in its sense the various applications and techniques that are being utilized in different specialties of medicine. For instance, with inflammatory bowel disease (IBD), endoscopy offers a superior assessment and monitoring of the ileocolonic mucosa, which overcomes the technicality of this chronic illness (van der Laan et al., 2020). With molecular imaging and other emerging techniques, endoscopy is evolving to emerge as an end-to-end diagnostic method capable of advancing deeper into biology at the cellular level. This multifaceted perspective lends credence to the worth of endoscopy as not just a diagnostic tool but as a useful part of treatment planning in diverse clinical contexts, ultimately leading to increased patient care and therapeutic outcome (Figure 1.1).

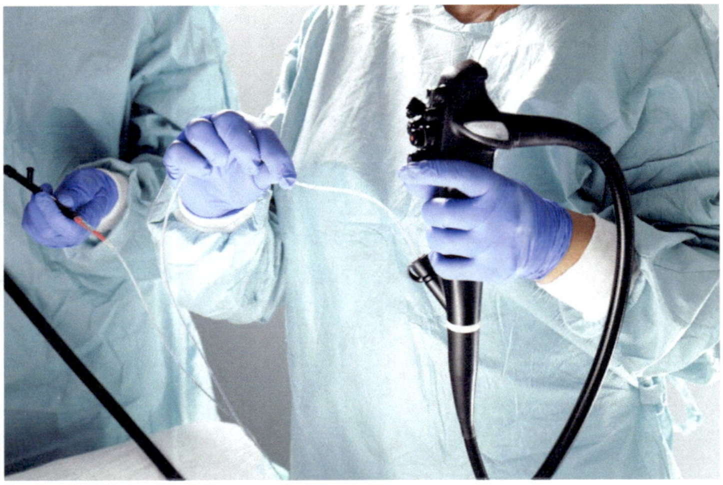

Figure 1.1. Endoscopy.

Source: https://healthtian.com/wp-content/uploads/2020/08/Endoscopy1-1536x1023.jpg.

Definition of the Term "Endoscopy"

Endoscopy can be defined as a medical procedure where a specialized instrument known as an endoscope is used. This handy tube is also equipped with a light and a camera, allowing physicians to observe the inner walls of cavities and organs within the body. Most commonly utilized in the examination of the gastrointestinal system, endoscopy helps to diagnose various conditions ranging from ulcers and tumors to gastrointestinal tract bleeding. The method not only makes direct visualization possible but also the return of tissue samples via biopsy, providing excellent information regarding the condition of the patients. Furthermore, advances in endoscopic technology have persistently improved its application and utility, and it is presently a must-have tool in modern medicine for both therapeutic and diagnostic purposes. The role of endoscopy in modern healthcare cannot be overstated with regard to the advancement of medical science. Due to its least invasive nature, endoscopy poses a reduced risk of complications compared to the traditional surgical methods. The patients also experience fewer postoperative complications, less pain, and shorter recovery periods. This efficiency is particularly beneficial during procedures , such as standard gastrectomy, whose intention is to facilitate successful resection of gastric cancer while ensuring the highest level of patient safety and comfort. In addition, endoscopy's role is not only for viewing but also covers therapeutic uses , such as stricture dilation and foreign body extraction, thus further enhancing its applicability across various clinical settings.

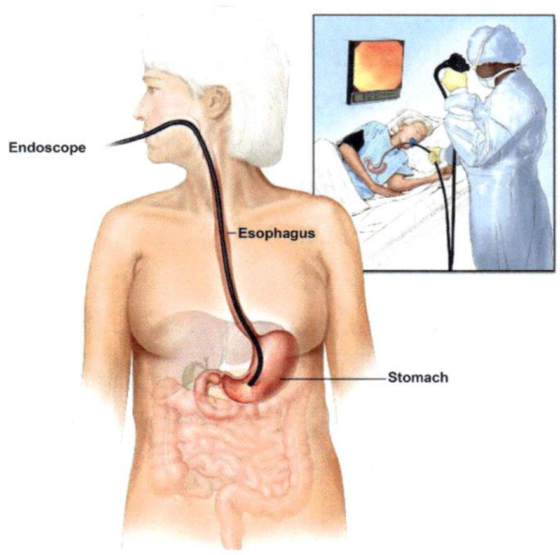

Figure 1.2. Upper endoscopy.

Source: https://nci-media.cancer.gov/pdq/media/images/433287.jpg.

Thus, the integration of endoscopy into conventional clinical practice is a sign of the ongoing evolution of diagnostic methods and the relentless search for optimizing patient outcomes. Endoscopy plays a central role in the treatment of gastrointestinal illnesses, one of the leading public health concerns. Conditions , such as gastric cancer highlight the value of early diagnosis and treatment because its early detection is associated with improved survival (Rawla & Barsouk, 2019). Endoscopy allows for detailed evaluation, which facilitates accurate staging and treatment planning. Also, as our understanding of the epidemiology of gastric cancer evolves, so does the relevance of adding endoscopy to preventive and surveillance strategies, eventually minimizing incidence and mortality for this disease. In general, the term endoscopy refers to an important division of clinical practice that has totally reshaped the practice of diagnosis and treatment across many specialties, underscoring its ongoing preeminence in modern medicine (Figure 1.2).

Overview of the Procedure and its Purpose

Endoscopy is a highly safe and minimally intrusive medical intervention that employs an endoscope, a flexible tube with a light and a camera, to examine the interior mechanisms of the body. The procedure is largely applied in the diagnosis and treatment of different gastrointestinal ailments, but its application isn't confined to the digestive tract. The endoscope is inserted through natural channels, such as the mouth or rectum, so that medical staff may view organs , such as the esophagus, stomach, and intestines in real time. Endoscopy possesses one of its stronger assets in that it is able to provide direct visualization to recognize abnormalities , such as tumors, inflammation, or infection. The technique can be applied therapeutically as well, allowing procedures , such as biopsy harvesting or removal of a polyp to be conducted, making it a crucial tool in modern medicine. The primary application of endoscopy is its double role as both a treatment and diagnostic modality. By visualization of organs from the inside, endoscopy enhances the reliability of diagnosis and minimizes the need for other invasive surgical techniques. This technique shortens patient recovery periods and complications of normal surgery. For instance, in gastrointestinal disorder conditions, the procedure is capable of detecting early cancer signs, thereby optimizing the response of patients through successful intervention at the appropriate time. Additionally, endoscopy's minimal invasiveness also means less postoperative discomfort and shorter hospital stays, further highlighting its importance in the broader regime of patient-centered care. The advancing technologies of endoscopy, with enhanced imaging modalities and devices for interventional therapies, work to further expand its use in a variety of clinical disciplines. The ongoing attempt to refine the process of endoscopy is exemplified through the newer advances in endoscopic technology, such as the innovation of endoscopic ultrasound (EUS) and capsule endoscopy. EUS marries endoscopy and ultrasound imaging in order to facilitate the precise assessment not just of the lining of the gastrointestinal tract but of structures around it, significantly augmenting diagnostic capability. Capsule endoscopy involves swallowing an ingestible camera about the size of a pill, which photographs the digestive system without invasiveness, providing a helpful alternative in patients who are unable to undergo standard endoscopy and to visualize areas that are beyond traditional endoscopy reach, like the small intestine. These advances not only improve diagnostic accuracy but also facilitate earlier disease detection, as shown in current research in the use of artificial intelligence and image analysis for the better optimization of diagnosis from imaging data (Singhal et al., 2023). With the technology continuously advancing, endoscopy is well placed to continue being a cornerstone in clinical practice, facilitating effective management of patients for a variety of health conditions (Wang et al., 2021).

Types of Endoscopic Procedures

Endoscopy is a set of procedures employed to allow doctors to see and treat interior structures of the body through minimal invasion. Colonoscopy, one of the most common endoscopic interventions, is done by introducing a flexible tube with a camera into the colon in order to diagnose and treat. The process not only makes detection of colorectal cancer and polyps easier but also builds a platform for therapeutic procedures, such as polypectomy. The increasing emphasis in the past few years on colorectal cancer screening programs has indicated the role of colonoscopy in the improvement of patients' outcomes and reducing surgical interventions, with the developing methods enhancing the detection and removal of polyps (Arebi & Saunders, 2005). As a result, colonoscopies are now part of the routine preventive health care measures. Upper gastrointestinal endoscopy, or esophagogastroduodenoscopy (EGD), as it is also known, is another major category. Through EGD, the esophagus, stomach, and duodenum can be visualized, which helps in diagnosing many diseases of the gastrointestinal tract, including ulcers, inflammation, and cancers. EGD has been advanced to incorporate new techniques, one of which is chromoendoscopy, where special dyes are used to identify abnormalities, making the diagnosis more accurate. The employment of modern imaging techniques has enabled easier identification of many tiny lesions that would otherwise have gone undiagnosed. Furthermore, in addition to being applied for diagnostics, EGD also enables therapeutic maneuvers , such as stent placements and stricture dilations, thereby reducing subsequent surgery (Septimiu et al., 2018). As a result, EGD is a valuable resource in modern gastrointestinal medicine. Other than these interventions, endoscopic retrograde cholangiopancreatography (ERCP) plays a key role in the diagnosis and treatment of pancreatic and bile duct disorders. Using fluoroscopy in conjunction with endoscopic techniques, ERCP allows examination and treatment of conditions , including biliary stricture, gallstones, and pancreatitis. This dual modality employs the instruments of visualization and intervention, facilitating procedures like stone removal and stent placement in one procedure. Advances over the last few years have contributed to the success of ERCP, further enhancing patient safety and outcomes. As endoscopic technology advances, ERCP is perhaps one of the best demonstrations of how endoscopy is not merely a diagnostic tool but also increasingly therapeutic in purpose, indicative of its becoming progressively more central to all medical disciplines (Arebi & Saunders, 2005) (Figure 1.3).

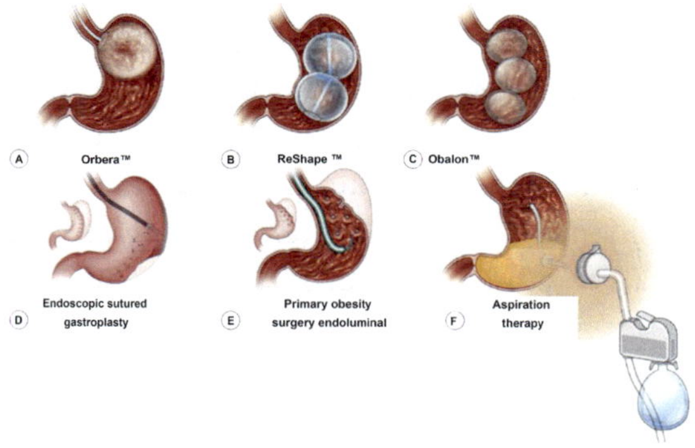

Figure 1.3. Endoscopic procedures types.

Source: https://www.e-ce.org/upload/thumbnails/ce-2018-148f1.jpg.

1.1. Historical Background

Endoscopy has a long history that dates back to ancient times when straightforward instruments , such as tubes and mirrors were employed to explore internal structures. Endoscopy is derived from the Greek terms endo, meaning within, and skopein, meaning to see. This concept was expanded in the 19th century with the discovery of the advancements in optics and illumination, attributed primarily to scientists , such as Anton van Leeuwenhoek and his microscopic observations. These advances led to the development of even more sophisticated endoscopic devices, which would allow one to view the interior of the human body directly, transforming diagnostic and therapeutic procedures in medicine. The development of endoscopy has not only been marked by technological innovations but also by increasing knowledge of human anatomy and physiology, such that it is now used in all the major medical specialties. The 20th century alone saw a decisive turning point in endoscopic technology, in particular through the arrival of fiber optics in the 1950s. Fiber optic endoscopy gave unprecedented flexibility and light, a process much safer and more efficient. Subsequently, various endoscopic techniques were created, such as gastrointestinal endoscopy, which turned out to be a primary diagnostic tool for gastrointestinal ailments. The work of clinicians like Dr. Rudolf Schindler and Dr. Georgios Kelling further solidified endoscopy's position in clinical practice. In addition to all these advancements, progress in minimal invasive surgical techniques also assisted in driving the adoption of endoscopy to other branches of medicine, such as urology and gynecology. It turned out that endoscopy not only served as a diagnostic method but also as an essential instrument for therapy, a revolution in surgery. The interlink between endoscopy and minimally invasive surgery is a sign of the revolutionary techniques used in modern medicine. In association with minimally invasive procedures, endoscopy evolved, and physicians began exploring the possibility of it being able to heal diseases without large cuts and lengthy recuperation periods. For example, the anterior transcorporeal method has been adapted in cervical spine surgery and has provided a less invasive alternative for certain pathologies, demonstrating how endoscopic techniques can lead to less traumatic procedures with better patient outcomes (Liu et al., 2024). Additionally, the study of residency program performance emphasizes the need for trainees to master these new methods in order to achieve high standards of care in endoscopic procedures (Karimian et al., 2024). This past gives rise to contemporary endoscopy that keeps expanding its scope and improving healthcare delivery through acquisition and innovation (Figure 1.4).

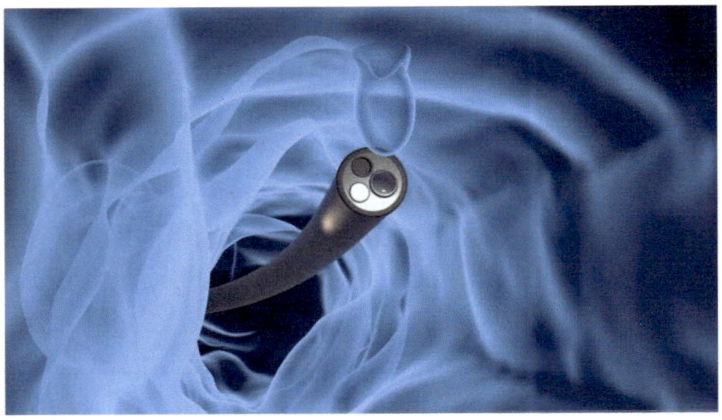

Figure 1.4. The first endoscopic equipment.

Source: https://lh7-rt.googleusercontent.com/docsz/AD_4nXdAbE7uTE5U8Vf-qIGAcMqab1YXFjuTqzbiBCysbXCouZcv7wEXk2QlUXGbK3qME35z8l-q1QIUTncsHvr6AOaffFUEXQnpzIcH8AcOok4-dGYB0kDxqevYtDzp3vuOeDjEbz9Ap2gzekYf6jxCSzwX1alu?key=tVczLubDLosGnEvOOw1fZQ.

1.1.1. Early Developments in Endoscopic Techniques

The evolution of endoscopic methods started in the 19th century, marked by groundbreaking innovations that revolutionized medical diagnosis and interventions. Early attempts at this were primitive and used mainly rigid tubes and primitive illumination systems to examine internal organs. The first breakthrough was with the development of the fibroscope in the 1960s, which brought in the idea of flexible endoscopy.

This technology made the patient's experience more enjoyable and allowed physicians to probe the gastrointestinal tract's intricate anatomy with greater ease. The employment of fiber-optic technology, in addition to enhancing visibility, opened the door to countless therapeutic interventions, heralding a revolutionary shift in practice. The pioneering foundational research set the stage for the advanced endoscopic techniques used in medicine today. Continued advancement of technology in endoscopic sciences saw the inclusion of video imaging optimized the field and enhanced procedures to be more effective and safer. Video endoscopy made real-time imaging possible, allowing clinicians to take high-level examinations of body structures and to capture results for subsequent analysis. This advance in technology improved the accuracy of diagnosis, particularly in gastrointestinal disease, where visual observation is of maximum concern. More importantly, the activities of various organizations like the British Society of Gastroenterology have brought to light the formation of guidelines that are based on evidence-based treatment of illnesses like ulcerative colitis and Crohn's disease. These developments in diagnostic application were complemented by expansion in therapeutic endoscopy, including biopsies and polyp removal, further cementing endoscopy's status as an omnipresent gadget in modern medicine (Lamb et al., 2019). The first two decades of the 21st century witnessed expansion in the use of endoscopy with new methods , such as endoscopic mucosal resection (EMR) and endoscopic submucosal dissection (ESD). These minimally invasive procedures made it possible to remove lesions through few surgeries, which left patients with quick recovery and less risk. As soon as these technologies gained pace, guidelines like the JSCCR guidelines 2019 were formulated, which provided standard methodologies for disease management, including colorectal cancer, as well as reducing discrepancies in treatment protocols among institutions (Hashiguchi et al., 2019). This time also saw the development of high-tech imaging techniques , such as chromoendoscopy and narrow-band imaging, which made the small lesions more visible. The consistent development of endoscopic techniques signals their central role in influencing future medical practice trends and ongoing efforts to improve patient outcomes (Figure 1.5).

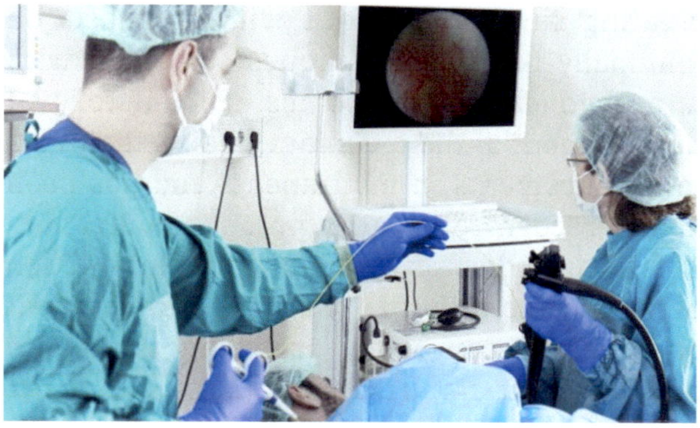

Figure 1.5. The evolution of endoscopy: From early techniques.

Source: https://www.dailyhealthideas.com/wp-content/uploads/2024/01/The-Evolution-of-Endoscopy-From-Early-Techniques-to-Modern-Advancements-750x460.jpg.

1.1.2. Key Figures in the Evolution of Endoscopy

Endoscopy cannot be understood without recognition, though, of the accomplishments of great figures of history who opened the door for today's practice. Among these pioneers is Philipp Bozzini, a German doctor credited with the invention of the Lichtleiter (light conductor) in 1806. His pioneering achievement saw candlelight used to illuminate cavities within the body, with the very first glimpses of the human body. Although small in scale compared to today's standards, Bozzini's innovation was a turning point in technological development. This precursor to endoscopy set the stage for later developments and underscored the importance of continued advances in visualization techniques, eventually paving the way for developments in flexible endoscopy during the 20th century. The 20th century saw unprecedented developments in endoscopic procedures driven by pioneering figures , such as Rudolf Schindler and his creation of the first flexible fiber optic endoscope in the 1950s. Schindler's breakthrough revolutionized the manner in which doctors could visualize the gastrointestinal tract. Through marrying fiber optic technology, he made images sharper and more mobile than with rigid equipment. This innovation not only expanded diagnostic capability but also provided therapeutic intervention. The advent of flexible endoscopes represented a paradigm shift that reduced the procedure to less invasive and patient-friendly levels. Upon gastroenterologists' acceptance of the instruments, the practice began expanding, with more options for treatment being added and eventually culminating in minimally invasive procedures. Yet another essential figure in endoscopy's development is Dr. Hiromi Shinya, who made EMR popular and played a significant part in disseminating cutting-edge endoscopic technology.

His research, particularly in the 1980s, demonstrated that cancers at early stages could be excised with endoscopic interventions, opening up the potential of treatment without invasive surgeries.

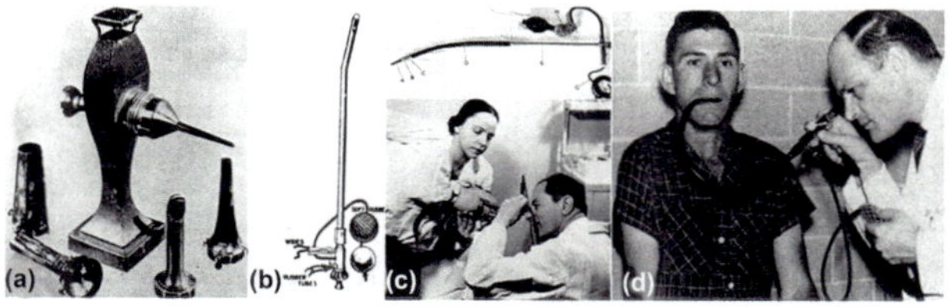

Figure 1.6. Evolution of the endoscope: (a) Lichtleiter endoscope (1806), (b) Mikulicz gastroscope (1881), (c) Schindler's gastroscope (1932) and (d) Hirschowitz fibrescope (1957).

Source: https://www.researchgate.net/publication/347513996/figure/fig1/AS:11431281133261826@1680274648589/Evolution-of-the-endoscope-a-Lichtleiter-endoscope-1806-b-Mikulicz-gastroscope.tif.

With these advances emerged Shinya's clinical studies on patient outcomes and comfort during procedures, ultimately transforming the field to an era that was not merely focused on diagnosis but also on effective therapeutic care. The evolution of endoscopy has, therefore, been shaped by these pioneers, whose contributions have made it a pillar of current clinical practice, an indication of the ongoing interaction between innovation and patient management in gastroenterology (Figure 1.6).

1.1.3. Milestones in Technology and Instrumentation

Advances in endoscopic technology have significantly transformed the landscape of medical practice, with minimally invasive techniques becoming the hallmark in most specialties. One of these advances has been the integration of robotic-assisted systems into operations, a case in point being improvements in spine surgery. Robotic systems like the Mazor X Stealth Edition have transformed the precision in techniques , such as minimally invasive transforaminal lumbar interbody fusion (MI-TLIF). These systems allow for increased precision in such critical procedures as pedicle screw fixation and facet joint decortications, ultimately reducing blood loss and pain postoperatively. The implementation of such advanced instrumentation marks a significant benchmark in that it diverts surgical focus toward automation, thereby eliminating the risks inherent in conventional methods while guaranteeing enhanced recovery profiles for patients. These developments point to the very important position of technology in defining surgical methods and how best to enhance patient care within the endoscopic field (Altorfer et al., 2024). Another turning point in endoscopic technology is the ongoing development of minimally invasive surgical techniques for operations on the cervical spine, and in particular, the anterior transcorporeal method. The method utilizes advancements in endoscopy to facilitate better-intervention therapy for curing pathologies leading to radiculopathy or myelopathy. As medical equipment evolves, the methods become more refined and, hence, surgical interventions more efficient. The anterior transcorporeal method is the ultimate result of efforts directed towards creating surgical methods with emphasis on minimally invasive techniques combined with improved clinical outcomes. The history of development of the technique is directly linked to advancements in instruments and has been highly recognized for its potential outcomes. This is an indicator of the ongoing interaction between genomics change and the development of surgery in endoscopy, propelling the two to better patient care (Liu et al., 2024).

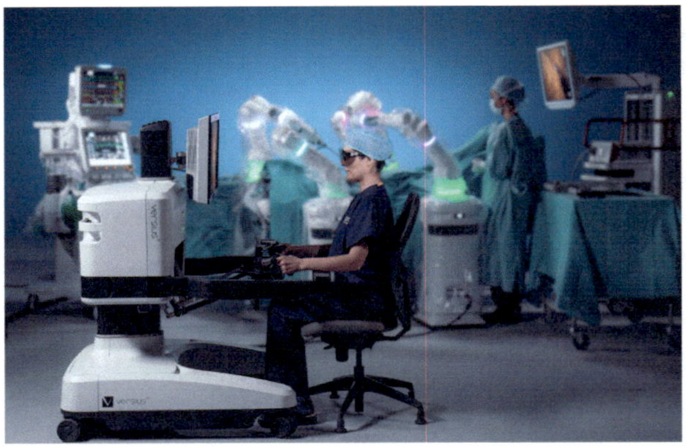

Figure 1.7. Minimally invasive robotic surgery systems.

Source: https://www.surgicalroboticstechnology.com/wp-content/uploads/2022/02/minimally-invasive-robotic-surgery.png.

The future of endoscopy will most likely witness still more landmarks as a result of the continuous progress in technology and instrumentation. New technologies and techniques, such as machine learning and augmented reality, are in the pipeline to upgrade the performance of traditional endoscopic methods and extend their application. Robotic interventions, already proving themselves in specialties like spine surgery, are set to evolve into more widespread forms, providing greater precision and dexterity in complex procedures. Furthermore, the integration of advanced imaging modalities with endoscopic platforms may render real-time data analysis a reality, facilitating improved surgical decision-making.

These innovations speak not only to progress in the field but also to promise new frontiers in medicine. As technology continues to evolve, the future of endoscopy will likely be characterized by greater precision, safety, and beauty in surgical procedures, culminating in improved outcomes for patients across most medical specialties (Figure 1.7).

1.2. Types of Endoscopic Procedures

Endoscopic procedures have revolutionized diagnosis and treatment in medicine by offering minimally invasive methods for visualization and control of numerous internal diseases. Upper gastrointestinal endoscopy, or esophagogastroduodenoscopy (EGD), is the most common type of endoscopic procedure.

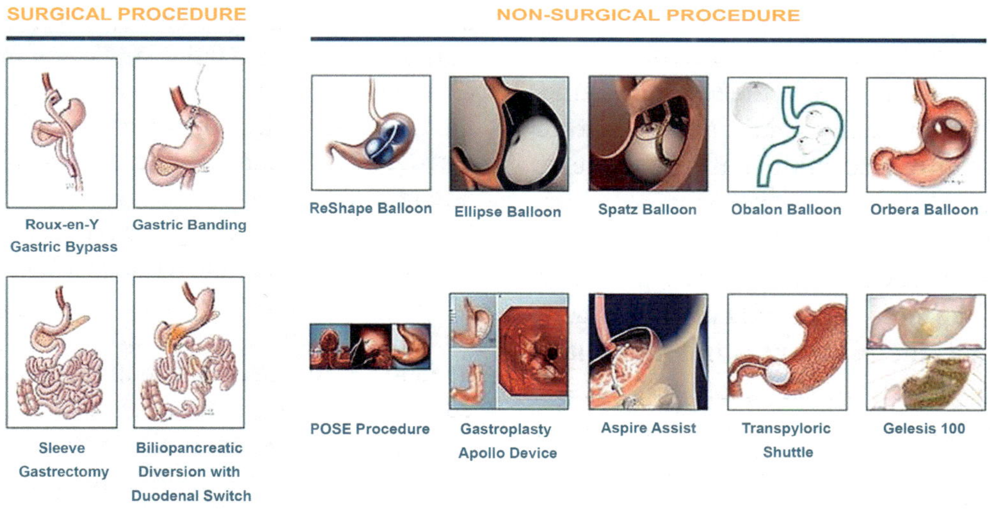

Figure 1.8. Current surgical and endoscopic bariatric procedures.

Source: https://www.researchgate.net/profile/Richard-Lindquist/publication/337027929/figure/fig3/AS:821886963433474@1572964530898/Current-Surgical-and-Endoscopic-Bariatric-Procedures-The-four-surgical-procedures-shown.jpg.

The procedure allows for visualization of the esophagus, stomach, and duodenum. It is extensively used for diagnosing diseases , such as gastroesophageal reflux disease, ulcers, and tumors. The procedure frequently involves insertion of a flexible endoscope through the mouth, enabling real-time visualization of the upper GI tract, allowing health care providers to obtain biopsies or even intervene with procedures like stricture dilation or foreign body removal. Such features identify the key place of EGD in the continuum of patient care and solidify its place as a cornerstone of gastroenterological practice (Nehme et al., 2021). Besides upper GI endoscopy, colonoscopy is another important endoscopic procedure that is used to investigate the large intestine. The technique is responsible for colorectal cancer screening and diagnosing other gastrointestinal conditions, such as inflammatory bowel disease. During a colonoscopy, a flexible endoscope is inserted through the rectum, through which physicians can investigate the lining of the colon and identify abnormalities. The method not only facilitates visualization but also therapeutic interventions like polypectomy, where the polyps can be excised to avoid their development into cancers. Apart from this, colonoscopy preparation may include diet restriction and bowel purging in some cases, and thus, patient compliance and preparation are indicated for the best possible outcome. As increasing awareness of colorectal well-being continues to make colonoscopy a central preventive measure in healthcare systems (Gershman & Ament, 2021), capsule endoscopy has been a revolutionary innovation in the area of endoscopic examinations, particularly in the imaging of the small intestine, which was once really challenging due to its length and inaccessible nature. Folkerts has also clarified capsule endoscopy, which was introduced in 2001. Capsule endoscopy involves a patient swallowing a small, pill-sized camera that captures thousands of images as it travels through the gastrointestinal tract. It is particularly valuable in diagnosing diseases , such as Crohn's disease and small bowel tumors because it is less invasive than enteroscopy. Due to the high-resolution imaging technology employed, clinicians can obtain an extensive visual assessment of the small bowel, and diagnostic yield is greatly improved. Advances in this technique are a significant milestone in gastroenterology, demonstrating the continued evolution of endoscopic technology and its implications for patient management (Gershman & Ament, 2021; Nehme et al., 2021) (Figure 1.8).

1.2.1. Gastrointestinal Endoscopy

The role of gastrointestinal endoscopy in modern medicine cannot be underestimated since it is a critical diagnostic and therapeutic procedure to employ within the gastrointestinal tract. It is a minimal invasiveness procedure that allows for direct visualization of the esophagus, stomach, and intestines and has proven highly valuable in the diagnosis of ailments , such as gastroesophageal reflux disease (GERD), ulcers, and various forms of gastrointestinal bleeding. During the past decades, development in technology has enhanced the efficacy and safety of endoscopic interventions through the provision of improved imaging and higher precision interventions. Gastrointestinal endoscopy became pivotal in diagnostic procedures as well as therapeutic interventions, including polypectomy and stent placement, illustrating the advancement in this area in contemporary gastroenterology. Despite numerous benefits associated with gastrointestinal endoscopy, patient safety, in particular issues of radiation exposure during fluoroscopy-guided procedures, has become a first-order concern. Endoscopic retrograde cholangiopancreatography (ERCP) and interventional endoscopic ultrasound (EUS) both routinely employ fluoroscopy, which is dangerous to both patients and doctors due to radiation exposure. Gastroenterologists tend to be poorly trained in radiation safety, and the need for formalized dose management and safety education is highlighted. As outlined in current literature, adherence to current guidelines of organizations like the American Society for Gastrointestinal Endoscopy (ASGE) and European Society of Gastrointestinal Endoscopy (ESGE) can promote a safety culture, with practices like reducing fluoroscopy time and employing protection in endoscopy being crucial (Nishida et al., 2025). The psychological and emotional aspects of undergoing gastrointestinal endoscopy have gained increasing attention in recent studies, particularly regarding the anxiety levels of patients undergoing such procedures. Research has proven that pre-procedure anxiety can significantly impact patients' experiences and outcomes. Anxiety-reducing interventions, such as relaxation therapy and psychological preparation, have proved to be effective in alleviating patient discomfort before and during an endoscopic procedure. The results of studies have also indicated that the implementation of such strategies is capable of reducing state and trait anxiety in patients by a significant extent, enhancing the quality of their experience and satisfaction with care (Kaur & Williams, 2022). As the application of gastrointestinal endoscopy widens, the psychological dimensions of care will be critical in the provision of care to ensure patients' physical and psychological safety during the endoscopy procedure (Figure 1.9).

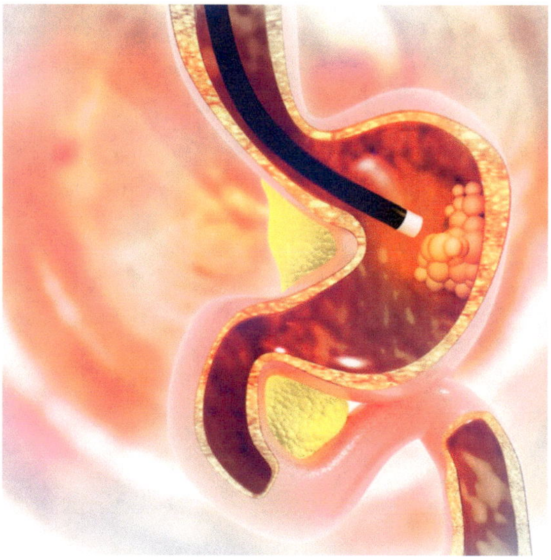

Figure 1.9. Upper Gi endoscopy procedure.

Source: https://ocgastroclinic.com/wp-content/uploads/2019/12/endoscopy-illustration-Orange-County-Gastro-Clinic.jpg.

1.2.2. Bronchoscopy

Bronchoscopy is a highly significant technique within the purview of endoscopy, applied particularly for observing airways and lungs. With a thin, flexible tube equipped with a camera and light source, physicians are able to examine the bronchial tubes for the kind of abnormalities that include tumors, infection, or obstruction. Perhaps the greatest advantage of bronchoscopy is that it is a minimally invasive procedure, allowing diagnostic and therapeutic interventions , such as biopsies or removal of foreign bodies. With advancing medical technology, bronchoscopy procedures are being pushed forward as well, with the addition of robotic aid, which will be able to improve precision and reduce patient discomfort. This transition to robotic bronchoscopy reflects a broader trend towards minimally invasive surgery with the theoretical advantages of decreased recovery periods and decreased complication rates that many clinicians and patients wish to explore (Runciman et al., 2019). The core of the evolution of bronchoscopy lies in increasing usage of artificial intelligence (AI) and imaging technology, which is being developed to augment the advantages of traditional bronchoscopy. AI will assist in identifying pathological change within lung tissue and provide physicians with important information that might not be visually discernible on a routine inspection. To this end, advances in imaging technology , such as high-definition scopes and augmented reality software, enable more precise visualization of complex lung anatomical structures. Such advances in technology promise to enhance diagnostic accuracy and unlock wider therapeutic potential of bronchoscopy, enabling clinicians to make improved treatment choices for patients. Secondly, ethical standards and regulatory guidelines overseeing the use of AI in bronchoscopy play an important role in advancing patient safety as this technology is applied to clinical use (Shane O'Sullivan et al., 2018). Bronchoscopy involves implications that extend beyond therapy and diagnosis; it also plays a critical role in research and training in pulmonary medicine. Through the use of bronchoscopy, researchers can gather valuable information on respiratory illness, which will facilitate a better comprehension of asthma, COPD, and lung cancer. The knowledge gained from interventions can be utilized to formulate clinical guidelines and enhance education programs for healthcare professionals. With the development of new procedures in bronchoscopy, it will be essential to establish an environment of interprofessional collaboration among pulmonologists, radiologists, and biomedical engineers. This collaborative model will ensure innovation and impose stringent standards in the practice of endoscopy, ultimately advancing patient outcomes in respiratory medicine (Runciman et al., 2019) (Figure 1.10).

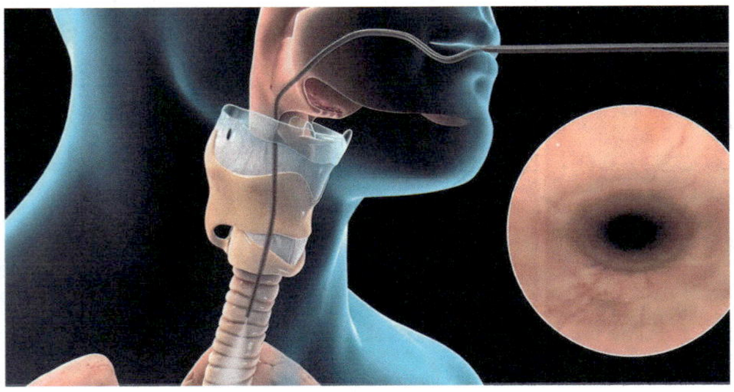

Figure 1.10. Bronchoscopy.

Source: https://hospitalpharmacyeurope.com/wp-content/uploads/2023/01/Dextromethorphan-premedication-decreases-self-rated-cough-in-bronchoscopy.jpg.

1.2.3. Urological Endoscopy

The urological endoscopy sector has evolved a great deal, a revolutionary progression that testifies to the changing nature of medical technology. The minimally invasive technique allows direct visualization of the urinary system, comprising the bladder, ureters, and kidneys. With the aid of advanced machinery, urologists can diagnose and also manage many conditions, such as urinary tract infections, bladder tumors, and kidney stones. More frequent use of endoscopic techniques over traditional open surgery has led to better patient outcomes, reduced recovery times, and fewer complications. With advances in imaging technology and instrumentation, not only does urological endoscopy enhance diagnostic effectiveness, but also provides ease in therapeutic maneuvers, and thus becomes a major contribution to the practice of contemporary urology. An example of such a remarkable procedure under urological endoscopy is the percutaneous nephrolithotomy (PCN), a procedure for the treatment of kidney stones. With the introduction of minimally invasive methods, open renal calculi surgery has become less frequent, as evidenced by statistics presented by the Department of Urology and Urological Endoscopy of St. Luke's Hospital. The hospital achieves a remarkable 90% success rate with PCN, along with anecdotal reports establishing zero mortality rates for these procedures (Cutajar, 1989).

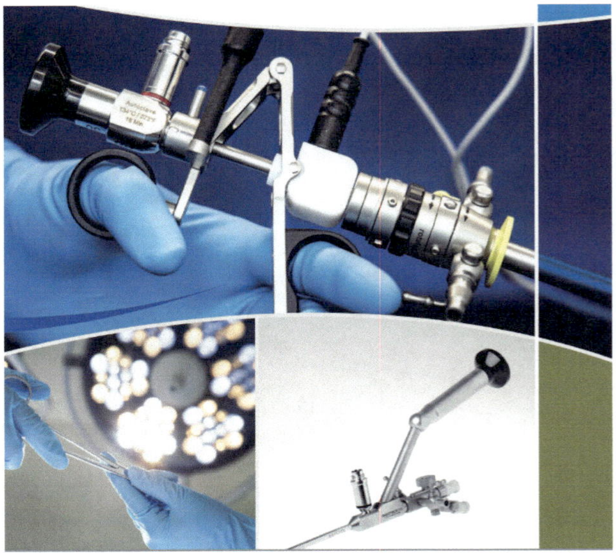

Figure 1.11. Endoscopy urology installation.

Source: https://edisondutasarana.co.id/bivocel/2023/03/Screenshot-2023-03-30-at-01.24.25.png.

Such statistics prove the efficiency of urological endoscopy in the management of recurrent yet complex urinary complications, and call for sustained learning and adoption of such procedures in urological practice. Additional commitment to ongoing research and practice in the application of urological endoscopy is also necessary to enhance further medical progress. Acknowledgment of contributions from all parties involved, including patients and physicians, is crucial in the enhancement of such procedures. Grant-funded research investigations, such as funding from the Big Lottery Fund, play an important role in evaluating and maximizing the effectiveness of urological procedures (Kazimierczak et al., 2015). With the vision of enhanced patient care by the medical community, such investigations support the development of best practice and awareness of complications, finally towards an evidence-based approach to urological endoscopy. Therefore, training programs emphasizing the values and benefits of this specialty not only inform practitioners but also empower patients with their treatment journey (Figure 1.11).

1.3. Indications for Endoscopy

The reach of endoscopy usage has gone far beyond due to its critical role in the diagnosis and treatment of gastrointestinal illnesses. Initially, endoscopy was primarily applied for diagnostic purposes, allowing physicians to visualize the esophagus, stomach, and intestines directly. However, its uses expanded to therapeutic interventions, such as tissue biopsy, polypectomy, and the management of gastrointestinal bleeding. By enabling practitioners to give visual feedback in real time, endoscopy makes possible interventions that would otherwise have to be achieved through invasive surgical methods, and hence reduces recovery and hospitalization times. This is evidence of the growing utilization of minimally invasive techniques in modern medicine, where patient outcomes are maximized and the physical cost of treatment is kept to an absolute minimum. With advances in endoscopic technology, its application range is likely to broaden further, making it even more useful in clinical practice. For inflammatory bowel diseases (IBD), endoscopy indications are immensely significant. With the growing know-how about IBD, appreciation of its associated neoplastic and structural complications that can arise has also grown. Endoscopic therapies are increasingly being employed to manage colitis-associated dysplasia, reflecting their utility in preventing disease progression. Endoscopic submucosal dissection is one of the methods that is increasingly becoming the frontline in managing such complex cases, though the evidence base is still emerging. A recent overview emphasized that advances in endoscopic technology have encouraged minimally invasive methods to erstwhile surgical conditions, citing a paradigm shift in the treatment of IBD patients. These advances are a measure of the augmenting demand for endoscopy, not merely in diagnosis but also in managing pesky complications of long-standing gastrointestinal illness (Clement & Reyes, 2024).

Aside from therapeutic and diagnostic intervention in IBD, endoscopy is better known for its use in the treatment of complicated, advanced gastrointestinal disease. These include future uses in the management of fibrostenotic disease complications, such as balloon dilation, with encouraging results. Incorporation of augmented reality (AR) into endoscopic interventions is also gaining traction, permitting improved navigation for operators during difficult interventions. While AR systems are as yet in an early stage in clinical practice, they offer exciting prospects for improved outcomes in gastrointestinal endoscopy with regard to real-time visualization and guidance, especially in complex cases (Metzger et al., 2024). Since endoscopic techniques are becoming more sophisticated and universally accepted, the field of endoscopy indications includes an expanded list of gastrointestinal ailments, reshaping the norm of how practitioners make diagnoses, treat, and intervene in this field.

1.3.1. Diagnostic Purposes

The diagnostic capability of endoscopy has revolutionized the scope of practice in the field of gastrointestinal medicine with direct visualization inside and with the option of procuring tissue specimens for histological analysis. The importance of this technique is underscored by the fact that it is employed to identify abnormal growths, inflammatory bowel disease, and other serious gastrointestinal illness. In addition to aiding in diagnosis, endoscopy plays a crucial role in disease follow-up and response to treatment. Practitioners are thus capable of tailoring treatment based on concrete, visible facts. With the use of advanced endoscopic technology, such as endoscopic ultrasound and video capsule endoscopy, there is greater diagnostic accuracy that can allow for examination of conditions not readily predictable from traditional imaging studies. Beyond direct visualization, the growing research into biomarkers that indicate digestive well-being becomes more emphasized in endoscopic diagnosis. For instance, fecal volatile organic compounds (VOCs) analysis has been suggested as one possible non-invasive diagnostic method for the detection of some gastrointestinal disorders. Experiments show that lifestyle parameters , such as body mass index, diet, and smoking status heavily influence the content of fecal VOCs, making it theoretically challenging to decode the biomarkers for use as diagnostic markers (Bosch et al., 2019). The combination of VOC analysis with endoscopic evaluation has the potential to streamline patient evaluation, provide more substantial diagnostic insight and hence improve clinical outcomes in the treatment of gastrointestinal diseases. The other significant role of endoscopy in diagnostic practice is that it is able to differentiate noncardiac chest pain (NCCP) from other more lethal conditions. NCCP patients usually undergo a series of interventions, including endoscopic testing to exclude gastrointestinal disorders , such as GERD and dysmotility of the esophagus (Yamasaki & Fass, 2017). The introduction of novel diagnostic approaches, including high-resolution esophageal manometry and pH-impedance testing, has enhanced understanding of NCCP and its pathophysiology. By combining these diagnostic modalities with endoscopic findings, clinicians are able to deliver targeted interventions addressing the root causes of patient distress, thereby allowing for both diagnostic sensitivity and therapeutic efficacy in the management of complicated cases seen in contemporary gastrointestinal practice (Figure 1.12).

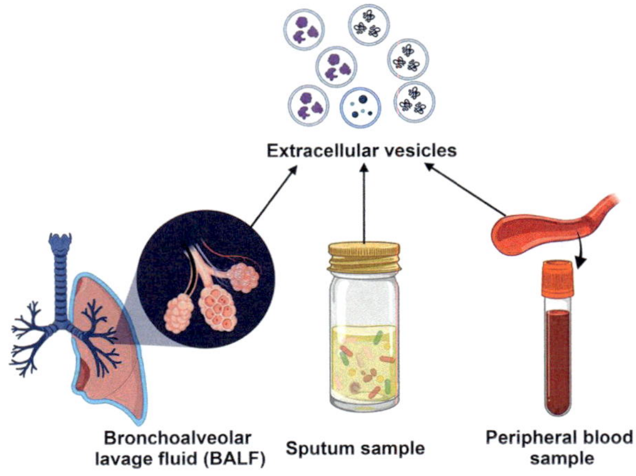

Figure 1.12. Three sources of possible extracellular vesicles (EVs) for diagnostic purposes.

Source: https://www.researchgate.net/publication/370558997/figure/fig3/AS:11431281156036738@1683340008292/Three-sources-of-possible-EVs-for-diagnostic-purposes-created-with-BioRendercom.png.

1.3.2. Therapeutic Interventions

The introduction of endoscopic technology has greatly transformed therapeutic interventions in the gastrointestinal space. Traditionally, invasive treatments commonly involved large incisions, permitting brief periods of recovery and greater patient discomfort. However, endoscopy has shifted this model by enabling minimally invasive treatments that address many different gastrointestinal conditions. This evolution involves the application of advanced methods , such as EMR and ESD, which enable the resection of early cancers and other lesions with preservation of the integrity of the surrounding tissue. These procedures are a reflection of the growing emphasis on methods that facilitate effective treatment with less post-procedure recovery needs, and thus enhance patient care and postoperative recovery in general (Ana-Maria Sîngeap et al., 2023). Moreover, therapeutic intervention via endoscopy encourages a more precise approach to disease management. With evolving knowledge regarding gastrointestinal diseases, endoscopic procedures are increasingly being applied not just for diagnostic purposes but also to bring about direct therapy. Techniques , such as balloon dilatation for strictures or stent placements have laid the foundation for remarkable improvement in therapeutic results. For instance, therapeutic intervention within the small intestine has traditionally been limited by the complexity of the area, informally known as the black box of the GI tract. But the combination of capsule endoscopy and enteroscopy allows for a complete evaluation and management of disease in this enigmatic region, greatly aiding clinical decision-making (Ana-Maria Sîngeap et al., 2023). The combination is an expression of greater capacity toeffectively treat complex gastrointestinal disease. The prospect of endoscopic treatment appears ever brighter, with continuous innovation offering better therapeutic outcomes. Video and robot-assisted techniques are also becoming integral to endoscopy, with hybrid surgical techniques progressively diminishing invasiveness. Super minimally invasive surgery (SMIS) is particularly noteworthy, with its goal of treating diseases in a manner that cures without impairing the functioning of the organ or anatomical structure. This new technique is shared with ongoing work on screening for the common complications of open and even minimally invasive surgery (Linghu, 2021). As the field of medicine continues to refine and perfect these techniques, the future potential for endoscopic therapeutic procedures to guide the way for new treatment paradigms is significant; its promise to simplify patient outcomes across a broad range of gastrointestinal disease is encouraging.

1.3.3. Screening for Diseases

The role of endoscopy in the detection of disease is significant, particularly in the early diagnosis of gastrointestinal disease. The endoscopic techniques allow direct visualization of the gastrointestinal tract, which is much better in its ability to identify abnormalities , such as polyps, tumors, and lesions that are not readily visible using non-invasive imaging modalities. For instance, screening for colorectal cancer increasingly relies on procedures , such as colonoscopy, where adenoma detection rates become key indicators of ongoing surveillance and prevention programs. As guidelines on screening evolve, the emphasis on the value of early intervention by these measures comes into focus, affirming the necessity of effective screening protocols in clinical practice. Advances in endoscopic devices have also improved the efficiency of disease screening, leading to improved patient outcomes. Techniques like water-assisted colonoscopy (WAC) offer the important advantage of eliminating pain in patients, which is an important consideration that can influence adherence to screening and patient compliance with follow-up recommendations. WAC not only enhances bowel cleanliness, hence procedural visibility, but also enables more accurate identification of important lesions important for the early diagnosis and treatment of disease, particularly in IBD patients. These technologies show an unmistakable drift toward decreased procedural pain at the cost of greater diagnostic accuracy, emphasizing the pivotal role that endoscopic technology plays in disease screening. Moreover, the introduction of AI in endoscopy will revolutionize screening by enabling more precise detection and evaluation of gastrointestinal disease. With continued research that identifies applications for AI in interpreting endoscopic images, the worth of reducing false negatives and enhancing diagnostic confidence is multiplying exponentially. According to existing literature, the application of AI technologies in screening processes can aid gastroenterologists in the identification of low-risk neoplastic lesions and the overall quality improvement of gastrointestinal screening. This enhances patient safety as well as optimizes resource allocation in the healthcare system through targeted interventions directed at individuals with a higher risk of severe conditions, thereby optimizing the overall process of disease screening (Falt et al., 2023).

1.4. Preparation for Endoscopy

Preparation is necessary before endoscopy for the purposes of obtaining safety and efficiency in the process. It is a process consisting of a set of protocols that patients must follow in an attempt to optimize their preparation for gastrointestinal examination. Preparation takes the form of dietary restriction, bowel preparation, and consultation for medication adjustment. Patients are normally requested to have a clear liquid diet for some period of time before the procedure to reduce any food residues that may obscure the field of vision during endoscopy. Laxatives may also be administered to enhance bowel cleansing, diminish complications, and enhance diagnostic yield. This preparation phase has a crucial function in patient outcomes through minimizing procedural risk and enhancing the visual delineation of the gastrointestinal tract during endoscopy, consistent with the broader goal of value creation in healthcare as described in recent work on patient-centred strategies (Böbel & Martis, 2009). Apart from dietary changes, patients need to be educated about the need to reveal their medical history, particularly previous gastrointestinal complaints and current medications. Some drugs, notably anticoagulants, may pose a risk of bleeding during the procedure, and their handling should be dealt with before endoscopy. In this regard, patient-physician communication is crucial. It facilitates customization of care and preparation to the individual needs of the patient, providing a setting that is centered on high-value delivery of medical care.

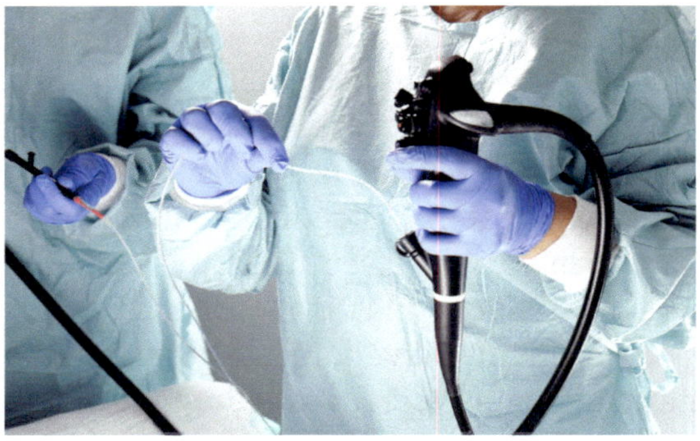

Figure 1.13. Prepare for your endoscopy procedure.

Source: https://www.dhcoftx.com/wp-content/uploads/2020/03/endoscopy-procedure-scaled.jpg.

In addition, patient education about what to expect, for example, sedation options and related discomfort, can minimize anxiety and enhance overall satisfaction with the endoscopic process, thus stimulating both better patient compliance and positive health outcomes (Bloor et al., 2009). Finally, awareness of the part to be played by medical workers conducting the endoscopy is important at the point of preparation. Nurses as well as physicians receive training for such procedures, but the expanding role of the nurse practitioner in gastro-endoscopy has been established in current literature. Evidence proves that trained nurses not only provide care effectively and safely but can also enhance patient satisfaction by a thorough examination. This shift to an interdisciplinary approach to preparing and conducting endoscopies highlights the potential for integrating care for patients while maintaining high degrees of quality and efficiency (Bloor et al., 2009; Böbel & Martis, 2009). With their experience and patient-focused practices, healthcare teams can generate a supportive system that maximizes effective endoscopic outcomes (Figure 1.13).

1.4.1. Patient Assessment and Medical History

Medical history and patient assessment are crucial to understanding the endoscopy practice as the foundation for effective diagnosis and treatment planning. A thorough patient history is information related to symptoms, previous illnesses, medications, and family health history, all of which provide insight to the endoscopist about risks and conditions that may affect the process. The information obtained in this assessment allows clinicians to anticipate complications and modify their approach accordingly. A patient with underlying gastrointestinal conditions or prior adverse reactions to sedation, for instance, requires specific considerations that can dramatically alter the management course. Hence, the inclusion of comprehensive patient histories is not just a check-box exercise; it is an integral component in patient outcome optimization, particularly in endoscopic interventions that could be fraught with risks involved with working in the gastrointestinal tract (Essaidi et al., 2025). In addition to traditional methods of obtaining medical histories, emerging technologies like the use of AI and large language models (LLMs) are transforming the manner in which healthcare practitioners can assess patient histories. One recent paper demonstrates the ability to use a GPT-capable chatbot to help administer history, demonstrating that technology can automate the stress previously inherent with patient encounters (Holderried et al., 2024). By providing medical students and practitioners a low-stress environment in which to hone their communication skills, these machines not only enhance test validity but provide a way of repeated practice in an environment of control. The ability of the chatbots to imitate a list of responses ensures that healthcare providers can prepare for various patient scenarios, leading to improved patient assessments which are crucial before endoscopic procedures.

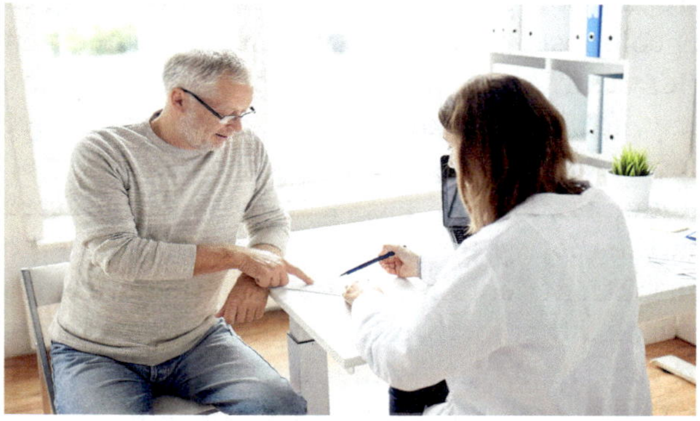

Figure 1.14. Patient assessment.

Source: https://images.squarespace-cdn.com/content/v1/5b9ad4b631d4df982a3a2ebe/1575301057313-XFFH9I1HCT67RSDYUKGI/provider_patient_asssessment.png.

In addition, the potential use of LLMs consists of speeding up and improving documentation within patient assessments. Improved documentation has been directly linked to better patient safety results, particularly in complex procedures like endoscopy where communication is absolutely imperative. As digital technologies continue to advance, the integration of AI-driven solutions into clinical work might make documentation easy while ensuring all patient information that needs to be gathered is captured firmly (Essaidi et al., 2025). This development emphasizes ongoing research and training with regard to these technologies because they represent an innovative step toward improving patient assessment procedures. In the long term, the use of AI in the form of patient history not only saves time but also enhances the overall safety and efficiency of medical care in the context of endoscopy (Figure 1.14).

1.4.2. Pre-Procedure Instructions

Effective pre-procedure counseling is a key to the success of endoscopic procedures as it influences patient outcomes and procedure efficiency. Such counseling typically includes dietary modifications aimed at optimal preparation of the bowel in procedures , such as colonoscopy. Recent evidence indicates that diet restrictions in the pre-procedure period may not be standardized in nature and hence necessitate the application of evidence-based guidelines. For instance, a study was conducted on the dietary intake of patients who undergo outpatient colonoscopy, and the findings revealed that food restriction compliance tends to vary. Importantly, the findings showed that patients would not necessarily need to adhere to rigid fiber restriction on the day before the procedure, favoring greater flexibility in diet choices to enhance patient comfort without risking bowel preparation quality (Jacobson et al., 2018). These strategies not only help manage pre-procedure anxiety but also improve overall patient satisfaction. Other than dietary requirements, pre-procedure instructions for endoscopy also involve significant recommendations regarding medications and lifestyle considerations. Patients typically are instructed to discontinue certain medications, namely anticoagulants and antiplatelet drugs, in an attempt to decrease the risk of bleeding during and after the procedure. Furthermore, preprocedural instructions may extend to counsel regarding abstaining from alcohol or cigarettes, as these inversely impair sedation effectiveness and integrity of the gut mucosa. Adherence to such instructions is paramount for facilitating safe and effective procedures. As noted in volumetric laser endomicroscopy research, adherence to such guidelines will have significant impacts on diagnosis outcomes, influencing the identification of tissue pathology and the implementation of suitable intervention strategies (Smith et al., 2019). Detailed pre-procedure counseling is thus critical in patient preparation for an effective endoscopy. Moreover, patient education is a fundamental component of pre-procedure education aimed at demystifying endoscopy and eliminating any fears the patient might have. Providing patients with clear, succinct information on what to expect during the procedure, including sensations, duration, and risk factors, empowers patients to become actively involved in their health care decisions. Educational outreach can be facilitated through the use of brochures, videos, or direct one-on-one interaction with healthcare workers to effectively transmit this information. These interventions enhance patient comprehension, providing a setting for teamwork that ultimately leads to optimal follow-through on pre-procedure instructions and increased procedural preparedness. Overall, a thorough pre-procedure preparation involving dietary advice, management of medications, and patient education is the cornerstone of a successful endoscopic procedure, emphasizing the importance of correct preparation in achieving maximum outcomes.

1.4.3. Importance of Informed Consent

Informed consent is a central component of the ethical model in healthcare generally and of endoscopic procedures in particular. This critical process facilitates that patients are appropriately informed about the nature, risks, and benefits of the procedure to be undertaken. In the case of endoscopy, where therapeutic and diagnostic interventions take place within the gastrointestinal tract, the stakes are high; hence, patient comprehension of options is vital. By requiring that the patients are well-informed and by voluntarily consenting to the procedure, medical practitioners not only comply with lawful criteria but also establish a trusting relationship with the patients. Recent research conducted at the Nishtar Hospital Multan, presents evidence to the fact that nurses recognized patient information as an important aspect while undergoing endoscopy procedures and stressed the involvement of the nurses in making informed consent a part of holistic patient care (Parveen et al., 2023). The COVID-19 crisis has once again highlighted the significance of informed consent for endoscopic practice. As clinics evolve with new challenges and guidelines, the need to convey risks more effectively has become imperative. Endoscopic procedures fall under the category of aerosol-generating procedures and carry their own set of challenges requiring transparent communication regarding other risks pertaining to viral transmission. Informed written consent involving relevant information regarding the pandemic must be obtained from the patient's family and him. This not only ensures compliance but also harmonizes patient expectations with the facts of their clinical situation in times so unprecedented. Appropriate conversation about the implications of having procedures done during a pandemic demonstrates how informed consent plays a crucial role in patient and healthcare provider health (Pate et al., 2020). Furthermore, informed consent also allows for greater patient satisfaction and adherence to follow-up care. When patients are empowered to feel included in their process of care and are well-informed about their treatment, they are more likely to follow medical advice and achieve favorable outcomes. The technical nature of endoscopy is likely to instill fear; therefore, detailed explanation and resolution of patient concerns becomes the norm. Continuous education of healthcare professionals about the practice of effective consent ensures that patients feel respected and valued. Since the study's results have indicated, ongoing training of the medical personnel, especially nurses, significantly helps to enhance the process of informed consent and thereby patient overall safety and satisfaction during endoscopic treatment (Parveen et al., 2023) (Figure 1.15).

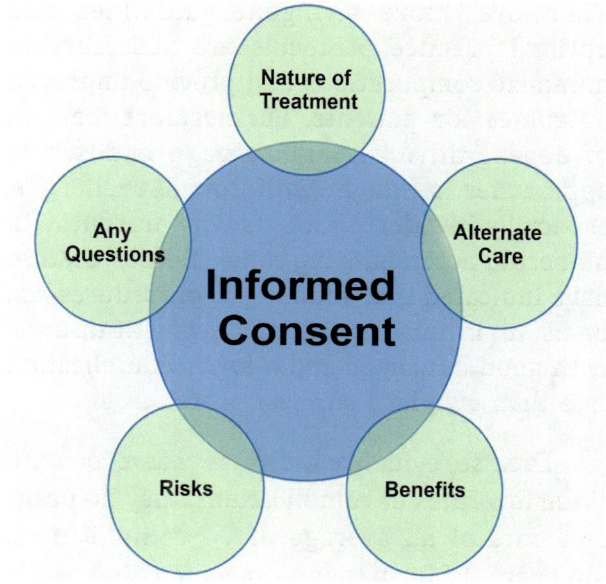

Figure 1.15. Informed consent.

Source: https://postgraddc.com/wp-content/uploads/2022/08/Informed-Consent-2048x1408.png.

1.5. Risks and Complications

The endoscopy procedure, while sophisticated and extensively used, is not free of risk and complications and must be faced by the practitioners. One of the serious hazards is neurological deterioration, particularly with fluid insufflation. These accidents, though infrequent, can have calamitous implications for the patient, including heightened intracranial pressure and trauma secondary to durotomy, as highlighted in recent surveys. A case series documented transient ipsilateral weakness and lumbosacral plexopathy, both secondary to high irrigation pressures with uniportal spine endoscopy. These complications underscore the paramount importance of properly managing pressures for irrigation to minimize related risks and enhance patient safety during endoscopic interventions (Liu et al., 2025).

Therefore, more stringent guidelines and optimal practice protocols are necessary to minimize complications and provide improved outcomes for patients. Furthermore, control of degenerative disease through endoscopic approaches is fraught with unique challenges, especially in elderly patients who present with numerous accompanying comorbidities. Studies have indicated that endoscopic procedures can be useful in treating adjacent segment disease, with good outcomes and a lower complication rate than standard surgical procedures.

Even so, evidence indicates that, even with these low rates of complications, they do occur at a rate of an average of 94 complications for every 1,000 patients, meaning that while endoscopy might significantly benefit clinical outcomes, caution is still the key with this vulnerable population. The search for ways to enhance postoperative recovery while concurrently minimizing complications is critical in advancing endoscopic procedures (Evangelista et al., 2025). Thus, research needs to continue to evaluate the effectiveness and safety of such methods. In conclusion, education and resolution of the complications and risks associated with endoscopic procedures are critical in enhancing patient care. As the field advances, additional study of complications arising from various techniques and patient populations will be needed to direct optimal practice. By examination of the mechanisms by which complications develop, particularly in areas like neurological decline and management of degenerative disease, clinicians may start to develop more effective prevention strategies. The ongoing evolution in endoscopic methods necessitates an ongoing equilibrium among clinical efficacy and patient safety, which emphasizes the need for ongoing high-quality studies with the focus of illuminating the entire spectrum of risks present in the procedures (Evangelista et al., 2025; Liu et al., 2025).

1.5.1. Common Risks Associated with Endoscopy

Endoscopy, being a valuable diagnostic and therapeutic tool, carries intrinsic risks that cannot be avoided. Some of the most common complications are hemorrhage and perforation, either of which can be caused during the procedure. Perforation is caused by the endoscope unintentionally breaking through a nearby organ, leading to possible intra-abdominal infections or needing surgery. Clinical studies indicate that risk of perforation, although small, is determined by the type of procedure as well as the existing diseases of the patient.." Apart from this, bleeding from the polypectomy or biopsy site can also occur, and though generally manageable, may become a serious condition requiring blood transfusion or further operation. The importance of understanding these risks is pivotal to health care providers and patients alike as they attempt to navigate the complex field of endoscopic procedures. Apart from these risks, there is also sedation-related complication to be performed during endoscopy. Procedures are usually done with moderate sedation to make the patient more comfortable and cooperative, but it is also risky. Side effects of sedative drugs can range from respiratory depression to cardiovascular instability, particularly in comorbid patients. Observational evidence indicates that older patients or comorbid diseases patients, like heart disease, are at greater risk of facing these complications. Further, the potential for solving sedation issues requires trained personnel and observation, again highlighting the complications inherent in the endoscopic technique. Thus, the sedation aspect of endoscopy must be approached with care, yet keeping patient safety foremost during the procedure. Finally, infection is also a specific risk associated with endoscopic techniques. While infrequent, the introduction of instruments into clean sites provides channels for bacterial penetration. Endoscope reprocessing guidelines attempt to minimize this risk, but there can be failures and nosocomial infections can ensue. Research indicates that such nosocomial infections can appear in the form of loose cases of gastroenteritis or, in severe instances, lead to systemic infection requiring extended hospital stay and even intensive care unit admission. Certain procedures, such as ERCP, have been found to be most often linked with post-procedure pancreatitis as a complication. Although the rate of occurrence of these complications is fairly low, the potential consequence makes it important to ensure meticulous procedural protocols and patient education regarding the risks involved with endoscopic interventions (Vasireddy et al., 2021; Marinov et al., 2024) (Figure 1.16).

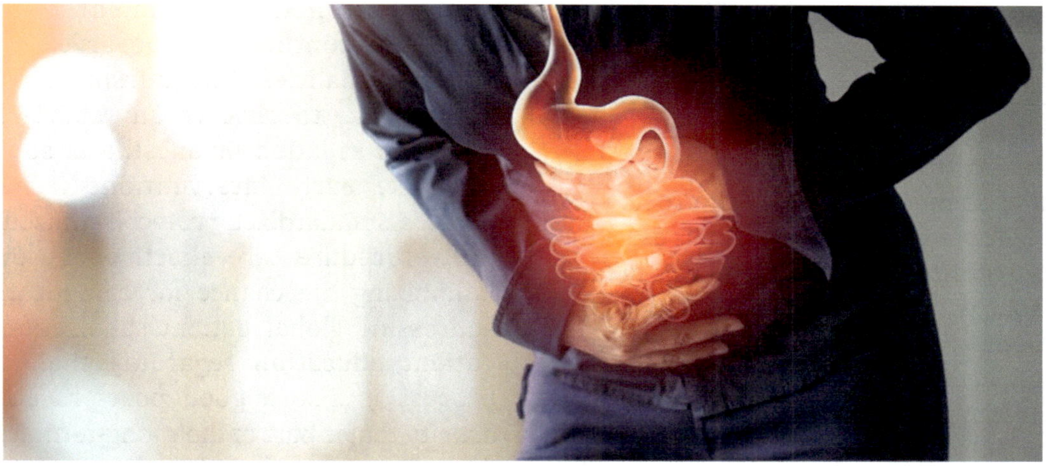

Figure 1.16. Common risks associated with endoscopy.

Source: https://clinicbooking.com/uploads/users/33/articles/blog-single-1728917901-shutterstock_1185264241.jpg.

1.5.2. Potential Complications During the Procedure

Endoscopic tests, as helpful as they are in making the interior of the gastrointestinal tract visible, are accompanied by a set of possible complications. Hypoxemia, a risk otherwise, is one such possible complication, particularly in those involving sedation. Patients undergoing endoscopy may exhibit fluctuations in levels of oxygen saturation, which causes severe respiratory distress unless monitored and treated promptly, can result. Existing research emphasizes the importance of employing advanced monitoring techniques to detect hypoxemia early. Such circumstances have seen growth in automated anesthesia systems, which have been helpful in maintaining oxygen levels at bay. The AAS-GE trial, for instance, will determine if an AI-assisted anesthesia system can reduce episodes of hypoxemia by adjusting anesthetic delivery automatically based on real-time information, which could enhance patient safety while undergoing gastrointestinal endoscopy (Bing et al., 2025). One other complication that may arise during endoscopic procedures is hemodynamic instability, an episode caused by changes in vascular response after sedation or mechanical manipulation during the procedure. Unpredictable hypotensive attacks can occur, and prompt intervention by the anesthesia team is indicated. Close observation of hemodynamic parameters is to be emphasized, especially in patients with underlying cardiovascular illness. Application of AI in the management of anesthesia, as discussed in the AAS-GE trial, could provide an active approach. By fine-tuning anesthetic agents according to the individualistic features of patients and maintaining diligent observation on vital signs, the risk of hemodynamic instability can be significantly reduced, resulting in safer procedural outcomes (Bing et al., 2025). Hemodynamic stability remains an essential issue in endoscopic practice, reinforcing the requirement of advanced monitoring and experience. In addition to respiratory and hemodynamic complications, procedural failures remain a problem in endoscopy. Whereas procedures such as capsule endoscopy have been utilized for home use, seen with the ACE service, issues like poor preparation can enable the success of such procedures to be thwarted. Data from the UCLH's ACE service indicated high rates of completion, but failed procedures reveal that proper bowel preparation is essential for success. Understanding the etiology behind complications will aid protocol adjustments and patient counseling. Of note, low complication rates in ACE, in addition to high scores of patient satisfaction, suggest that new methods are able to surmount traditional risks while enhancing patient compliance and tolerance for endoscopic assessment (Figure 1.17).

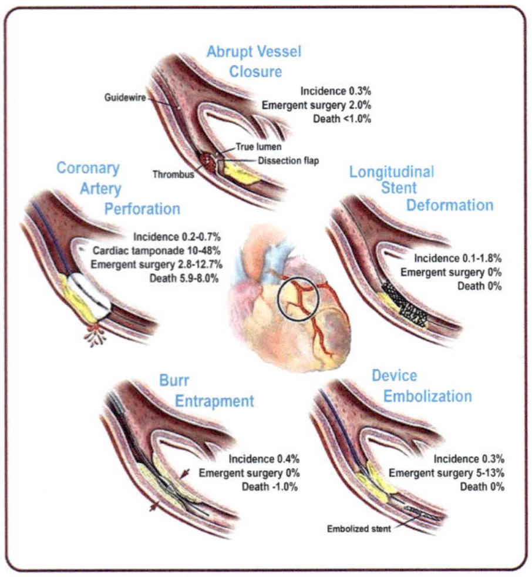

Figure 1.17. Complications during the procedure.

Source: https://cdn.medizzy.com/2W4xymdl0OIYsPjFbXM2w3PuU6Q=/680x669/img/posts/dc5ce465-22fd-49d9-9ce4-6522fd69d9bd.

1.5.3. Post-Procedure Care and Monitoring

Post-procedure monitoring and follow-up are crucial to ensure patient protection and optimal results following endoscopic interventions. Recovery must be closely observed for the development of complications like bleeding, perforation, or infection. Monitoring is done in a controlled environment where vital signs are continuously observed to search for abnormalities. The nursing staff should be attentive to observe any short-term side effects of sedation or anesthesia so that they can take early interventions if necessary. Besides, standardized protocols utilized enhance post-procedure care effectiveness, eventually minimizing the chance for complications and addressing global patient satisfaction. Proper patient education regarding their recovery process is also a good post-procedure care activity that is part of their long-term well-being.

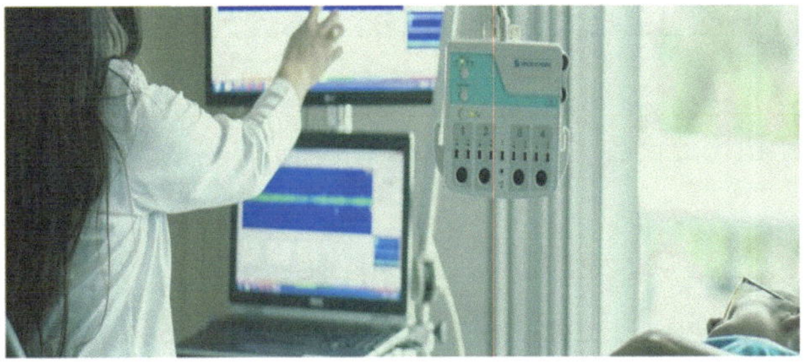

Figure 1.18. Post-procedure care and monitoring.

Source: https://www.slideteam.net/media/catalog/product/cache/1280x720/p/o/post_procedure_care_and_monitoring_myelogram_ppt_template_st_ai_ss_slide01.jpg.

Patients must be instructed on potential symptoms that will require immediate medical attention, like severe abdominal pain or excessive vomiting, which may not be complications following gastrointestinal endoscopy. In addition, giving patients detailed discharge instructions, including dietary restriction guidelines and how to take medication, allows them to be actively engaged in their postprocedure recovery. Clear communication is essential, as it leads to a sense of reassurance and confidence, which affects the patients' experience and follow-up care adherence significantly.

While under continuous surveillance, the implementation of performance measures that have been set by organizations , such as the European Society of Gastrointestinal Endoscopy is required to enhance the quality of endoscopy service care. Of all these measures, the adenoma detection rate and bowel preparation adequacy are sentinel markers of procedural and patient outcomes success. As brought into focus in updated guidelines, appropriateness of post-polypectomy surveillance recommendations is not only critical for the identification of patients at risk for potential complications but also for facilitating timely intervention plans. Continuous quality improvement programs founded on these performance measures can lead to optimized patient management, where the patient receives maximum care during their endoscopic process (Kamiński et al., 2017; Joshi & Badgwell, 2021) (Figure 1.18).

1.6. Advances in Endoscopic Technology

The endoscopy technology has experienced remarkable advancements that have positioned it as an advanced instrument in diagnosis and treatment. Advanced imaging technology, such as HD endoscopes and narrow band imaging (NBI), has significantly enhanced the visualization of anatomical structures and lesions. These technologies provide healthcare professionals with the ability to detect abnormalities at an early stage, which is crucial for conditions , such as gastrointestinal cancers. Furthermore, digital integration provides enhanced documentation and analysis of results, enabling specialists to collaborate. With the increasing demand for minimally invasive treatments, the continuous development of endoscopic equipment, such as cutting-edge EUS and robot-assisted platforms, highlights the position that technology holds to drive forward in this area. Not only does this improve the patient's outcomes, but also the efficiency of clinical pathways, such that endoscopy becomes the centerpiece of contemporary medicine.

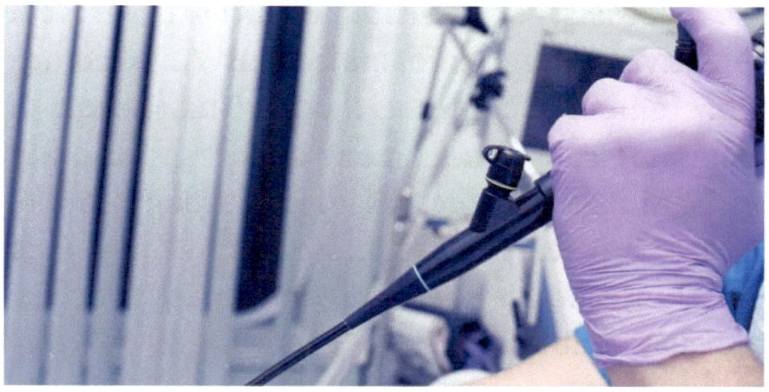

Figure 1.19. Advances in endoscopy.

Source: https://smarttechmed.com/wp-content/uploads/2024/12/BLOG5-1440.720-21-1024x512.webp.

The second major endoscopic innovation is the incorporation of AI into the procedural setting. AI is beginning to influence training, diagnostic sensitivity, and post-procedure analysis in the world of endoscopy. As an illustration, machine learning algorithms will be applied to assist in detecting polyps on colonoscopy and, as such, potentially reduce the risk of missed diagnosis. The use of AI in image segmentation and computer-aided diagnosis has the potential to maximize clinical workflows by simplifying endoscopic image analysis. But that thrilling potential is offset by the challenges that come with AI integration, such as data security and ethical implications related to patient confidentiality. The takeaways based on Najjar (2023) point to the reality that while AI possesses revolutionary potential, it also requires careful oversight of data quality as well as ethical standards governing its application so that the confidentiality of patients is preserved in clinical settings. The future of endoscopic technology is promising for increased advancements as researchers and clinicians unite to utilize new tools. Sustaining advancements are designed to make minimally invasive treatments more precise, to advance personalized medicine. The data protection issues that (Khan et al., 2023) highlighted acknowledge the necessity of robust measures to protect sensitive patient information as AI becomes more embedded in healthcare. This fusion of technological advancement and responsibility will guide the direction of endoscopy in the future. As health care increasingly moves to more interactive and preventive approaches, the sustainability of these innovations will rely on ongoing cooperation between technologists, practitioners, and policymakers to guarantee that innovations in endoscopy are aligned with ethics while providing improved health outcomes for patients (Figure 1.19).

1.6.1. Innovations in Imaging Techniques

The technological progress in imaging modalities has, in effect, revolutionized endoscopy as a clinical practice to enhance the possibility of proper diagnosis and therapeutic interventions greatly. Advanced high-definition imaging modalities , such as NBI and chromoendoscopy enable visualization of minute mucosal changes that may represent neoplastic processes. These developments enable clinicians to visualize the gastrointestinal tract's vascular networks and surface anatomy with unprecedented degrees of resolution and detail, enabling the earlier diagnosis of conditions , such as gastric neuroendocrine tumors (G-NETs). As highlighted by newer literature, the addition of such imaging modalities to endoscopic exploration significantly improves the diagnostic yield and allows interventions, which are significant given the varied nature of G-NETs, Type I to Type III, with different treatment modalities and outcomes (Christodoulidis et al., 2025). Furthermore, the development of EUS is a valuable innovation in abdominal imaging that offers an endoscopic view with ultrasonographic capability. EUS not only has utility in the assessment of gastrointestinal wall layers but also for the evaluation of nearby structures and metastatic detection in diseases , such as G-NETs.

Modality-two approach enhances the quality of tumor staging and grading, thereby making treatment planning more suitably personalized. The impact is enormous in clinical practice; with enhanced staging accuracy, the management of G-NETs is more evidence-based, ultimately culminating in optimal patient outcomes. The requirement for endoscopic ultrasound in clinical practice necessitates constant learning and training of health professionals to effectively use these advanced devices (Hill et al., 2024). Finally, imaging technologies are not only useful for diagnosis but also for treatment procedures. Techniques , such as laser endoscopy and radiofrequency ablation have been developed to offer minimally invasive tumor treatment, which is particularly suitable for gastric tumor patients. These techniques have the potential to reduce recovery periods and the associated risks of more aggressive procedures, such as partial or total gastrectomy for Type III G-NETs. The evolution of these imaging modalities underscores the necessity for continued education for gastrointestinal (GI) nurses, since they continue to play a critical role as members of procedural and post-procedural patient care teams. Keeping in line with the latest developments makes nursing responsibilities catch up with innovations in technology, ultimately leading to enhanced patient safety and care (Hill et al., 2024).

1.6.2. Development of Minimally Invasive Tools

The development of minimally invasive instruments revolutionized endoscopy, greatly enhancing diagnostic and therapeutic capabilities. Absent these technologies, traditional surgical approaches consisted of big cuts and lengthy recovery periods with substantial possibilities of complications. The development of endoscopic treatments has made it possible to use less invasive methods, reducing patient discomfort without compromising anatomical integrity. Procedures , such as laparoscopy and endoscopic mucosal resection involve minimal cuts or natural orifices and are responsible for enhanced cosmetic results and shortened hospital stays. Moreover, improvements in imaging technology, including high-definition visualization and fluorescence imaging, have enhanced the visibility and precision of endoscopic procedures, enabling practitioners to identify pathologies more efficiently. This transition to minimally invasive techniques is part of an overarching movement in medicine to optimize patient outcomes with minimal procedural risk, a sign of how technological innovation has come to critically influence the delivery of healthcare. Over the past decade or so, artificial intelligence and machine learning have become key drivers of innovation in the creation of minimally invasive devices. Methods , such as U-net, initially developed for image segmentation, have been found to be highly useful in the medical imaging community, even in the case of endoscopy. By their capacity to deliver quality segmentation of complex anatomical structures, these tools are facilitating improved training and performance of endoscopists, eventually leading to improved diagnostic performance. Integration of AI-based analysis into endoscopic systems allows for real-time feedback during procedures, which identifies potential abnormalities and supports decision-making. These technologies are a defining moment in endoscopic technology, merging advanced computing methods with traditional medical practice. The capacity for processing vast data sets of image data has maximized the speed of minimally invasive interventions, a watershed moment in the ongoing development of endoscopy and patient care. In addition, the application of minimally invasive devices has been found to have a significant impact on outcomes of surgery, particularly in colorectal cancer screening and management. According to the American Cancer Society, the introduction of high-sensitivity stool-based tests and visual examination procedures has allowed for early detection of colorectal cancer, drastically reducing death rates of the prevalent disease. Because these measures encourage habitual screening at age 45, they place emphasis on the employment of minimally invasive methods to facilitate patient compliance and success. The capacity to detect adenomatous polyps and precancerous lesions using endoscopic methods has underscored the role of these instruments in preventive medicine. By decreasing interventions required, yet enhancing screening methods, minimally invasive devices have transformed the treatment of colorectal cancer, promoting patient-centered care along with stringent clinical guidelines as outlined in recent studies (Wolf et al., 2018).

1.6.3. Future Trends in Endoscopic Research

The future of endoscopic research stands on the verge of dramatic advances brought about by technology and increasing understanding of gastrointestinal disease. One of the prime trends is the expansion of sophisticated imaging technology that will enhance visualization in endoscopy. Technologies , such as high-definition optical coherence tomography and narrow-band imaging will enable earlier and more accurate diagnosis of diseases , such as colorectal cancer and inflammatory bowel disease. As noted, colorectal cancer (CRC) is the second most common cause of cancer mortality globally, and early detection is of critical significance to effectively treat and manage (Hossain et al., 2022). The evolution of such imaging modalities underscores the importance of further research in developing and utilizing these technologies in clinical practice, culminating in better patient outcomes and survival rates. Moreover, AI and machine learning integration into endoscopy is a transformative trend that can revolutionize diagnostic capability. Algorithms that can decipher endoscopic images can assist doctors in detecting abnormalities more efficiently, reducing the risks of missed diagnosis and misdiagnosis. This technology is also supplemented by newer proposals for the use of small-bowel capsule endoscopy to optimize diagnostic accuracy for suspected gastrointestinal bleeding, again marking the influence of AI on procedural efficiency (Hossain et al., 2022). The capability of AI to examine large data sets in real-time would speed up diagnosis, streamline workflow, and tailor patient care, and thus is a promising advance in the future of endoscopic procedures. Lastly, the shift toward minimally invasive procedures is remodeling the future of endoscopic practice and research. Techniques , such as device-assisted enteroscopy allow for both therapy and diagnosis without the need for major surgery, which can be particularly beneficial for sick patients. The endorsement recommendation for these techniques underscores their place in managing complications , such as foreign body obstruction and life-threatening gastrointestinal bleeding (Pennazio et al., 2022). With more knowledge about the application of minimally invasive technologies, more and more of these technologies will be embraced and utilized in clinical settings, leading to improved patient experiences, reduced recovery times, and overall improved healthcare delivery.

SUMMARY

In conclusion, the development of endoscopy is a milestone in the medical field, especially in minimally invasive methods that improve patient care. The evolution of flexible endoscopes throughout history shows a trend towards increasing functionality and adaptability in diagnostic and therapeutic procedures. As the literature has outlined, with traditional designs stuck around for decades, the future of automation in endoscope navigation is a promising future for both maximizing procedure effectiveness and expanding fields of application. This advance highlights the ongoing requirement for research and development, as automated systems remain far from commercial feasibility, and invites research into cheap navigation algorithms as well as mechatronics addressing contemporary challenges in the field (Van der Stap et al., 2013). Additionally, the integration of advanced image-based navigation techniques offers considerable promise for advancing beyond contemporary limits. The most significant challenge remaining is determining strong steering algorithms that are capable of dealing with various forms of visual occlusions , such as bubbles and motion blur. These will be vital in ensuring that the autonomous navigation systems work efficiently and effectively during procedures, which will further enhance the surgeon's capability to carry out intricate operations. With the development of the area, it will become all the more essential for researchers to engineer systems that are not only technically skilled but also affordable and accessible to a greater number of healthcare centers (Van der Stap et al., 2013). The search for these additional functionalities and software development avenues will be critical to address the pressing demand for innovative solutions in endoscopy. Lastly, the future of endoscopy is closely tied to the provision of persistent funds and research inputs, as witnessed with initiatives , such as the Derek Willoughby Fund for Inflammatory Research, providing funding to the work of researchers in developing novel ideas. The advances, in addition to robust financial backing, put the discipline in good standing for radical growth. This support draws attention to the necessity for continued investment in the creation of low-cost, innovative technologies that can upgrade the functionality of flexible endoscopes. Overall, the combination of technological advancement, facilitative finance, and focused research will be the most important factors in ensuring the successful formulation of endoscopic practices and ultimately improved patient outcomes through diverse diagnostic and therapeutic procedures.

The evolution of endoscopy has been marked by major advances, particularly in the development and application of flexible endoscopes. While there has been no major modification in their design for half a century, there has been a remarkable shift towards applying flexible endoscopes in more complex therapeutic interventions. The trend points to the potential of expanded applications in clinical practice. However, current control systems of such endoscopes have been referred to as nonintuitive and nonergonomical at times, limiting their function in a broad spectrum of medical cases. Writers are convinced that endoscope navigation can be automated to counter such limitations, mentioning recent improvements in image-based algorithms for navigation. These new approaches are trying to optimize the control and dexterity of endoscopes during procedures, with the potential to revolutionize both the patient and practitioner experience in the field of flexible endoscopy (Van der Stap et al., 2013). The development of new endoscopic technologies was also catalyzed by the advent of wireless capsule endoscopy, providing a less invasive alternative for examining the GI tract. This new diagnostic tool offers complete probing of the entire GI tract, making it possible to diagnose various pathologies and diseases. Challenges still remain as the field develops to more advanced applications. The evolution from passive to active robotic capsule endoscopes is particularly noteworthy, with manufacturers working to add functionalities comparable to those of regular flexible endoscopes. Key to this shift is the need for precise localization of the active capsule devices within an anatomical three-dimensional space, which is critical to useful mapping and natural diagnosis (Turan et al., 2017). Moreover, advancing technological capabilities continue to extend endoscopic systems' capabilities. Among the most groundbreaking developments is the presence of visual simultaneous localization and mapping (SLAM) made custom for endoscopic capsule robots. The RGB-Depth SLAM technique is an engineering innovation in the sense that it enables real-time dense, globally consistent mapping of organs inside the body. Such precision not only helps ease healthcare practitioners through the complex anatomical landscape but also helps improve diagnostics. Incorporation of sophisticated tracking and modeling techniques makes these endoscopic robots capable of accommodating non-rigid surface deformations within the body, thereby improving overall efficacy and safety while inspecting. Emerging research in these technologies indicates a promising future for endoscopy, with the potential to enhance patient outcomes and diagnostic potential (Turan et al., 2017).

CLOSER LOOK

AEROSOL-GENERATING PROCEDURES:

Aerosol-generating procedures (AGPs) are medical or dental interventions that can produce tiny airborne particles capable of remaining suspended in the air for extended periods. These particles may contain infectious agents such as viruses or bacteria, which makes AGPs an important focus in infection-prevention planning, especially in the context of respiratory diseases. While many healthcare activities produce some degree of droplets, AGPs differ in that they create fine aerosols that can travel farther and persist longer, increasing the potential for airborne transmission.

Commonly recognized AGPs include procedures that manipulate a patient's airway or respiratory tract. Examples often cited in clinical literature include endotracheal intubation, bronchoscopy, open suctioning of airways, and certain forms of non-invasive ventilation. Dental interventions that rely on high-speed instruments can also generate aerosolized particles. Although the degree of risk varies across procedures, the shared characteristic is the potential for producing respirable particles that may carry infectious material.

Understanding AGPs requires considering three key factors: the method by which aerosols are produced, the environment in which the procedure occurs, and the pathogen involved. Mechanical forces—such as high-velocity airflow or rapidly moving instruments—can disperse secretions into fine particles. Enclosed or poorly ventilated spaces can allow these particles to accumulate, increasing exposure risk. Additionally, some pathogens are more efficiently transmitted through aerosols, meaning the same procedure may pose different levels of concern depending on the infectious agent present.

Because of these dynamics, AGPs have implications for how healthcare systems design protective strategies. Institutions typically evaluate room ventilation, airflow patterns, and the timing of room clearance after certain procedures. Protective measures—such as appropriate respiratory protection for staff—are chosen based on established risk assessments. While frontline workers often follow detailed procedural guidelines, the broader principle is that AGPs call for heightened awareness of airborne exposure pathways.

AGPs have also become a topic of discussion in public health policy. Outbreaks involving airborne or potentially airborne pathogens have prompted updates to guidance on which procedures should be categorized as aerosol-generating and how to mitigate associated risks. Ongoing research continues to refine these classifications, examining not only particle generation but also the infectious potential of the aerosols produced.

REFERENCES

1. Septimiu A, Ungureanu FD, Reka KI, Moldovan AC. A Proposed Therapeutic Algorithm for Colorectal Cancer Prevention, Based on Endoscopic Polypectomies in Patients with Multiple Colonic Polyps. *Journal of Mind and Medical Sciences.* 2018; 5(2):261-269. https://doi.org/10.22543/7674.52.P261269.pdf (accessed on 15th July 2025).
2. Turan, M., Almalioglu, Y., Araujo, H. *et al.* A non-rigid map fusion-based direct SLAM method for endoscopic capsule robots. *Int J Intell Robot Appl* **1**, 399–409 (2017). https://doi.org/10.1007/s41315-017-0036-4 (accessed on 15th July 2025).
3. Altorfer, F., Avrumova, F., & Lebl, D. (2024). Robotic-assisted decompression, decortication, and instrumentation for minimally invasive transforaminal lumbar interbody fusion. *JBJS Essential Surgical Techniques, 14*(4). https://www.semanticscholar.org/paper/2a0142d6a37d5c6c1beaf931b8a7690bf647a25c (accessed on 15th July 2025).
4. Arebi, N., Saunders, B. P., & Surgical Procedures, Endoscopic. (2005). *Endoscopy: An Evolving Specialty.* https://core.ac.uk/download/46602009.pdf (accessed on 15th July 2025).
5. Aziz, M., Haghbin, H., Sayeh, W., Alfatlawi, H., Gangwani, M. K., Sohail, A. H., Zahdeh, T., et al. (2022). Comparison of artificial intelligence with other interventions to improve adenoma detection rate for colonoscopy. *Journal of Clinical Gastroenterology, 58,* 143–155. https://doi.org/10.1097/mcg.0000000000001813 (accessed on 15th July 2025).
6. Smith, M. S., Cash, B., Konda, V., Trindade, A. J., Gordon, S., DeMeester, S., Joshi, V., Diehl, D., Ganguly, E., Mashimo, H., Singh, S., Jobe, B., McKinley, M., Wallace, M., Komatsu, Y., Thakkar, S., Schnoll-Sussman, F., Sharaiha, R., Kahaleh, M., Tarnasky, P., ... Chang, K. (2019). Volumetric laser endomicroscopy and its application to Barrett's esophagus: results from a 1,000 patient registry. *Diseases of the esophagus : official journal of the International Society for Diseases of the Esophagus, 32*(9), doz029. https://doi.org/10.1093/dote/doz029(accessed on 15th July 2025).
7. Bing, H. L., Li, S. Y., Li, Y. W., Wang, Q. M., Wang, Y., Li, L. M., Liu, S. Q., et al. (2025). Automated anesthesia systems–gastrointestinal endoscopy (AAS-GE): Protocol for a single-center, randomized controlled trial. *Intelligent Anesthesia.* https://www.semanticscholar.org/paper/0d352131b2c7da81357f54bc58d0bf8bb824a9cd (accessed on 15th July 2025).
8. Bloor, K., Cheung, W. Y., Coulton, S., Durai, R., et al. (2009). *Effectiveness of nurse delivered endoscopy: Findings from randomized multi-institution nurse endoscopy trial (MINuET).* https://core.ac.uk/download/50820.pdf (accessed on 15th July 2025).
9. Böbel, Ingo & Martis, Amrita, 2009. "**Value Creation in Health Care: The Case of the Princesse Grace Hospital (CHPG) Monaco**," MPRA Paper 19689, University Library of Munich, Germany.(accessed on 15th July 2025).
10. Bosch, S., Lemmen, J., de Menezes, R. X., van der Hulst, R. R. W. J., Kuijvenhoven, J., Stokkers, P., de Meij, T. G., et al. (2019). The influence of lifestyle factors on fecal volatile organic compound composition as measured by an electronic nose. *Journal of Breath Research, 13,* 046001–046001. https://doi.org/10.1088/1752-7163/ab2775 (accessed on 15th July 2025).
11. van der Stap, N., van der Heijden, F., & Broeders, I. A. (2013). Towards automated visual flexible endoscope navigation. *Surgical endoscopy, 27*(10), 3539–3547. https://doi.org/10.1007/s00464-013-3003-7(accessed on 15th July 2025).

12. Christodoulidis, G., Kouliou, M. N., Ragias, D., Chatziisaak, D., Agko, E. S., Schizas, D., & Zacharoulis, D. (2025). Last decade of advances in gastric neuroendocrine tumors: Innovations, challenges, and future directions. *World Journal of Clinical Oncology, 16*. https://www.semanticscholar.org/paper/7420d51562d29763824bab582d24ff820b48bd33 (accessed on 15th July 2025).

13. Clement, B., & Reyes, G. J. (2024). Interventional inflammatory bowel disease: Current and future practice. *Current Opinion in Gastroenterology.* https://www.semanticscholar.org/paper/24356b53809d235018a14e55ac77b76e60d5fca1 (accessed on 15th July 2025).

14. Cutajar, L. (1989). *New methods for the treatment of renal calculi: The St. Luke's Hospital experience.* https://core.ac.uk/download/46601744.pdf (accessed on 15th July 2025).

15. Essaidi, Z., Elkinani, S., Jamaleddine, K., Ettaoussi, A., Kamal, K., Majd, A., Bouali, M., et al. (2025). Ingestion of a metallic foreign body in an adult patient with psychosis: Case report. *European Journal of Medical and Health Research.* https://www.semanticscholar.org/paper/fb9f9b0457fa4481471136db2fa4321563c2bd2e (accessed on 15th July 2025).

16. Evangelista, P. F. D. R. R., Silva, A. G., Donatangelo, F., & Herval, L. M. D. A. (2025). Endoscopy in lumbar adjacent level disease – Systematic review and meta-analysis. *Coluna/Columna.* https://www.semanticscholar.org/paper/f985af9b0f43690034d9c8312cdb05581310713c (accessed on 15th July 2025).

17. Falt, P., Uricová, D., Fejfar, T., Šembera, Š., & Tachecí, I. (2023). News in gastroenterology, hepatology and digestive endoscopy. *Vnitrni Lekarstvi, 69*(3), 198–206. https://www.semanticscholar.org/paper/88f4421d8b142b29c142d0746d8816e6941f85f9 (accessed on 15th July 2025).

18. Gershman, G., & Ament, M. E. (2021). *Practical Pediatric Gastrointestinal Endoscopy.* Wiley eBooks. https://doi.org/10.1002/9781119423492 (accessed on 15th July 2025).

19. Hart, A. L., Askari, A., Bernstein, C., Blackstone, M., Braakhuis, B., Saunders, B. P., Choi, C. H. R., et al. (2015). *Forty-year analysis of colonoscopic surveillance program for neoplasia in ulcerative colitis: An updated overview.* https://core.ac.uk/download/30697713.pdf (accessed on 15th July 2025).

20. Hashiguchi, Y., Muro, K., Saitō, Y., Ito, Y., Ajioka, Y., Hamaguchi, T., Hasegawa, K., et al. (2019). Japanese Society for Cancer of the Colon and Rectum (JSCCR) guidelines 2019 for the treatment of colorectal cancer. *International Journal of Clinical Oncology, 25*, 1–42. https://doi.org/10.1007/s10147-019-01485-z (accessed on 15th July 2025).

21. Hill, B., Wamburu, A., & Clarke, F. (2024). Technological advancements in endoscopy and their impact on gastrointestinal nursing. *Gastrointestinal Nursing.* https://www.semanticscholar.org/paper/1d85c705f4234e2e1342efa811c95e4d5503f3f6 (accessed on 15th July 2025).

22. Holderried, F., Stegemann-Philipps, C., Herschbach, L., Moldt, J. A., Nevins, A., Griewatz, J., Holderried, M., et al. (2024). A generative pretrained transformer (GPT)–powered chatbot as a simulated patient to practice history taking: Prospective, mixed methods study. *JMIR Medical Education, 10*. https://www.semanticscholar.org/paper/0f3bc7bd909d7f8b0d9e1ffc8237dd51eb19abe8 (accessed on 15th July 2025).

23. Hossain, M. S., Karuniawati, H., Jairoun, A. A., Urbi, Z., Ooi, D. J., John, A., Lim, Y. C., et al. (2022). Colorectal cancer: A review of carcinogenesis, global epidemiology, current challenges, risk factors, preventive and treatment strategies. *Cancers, 14*, 1732–1732. https://doi.org/10.3390/cancers14071732 (accessed on 15th July 2025).

24. Jacobson, B. C., Leszczynski, A. M., MacArthur, K. L., Nelson, D., et al. (2018). *The association among diet, dietary fiber, and bowel preparation at colonoscopy*. https://open.bu.edu/bitstream/2144/40924/3/nihms981651.pdf (accessed on 15th July 2025).

25. Japanese gastric cancer treatment guidelines 2018 (5th edition). (2020). *Gastric Cancer, 24*, 1–21. https://doi.org/10.1007/s10120-020-01042-y (accessed on 15th July 2025).

26. Joshi, S. S., & Badgwell, B. D. (2021). Current treatment and recent progress in gastric cancer. *CA: A Cancer Journal for Clinicians, 71*, 264–279. https://doi.org/10.3322/caac.21657 (accessed on 15th July 2025).

27. Kamiński, M. F., Thomas-Gibson, S., Bugajski, M., Bretthauer, M., Rees, C., Dekker, E., Hoff, G., et al. (2017). Performance measures for lower gastrointestinal endoscopy: A European Society of Gastrointestinal Endoscopy (ESGE) quality improvement initiative. *Endoscopy, 49*, 378–397. https://doi.org/10.1055/s-0043-103411 (accessed on 15th July 2025).

28. Karimian, M., Rahmatizadeh, S., Kohzadi, Z., Kohzadi, Z., Madadi, F., Dabbagh, A., & Daccpm Department of Anesthesiology Critical Care and Pain. (2024). Analyzing patterns in anesthesiology residents' exam performance using data mining techniques. *Anesthesiology and Pain Medicine, 14*. https://www.semanticscholar.org/paper/67ee1fcf87843328ab231289ae764c09d7e55883 (accessed on 15th July 2025).

29. Kaur, M., & Williams, A. (2022). Effectiveness of relaxation technique on level of anxiety before upper gastrointestinal endoscopy (UGE). *International Journal of Nursing Education*. https://www.semanticscholar.org/paper/c38ab8205c3f9e5f68231f3d176ec23bc347f010 (accessed on 15th July 2025).

30. Kazimierczak, K. A., & Skea, Z. C. (2015). *'I've used the word cancer but it's actually good news': Discursive performativity of cancer and the identity of urological cancer services*. https://core.ac.uk/download/42130404.pdf (accessed on 15th July 2025).

31. Khan, B., Fatima, H., Qureshi, A., Kumar, S., Hanan, A., Hussain, J., & Abdullah, S. (2023). Drawbacks of artificial intelligence and their potential solutions in the healthcare sector. *Deleted Journal, 1*, 731–738. https://doi.org/10.1007/s44174-023-00063-2 (accessed on 15th July 2025).

32. Lamb, C. A., Kennedy, N. A., Raine, T., Hendy, P., Smith, P. J., Limdi, J. K., Hayee, B., et al. (2019). British Society of Gastroenterology consensus guidelines on the management of inflammatory bowel disease in adults. *Gut, 68*, s1–s106. https://doi.org/10.1136/gutjnl-2019-318484 (accessed on 15th July 2025).

33. Linghu, E. (2021). A new stage of surgical treatment: Super minimally invasive surgery. *Chinese Medical Journal, 135*, 1–3. https://doi.org/10.1097/cm9.0000000000001534 (accessed on 15th July 2025).

34. Liu, D., & Mobbs, R. (2025). Risk analysis of neurological deterioration associated with fluid insufflation in uniportal spine endoscopy: A case series and literature review. *International Journal of Spine Surgery, 19*, 279–287. https://www.semanticscholar.org/paper/fe08c6a5c2ab3c0f1cfa8a27500452b6c8a62cb7 (accessed on 15th July 2025).

35. Liu, Y., Suvithayasiri, S., Van Isseldyk, F., Kotheeranurak, V., Jitpakdee, K., Choi, K. C., Choi, G., et al. (2024). Evaluating the effectiveness of the transcorporeal approach in minimally invasive spine surgery for cervical spinal disease: A comprehensive review and technical insights. *BMC Surgery, 24*. https://www.semanticscholar.org/paper/505f30727dbe210eac7

8c1bb9c62d8a5457e8b79 (accessed on 15th July 2025).

36. Marinov, V., Karagyozov, P., Kostov, K., Emilova, N., Ivanova, S., Chaneva, M., Atanasova, V., et al. (2024). Complicated intraductal papillary mucinous neoplasia requiring a two-stage operation. *Pharmacia.* https://www.semanticscholar.org/paper/ada651f7fbb7ac456e07b2d83d34435e4c7d221c (accessed on 15th July 2025).

37. Martínek, J., Husťák, R., Mareš, J., Vacková, Z., Špičák, J., Kieslichová, E., Buncová, M., et al. (2022). Endoscopic pyloromyotomy for the treatment of severe and refractory gastroparesis: A pilot, randomised, sham-controlled trial. *Gut, 71*, 2170–2178. https://doi.org/10.1136/gutjnl-2022-326904 (accessed on 15th July 2025).

38. Mégraud, F., Bruyndonckx, R., Coenen, S., Wittkop, L., Huang, T. D., Hoebeke, M., Bénejat, L., et al. (2021). *Helicobacter pylori* resistance to antibiotics in Europe in 2018 and its relationship to antibiotic consumption in the community. *Gut, 70*, 1815–1822. https://doi.org/10.1136/gutjnl-2021-324032 (accessed on 15th July 2025).

39. Metzger, R., Suppa, P., Li, Z., & Vemuri, A. (2024). Augmented reality navigation systems in endoscopy. *Frontiers in Gastroenterology.* https://www.semanticscholar.org/paper/ef9446a682e85a83364c5367c1dc8cc4d9ce620a (accessed on 15th July 2025).

40. Najjar, R. (2023). Redefining radiology: A review of artificial intelligence integration in medical imaging. *Diagnostics, 13*, 2760–2760. https://doi.org/10.3390/diagnostics13172760 (accessed on 15th July 2025).

41. Nehme, F., Goyal, H., Perisetti, A., Tharian, B., Sharma, N., Tham, T., & Chhabra, R. (2021). The evolution of device-assisted enteroscopy: From sonde enteroscopy to motorized spiral enteroscopy. *Frontiers in Medicine, 8.* https://doi.org/10.3389/fmed.2021.792668 (accessed on 15th July 2025).

42. Nishida, T., Hayashi, S., Ikezawa, K., Matsumoto, K., Takenaka, M., & Hosono, M. (2025). Radiation safety and dose management in fluoroscopy-guided gastrointestinal procedures: Current evidence and future perspectives. *Expert Review of Gastroenterology & Hepatology.* https://www.semanticscholar.org/paper/3fa919fb79e8732803d3eba67a7485e8b405375f (accessed on 15th July 2025).

43. O'Sullivan, S., Nevejans, N., Allen, C., Blyth, A., Léonard, S., Pagallo, U., Holzinger, K., et al. (2018). Legal, regulatory, and ethical frameworks for development of standards in artificial intelligence (AI) and autonomous robotic surgery. *International Journal of Medical Robotics and Computer Assisted Surgery, 15.* https://doi.org/10.1002/rcs.1968 (accessed on 15th July 2025).

44. Parisi, I., Badat, S., El-Husseiny, M. H., Seward, E., & Wagner, C. (2022). *P149 Evaluation of the at-home capsule endoscopy (ACE) service at UCLH: Preliminary findings.* Poster presentations. https://www.semanticscholar.org/paper/94a454c35ef477e9181d6a64bf2d38e120f992aa (accessed on 15th July 2025).

45. Parveen, K., Parveen, M. K., & Parveen, R. (2023). Knowledge attitude and practices about endoscopy procedures among nurses of Nishtar Hospital Multan. *Biological and Clinical Sciences Research Journal, 2023*, 480–480. https://doi.org/10.54112/bcsrj.v2023i1.480 (accessed on 15th July 2025).

46. Pate, B. S., Yeola, M., Gawande, A. A., Singh, A., & Tayade, H. (2020). Best practices for endoscopic procedures in COVID-19 pandemic. *Journal of Evolution of Medical and Dental Sciences, 9,*

3760–3766. https://doi.org/10.14260/jemds/2020/825 (accessed on 15th July 2025).

47. Pellegrino, R., Palladino, G., Izzo, M., De Costanzo, I., Landa, F., Federico, A., & Gravina, A. (2024). Water-assisted colonoscopy in inflammatory bowel diseases: From technical implications to diagnostic and therapeutic potentials. *World Journal of Gastrointestinal Endoscopy, 16*, 647–660. https://www.semanticscholar.org/paper/e833b4e893ec4f314dcd41a98068c9e30252527a (accessed on 15th July 2025).
48. Pennazio, M., Rondonotti, E., Despott, E. J., Dray, X., Keuchel, M., Moreels, T. G., Sanders, D. S., et al. (2022). Small-bowel capsule endoscopy and device-assisted enteroscopy for diagnosis and treatment of small-bowel disorders: European Society of Gastrointestinal Endoscopy (ESGE) guideline – Update 2022. *Endoscopy, 55*, 58–95. https://doi.org/10.1055/a-1973-3796 (accessed on 15th July 2025).
49. Rawla, P., & Barsouk, A. (2019). Epidemiology of gastric cancer: Global trends, risk factors and prevention. *Gastroenterology Review, 14*, 26–38. https://doi.org/10.5114/pg.2018.80001 (accessed on 15th July 2025).
50. Runciman, M., Darzi, A., & Mylonas, G. (2019). Soft robotics in minimally invasive surgery. *Soft Robotics, 6*, 423–443. https://doi.org/10.1089/soro.2018.0136 (accessed on 15th July 2025).
51. Siddique, N., Paheding, S., Elkin, C., & Devabhaktuni, V. (2021). U-Net and its variants for medical image segmentation: A review of theory and applications. *IEEE Access, 9*, 82031–82057. https://doi.org/10.1109/access.2021.3086020 (accessed on 15th July 2025).
52. Sîngeap, A. M., Sfarti, C., Minea, H., Chiriac, Ş., Cuciureanu, T., Năstasă, R., Stanciu, C., et al. (2023). Small bowel capsule endoscopy and enteroscopy: A shoulder-to-shoulder race. *Journal of Clinical Medicine, 12*, 7328–7328. https://doi.org/10.3390/jcm12237328 (accessed on 15th July 2025).
53. Singhal, K., Azizi, S., Tu, T., Mahdavi, S. S., Lee, J., Chung, H. W., Scales, N., et al. (2023). Large language models encode clinical knowledge. *Nature, 620*, 172–180. https://doi.org/10.1038/s41586-023-06291-2 (accessed on 15th July 2025).
54. van der Laan, J. J. H., van der Waaij, A. M., Gabriëls, R. Y., Festen, E. A., Dijkstra, G., & Nagengast, W. B. (2020). Endoscopic imaging in inflammatory bowel disease: Current developments and emerging strategies. *Expert Review of Gastroenterology & Hepatology, 15*, 115–126. https://doi.org/10.1080/17474124.2021.1840352 (accessed on 15th July 2025).
55. Vasireddy, A., Watson, C., Safinia, N., Stevens, S., & Hicks, L. (2021). *P282 A study of nasojejunal tube placement and outcomes in a tertiary NHS trust.* Posters. https://www.semanticscholar.org/paper/e640504df74c447e3d98c3279a8c88f2cd06b0d4 (accessed on 15th July 2025).
56. Wang, S., Kang, B. K., Ma, J., Zeng, X., Xiao, M., Guo, J., Cai, M., et al. (2021). A deep learning algorithm using CT images to screen for coronavirus disease (COVID-19). *European Radiology, 31*, 6096–6104. https://doi.org/10.1007/s00330-021-07715-1 (accessed on 15th July 2025).

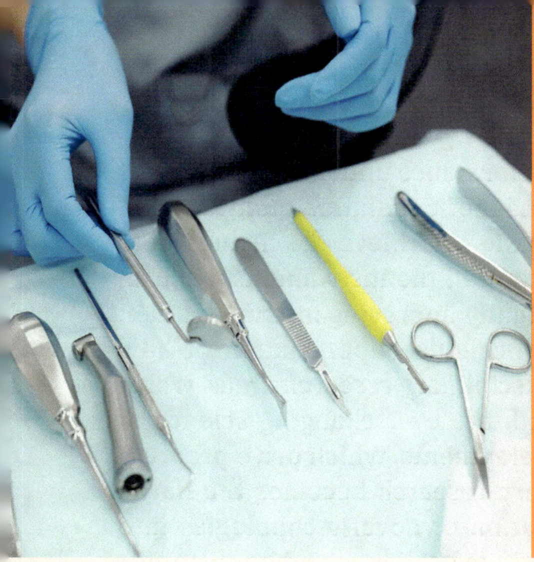

Chapter 2

INSTRUMENTATION AND EQUIPMENT

Contents

Introduction....35

2.1. Types of Instrumentation....38

2.2. Common Equipment in Laboratories....42

2.3. Instrumentation in Medical Applications....45

2.4. Industrial Instrumentation....48

2.5. Advances in Instrumentation Technology....52

2.6. Maintenance and Calibration of Equipment....55

Summary....59

References....62

Introduction

In the identification of equipment and instrumentation, knowledge of the technical equipment used in the collection, processing, and analysis of data is needed. Instrumentation not just involves the equipment employed but also the systematic processes behind their use. Various fields rely on precise instrumentation to support the collection of empirical data that informs research and enhances operational efficiency. For instance, in meteorology, the integration of sophisticated equipment allows for the tracking and analysis of weather patterns, thereby increasing predictive ability and response processes in extreme weather. It is thus important to study the design, characteristics, and applications of such equipment to analyze their impact on scientific research and real-world use, particularly in fields , such as atmospheric science, engineering, and environmental monitoring. Beyond the subject comes the reality that instrumentation is usually created on the basis of specific operational needs and scientific research. Design requirements interface with performance properties in a most critical way, as evidenced by many field tests conducted to assess instrument performance under conditions. For example, the deployment of airborne and surface units for electromagnetic radiation monitoring in extreme weather conditions shows the nuanced design choices made to achieve the highest data quality and accuracy. The tests not only provide an insight into how well the instruments perform but also into where there is potential for improvement, thereby constantly improving instrumentation technologies. Understandings of these dimensions develop a well-rounded appreciation of how equipment technologies can lead to important milestones in multidisciplinary research areas, which are in alignment with present-day scientific requirements. Second, the ever-changing science of instrumentation is also increasingly governed by technological developments, which drive progress in both hardware and software. As more and more interdisciplinary research becomes the norm, blurring concepts among different fields stimulates the incorporation of novel technologies into established instrumentation frameworks. This progress creates a unique challenge and opportunity, as scientists must navigate the innovations of new technology while being compatible with traditional approaches. Advances in computer power and data analysis have transformed the analysis and interpretation of data, creating a feedback loop in which more instrumentation yields more precise datasets and thus more insight. Thus, ongoing debate pertaining to equipment and instrumentation remains pivotal for promoting scientific knowledge and practical application in a broad variety of fields (Figure 2.1).

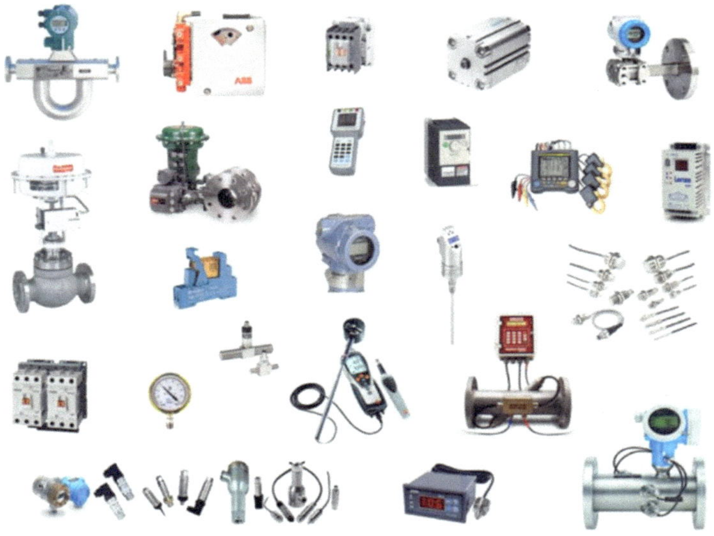

Figure 2.1. Instrumentation and equipment.

Source: https://www.parskhorshid.com/upload/img_1651906220_1.png.

Definition of Instrumentation

Instrumentation refers to the collective science and art of designing and utilizing instruments or equipment necessary to measure, monitor, and control physical quantities in various disciplines, including engineering, medicine, and environmental science. At its core, instrumentation is a wide variety of technologies and methods that allow precise data gathering, upon which informed decisions in research and industry can be made. It has transformed the instrumentation field significantly with advanced sensors and data acquisition systems, allowing for real-time analysis as well as improved accuracy. The convergence of software improvements also supports increased data interpretation, rendering instrumentation an essential component of current scientific inquiry and industrial applications. Instrumentation is not only defined as measurement but also as the processes that go into interpreting and regulating variables from the derived data. In most applications, particularly in those handling complex systems, instrumentation plays a key role in improving efficiency and safety of operation. This can be seen in the situation of sophisticated systems where system performance is directly influenced by instrumentation. In Saturn IB hardware, for instance, passive instrumentation not only senses but also generates stimuli needed in nondestructive tests, illustrating the two-functionality that can be possessed by instrumentation in other industries (Kaushagen & Skinner, 1966). This subtle understanding of instrumentation underscores its significance as both an analytical and control instrument, central to the integrity of systems in the current technological setting. Furthermore, the continued evolution of instrumentation is marked by advances toward making experimental results more reliable and improving operational efficiencies. A good example is that of the development of Thick Gas Electron Multipliers (THGEM), where gain stability over time has become increasingly important in detector functionality. With utmost caution in simulations, the impacts of charging-up processes have been examined, finding the relationship of electrode thickness and applied voltage on gain stabilization (Azevedo et al., 2017). This indicates that modern instrumentation not only attempts to obtain accurate measurements but also achieves more understanding about the underlying physical processes governing these measurements. Therefore, the concept of instrumentation encompasses a dynamic interplay of design, deployment, and ongoing optimization, required to drive technology forward in experimental as well as operating conditions (Figure 2.2).

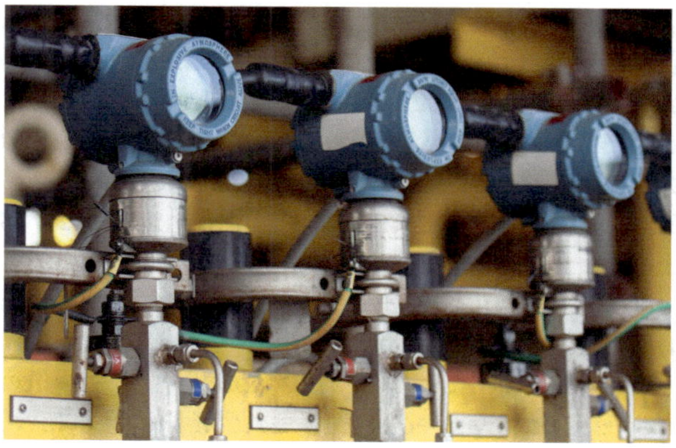

Figure 2.2. Instrumentation.

Source: https://icss.engineer/wp-content/uploads/2022/01/instrumentation.jpg.

Importance of Equipment in Various Fields

The function of specialized equipment in contemporary society is multiplied in most industries, primarily in scientific research and exploration. NASA, for instance, employs advanced instrumentation to a high degree to achieve its mission of space exploration and scientific research. They actively seek inclusion of diversified research output, such as conference papers and doctoral dissertations, which are very crucial in augmenting their scientific horizon. This brings to the fore the issue that advanced devices not only help in conducting research but also facilitate the greater achievements of institutions dedicated to advancing human knowledge and abilities. The quality of gadgets used in these efforts frequently determines the accuracy and reliability of outcomes, thus making machinery a primary foundation of achievement in high-risk fields , such as aerospace and environmental science (Kaushagen & Skinner, 1966). The healthcare sector provides a traditional case of the transformative impact that equipment has in determining outcomes and efficiencies in patient care. Medical equipment, from MRI machines to portable diagnostic devices, is essential to disease diagnosis and disease management. Accurate measurement and reliable data are required to develop successful treatment plans. Thus, the addition of advanced instrumentation introduces a more comprehensive and individualized system of healthcare. Also worth noting is the educational implication of such technologies, as they harmonize theory with practice in synergy for current and future health practitioners. In an era where precision medicine is gaining traction, equipment quality and sophistication are essential aspects that determine the level of care and outcomes in the healthcare industry (Kaushagen & Skinner, 1966). Metrology, the science of measurement, is a critical though sometimes forgotten part of varied disciplines like engineering and manufacturing.

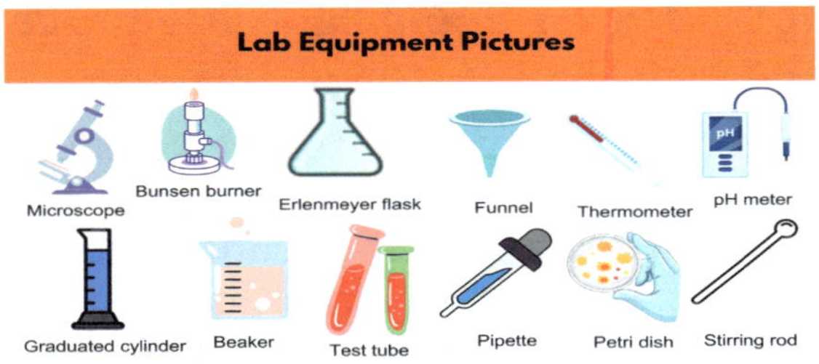

Figure 2.3. Lab Equipment.

Source: https://grammarvocab.com/wp-content/uploads/2023/04/Lab-equipment-names-and-pictures-feat.png.

The criticality of precise measurement in making quality control possible cannot be overstated; efficient production processes rely on sound data from high-technology measuring instruments. However, as new fields of science and technology emerge, metrology education has to fight for attention. Despite this, the fundamental foundation of measurement remains priceless, ensuring that innovations are established with accuracy to some degree. Having the ability to utilize the latest equipment provides scientists and engineers with the confidence to approach measurement with increased confidence, hence allowing them to push the boundaries of innovation. A critical perspective towards the measurement of practice adds depth to this branch, drawing from the understanding that technology can make processes easy, but not the value of systematic analysis of measurements (Kaushagen & Skinner, 1966) (Figure 2.3).

2.1. Types of Instrumentation

Instrumentation encompasses a vast array of tools and equipment used to measure, monitor, and control various physical properties. Some of the most significant types of instrumentation include analytical equipment, which plays a very important role in material characterization for use in fields , such as chemistry and biology. Equipment , such as spectrophotometers and chromatographs, enable scientists to precisely analyze the properties and make-up of chemicals. Apart from this, they also facilitate critical applications like environmental monitoring and quality control in manufacturing. The importance of such instruments is also boosted by bodies , such as NASA, which calls for research reports in consonance with the evolution of instrumentation technology pivotal to its mission and objectives (Kaushagen & Skinner, 1966). This ensures instrumentation used in research science is not only effective but also in line with contemporary models of research. Aside from analytical instruments, process control instrumentation is similarly significant for industrial use. Included in this category are devices , such as pressure sensors, flow meters, and temperature controllers, which are utilized to monitor and regulate physical states within various systems. Through the provision of ideal parameters, the instruments enhance efficiency in operations and provide safety in applications of varied nature, from chemical processing to food manufacturing. The integration of instrumentation and control systems has revolutionized industries to facilitate real-time data acquisition and automated tuning based on pre-defined criteria. A particularly fascinating example of this blending is evident in initiatives like that of the UC Berkeley research team, where a combined testbed was created to optimize energy flows in a building and thereby advance the multi-faceted applications of instrumentation to maximize control of resources (Peffer, 2010).

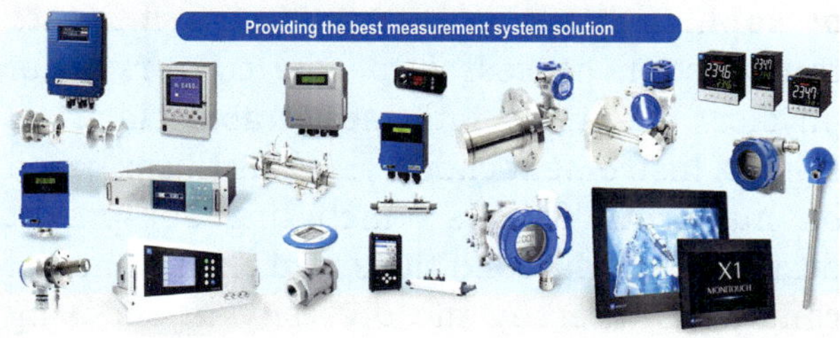

Figure 2.4. Instrumentation.

Source: https://www.fujielectric.fr/wp-content/uploads/2024/07/instruments-et-appareils-de-mesure-en.png?x39279.

Moreover, fields of environmental and biomedical instrumentation are becoming progressively more sophisticated, reflecting the growing complexity of modern issues. Environmental sensors, remote sensing instruments, and air quality sensors help to measure ecological patterns and human impacts on the environment. In the biomedical field, electrocardiograms and imaging devices serve as key players in diagnostic processes, providing critical details regarding patients' health. As these devices become better, vast amounts of data are generated as well that need advanced analytics for meaningful interpretation. Since the world still grapples with such highest-order issues as climate change and health, continued progress and development of many forms of instrumentation are essential. This is a testament to the complex role of instrumentation in advancing the knowledge of natural processes and human health (Figure 2.4).

2.1.1. Analytical Instrumentation

The growth of analytical equipment has had a tremendous influence on a broad range of areas, including materials science, environmental monitoring, and preservation of cultural heritage. The new equipment allows chemists to accurately measure and identify chemical components in complex samples to gain information that cannot be obtained using other techniques. For instance, techniques , such as Raman spectroscopy and X-ray fluorescence spectrometry allow researchers to analyze material *in situ* without destroying the inherent nature of the material. Such non-destructive methods are especially crucial in fields like archaeometry, in which the integrity of old artifacts must be preserved at all costs. The use of mobility instrumental techniques makes it possible for researchers to directly analyze artifacts in archaeological sites or museums, thus circumventing the risks involved in moving delicate objects (Donais et al., 2016). Consequently, the advancement of analytical instrumentation continues to expand beyond the traditional laboratory setting, facilitating greater interdisciplinary research and greater insight into various properties of materials. In particular, handheld analytical instruments have become more popular due to the fact that they can provide instantaneous and on-site results. This focus on instrument mobility is part of a greater trend in scientific inquiry to provide greater efficiency while still upholding strict preservation standards. For example, Fourier transform infrared spectrometry and laser-induced breakdown spectroscopy have been adapted for field use, leading to more rugged data acquisition at the expense of no conservation of valuable material. As analytical methodology is improved, application of high-end analytical methods not only ensures the quality of data gathered but also makes high-end analyses affordable to more scholars and practitioners, facilitating breadth in terms of the number of experts (Donais et al., 2016). Increased reliance on such mobile machines underscores the core significance of analytical tools in today's science and heritage research. Furthermore, the calibration of analytical equipment with real-world applications addresses industrially encountered problems of a complicated nature in industries like healthcare and aviation. The operation of rotorcraft icing test methods, for example, demonstrates the need for accurate instrumentation to ensure safety and compliance with standards in aerospace applications. Real-world ice protection technology from solid analytical assessment facilitates decision-making in industrial standards. With such programs evolving, they highlight the necessity of sustained research and innovation in instrumentation to match the evolving requirements of various industries. Ultimately, the focus on enhancing analytical instrumentation not only enhances technological advancement but also strengthens the fundamental foundations of scientific research to equip practitioners with capabilities to confront future challenges (Figure 2.5).

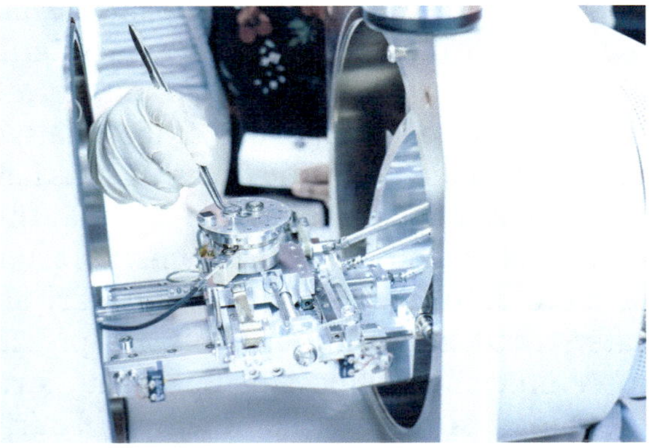

Figure 2.5. Analytical instrumentation.

Source: https://www.inficon.com/uploads/media/1000x670/01/1261-Analytical%20Instrumentation%201.jpg?v=1-0.

2.1.2. Measurement Instrumentation

In technical application and engineering, measurement instrumentation is the core component that ensures accuracy and precision in most areas of application. Quantification of physical phenomena is the foundation of technology and science progression where solid instrumentation is required for design and hypothesis validation and verification. For instance, in the automotive and power generation sectors, torsional vibration has to be measured to improve performance and safety. This process not only involves the use of sophisticated sensors but also intricate transduction processes for the conversion of physical quantities into measurable electrical signals. Instrument choice , such as this is based on numerous factors , including equipment design, operating conditions, and environmental conditions, thereby the diversity in choosing the right measurement means to suit the intended application (Marín et al., 2014). In highly specialized applications, particularly when dealing with radio-frequency (RF) and microwave technology, highly specialized measurement equipment becomes inevitable. With the use of RF applications becoming more prevalent in communications and industrial applications, the need to properly characterize signals has become a demand met by specialized equipment for use with such frequencies. Understanding the basics of RF signal processing allows for the ability to design effective measurement systems that can properly acquire, analyze, and interpret data. This needs theoretical education and practical skill sets, a holistic approach to training and education in fields , such as accelerator physics. Subjects , such as courses offered in the CERN Accelerator School emphasize the need for complex RF measurement techniques, marrying academic education with the applied learning of skills in real environments (Wendt, 2020). The meeting of high-precision measurement equipment with the contemporary technological wave marks an era of innovation and precision. As industries make their choice based on data increasingly, measurement devices take on an even more vital role. The improvement in sensor technology, data capture systems, and signal processing algorithms contributes to an enhanced capability to monitor and assess dynamic systems in real time. Moreover, the integration of measurement devices into automation and control systems provides a means of feedback loops to be employed towards optimizing performance continuously. As such, field practitioners are not only tasked with the selection of appropriate measurement devices but also the interpretation of and reaction to resultant data, thereby promoting innovation and efficiency in various industries. This intricate relationship between measurement, analysis, and application highlights the crucial role instrumentation has played in the technology of the time (Figure 2.6).

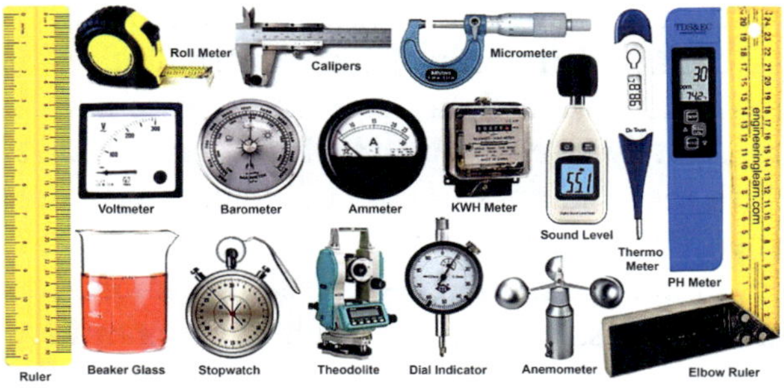

Figure 2.6. Measurement instrumentation.

Source: https://engineeringlearn.com/wp-content/uploads/2021/11/Measuring-Instruments-1024x539.jpg.

2.1.3. Control Instrumentation

Control instrumentation plays a crucial role in modern engineering and science applications, particularly in environments that need high accuracy and dependability. Control instrumentation includes a number of devices and systems that monitor and regulate processes and ensure they operate within predetermined parameters. This applies especially in real-time systems, where millions of points of data, generated sequentially at high rates, need to be processed and answered to immediately. In, say, spacecraft applications, the coupling of digital processors and analog sensors is crucial since it provides synchronized data capture and control, responding to inputs at stunning speed and accuracy. Such top-level control is important in applications where even small fluctuations lead to disastrous failures, showing how robust control systems can significantly enhance the security and efficiency of processes (Lux et al., 2004). The application of Nuclear Instrumentation Modular (NIM) and Computer Automated Measurement Control (CAMAC) systems is indicative of the universality of control instrumentation across various disciplines. These systems are designed to satisfy specific data acquisition and control requirements in scientific payloads. A review of some sample payloads shows the commonality and feasibility of these equipment types for applications that need to collect precise data and observe. Through a representative set of payloads, researchers can determine the extent to which NIM and CAMAC manage to resolve the issues of instrumentation in sciences , such as astrophysics, environmental monitoring, and medical imaging. This is critical to the optimization of instrumentation choice and data reliability as control instrumentation plays a role in the interpretation of scientific phenomena and in the development of technology (Kaushagen & Skinner, 1966). Secondly, trends in control instrumentation are towards more integrated systems due to advancements in software and computer technology. A case in point is the use of scalable multiprocessor computing systems, particularly for hard real-time systems. Such systems consist of clusters of digital-signal-processing computers that are linked with high-speed serial links and support flexible and parallel task distribution. The ability to coordinate functions through a master/slave control scheme enhances processing performance and responsiveness to input. As the technology develops further, control instrumentation will be yet more sophisticated, with better performance and enabling increasingly complex applications across a broad range of industries. This evolution highlights the critical importance of continued innovation in control instrumentation to respond to the growing demands of modern processes (Lux et al., 2004).

2.2. Common Equipment in Laboratories

Lab facilities are shared with a vast range of equipment that is crucial for conducting scientific experimentation and research. General equipment , such as pipettes, spectrophotometers, and centrifuges, serves fundamental roles in most disciplines, such as physics, chemistry, and biology. Pipettes, for instance, enable the accurate measurement and transfer of liquids and support accurate experimental practice. Spectrophotometers are vital for understanding the light absorption and transmission, a factor that is very important in chemical reaction research and concentration analysis. Centrifuges, further, facilitate the separation of materials based on their density, a factor vital for protein purification and cell analysis. The merging of these devices creates a single ecosystem that enables rigorous scientific investigation and encourages reproducibility in research outcomes. Lab equipment has a value beyond performance; it is a union of technology and methodology for a specific research objective. With progressing scientific investigation, the demand for specific equipment builds up, hence propelling the formation of standard laboratory equipment. For instance, the development of advanced spectroscopic techniques has improved the accuracy and sensitivity of measurements, such that new chemical phenomena heretofore not examined have been made accessible to investigation. Instrumentation like automated liquid handlers also streamlines repetitive operations, such that scientists can focus on hypothesis testing and data interpretation. Mixing up historical and contemporary instrumentation reveals the dynamic nature of the laboratory setting and emphasizes the importance of technicians and scientists understanding deeply the instrumentation and its mechanisms. Maintenance and calibration of equipment in the laboratory are crucial in maintaining the integrity and validity of data in research results. Standard calibration procedures must be done to satisfy set standards and procedures, typically by intercomparison with standard equipment. This is particularly important for equipment , such as mass spectrometers and chromatographs, where small differences can lead to huge amounts of errors in analytical information. Finally, new methods and technologies require constant training and adaptability of laboratory personnel. For example, the introduction of computer-based data acquisition systems has completely overhauled traditional workflows. With the dynamics of lab equipment, optimum operating integrity—both user capability and equipment proficiency—is becoming more and more necessary, fostering a culture of innovation and accuracy in scientific discovery (Figure 2.7).

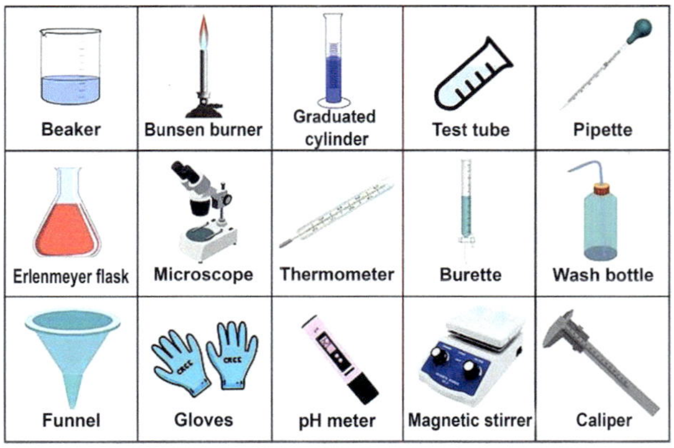

Figure 2.7. Common equipment in laboratories.

Source: https://i.pinimg.com/originals/aa/2e/c7/aa2ec7570bf6d12e9f4515818ebd8eb8.jpg.

2.2.1. Spectrophotometers

The role of spectrophotometers in scientific research is of utmost significance, in light of the fact that they are able to quantify and determine the type of substance properties through light absorption. The instruments operate based on the fact that different substances absorb light of different wavelengths, thus enabling one to derive concentration and identification in a sample. The spectrophotometer quantitatively measures the intensity of light both before and after passing through a sample by allowing a beam of light to pass through it. The data is then used to plot absorbance spectra, which can potentially provide information on the molecular structure of the sample and on the concentration of the individual components. The sensitivity and accuracy of spectrophotometers make them invaluable in applications , such as biochemistry, environmental monitoring, and the pharmaceutical industry, where accurate measurement will decide critical research outcomes and industrial operations. In institutions of higher learning, placing spectrophotometers in laboratory instruction has the effect of complementing the learning process for chemistry students by making laboratory application fundamental to understanding theoretical concepts. Facilities that focus on access to state-of-the-art equipment, such as spectrophotometers, can significantly enrich their curriculum so that students are able to conduct hands-on experiments that link theory and practice. Research opportunities are also enhanced when students can utilize advanced equipment to conduct independent studies, promoting a culture of inquiry and innovation. Notably, it was found that more than 90% of the historically Black colleges were well-equipped with laboratory instruments, such as spectrophotometers, facilitating the expansion of the undergraduate programs and contributing towards a better-skilled workforce in the sciences (Wear & Shastri, 1974). Such investment results in academic intensity and ingenuity and the general quality of the education system. In addition, technological advances in spectrophotometry also assist in the level of precision and range of analysis methods available in most fields. Recent advances have improved miniaturization and mobility, such that field-based and remote applications are now realized. For instance, field spectrophotometers are applied in environmental science for real-time water quality measurements, thus allowing researchers immediate data required for public safety and health. This ability to use testifies to the universal relevance of spectrophotometers beyond traditional laboratory settings, which speaks to their suitability in contemporary research and practice (Fischer et al., 1961). Spectrophotometers are, therefore, not just a pillar of laboratory instruments but also an exemplary model of innovation and usefulness, shaping the direction of scientific inquiry in a number of fields (Figure 2.8).

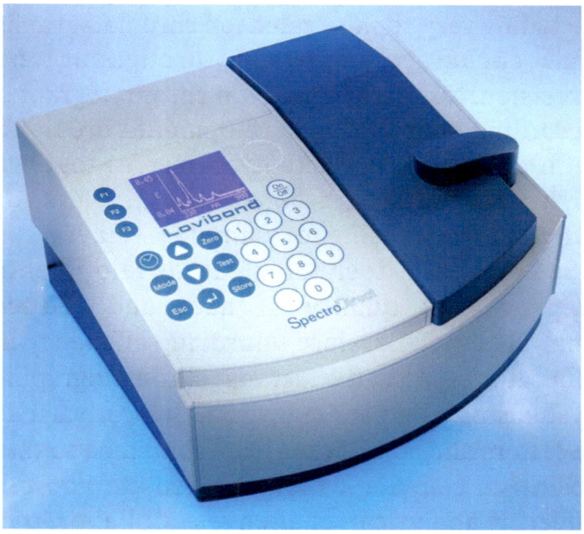

Figure 2.8. Spectrophotometers.

Source: https://www.unitedscientific.co.za/templates/yootheme/cache/spectrodirect_mb2_01-f077a16c.jpeg.

2.2.2. Chromatographs

Chromatography is an important analysis technique that facilitates the resolution and detection of components in complex mixtures and has rendered chromatographs indispensable tools in many branches of science. Chromatographic operation is based on the interaction between the stationary phase and the mobile phase, enabling analyte migration along a medium. The distinct chemical characteristics of each constituent define its displacement, hence ensuring separation based on size, charge, or affinity. This separation allows for quantitative and qualitative sample analysis, which is crucial in applications ranging from environmental monitoring to pharmaceuticals. With different types of chromatography, such as gas and liquid chromatography, researchers are able to adjust techniques to suit the specific analytical requirements, thereby making the chromatographs even more versatile in laboratory work. Technological innovations in chromatographic equipment have seen the development of very sophisticated equipment, including very sophisticated ion chromatographs that encourage analytical throughput and precision. Newly designed ion chromatographs, according to emerging developments, are fitted with advanced conductivity detectors that are highly sensitive with allied autosamplers for efficient processing of samples (Mayewski, 2001). These technological developments improve the quality of data and reduce analysis time, therefore improving efficiency in laboratories. Also, the fact that chromatographic systems may be personalized allows for various detectors and approaches to be combined so that scientists can adapt their methods to address specific analytical challenges. Collaborative efforts in equipment upgrade in processing have also demonstrated the fundamental role chromatographs play in contemporary research. Portable chromatographs, particularly gas chromatographs, have also played leading roles as they are portable and need minimal power, making them suitable for field applications. As outlined in recent studies, the development of miniaturized gas chromatographs has provided a new opportunity for on-site and environmental analysis, complementing their application in real-world applications (Kunwar, 2011). The devices allow real-time determinations and more rapid decision-making, particularly in applications , such as environmental science and the production of biofuels. Furthermore, the integration of such mobile devices into learning packages allows students to see the practical application of chromatography, providing a higher appreciation of analytical chemistry. The ongoing evolution of chromatographic technology also serves to underscore its vital contribution to scientific research and industry, further reinforcing the position that effective equipment is instrumental in propelling knowledge and innovation (Figure 2.9).

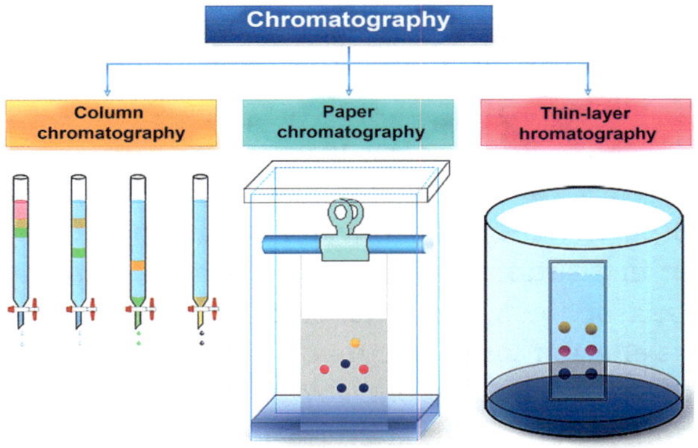

Figure 2.9. Chromatography.

Source: https://www.priyamstudycentre.com/wp-content/uploads/2021/11/chromatography-techniques.png.

2.2.3. Microscopes

The development of microscopes has actually revolutionized scientific research by allowing material to be studied at resolutions that were unavailable before. Initially conceived in the late 16th century, the microscope has developed with better models, including the electron microscope and scanning probe microscope. The more advanced models function on different principles; for example, electron microscopy uses electron beams to deliver atomic-level imaging. This level of precision enables scientists to examine the structure and morphology of biological samples, materials, and nanostructures with accuracy. The significance of these breakthroughs is underscored by their interdisciplinary application from biology to materials science, thus broadening the area of study and adding depth to our understanding of the microscopic universe. In materials science, microscopes play an important role in characterizing the properties and behavior of materials under various conditions. For instance, optical coherence tomography (OCT) is utilized as an effective tool to investigate metallic surface topography under various types of fracturing. With the application of this non-destructive imaging technique, scientists can produce high-resolution height profiles of materials that are informative of their structural integrity without having to remove samples, unlike with standard techniques like scanning electron microscopy (SEM) (Camacho et al., 2014). This capability proves particularly valuable when measuring machinery components and determining failure mechanisms, offering real-time analysis that would be impossible otherwise. Consequently, the synergy of the advanced microscopy techniques continues to increase the efficiency and the research level in material properties. Additionally, the use of microscopes goes beyond looking; they are a crucial component of laboratory equipment in various scientific fields. For instance, in proposed microgravity labs, microscopes will be at the center of studying low-speed particle collisions and how geologic materials are put together (Bridges et al., 2025). These experiments require high-resolution imaging to find out what is going on at the microscopic scale of interaction and transformation, which in turn might give information usable for general phenomena, such as planetary assembly or material synthesis in space environments. The modification of microscope design to accommodate certain experimental needs illustrates the flexibility and importance of microscopes in facilitating scientific knowledge through a wide range of research fields, highlighting the intermediacy of instrumentation and apparatus in the establishment of modern science (Figure 2.10).

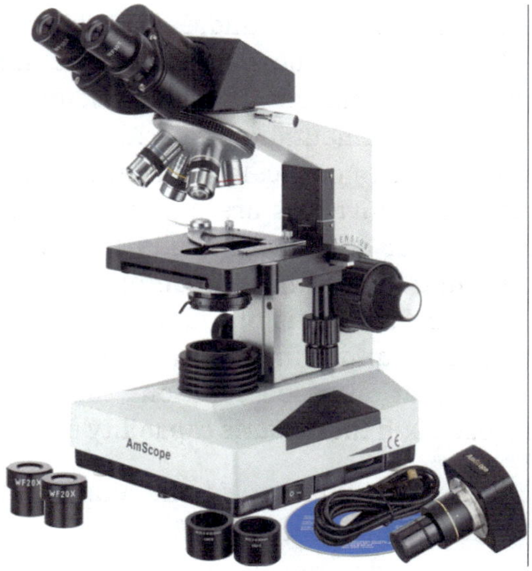

Figure 2.10. Microscopes.

Source: https://www.microscopemaster.com/images/AmscopeB490B-3Mdigitalcompoundmicroscope.jpg.

2.3. Instrumentation in Medical Applications

Instrumentation plays key significance in medical applications for diagnosis and treatment of varied illnesses. The technology employed in this field involves a wide variety of technologies, ranging from simple tools to electronic equipment. For instance, imaging devices like MRI and CT scanners allow for the visualization of internal body structures, significantly enhancing a clinician's ability to make sound decisions. Moreover, advancements in sensor technology have revolutionized patient monitoring systems, enabling real-time gathering and analysis of data. This continuous vigilance aids in the early detection of health status, demonstrating the huge potential of precise instrumentation in the enhancement of patient care in clinics. Moreover, the incorporation of biomedical engineering concepts into instrument design has facilitated the development of specialist devices that are specifically designed to address specific medical needs. Devices , such as automated insulin pumps and advanced prosthetics demonstrate the way instrumentation can address patient requirements in particular and enhance quality of life. Such advances are due not only to the technological accomplishments but also to a better understanding of complex biological processes. In addition, dialogue between researchers and clinicians has brought new instrumentation-based solutions that enhance diagnostic and therapeutic capability even more.

Interdisciplinarity of the contributions is essential in the establishment of cutting-edge instrumentation in medical applications, exemplifying symbiotic interactions between technology and medicine. NASA also possesses a strong legacy of advancing instrumentation in medical applications, primarily in the form of cardiovascular monitoring research. The organization's commitment to exploring how environmental factors affect human health adds validity to its work in designing advanced monitoring technologies (Jones et al., 2025). Besides, NASA hopes to include diverse scientific studies, like research studies and conferences, as per its goals in the release of technical information (Lux et al., 2004). These activities not only increase our understanding of cardiovascular function in space-like environments but also promote advancement in instrumentation applicable more widely in the practice of medicine. The use of aerospace-inspired observations for medical equipment brings into focus the interconnectedness of various domains of knowledge, bringing to mind the multidisciplinary nature of healthcare improvement through the assistance of technological breakthroughs.

2.3.1. Diagnostic Equipment

The evolution of diagnostic equipment has revolutionized the landscape of medical practice, making disease detection possible at an earlier and more accurate stage. Among the various tools employed, imaging technologies , such as MRI and CT scans are highly regarded for their capability to provide clinicians with a precise inner view of the human body. Not only do these advanced modalities helpdx enhance diagnosis functions, but they also enable clinicians to monitor disease progression and response to treatment in real time. The application of such state-of-the-art equipment illustrates the central importance that instrumentation assumes in the practice of diagnosis, advancing patient treatment by furnishing targeted therapeutic treatments. With the constant evolution of technology and software, there are even further possibilities for the diagnostic tools to become even more precise and efficient, so that routine tests could be revolutionized in the future. Alongside this is the intersection of automation and artificial intelligence in diagnostic equipment, a new era in laboratory testing. Automated analyzers, which streamline procedures , such as blood and urine analysis, not only increase throughput but also reduce margins of human error, leading to more precise results. In addition, AI algorithms used for imaging assist radiologists by drawing attention to abnormal findings, thus accelerating diagnosis. This combination of technology and practice in diagnostics is a prime example of the function that instrumentation serves to improve analytical capability. As termed in recent publications on laboratory medicine, including opinion from Culclasure and Wall (1970) and Fortina et al. (2015), the convergence of technology and diagnostic equipment has implications suggesting future innovations will continue to advance boundaries of normal practices into the future, positioning healthcare practitioners at the vanguard of diagnostic accuracy and efficacy. The horizon of diagnostic devices lies in their further development to cope with the intricacies of medicine and patient care today. As medicine advances further, there will be greater demands for devices that can offer instant and correct information. Trends point to diagnostic instruments not only functioning with physical measurements but also with genomics and personalized medicine modalities. This shift to individualized care demands diagnostic instruments to evolve away from traditional forms towards merged platforms better attuned to the provision of comprehensive analyses. With progress in this field, continuous research and investment will play a crucial role in ensuring that diagnostic machines not only keep pace with the technology developments but also address the evolving needs of the healthcare system, thus encouraging an integrative methodology in the management and treatment of patients and the quality of treatment (Figure 2.11).

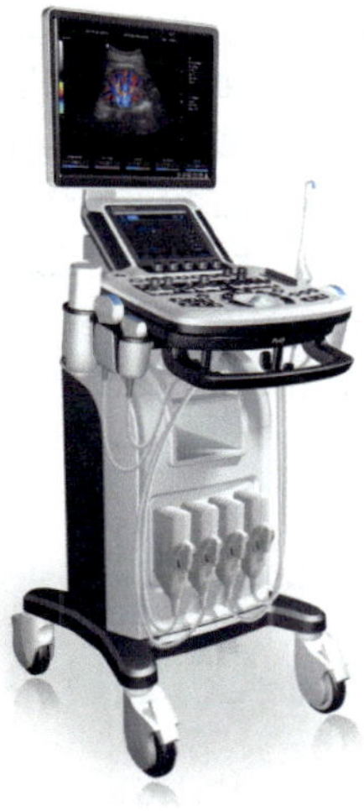

Figure 2.11. Medical diagnostic equipment.

Source: https://image.made-in-china.com/2f0j00yvcfIGpEaSbz/Medical-Diagnostic-Equipment-4D-Color-Doppler-Ultrasound-Imaging-System.jpg.

2.3.2. Monitoring Devices

Monitoring devices form part of the instrumentation and equipment and serve as principal tools for data collection and analysis in most fields. Monitoring devices are made up of a series of sensors and meters that are applied in the observation of environmental aspects, energy usage, and equipment performance. Being included in systems enhances effectiveness in operations through real-time feedback that is used to guide decisions. For example, in an undertaking at UC Berkeley, researchers utilized high-tech equipment to monitor energy flows in Cory Hall and created a Building-to-Grid testbed. The methodology used not only high-tech sensors but rigorous analysis to tailor the monitoring component network appropriately and hence capture the complex interplay between technology and actual application in monitoring systems (Peffer, 2010). The installation and design of monitoring devices involves a process with selection, setup, and testing. As regards UC Berkeley's project, that various institutions participated in the work pointed to the importance of multidisciplinary action in calibrating monitoring systems. Firstly, scientists defined appropriate types of sensors and meters to be employed, drawing on the premise that the chosen technology would be able to capture the required information appropriately (Peffer, 2010). The second phase was the planning and analysis of the energy requirements of the buildings so that a steady network of metering devices could be created. Such meticulous exercise of calibration allowed the creation of an effective data storage and display system, demonstrating that the successful implementation of monitoring devices is not only a matter of technological expertise but also an understanding of actual-world conditions under which such devices shall operate. Moreover, long-term success for monitoring devices is connected with their capacity to keep pace with evolving technologies and operational needs. As noted in the UC Berkeley project, analysis entailed establishing communication links between buildings and utilities, which demonstrates how monitoring devices contribute to greater systems integration efforts. This aspect is particularly significant in modern applications, where passive instrumentation and stimulus generation are utilized to ensure equipment reliability and safety in test phases. With constant evaluation and updating of monitoring techniques, engineers and researchers have the capability to enhance the field of knowledge concerning energy management and the efficiency of equipment. Thus, the role of monitoring equipment is pivotal not only for short-term data collection but also to foster long-term innovations and developments in instrumentation and equipment management.

2.3.3. Therapeutic Instruments

The evolution of therapeutic instruments is a serious branch of contemporary healthcare, exhibiting development in both technology and patient care practices. These gadgets are part of a broader range of devices meant to diagnose, cure, and observe medical conditions, often complementing the therapeutic interventions' overall efficacy. For instance, there is equipment like robot-assisted surgery equipment and telemedicine platforms, which have revolutionized treatment by allowing surgeons to perform procedures with greater accuracy and monitor patients. While medicine continues to emphasize evidence-based practice, there has been the need for innovative tools to demonstrate quantifiable outcomes, keeping with the drive of continued research and technology transfer as seen in efforts , such as those being undertaken in NASAs Biomedical Application Team (Culclasure and Wall, 1970). Even beyond conventional medical gear, introducing robotics into therapeutic treatment is transforming the long-held paradigms in medicine. Robots can assist health workers in various activities , such as surgery, rehabilitation, and patient monitoring, consequently improving the health benefits and organizational efficiency. These advanced systems not only address the specific needs of individual patients but also supplement care deficits by supporting caregivers and healthcare teams. But their deployment is hindered by enormous obstacles, including regulatory hurdles and the necessity for strong evidence of their effectiveness. These are obstacles to overcome in designing a healthcare system where robotics is given the setting to thrive, as outlined in implementation discussions (Riek et al., 2017). The meeting of therapeutic devices and patient-oriented medicine is also of special interest; with changing healthcare, individualization is on the rise. Adaptive instruments that respond to the individualized needs of every patient complement the healing process and enable providers to provide interventions more closely aligned with patient-specific goals and preferences. This approach not only increases patient compliance with treatment plans but also encourages increased participation in self-management. As technology continues to progress, there is a need to track the impact of such devices on the end result for the patient and ensure that they are complementing the human elements in treatment. The construction and application of therapeutic instruments, thus, must be continuously examined to assist in refining treatment methods and address the complex demands of the contemporary, diverse patient population adequately.

2.4. Industrial Instrumentation

Industrial instrumentation plays a significant role in maximizing the efficiency and accuracy of various processing and manufacturing operations. It describes a set of devices and systems that are designed to monitor and control industrial processes to ensure safety levels and operational efficiency. The instruments are applied in the measurement of various parameters , such as pressure, temperature, flow, and level, and all play a significant role in ensuring proper conditions within industrial processes. By employing sensors and transmitters, real-time data are obtained for immediate changes and reduced risk for accidents or process failure. On top of this, cutting-edge technologies in data analytics enable integration of such devices in more sophisticated control systems, therefore maximizing industrial processes and being more sustainable in managing resources. Thus, it is critical that engineers and technicians engaged in productivity improvement for various industries should be well informed of industrial instrumentation principles and applications. The integration of sophisticated technologies into industrial instrumentation is driving tremendous developments in the field, ultimately transforming traditional approaches. One of the strong means through which image and equipment performance can be enhanced is by methods like edge illumination X-ray phase-contrast imaging (XPCI). It has shown enormous potential for use as varied as materials science and medical imaging. Above all, its ability to be used with common lab equipment reduces the need for microfocal-source-specific equipment, rendering it suitable for regular research environments. Innovations , such as photon-counting energy-resolved detectors have enabled scientists to improve imaging quality in laboratory use. As in most of the studies, such as the findings on XPCI, the constant evolution in instrumentation technologies contributes to increasing accuracy and efficiency in industrial processes, thereby indicating the ongoing use of instrumentation in innovation in the industrial processes (Basta et al., 2015). The implementation of large-scale projects , such as the Building-to-Grid testbed at UC Berkeley, is also indicative of the importance of instrumentation in energy management as well as sustainability practices. This project involved a comprehensive strategy of mapping the energy flows within a building and coordinating with other prominent institutions to develop an efficient network of metering components and data visualizing systems. Together, the team undertook a number of assignments varying from building need analysis to the preparation of a vision plan for future energy management technologies. The findings from this project not only demonstrated the technical subtleties of energy monitoring but also how effective instrumentation can be employed to create communication between buildings and energy providers. Ultimately, these improvements are the indispensable role that precise instrumentation plays in bringing smarter energy solutions and encouraging sustainable practice into industrial environments (Peffer, 2010) (Figure 2.12).

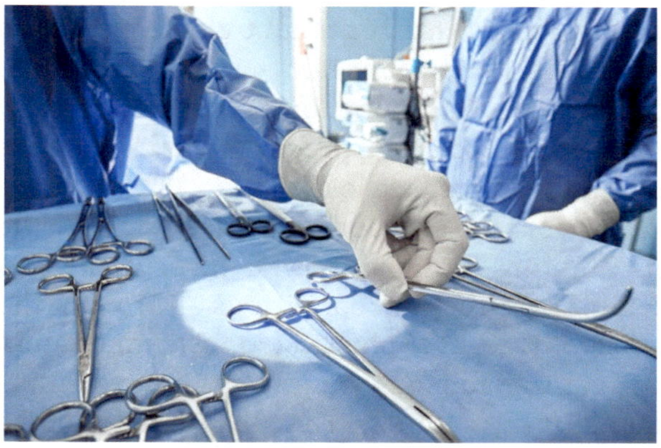

Figure 2.12. Industrial instrumentation.

Source: https://res.cloudinary.com/healthmanagement-org/image/upload/c_thumb,f_auto,fl_lossy,q_90/v1738301317/cw/00129159_cw_image_wi_48bbfa2077f3519f16aff5142a62f011.webp.

2.4.1. Process Control Systems

The role played by process control systems in modern industrial applications cannot be overstated, as they are a constituent part of the upkeep of the efficiency of operations and safety of advanced instrumentation and equipment. The systems operate through a sequence of automated controls that tend to constantly monitor and adjust parameters of operation. Automated responses under such circumstances make processes stable even with a varying external environment, minimizing equipment breakdown or safety hazards. For instance, in rocket engine test facilities, certain computer programs assess the performance of the various instruments, ensuring they meet stringent calibration levels. With the use of such automatic diagnostic tools, companies are capable of reducing downtime while maintaining a stable operating environment that meets specifications, as cited in Merewether et al. (1966). Besides, advancements in microtechnology have pushed the boundaries of currently available process control systems, particularly in high-end applications , such as medical device manufacturing. The integration of microfluidic technologies possesses unique challenges when scaled up from laboratory-scale research to industrial-level production. Nevertheless, new approaches, including precision hot embossing, have been created to close the gaps. This method allows for mass production of devices while maintaining minimal capital investment and flexible production conditions. Through the incorporation of sophisticated instrumentation to quantify forming conditions in real-time, manufacturers can exercise increased control over the production process. Such precise monitoring ensures the material property variation is promptly detected and, therefore, enhances the global quality control of the end product as described by Bageant & Hardt (2015). The incorporation of real-time sensing within process control systems enhances not only the ease of production but also optimizes resource utilization in the manufacturing industry. Real-time monitoring feedback control can inform decision-making, allowing manufacturers to dynamically change parameters to enhance yield and reduce waste. The correlation of force and displacement signals with functional outcome allows systems to implement closed-loop controls to maintain product integrity throughout the production cycle. These sophisticated strategies underpin the need to integrate advanced instrumentation into process control systems, validating the call for accuracy and adaptability in contemporary manufacturing operations. This level of control ultimately benefits the goal of achieving improved efficiencies and product quality, further highlighting the pivotal role instrumentation plays in modern industrial processes.

2.4.2. Quality Assurance Tools

Necessary under the heading of instrumentation and equipment are tools for quality assurance to offer assurance of the reliability and quality of measurement and process. These tools consist of various methodologies and technologies that assist in the identification and assessment of instrumentation system errors. For instance, calibration tools play a major role in maintaining the integrity of equipment, with measurements held in predetermined parameters. Calibration ensures that equipment is optimized in performance, along with the attainment of compliance with industrial standards. Also, statistical process control (SPC) techniques can be utilized to control and check manufacturing processes such that equipment can function at its optimum level throughout its entire duration of usage. With the use of these tools of quality assurance, organizations can minimize risks associated with measurement errors by a significant amount, thereby improving overall operating efficiency. Also, the implementation of advanced quality assurance tools can trigger intricate benefits in aerospace applications, particularly for manufacturing and operating purposes. In this paradigm, tools , such as Six Sigma and Total Quality Management (TQM) have been of immense use in streamlining quality control mechanisms. These tools introduce systemic processes for the identification of defects and variances in equipment output so that organizations are able to use preventive measures proactively. For the aerospace sector, where precision is not an option, productivity gains in systematic quality assurance procedures translate into not only better product performance but higher levels of safety for users. Surprisingly, benefits to the use of aerospace technology do not end with the purely improved performance; they also generate significant manufacturing practice enhancement, creating operational excellence and competitive edge in a globalized marketplace (Lux et al., 2004). Lastly, good quality assurance solutions have an important function in equipment performance assessment and optimization throughout its life cycle. With the use of data analytics and machine learning procedures, organizations are able to predict equipment failure even before it occurs, thus enabling early intervention that enhances reliability.

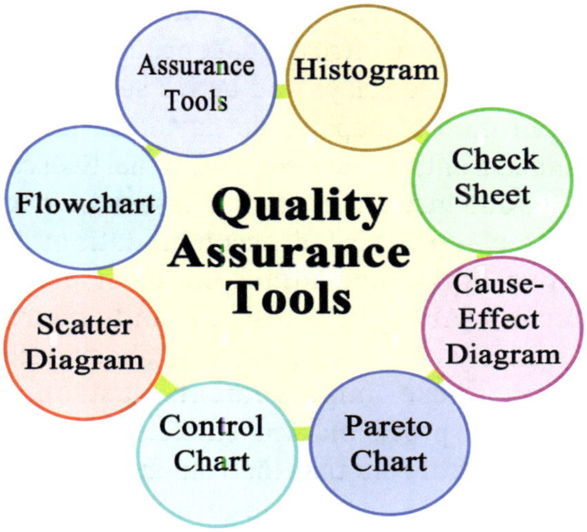

Figure 2.13. Quality assurance tools.

Source: https://c8.alamy.com/comp/2CCYWTG/tools-for-quality-assurance-2CCYWTG.jpg.

These predictive maintenance solutions are founded on quality assurance platforms that assess equipment parameters in real-time to make way for real-time feedback and correction mechanisms. Second, as exhibited in advancements on aerospace-related uses , such as improved compressor designs, these methodologies provide significant improvements in performance, e.g., fuel efficiency and reduced operations costs (Gaffin, 2025). Therefore, by integrating solid quality assurance instruments into instrumentation frameworks, organizations not only enhance their product outcomes but also create a culture of continuous improvement essential to sustaining long-term operational success (Figure 2.13).

2.4.3. Safety Instrumentation

The incorporation of safety instrumentation in advanced systems is crucial in guaranteeing the strength of functioning and safeguarding human life. With the increased reliance of industries on advanced technologies, safety instrumentation is the backbone of risk management strategies. This covers systems that aim to detect dangerous conditions, produce real-time data, and ensure automatic safety actions. For instance, monitoring equipment is able to detect pressure or temperature deviation, which is essential for the prevention of accidents within areas , such as chemical plants or nuclear facilities. Due care should be taken in the planning and design as well as the implementation of such instruments so that they are able to perform effectively under varying operating conditions, imposing the need for stringent testing , such as that conducted at UC Berkeley with their Building-to-Grid project, where widespread instrumentation was used to test energy flow and safety specifications (Peffer, 2010). Furthermore, safety instrumentation design is not limited to traditional industrial applications; it also applies in cutting-edge technology utilized for space exploration. Devices deployed in the International Space Station, for example, have safety instrumentation to monitor environmental conditions and manage waste effectively. Such systems enable astronauts to remain within safety working limits, thereby minimizing hazards associated with the space environment's unique challenges. As highlighted by research on spacecraft systems, such safety measures are core in managing critical components, such as resistojet systems for orbit control, and thereby showing the interdependence of safety instruments across disciplines (Abe & Greco, 1971). The need for continuous enhancements to safety instruments cannot be overstressed. With emerging technologies and increasing integration, such systems must themselves adapt to meet new challenges like cybersecurity weakness and artificial intelligence incorporation. Future developments will find themselves gravitating towards the creation of more robust, networked safety frameworks that operate in harmony within extended organizational networks. Injecting a proactive design philosophy for safety instrumentation—a philosophy looking ahead and anticipating impending failure and redundancy—can contribute a great deal to enhancing system robustness. Furthermore, while the industries evolve, sharing best practices and lessons learned from projects like the one at USC Berkeley will be instrumental in shaping the safety instrumentation of the future to put safety at the forefront of technological advancement.

2.5. Advances in Instrumentation Technology

Advances in instrumentation technology have been instrumental in shaping the context of scientific research and industrial applications. A prime example is the development of holography, which initially emerged in 1947 as a method for improving electron microscopy. It then underwent significant alterations, particularly in the 1960s, when engineer-scientists in classified research laboratories reanimated the technology. This development not only drove holography into mainstream optical engineering but also inspired a new collaborative relationship between scientists and artists, leading to the expansion of distinct communities. The divergent strategies of holography illustrate the complex interplay between technological innovation and user engagement, showing how various motivations can drive instrument development. Such dynamics reflect the practice of research-technologists and highlight the political forces that may decide the course of technological communities, both impacting instruments themselves and the culture that surrounds them (Johnston et al., 2005). The innovation of new multi-object instrument concepts also symbolizes the latest progress of instrumentation technology, particularly in astronomical studies. Through devising the Starbug focal plane positioning concept, researchers have developed a sequence of new instruments that enhance observation. These innovations comprise fiber positioners and deployable fiber-fed Integral Field Units (IFUs), allowing for more intricate data acquisition with improved image relays and active sensors. The incorporation of deployable payloads has also expanded frontiers between traditional telescope systems and instrumentation. These pairs create space for sophisticated accommodations like adaptive optics and atmospheric dispersion correctors (ADCs), which significantly improve the quality of astronomical observation. Through these improvements, astronomy reaps more precision and efficiency, pointing out the central role that instrumentation takes in heightening scientific discovery (McGrath & Haynes, 2006). The advancement in technology in the instrumentation not only enhances efficiency but also expands the scope of research potential through interdisciplinarity. One of the fascinating impacts of these technologies is evident in fields , such as materials science and biotechnology, where measurement and analysis precision has become increasingly critical. Modern instruments that incorporate advanced sensors and automation allow scientists to record data with unparalleled accuracy, leading to higher insight and discovery. Besides, with the improvement of technology in instruments every day, the integration of artificial intelligence in data processing operations has opened new avenues for real-time processing and interpretation. This convergence of cutting-edge technology and wise utilization does more than streamline efficiency; it fosters a culture of ongoing change and adaptation, ultimately bringing innovations beyond normal limits. These developments underscore the importance of ongoing investment in instrumentation technology to propel scientific and technological future endeavors.

2.5.1. Automation and Robotics

Automation and robotics are among the prime movers of equipment and instrumentation development, particularly in high-hazard environments , such as space exploration. With the advancements of these technologies, they significantly enhance productivity, precision, and safety of operations. For example, operations in the Space Station Freedom Program have illustrated how the integration of advanced automation and robotics technology can make operations that otherwise take human effort easier, thereby reducing risks to space missions. The development of technologies , such as flight telerobotic servicers illustrates the potential of robotics to perform difficult maneuvers remotely so that vital space operations may be continued even under challenging conditions. This sort of technology is not just an addendum to human effort; it is becoming increasingly a necessity to the operational framework of modern-day space exploration and a template for use in other fields. The Office of Aeronautics and Space Technology (OAST) has placed emphasis on the need to ensure automation and robotics as central factors in national space endeavors of the future. This ranking resulted from a workshop whose goal was to identify the most important technologies for validation in the space environment, which proved the industry's commitment to enhancing these areas. As far as instrumentation and equipment go, the integration of robotic systems can provide the capabilities for sophisticated data collection and analysis for enhanced scientific research capabilities. By addressing robotics and automation's fundamental technology needs, businesses can ensure their equipment is on the cutting edge, creating new solutions to complex problems. R&D within this industry today demonstrates that a cooperative relationship between business and academia is most effective in achieving breakthroughs in these technologies. Furthermore, advances in robotics and automation are reflected across broader trends going beyond space travel into numerous applications on Earth.

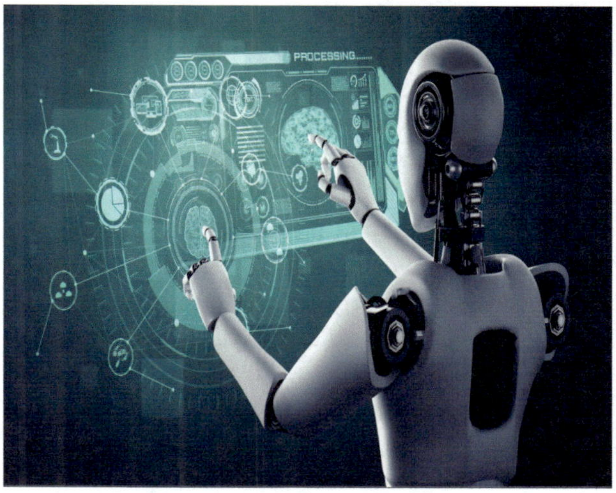

Figure 2.14. Robotic process automation (RPA).

Source: https://xcelacore.com/wp-content/uploads/2022/04/robotic-process-automation.jpg.

Merging cutting-edge robotic systems with various branches of business — from production to healthcare — indicates growing recognition of how capabilities can be augmented through automation. For instance, where accuracy and reliability are top priority, such as in medical equipment, robotics can enhance precision and reduce human error. As the terrestrial and extraterrestrial environments are extended, it is evident that automation and robotics will play a growing role in influencing the character of instrumentation and equipment to enable more challenging endeavors than ever before. It is thus crucial for high-efficiency operations and human knowledge advance in terrestrial and space environments that there be a synergistic interaction among the instrumentation and technologies (Figure 2.14).

2.5.2. Digital vs. Analog Instrumentation

Analog vs. digital instrumentation is a result of the basic differences between these technologies in how they process and display data. Analog instrumentation employs continuous signals to measure physical properties, which can provide smooth, real-time readings. This approach is unfortunately prone to numerous forms of noise and distortion, which can corrupt measurement accuracy. For instance, environmental factors and conditions , such as electromagnetic interference have a very significant effect on analog systems. Digital instrumentation, of course, converts signals into discrete numbers, where there is greater accuracy and ease with which data can be handled. With the ability to filter noise and enhance signal quality, digital systems are better in cases where precision is most critical, such as in high-stakes applications of aerospace instruments. Furthermore, technological improvements in digital data acquisition systems have revolutionized data acquisition operations in a variety of different fields. An example is the National Transonic Facility at Langley Research Center, where high-speed digital systems originally produced data that included unacceptably large amounts of noise. Following a disciplined search for the cause of contributing noise sources—, such as electromagnetic interference and grounding issues—remedies upgraded system performance by more than five times. These advancements call out the function of digital systems in enhancing measurement reliability, especially in situations calling for fine calibration. While analog systems may continue to be helpful in some scenarios, the effective capabilities of digital equipment tend to outdo their analog counterparts, especially where precision and accuracy become the concern (McPhee, 1988). The second major distinction between analog and digital equipment lies in their operational flexibility and ease of integration into modern technologies. Digital equipment can seamlessly interface with computers and software for remote analysis, storage, and monitoring of data, broadening its application. In real-time data visualization applications, such as aviation, digital systems allow precise feedback that supports critical decision-making tasks. For instance, boresight camera images applied in aircraft angular tracking show how digital technology enhances measurement responsiveness and precision in high-performance environments (Britt et al., 2025). Beyond making data handling simpler, this integration supports more complex processing techniques , such as statistical analysis and simulation. Thus, with the increasing technological capabilities, the advantages of digital instrumentation increasingly render it the option over analog systems in most contemporary applications.

2.5.3. Integration of Artificial Intelligence (AI) in Instrumentation

The role of AI in instrumentation is revolutionizing many industries, particularly in sensor technology. The development is being driven by smart sensors, with their capacity to interpret data in real-time and adapt to fluctuating conditions. These sensors offer enhanced precision and precision, and are completely necessary for uses ranging from aerospace to medicine. For example, NASA's research on smart sensor technology demonstrates advanced applications in Life Sciences research to leverage the advancements onboard space stations , such as the Space Station Freedom (SSF) (Cooper et al., 2025). AI sensors' capacity to process vast volumes of data autonomously and make informed decisions significantly improves the effectiveness and efficiency of advanced systems and thus represents an instrumental turning point. Furthermore, AI's ability to augment predictive maintenance of instrumentation cannot be overstated. With machine learning algorithms, instrumentation systems are able to predict potential failures before they happen, reducing downtime and maintenance costs. This aspect is superior to regular sensors, as AI algorithms review past performance data to identify patterns, enabling proactive actions.

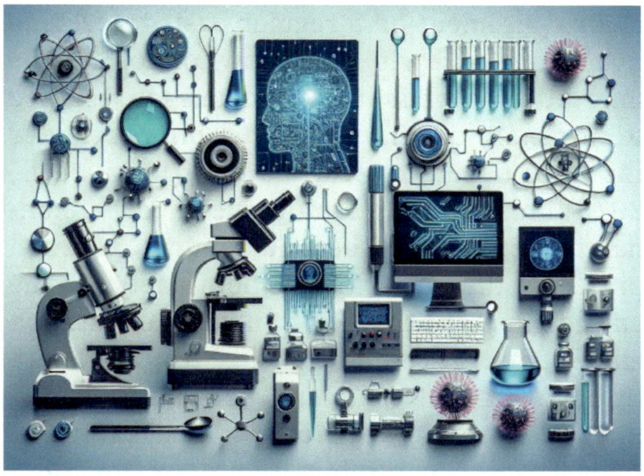

Figure 2.15. The transformative role of artificial intelligence (AI) in biomedical instrumentation.

Source: https://biomedicalengineering.io/_next/image/?url=https:%2F%2Fcdn.sanity.io%2Fimages%2Fcpgts12o%2Fproduction%2F04d55c5cafc966bceee0d44fc876937dc1f346e5-1792x1024.webp%3Fw%3D1792%26q%3D100%26auto%3Dformat&w=3840&q=100.

The OAST has identified automation systems and robotics as frontline areas where such technologies can be employed to facilitate the integration of AI into future technology development (Beck et al., 2025). Not only does this enhance the working reliability of instruments, but also their overall effectiveness in data collection and analysis, which is crucial to experimentation and research in multiple fields. Additionally, the combination of AI and instrumentation creates a highly innovative environment for increased research capabilities. An example is how AI algorithms are being used more to maximize the performance of fluid management and propulsion systems, which are central components in aerospace uses. By incorporating AI, scientists are well positioned to carry out experiments across a wide range of fields with a more efficient process, which previously required extensive manual intervention. The evolving climate of astute instrumentation provides real-time measurement and calibration, which is vital in life-critical operations. This integration finally makes scientific investigation possible by having more responsive and versatile instruments, which allow scientists to push the boundary of what can be achieved in instrumentation and equipment dynamics in different areas (Figure 2.15).

2.6. Maintenance and Calibration of Equipment

Equipment maintenance and calibration are crucial aspects in ensuring the functionality and accuracy of instrumentation across various disciplines. Regular maintenance checks help identify potential problems and make adjustment before equipment failure occurs, leading to costly downtime and erroneous data. For instance, in biomedicine, equipment , such as the Bedrest Muscle Stress Apparatus has to be maintained to ensure that its measurement of disuse muscle strength and tone is correct. Booher et al. (1979) observe that measurements made with this equipment correspond most significantly, which implies that even minimal variation of the function significantly affects research results. A good maintenance schedule, then, enhances reliability and precision, which are crucial in achieving accurate and consistent results in scientific research. Calibration is actually all about ensuring instruments provide measurements not only accurate but also consistent in the long run. Calibration is achieved by comparing the measurements an instrument provides with a known standard, thereby enabling adjustment where necessary. In remote sensing technology, as described in Lux (2004), external environmental degradation of equipment performance, e.g., contamination or stray light, necessitates stringent calibration protocols. Maintaining measurement integrity, especially to allow for infinitesimal variations over a long duration, helps make quality decisions from data. Therefore, calibration is not only a procedural ritual but an obligatory practice that guarantees that the measurement systems are scientifically sound and operationally efficient. Moreover, calibration and maintenance are complementary practices that feed on each other. Failure to keep equipment in proper condition can have an impact on the calibration process and, consequently, lead to erroneous measurements and compromised integrity of data. In high-risk settings, such as in space exploration or in clinical diagnostics, this coupling is even stronger. Equipment for deployment in mission-critical applications must be put through severe testing to ensure long-term stability and reliability, such as in the production of spectrally flat detectors for flight sensors. Organisations therefore, must adopt an integrated maintenance and calibration strategy, promoting diligence culture and quality assurance. This system-centric focus eventually results in the creation of reliable instrumentation and equipment across different areas of study, which increases research and operating results.

2.6.1. Importance of Regular Maintenance

Maintenance on a regular basis is crucial for instrumentation and equipment reliability and longevity in different industries. Preventive maintenance measures not only help to prevent failures but also enhance the system's overall efficiency. When equipment is regularly inspected and serviced, it becomes easier to detect and repair small issues before they lead to catastrophic failures. This kind of preventive approach drastically reduces downtime and repair costs, hence leading to increased levels of productivity. For example, in areas , such as the aerospace industry, where systems must meet stringent levels of safety, maintenance is a requirement on a regular basis to provide operational integrity and allow for continuous innovation , such as lunar missions for resource exploration, as the objectives offered under the First Lunar Outpost mission (Bartz et al., 2025) illustrate. In addition, the effects of non-maintenance extend beyond routine operation problems; they are critical to both safety and the environment. In the long run, instrumentation and equipment can lead to catastrophic failure through gradual wear and deterioration. For instance, failing to monitor and maintain critical parts may result in hazardous situations, particularly in plants that rely on precise measurements and control systems, such as nuclear power plants. Research has indicated that aging impacts in major components, including electrical cable and instrumentation, are bound to considerably weaken functionality and safety and identify the necessity of strategic maintenance frameworks (Golay & Moinzadeh, 1986). Hence, embracing holistic maintenance procedures not only protects personnel and equipment but is an inherent responsibility of organizations to adhere to industry standards and fulfill moral obligations. In addition, advancements in technology have transformed maintenance approaches, leveraging predictive analytics and IoT technology to achieve maximum performance. Technologies like condition-based monitoring and automatic alerting have been made available to assist organizations in taking a more data-driven maintenance approach. By constantly keeping track of equipment performance data, organizations can develop tailored maintenance calendars, maximizing lifecycle management and efficiency. The movement also highlights the importance of regular maintenance by providing opportunities for convenient proactive action that minimizes inconvenience. Furthermore, as industries are turning to sustainable operations, maintaining equipment at its peak further supports energy reduction and waste reduction, all towards conserving the environment. This diversified approach is based on the aspect that maintenance is not only an economic requirement but also a vital component of wise and sustainable working practice in the instrumentation and equipment field.

2.6.2. Calibration Procedures

Calibration procedures are the most important aspects for maintaining the accuracy and reliability of instrumentation and equipment used in various scientific and engineering disciplines. These activities involve controlling and testing equipment accuracy in a systematic way, resulting in their output being consistent with set standards. Calibration minimizes measurement errors to the lowest level that would lead to significant variations in data interpretation. For instance, if sensor readings fluctuate over time due to environmental factors or mechanical deterioration, calibration enables technicians to make adjustments so that the equipment remains as accurate as it was when new. This uniformity is not only imperative in the laboratory but also in field deployment, where data are usually collected under varying conditions. Adherence to these steps to the letter builds confidence in the validity of the data, which is important when empirical choices have to be made from instrument readings (Jackson, 2015). Calibration entails a number of methodologies, depending on the application and the specificity of the instruments employed. Techniques , such as direct calibration, where a standard reference is applied, or intercomparison with another unit that has been calibrated, are commonplace. For use in airborne research, where equipment will operate under conditions other than normal, strict calibration procedures become part of the design. The integration of airborne sensors highlights the requirement to establish procedures sensitive to special flight dynamics. On-board equipment is calibrated to ensure accurate measurement, commonly by a systematic process of both isolation and comparative measurement against other calibrated instruments. These rigorous methods not only assist in measurement accuracy but also in maintaining ongoing compliance with industry standards as well as safety legislation (Andrés-Hernández et al., 2012).

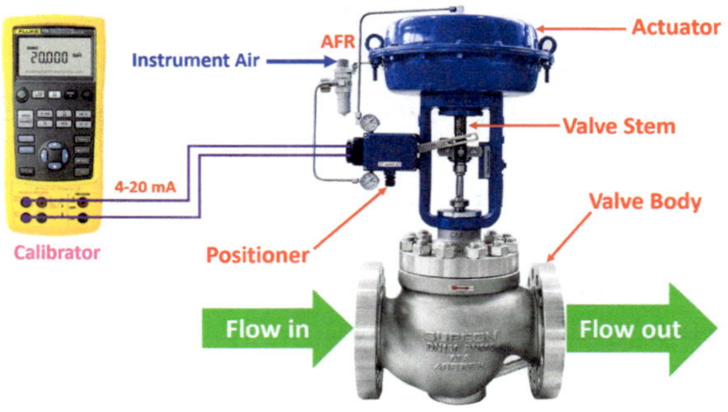

Figure 2.16. Calibration procedure of a control valve.

Source: https://automationcommunity.com/wp-content/uploads/2021/05/Calibration-procedure-of-a-Control-Valve-1536x887.png.

Moreover, the application of quality assurance controls within calibration activities is equally significant to financial as well as operational efficiency. Regular calibration processes can prevent costly equipment failure and false data by catching imminent issues early on. Calibration should be performed exhaustively and documented meticulously to maintain a traceable record for each instrument. Traceability ensures compliance with the regulation and makes it easier to troubleshoot processes upon observing any abnormalities. These calibration records can also be utilized by organizations as financial audit or certification records, illustrating their commitment to maintaining high standards of operation. Thus, the integration of good calibration procedures not only increases the research results' integrity but also enhances overall equipment performance management throughout its operational life cycle (Jackson, 2015) (Figure 2.16).

2.6.3. Troubleshooting Common Issues

Successful troubleshooting plays an important role in instrumentation and equipment maintenance and operation, particularly in high-risk environments , such as laboratories and aerospace engineering. Where things go amiss, there is a requirement for systematic intervention; this begins by acknowledging the symptoms of the failure. For instance, malfunctioning sensors can produce erroneous readings, leading to poor data that compromises experimental validity. Through diagnostic tools and visual inspections, technicians are able to identify anomalies that may suggest recalibration or replacement is warranted. Moreover, understanding the underlying principles of equipment operation facilitates more efficient troubleshooting, which, in turn, results in quicker and minimized downtime. Another problem usually encountered is electromagnetic interference (EMI), which could have a negative effect on the operation of sensitive instruments. Equipment operating in environments that are exposed to high-frequency fields, such as avionics systems, could be susceptible to interference that could go unnoticed due to the lack of rigorous EMC verification and validation activities. The importance of grounding, bonding, and shielding methodologies cannot be overemphasized in this context, as they are the main keystones for effective electromagnetic compatibility. A comprehensive approach to grounding methodologies not only minimizes EMI but also enhances the longevity and reliability of the equipment and instrumentation, ultimately contributing to operational requirements in commercial and research environments (Clarke & Larsen, 1987). In addition to environmental conditions, instrumentation operating and physical conditions may also produce common issues requiring troubleshooting. Equipment designed for use in microgravity environments, like that found on space stations, presents special conditions demanding unique design considerations. The Combustion Tunnel and the Advanced Modular Furnace, for example, are designed for optimized microgravity research capabilities but possess equally rigorous support systems to be used strictly for diagnostics and fault correction (Fiske et al., 2025). Failure detection in such specialized equipment is generally reliant on understanding how traditional methods of troubleshooting must reorient themselves to accommodate the nuances of the operational environment. Therefore, effective troubleshooting methods must evolve to handle the needs of both technological advancements and environmental conditions so that instruments are always operating optimally.

SUMMARY

In summarizing the observations in the course of researching instrumentation and equipment, it is evident that accuracy and adaptability are of utmost significance in modern research approaches. Instrument choice and calibration, as explained, define the validity of data obtained in most environmental and aerospace research. For instance, the use of airborne platforms, among other benefits, enables sensor positioning at appropriate heights but complicates the stability and reliability of the instruments. As noted, such research platforms require concentrated changes and constant calibration to keep them from losing functional integrity. Therefore, the efficacy of these instruments is facilitated by the meticulous process of calibration, exemplifying why methodological consistency in data collection is crucial (Andrés-Hernández et al., 2012). Moreover, instrument complexities are not limited to physical aspects; they permeate the operational systems in which the instruments function. Proper data collection relies on comprehensive organizational structures that enable regulatory clearances in order for complex research processes to proceed. Scientists have to work within these operational environments, making sure that their equipment not only complies with technical requirements but also with safety and quality assurance guidelines. It becomes imperative to understand the complex interplay between different instrumentation elements and environmental parameters, especially in complex applications like work with radionuclides in geochemical research. The various contexts in which the instruments are employed reflect a broad trend towards interdisciplinarity in research (Cizdziel et al., 2005). Lastly, what is to be learned from the battle over instrumentation and equipment is a scenario with continuous innovation and methodological evolution. Scientists find themselves more and more requiring innovative technologies and being sensitive to environmental variables that can largely influence experimental outcomes. As testaments to the complexity of tracking radionuclides and airborne science, the potential of instrumentation in the future lies in its ability to be flexible as research conditions evolve. The commitment to continuous calibration, operational performance, and multidisciplinary collaboration is paramount in tapping the capabilities of advanced instruments. This conservative approach not only delivers precision to the utmost degree but also gains a better understanding of complex environmental interactions, thereby extending the frontiers of scientific inquiry.

In the aspect of instrumentation and equipment, an extensive understanding of the main parts is required to enhance system functionality. Some of the noted points to emphasize include the significance of antenna system instrumentation in the provision of coherent communication, as well as signal integrity. Phase modulator development, for example, plays a great role in furthering the reception and transmission of signals in various applications. Furthermore, control systems of transmitters and motor generators enhance the performance and reliability of operation. These advancements underscore the inclusion of advanced technology in existing systems to attain maximum functionality and performance. As improvements are made over time, the instrumentation world gets better with more precise measurements and controlling ability that accommodates rising demands from various industries (Lux et al., 2004). Furthermore, passive instrumentation development continues to be an awe-inspiring aspect of equipment reliability enhancement. The incorporation of stimulus generation systems is particularly significant in the testing process of particular equipment, e.g., Saturn IB rocket systems. This type of nondestructive testing helps confirm equipment functioning without compromising the integrity of the instruments employed. Such methods play an important role in applications where failure would result in disastrous implications, and hence, the importance of articulated instrumentation strategies is further realized. Additionally, the inclusion of passive instrumentation systems assists in reducing potential errors during calibration or functioning. The evolution in this context serves to bring in further reliability as well as opportunities for safer working routines in various areas of engineering (Kaushagen & Skinner, 1966). Lastly, knowing how to calibrate and maintain instruments is part of what guarantees long-term working and reliability in any system. Routine calibration measures not only comply with industry standards but also safeguard against long-term deterioration in equipment performance. Appreciating the connection between maintenance and equipment life proves how important it is to embrace strategic maintenance practices. Besides, the potential for harmonizing instrumentation systems with evolving technological environments implies a necessity for continuous learning and training in the profession. This evolving nature of instrumentation and equipment confirms a collective responsibility among technologists and engineers to update themselves on advancing developments and better practices. Repeated exposure to this learning will eventually translate to greater innovation and operational excellence in the instrumentation field (Lux et al., 2004).

CLOSER LOOK

ENVIRONMENTAL MONITORING:

Environmental monitoring refers to the systematic collection, analysis, and interpretation of data about environmental conditions to identify changes, assess risks, and guide decision-making. It encompasses a wide range of activities intended to track the health of ecosystems, detect pollution, and evaluate the impact of human activities on natural resources. Because environmental systems are dynamic and interconnected, monitoring plays a crucial role in understanding how air, water, soil, and biological communities respond to ongoing natural and human-driven pressures. One central component of environmental monitoring is air quality assessment. This involves measuring pollutants such as particulate matter, nitrogen oxides, ozone, and volatile organic compounds. Air monitoring stations—both fixed and mobile—provide continuous data that can identify trends, support health advisories, and inform regulatory policies. Increasingly, satellite observations and low-cost sensor networks enhance traditional monitoring, allowing for broader spatial coverage and more real-time insights.

Water quality monitoring is another critical domain. It evaluates the chemical, physical, and biological characteristics of rivers, lakes, groundwater, and coastal areas. By tracking parameters like pH, dissolved oxygen, turbidity, nutrient levels, and microbial contamination, scientists can detect pollution events, assess ecosystem health, and ensure safe drinking water supplies. Long-term water monitoring reveals patterns linked to climate change, urbanization, agricultural runoff, and industrial activities.

Monitoring of soil conditions provides information essential for agriculture, land management, and contamination control. Soil sampling can detect heavy metals, pesticides, and other pollutants that may harm plants, enter food chains, or threaten human and animal health. Changes in soil structure, moisture, and nutrient content also offer early indicators of erosion, desertification, and land degradation. Biological monitoring adds another dimension by observing living organisms as indicators of environmental quality. Species diversity, population trends, and the presence of sensitive organisms—such as amphibians, lichens, or specific aquatic insects—can reveal subtle shifts in ecosystem health that chemical measurements alone may miss.

Environmental monitoring also increasingly relies on technological innovations. Remote sensing, geographic information systems (GIS), drones, automated sensors, and machine-learning models enable more precise, continuous, and wide-ranging surveillance. These tools allow faster detection of anomalies, from harmful algal blooms to wildfire smoke plumes.

Ultimately, environmental monitoring is vital for safeguarding public health, conserving ecosystems, and supporting sustainable development. By providing robust, evidence-based insights, monitoring programs help governments, industries, and communities make informed decisions that balance human needs with environmental protection.

REFERENCES

1. Abe, J. T., & Greco, R. V. (1971). *Resistojet systems studies directed to the space station/space base: Volume 2 – Biowaste resistojet system development program: Final report.* NASA CR-111878 MDC G2125 https://core.ac.uk/download/pdf/85235469.pdf (accessed on 15th July 2025).
2. Andrés-Hernández, L., Gawande, A., Glauert, A., Moore, B., Quant, M., Schmidt, L., & Sizoo, K. (2012). *Use of Airborne Vehicles as Research Platforms.* https://core.ac.uk/download/20496286.pdf (accessed on 15th July 2025).
3. Lux, D., et al. (2004). *Scalable Multiprocessor for High-Speed Computing in Space.* NASA Tech Briefs, October 200. https://core.ac.uk/download/pdf/10563724.pdf (accessed on 15th July 2025).
4. Bageant, M. R., & Hardt, D. E. (2015). *Measurement and Process Control in Precision Hot Embossing.* https://core.ac.uk/download/83232488.pdf (accessed on 15th July 2025).
5. Bartz, C., Cook, J., & Rusingizandekwe, J. L. (2025). *First Lunar Outpost Support Study.* https://core.ac.uk/download/pdf/42807793.pdf (accessed on 15th July 2025).
6. Basta, D., Bellazzini, R., Brez, A., De Ruvo, L., et al. (2015). *Laboratory implementation of edge illumination X-ray phase-contrast imaging with energy-resolved detectors.* https://core.ac.uk/download/29416333.pdf (accessed on 15th July 2025).
7. Beck, S. M., Breckenridge, R. A., Clark, L. G., Collier, R., et al. (2025). *Technology for the future: In-space technology experiments program, part 2.* https://core.ac.uk/download/pdf/42817270.pdf (accessed on 15th July 2025).
8. Bevan, A., Dadone, L., & Peterson, A. A. (2025). *Rotorcraft aviation icing research requirements: Research review and recommendations.* https://core.ac.uk/download/pdf/42860806.pdf (accessed on 15th July 2025).
9. Booher, C. R., Hooper, S. L., & Setzer, D. N. (1979). *Development of a Bedrest Muscle Stress Apparatus.* https://core.ac.uk/download/pdf/10339563.pdf (accessed on 15th July 2025).
10. Bridges, F., Gault, D., Greeley, R., Houpis, H., et al. (2025). *Planetary Science.* https://core.ac.uk/download/pdf/42833847.pdf (accessed on 15th July 2025).
11. Britt, C. L., Miller, L. S., & Thompson, W. S. (2025). *An analytical investigation of acquisition techniques and system integration studies for a radar aircraft guidance research facility.* https://core.ac.uk/download/pdf/85239191.pdf (accessed on 15th July 2025).
12. Camacho, R., Cernat, R., Duma, V. F., Goldstein, R., Heise, B., Honomura, T., et al. (2014). *Surface imaging of metallic material fractures using optical coherence tomography.* https://core.ac.uk/download/30708963.pdf (accessed on 15th July 2025).
13. Cizdziel, J., Van Luik, A., Stetzenbach, K. J., Williams, J., et al. (2005). *Impact of alteration phase formation and microbial activity on the fate and transport of the actinides and fission products: Alteration phase analysis.* https://digitalscholarship.unlv.edu/cgi/viewcontent.cgi?article=1111&context=yucca_mtn_pubs (accessed on 15th July 2025).
14. Clarke, C. A., & Larsen, W. E. (1987). *Aircraft Electromagnetic Compatibility.* DOT/FAA/CT-86/40 https://core.ac.uk/download/pdf/42836482.pdf (accessed on 15th July 2025).
15. Cooper, T. G., Costello, D. J., Davis, J. G., Horst, T., et al. (2025). *Advanced Sensors Technology Survey.* https://core.ac.uk/download/pdf/42810216.pdf (accessed on 15th July 2025).

16. Culclasure, D. F., & Wall, L. (1970). *Southwest Research Institute assistance to NASA in biomedical areas of the technology utilization program: Final report, 1 Feb. 1969 – 24 Aug. 1970.* https://core.ac.uk/download/pdf/85236539.pdf (accessed on 15th July 2025).
17. Donais, M. K., & Vandenabeele, P. (2016). *Mobile Spectroscopic Instrumentation in Archaeometry Research.* https://core.ac.uk/download/55846882.pdf (accessed on 15th July 2025).
18. Fischer, R. B. (1961). *Instrumentation in the Undergraduate Chemistry Curriculum.* https://core.ac.uk/download/76294068.pdf (accessed on 15th July 2025).
19. Fiske, M. R., Georgekutty, T., Uhran, M. L., Wear, R., et al. (2025). *Equipment concept design and development plans for microgravity science and applications research on space station: Combustion tunnel, laser diagnostic system, advanced modular furnace, integrated electronics laboratory.* https://core.ac.uk/download/pdf/42838809.pdf (accessed on 15th July 2025).
20. Fortina, P., Kricka, L. J., Park, J. Y., & Polsky, T. G. (2015). *The Future of Laboratory Medicine – A 2014 Perspective.* https://core.ac.uk/download/54509579.pdf (accessed on 15th July 2025).
21. Gaffin, W. O. (2025). *JT8D High Pressure Compressor Performance Improvement.* https://core.ac.uk/download/pdf/42858655.pdf (accessed on 15th July 2025).
22. Golay, M. W., & Moinzadeh, J. H. (1986). *Extending the life of nuclear power plants: Technical and institutional issues.* https://core.ac.uk/download/4385967.pdf (accessed on 15th July 2025).
23. McGrath, A. & Haynes, R. (2006). *Deployable payloads with Starbug.* https://core.ac.uk/download/44118427.pdf (accessed on 15th July 2025).
24. Jackson, M. D. (2015). *Instrumentation & data acquisition system (DAS) engineer.* https://core.ac.uk/download/pdf/42695417.pdf (accessed on 15th July 2025).
25. Johnston, S. F. (2005). *Shifting perspectives: Holography and the emergence of technical communities.* https://core.ac.uk/download/1393573.pdf (accessed on 15th July 2025).
26. Jones, W. J., & Simpson, W. C. (2025). *NASA Contributions to Cardiovascular Monitoring.* https://core.ac.uk/download/pdf/85250592.pdf (accessed on 15th July 2025).
27. Kaushagen, H. N., & Skinner, K. L. (1966). *Passive instrumentation and stimuli generation for Saturn IB equipment checkout: Volume I – Summary technical report: Final technical report, 26 Jun. 1965 – 31 May 1966.* D5 -1 32 68 -1 https://core.ac.uk/download/pdf/85250846.pdf (accessed on 15th July 2025).
28. Kunwar, B. (2011). *Miniature Gas Chromatography Development, Testing and Applications.* https://core.ac.uk/download/480810567.pdf (accessed on 15th July 2025).
29. Marín, F., Gómez, F. C., & Meroño, P. A. (2014). *Measurement Techniques of Torsional Vibration in Rotating shafts.* https://core.ac.uk/download/645584586.pdf (accessed on 15th July 2025).
30. Mayewski, P. A. (2001). *Acquisition of Ion Chromatographs and Related Glaciochemistry Equipment.* https://core.ac.uk/download/217121316.pdf (accessed on 15th July 2025).
31. McPhee, J. R. (1988). *Electrical noise reduction techniques contributing to improved data quality at the National Transonic Facility.* https://core.ac.uk/download/pdf/42831043.pdf (accessed on 15th July 2025).

32. Merewether, E. K. (1966). *Computer program determines performance efficiency of remote measuring systems.* https://core.ac.uk/download/pdf/10255097.pdf (accessed on 15th July 2025).
33. NPeffer, T. (2010). *UC Berkeley's Cory Hall: Evaluation of challenges and potential applications of building-to-grid implementation.* https://core.ac.uk/download/288432727.pdf (accessed on 15th July 2025).
34. Regtien, P. P. L. (2007). *Metrology as part and parcel of training programs for science and engineering.* https://core.ac.uk/download/pdf/11467917.pdf (accessed on 15th July 2025).
35. Riek, L. D. (2017). *Healthcare Robotics.* http://arxiv.org/abs/1704.03931 (accessed on 15th July 2025).
36. Wear, J. O. & Shastri, N. K. (1974). *Chemistry Departments in Predominantly Black Institutions.* https://core.ac.uk/download/84121128.pdf (accessed on 15th July 2025).
37. Wendt, M. (2020). *RF Measurement Techniques.* http://arxiv.org/abs/2005.09106 (accessed on 15th July 2025).

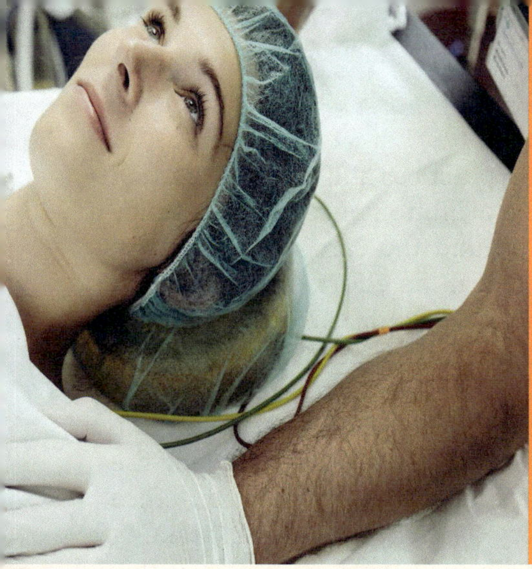

Chapter 3

PATIENT PREPARATION AND SEDATION

Contents

Introduction....65
3.1. Understanding Patient Preparation....68
3.2. Types of Sedation....72
3.3. Pre-Sedation Protocols....76
3.4. Monitoring During Sedation....78
3.5. Post-Sedation Care....82
3.6. Complications and Risks....85
Summary....89
References....92

Introduction

Patient sedation and preparation are key elements in the realm of modern medicine that have vital roles to play in determining the success of surgical procedures. Not only does the process guarantee the physical readiness of a patient, but it also guarantees that the emotional and psychological well-being of a patient is attended to. Good preparation can reduce anxiety levels, enhance cooperation, and finally lead to a successful procedure. Psychological factors typically play a major role, in view of accumulating evidence that preoperative anxiety can contribute negatively towards surgical recovery as well as patient satisfaction. The appropriate strategy for the preparation of patients is thus essential to attain a satisfactory healthcare experience, along with risk reduction in inappropriate procedures for sedation. Recent research has established the importance of correct sedation, especially in vulnerable individuals , such as the elderly. Interestingly, Lord et al. (2006) reveal disturbing patterns of benzodiazepine and opiate utilization in this population that have resulted in preventable morbidity and mortality. The information highlights re-prioritization of sedation practices and adherence to set standards calling for specific dosing according to patient profile. The evolution of sedation practice reflects greater knowledge regarding the complexity that exists around the care of the patient, and this would imply that the health profession needs to be attentive in its efforts to ensure that sedation is safe and effective. With regulation and formal instruction, health care professionals are better placed to deal with the subtleties of sedation. The preparation of the patient is more than the provision of sedation; it is an in-depth understanding of the unique patient anxiety and requirements. As seen in the review of literature in 1990–2002, Mitchell (2003) recognize the recurring issue with preoperative anxiety and a lack of official preoperative interventions for the same. Anxiety management strategies are therefore the core of preoperative preparation since they can significantly decrease patient distress and improve surgery outcomes. Universal training in anxiety management skills for healthcare practitioners would be well worthwhile since this would guarantee that both the physical and psychological demands of patient care are sufficiently addressed. Lastly, improved patient preparation habits and safe sedation habits provide a foundation for improved healthcare practice in operating theaters (Figure 3.1).

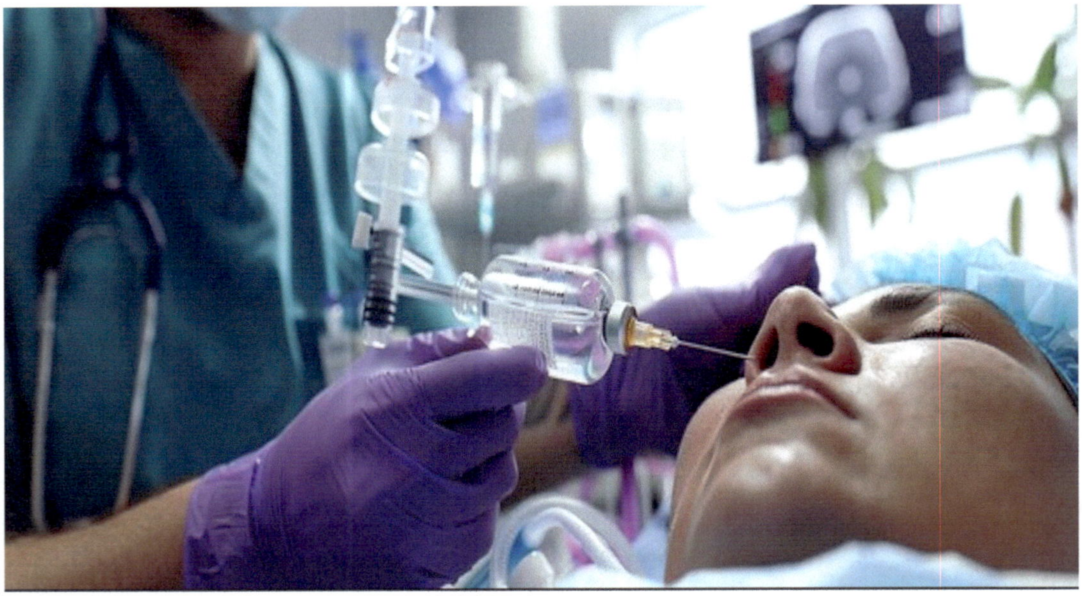

Figure 3.1. Anesthesia patient preparation.

Source: https://img.freepik.com/premium-photo/administering-anesthesia-patient-preparation-with-iv-line-setup_1168612-354606.jpg.

Definition of Patient Preparation

Patient preparation is an essential pillar in the healthcare environment, particularly where sedation will be required. Patient preparation is defined as a set of pre-procedure processes aimed at assuring and comforting the patient and maximizing the effectiveness of medical interventions. Some of these processes involve patient education, which involves educating individuals about the process, risks, and post-intervention care. This educational element not only decreases anxiety but also empowers patients, thereby encouraging cooperation among patients and healthcare providers. Effective patient preparation is closely linked to achieving optimal sedation results, as properly prepared patients have fewer complications and are more compliant with post-procedure care. Another essential function in patient preparation is the assessment of patients' medical history and current health status. Such evaluations include the discovery of underlying medical conditions, allergies, and medications that may influence the process of sedation. Through standardized assessment protocols, clinicians can reduce risk factors for sedation and enhance patient safety. Pre-procedure evaluation also assists in locating those patients who may require alternative methods, such as the integration of psychological interventions. As confirmed by recent research, hypnosis has proved to be a useful adjunct in procedural environments and has been shown to be effective in the control of acute pain and anxiety, especially for minor surgical procedures (Kendrick et al., 2016). As such, thorough patient assessment and preparation are essential in the process of tailoring sedation strategies to a specific patient's needs. Along with medical evaluation and education programs, preparation of the patient is also vital in creating a supportive environment. Creating a quiet and soothing atmosphere has a significant effect on patients attitudes towards the procedure that is to be done and towards the collaborative process as well. Methods , such as guided imagery, reassuring talks with the healthcare staff, and the utilization of collaborative sedation protocols can reduce pre-procedure anxiety. An empirical study highlights the importance of psychosocial interventions in supplementing the efficacy of pharmacologic agents in rapid tranquilization of agitated patients (Branford et al., 2008). By integrating these psychosocial variables into patient preparation, healthcare professionals can optimize the sedation process and make patients feel safe and certain about their interventions. Thus, the complex and multifaceted nature of patient preparation highlights its profound impact on the sedation process (Figure 3.2).

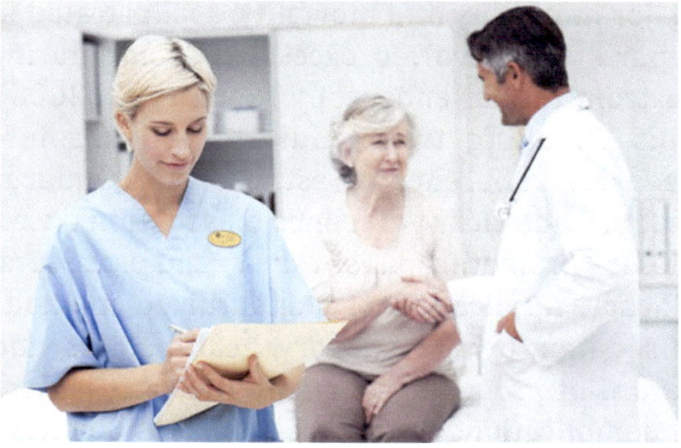

Figure 3.2. Patient preparation.

Source: https://winterhavendaysurgerycenter.com/wp-content/uploads/2016/12/welcome.jpg.

Importance of Sedation in Medical Procedures

Administration of sedation during the time of medical procedures helps to enhance patient comfort and alleviate anxiety. Patients are normally faced with a host of anxieties upon facing invasive procedures, from worries of pain to general experience within the hospital environment. Sedation not only minimizes pain physically but also helps to calm the patient psychologically, thereby enhancing cooperation throughout the procedure. It is particularly important in vulnerable groups, i.e., the elderly and children, who may become oversensitized to medical interventions. Studies demonstrate that children undergoing painful procedures most commonly rate them as the most distressing aspect of their illness and stress the importance of suitable sedation protocols to reduce their discomfort and anxiety (Liossi, 1999). Strategic use of sedation, therefore, becomes a key aspect of the patient-driven comprehensive medical care strategy. Moreover, the application of appropriate sedation techniques can significantly enhance procedural outcomes. In elderly patients, for example, inappropriate administration of sedation agents has previously led to side effects ranging from major morbidity and mortality, as illustrated in reports that involved excessive dosing during gastrointestinal endoscopy (Lord et al., 2006). This appalling trend indicates an absolute need for adherence to established standards that provide clear guidelines on sedation doses, thereby promoting patient safety and procedural efficacy. Application of standardized methods of sedation by age category, health status, and nature of procedure not only reduces the risk of complications but also establishes a culture of trust and safety, essential for successful patient outcomes. Therefore, a reflection with consideration of sedation's role is of paramount significance in conceptualizing interventions that cater to patient welfare.

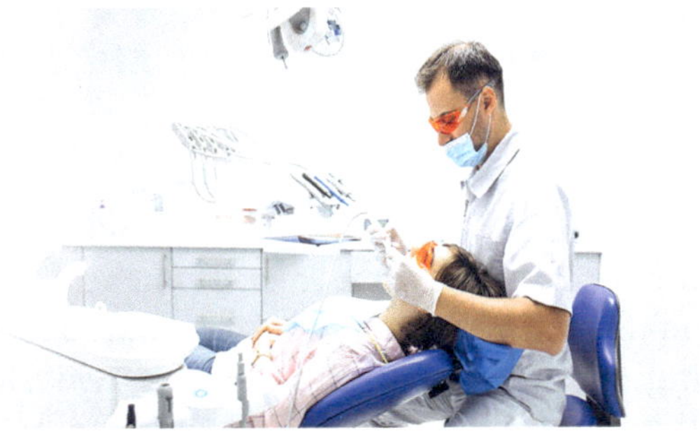

Figure 3.3. Enhancing patient comfort with sedation dentistry.

Source: https://adit.com/storage/files/enhancing-patient-comfort-with-sedation-dentistry.jpg.

Finally, regular training and continuing education for health care professionals in sedation methods must be sought to ensure safety and efficacy in practice. The medical procedure environment continues to evolve with evolving study findings and technological advancements, necessitating regular updates in sedation guidelines and approaches. With the inclusion of psychological interventions , such as cognitive-behavioral therapy and preparatory techniques, the sedative experience is further supported by creating a more holistic model of patient care (Liossi, 1999). By employing both pharmaceutical and psychological elements within treatment, medical teams can effectively address the multi-faceted aspects of painful procedures, thereby actually altering patient experiences. This sustained commitment to optimization of sedation practice is essential not only for short-term procedure success but also for long-term patient health and satisfaction in populations with wide demographics (Figure 3.3).

3.1. Understanding Patient Preparation

Effective clinical procedures, particularly those with sedation, significantly rely on effective patient preparation. It is the secret to obtaining cooperation from patients and healthcare professionals, ensuring that persons are well-educated and emotionally at ease before undergoing their treatment. Preparation is based on effective communication where healthcare professionals announce the intentions of the procedures and potential outcomes to lessen patient anxiety. In addition, understanding the background of the patients, such as their medical history and psychological makeup, enhances the individualization of pre-procedure instructions. For instance, patients with autism spectrum disorder (ASD) are likely to report challenging behaviors that complicate their healthcare process; hence, implementation of procedures tailored to these special needs is essential for effective interventions. Thus, patient preparation not only entails procedural preparedness but also the psychological as well as health environments that guarantee respect and responsiveness to patient needs (Johnson & Rodriguez, 2013). Ethical issues play a significant role in patient preparation, especially in child care with sedation. Most medical practitioners are faced with conundrums concerning decisions of priorities of sedative interventions, balancing priority with the ethical implications of such decisions. The case of restraining a child against his or her will for a procedure, while necessary at times for the processing of vital tasks, is an ethically questionable procedure. Parents and clinicians have reported feelings of moral distress about such conduct, highlighting the violation of the trusting relationship that ought to exist between caregivers and patients. Awareness of these ethical concerns is essential in producing more empathic models of care that prioritize pediatric patients' rights and well-being. Therefore, an ethos that values patient voice and respects their rights can conclusively enhance the process of preparation, making their best interests a priority in clinical decision-making (Bray et al., 2014).

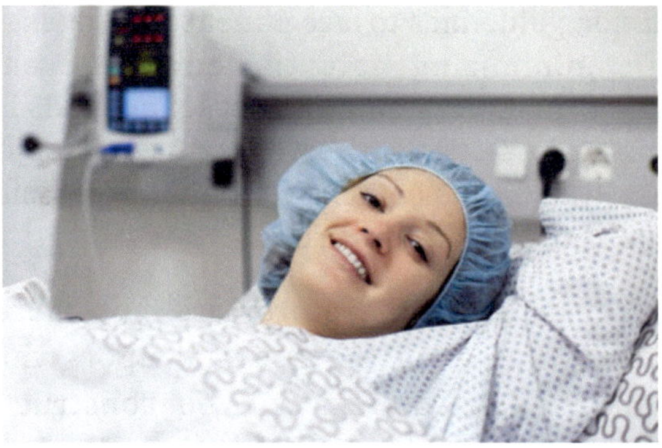

Figure 3.4. Understanding patient preparation.

Source: https://orchardsurgical.com/wp-content/uploads/2020/03/patient-preparation.jpg.

Moreover, the relationship between patient preparation and sedation not only impacts individual experiences but also has broader implications for the practice of healthcare. A systematic preparation strategy that incorporates interdisciplinary collaboration is worth it since it can allow for extensive assessments of the patients' needs. Family-centered practices with parents as active contributors to discussions and decision-making have the ability to enhance compliance with protocols and outcomes. This partnership model is particularly important in pediatrics, where children tend to be vulnerable and cannot fully comprehend the risks and implications of sedation and procedures. By embracing an inclusive practice that celebrates families and their knowledge, healthcare professionals can cope more effectively with the challenges surrounding patient preparation. In this context, it refers to the rise in the value of the necessity for ethical practice and individualized care when preparing patients for sedation, ultimately resulting in an improved and more humane health system (Figure 3.4).

3.1.1. The Role of Patient History in Preparation

Patient history assessment is an integral part of sedation preparation process since it offers individualized care that aligns with individual patient needs. Comprehensive patient history not only includes the medical history but also allergy, past reactions to anesthesia and any other medications, and psychological factors that can influence the sedation process. For instance, patients with a history of anxiety or claustrophobia can require special methods to overcome their state of anxiety during procedures. Having an understanding of these nuances allows medical professionals to devise an effective and safe sedation plan in terms of patient comfort and minimization of potential complications. Careful history taking is therefore a critical first step in the sedation process, resulting in good outcomes and instilling confidence in patients in medical procedures. Furthermore, patient history is not just in the form of short-term medical conditions but also lifestyle factors, medications, and comorbidities that may affect the success of sedation. Certain medications, particularly those with adverse interactions with anesthetic agents, have significant implications for procedures. An example would be patients on anticoagulants, who may develop complications if their history is not properly screened before being sedated. Similarly, chronic illnesses , such as cardiovascular or respiratory issues need to be met with an individualized technique of sedation so that professionals apply procedures that are both safe and effective for the patient. Thus, precise historical recording enhances readiness among medical teams, ultimately safeguarding against side effects and maximizing the success of the procedure.

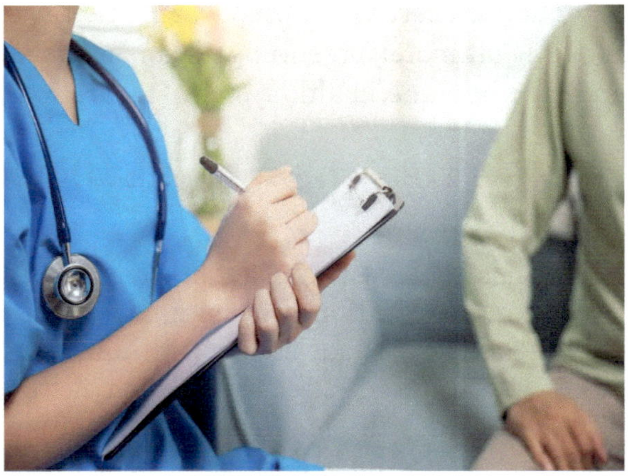

Figure 3.5. The importance of patient's medical history.

Source: https://simplenursing.com/wp-content/uploads/2023/08/iStock-1434595001-scaled.jpg.

With this background, it should be noted that taking patient history is not a fixed event and can vary with each patient presentation. Ongoing conversation about medical history, evolving conditions, and novel lifestyle concerns can offer useful information that determines preparation for sedation. For instance, patients may begin new medications or therapies that could affect their sensitivity to sedation; omitting to revise this history could be fatal. In addition, education and communication become a decisive aspect of such interaction. Educating patients about the value of providing a comprehensive history enables them to actively engage in their healthcare. By putting great emphasis on patients' correct medical history, healthcare providers can solidify trust and enhance collaborative decision-making, thus bringing about enhanced patient success in sedation scenarios (Figure 3.5).

3.1.2. Physical Assessments Before Sedation

Pre-sedation physical assessment has a central role in ensuring patient safety and success during various medical procedures. This assessment is a thorough examination of the patients' general health, enabling healthcare providers to identify any covert illness that could complicate sedation. Age, weight, allergies, comorbidities, and recent medications must be reviewed carefully. Gaining this information enables practitioners to tailor sedation guidelines to face patient heterogeneity while minimizing potential adverse events. Further, an understanding of baseline vitals like respiratory status and cardiovascular stability is essential in the context of predicting possible responses to sedative drugs.

These tests, therefore, are not merely routine; they form the pedestal upon which an individualized plan will be constructed that optimizes best practices in patient care and procedure success. In addition to the evaluation of overall physical health, ongoing communication with the patient during the pre-sedation assessment must occur. This conversation allows health care professionals to address patient concerns alongside educating them on the sedation process and its effects. Effective communication allows for the trust and cooperation of the patient in his or her care, which may enhance compliance and outcomes. Furthermore, discussion of the specific sedation plan, such as the depth of sedation, the time it is given, and side effects, can lessen anxiety significantly. Also effective is the incorporation of patient feedback into the sedation plan, promoting cooperation and bringing in a more patient-centered approach to care. The ultimate objective of this interactive process is to make patients feel safe and well-informed, thereby maximizing their readiness for sedation without giving rise to attendant risks. Evidence-based practices for sedation are continuous, incorporating learning from quality improvement programs that are aimed at optimizing patient evaluations. For instance, studies have shown that the implementation of standardized testing protocols enhances streamlining the process as well as maintaining consistency in evaluating patients across settings. Quality improvement initiatives emphasize the need for evidence-based management practices to guarantee the adoption of practices , such as the ABCDE bundle in critical care units (Hamilton, 2015). These bundles are designed to enhance patient outcomes, including efficient control of pain and minimization of risks during sedation (Beard et al., 2019). Embracing this evidence-based approach, healthcare providers can significantly amplify the precision and effectiveness of physical examination before sedation, which ultimately contributes to enhanced patient safety and satisfaction during medical care (Figure 3.6).

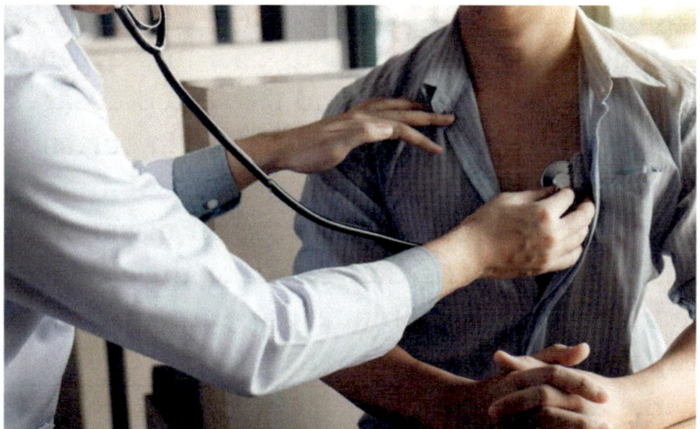

Figure 3.6. Physical exam.

Source: https://cdn-prod.medicalnewstoday.com/content/images/articles/325/325488/doctor-performs-physical-examination-on-patient-with-stethoscope.jpg.

3.1.3. Psychological Considerations for Patients

Understanding the psychological issues in patient care is imperative during sedation preparation. Medical procedures, including sedation, are normally identified by patients with fear and anxiety, which in turn enhances their distress. Psychological preparation of patients entails describing procedures, sensations to be anticipated, as well as outcomes expected in depth. Educating patients on procedures undertaken in their care de mystifies the process and can contribute immensely to reducing anxiety levels. Further, the implementation of relaxation skills and cognitive behavior techniques, such as guided imagery or mindfulness, may help in patient expectation management and emotional responses. Management of these psychological factors not only makes for a less stressful experience but also for a more cooperative and trusting encounter between patient and practitioner, ultimately leading to safer procedural outcomes. The significance of pain during procedures cannot be denied, particularly in sedation cases among pediatric patients. Children who experience painful procedures often describe these experiences as the worst part of their illness, indicating that there is an overwhelming demand for comprehensive emotional support during them. Effective management of procedure-related pain involves integrating pharmacological treatment with psychological interventions. Techniques , such as preparation and cognitive-behavioral therapy have proven to be helpful in helping children manage the distress of painful procedures. By incorporating these psychological considerations into patient care, healthcare providers can enhance overall satisfaction for sedated pediatric patients. Emphasis on a comfortable and calming presence is significant since it can actually influence the child's perception of pain and future coping processes, demonstrating the interconnectedness of psychological and physical health in medical settings (Liossi, 1999). Sleep disturbance has a major impact on the recovery of patients in critical care environments, influencing their psychological well-being and overall health outcomes. Recent research has suggested that poor sleep quality in critically ill patients tends to be associated with greater irritability, stress levels, and longer recovery times. Healthcare workers attempt to monitor and enhance patients' sleep quality, but standard assessment methods have been found to be ineffective. Instead, with the simple, patient-focused tools of assessment, patients' sleep experience perceptions can be better measured, as shown in recent research. With these results incorporated into practice, carers can develop strategies that minimize interruptions and encourage soothing surroundings. Lastly, an examination of the nuanced interaction between psychological elements and the quality of sleep forms the groundwork for more effective sedation practice, enabling optimal recovery and improved positive patient outcomes for critical care cases (Coghill et al., 2007) (Figure 3.7).

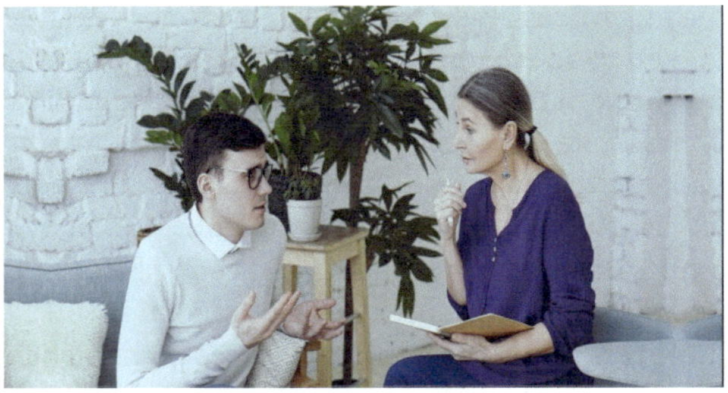

Figure 3.7. Providing psychological support.

Source: https://amandeephospital.org/wp-content/uploads/2022/09/Emotional-Support-for-Patients-min.jpeg.

3.2. Types of Sedation

Sedation is an extremely crucial patient preparation and procedure control component, particularly in the management of anxiety and discomfort during health procedures. Sedation can be conveniently categorized as mild, moderate, and deep sedation, each having a particular objective based on the procedure requirements and the patient's condition. Mild sedation, referred to in everyday language as anxiolysis, increases comfort with the patient remaining awake and cooperative. This category is most commonly used with less invasive procedures, enabling practitioners to function successfully while keeping the patient's cognitive. Alternatively, moderate sedation renders patients somewhat less aware of their surroundings, yet still responsive to verbal command. This level can be employed for more invasive diagnostic or treatment procedures, discovering a happy medium between comfort and responsiveness, which serves both patient comfort and procedure success. Deep sedation is the most profound alteration of consciousness, with patients being least responsive to the outside world, and this requires monitoring to control potential airway and cardiovascular complications.

Deep sedation is primarily used in invasive and complicated procedures or painful interventions and requires complex planning and preparation, such as patient health status, allergies, and history of previous sedation. Clinicians need to take into account pharmacologic profiles and suggested dosages to prevent complications, placing importance on careful pre-procedure assessments. Of particular interest, administration of sedation has inherent risks that reiterate the value of individualized techniques so that providers can achieve effective patient management while also assuring safety. This is a view that necessitates ongoing attention in monitoring patients undergoing deep sedation to achieve favorable outcomes and prevent adverse effects. In pediatric patients, particularly in oncology patients, procedural pain relief is prioritized and can often overlap with complex sedation methods. Children subjected to many painful procedures may benefit not just from sedation to alleviate pain but also from treating the psychological impacts of these procedures. Hypnosis has been discovered to have a significant impact on reducing procedural pain as an adjunct approach to support pharmacological sedation interventions. Although evidence demonstrates that hypnosis is highly effective, particularly in minor surgical environments, it also points to , including both psychological as well as behavioral therapies to optimize pain control (Liossi, 1999; Kendrick et al., 2016). This multi-faceted strategy not only enhances the patient's overall experience but also guides clinicians to formulate well-balanced care plans tailored to individual patients, particularly in pediatric patients, where procedural anxiety is prevalent (Figure 3.8).

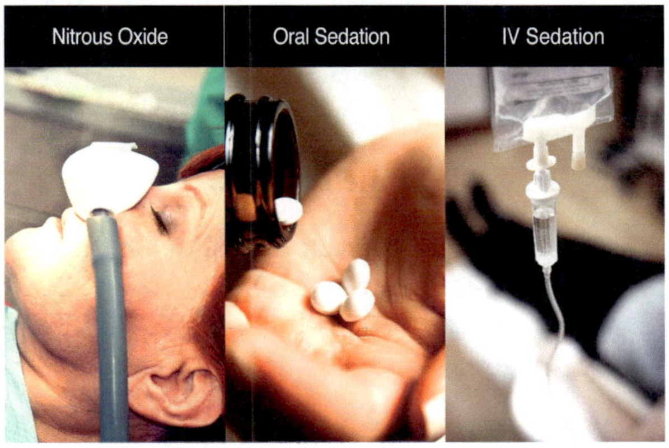

Figure 3.8. Types of sedation.

Source: https://d3b3by4navws1f.cloudfront.net/sedation4.jpg.

3.2.1. Minimal Sedation and Its Applications

Minimal sedation plays a central role in patient care by ensuring patients are comfortable and anxiety-free during certain medical procedures. This form of sedation, where patients can stay awake but respond less to stimuli, is commonly practiced in outpatient settings and diagnostic testing. The most significant aim of minimal sedation is to find a point at which the patient is comfortable, allowing for greater comfort in procedures and potentially quicker recovery. Also, minimal sedation reduces the need for general anesthesia, thereby making it relevant in cost-effective care and efficient patient management. A central aspect of the effective use of minimal sedation is thorough patient preparation and assessment to ensure safety and maximal benefit. Part of this preparation is for the healthcare providers to evaluate the patients' medical background, present condition, and potential airway management risk factors. Proper airway assessment and management techniques are crucial to prevent complications that arise during sedation, particularly for patients with challenging airway anatomical features.

Enhanced training and education of airway assessment, as discussed in a recent article, emphasize the importance of respecting the complexity included in patient readiness as much as the sedation process itself (Euliano et al., 2003). Through the focus on these factors, providers can ensure that minimal sedation is safely and successfully applied. The applications of minimal sedation extend beyond the procedural settings, affecting other specialties , such as dentistry and dermatology. For instance, in cosmetic treatments, minimal sedation allows patients to be treated with less pain and maintain as responsiveness. This is especially true for procedures that need to be executed accurately and require patient compliance, e.g., those involving injectables or stitches. Additionally, low-level sedation can improve the quality of care through improved communication between the physician and the patient during the treatment process. As evidenced by recent clinical studies, minimal sedation not only serves its purpose of utility in procedures but also in improving patient satisfaction and overall treatment experience (Carella et al., 2016). Thus, healthcare clinicians should consider minimal sedation as an alternative in many clinical scenarios, thus enhancing patient-centered care (Figure 3.9).

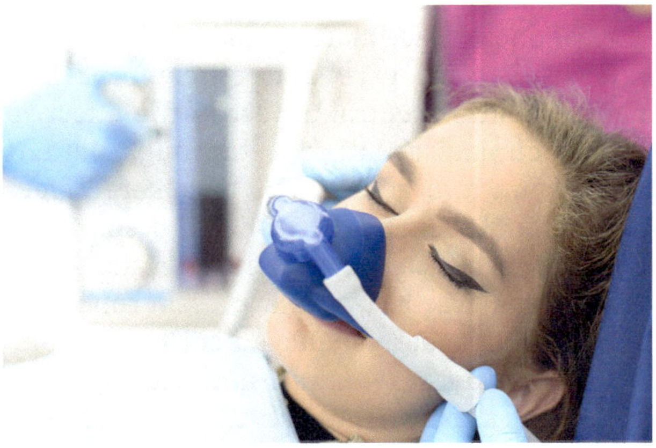

Figure 3.9. Minimal sedation.

Source: https://aegisdentalcentre.com/wp-content/uploads/2023/05/sedation-1024x684.jpg.

3.2.2. Moderate Sedation and Its Benefits

Moderate sedation is an integral aspect of patient preparation for contemporary medical interventions. The degree of sedation provides a state that makes patients conscious but relaxed and less responsive to their immediate surroundings, alleviating anxiety and discomfort during procedures. Several patients experience preoperative anxiety, which may have a substantial impact on their experience and recovery (Mitchell, 2003). By means of moderate sedation, healthcare providers are able to comfortably manage such psychological components, creating the doorway for a smoother procedural process. Not only does this heightened comfort contribute to satisfactory patient satisfaction, but it can also be found to lead to improved clinical results due to diminished stress responses. In addition to psychological benefits, moderate sedation also prioritizes the provision of safety and efficiency with medical interventions. Experiments confirm that employing agents , such as propofol and etomidate can achieve optimal levels of sedation with patients' vital signs kept stable throughout the procedure (Meng et al., 2016). This is particularly crucial in the case of older patients or those with comorbidities who are most likely to be susceptible to negative outcomes. By employing correct drug regimens, medical practitioners can minimize risks involved in sedation, including respiratory depression or prolonged recovery.

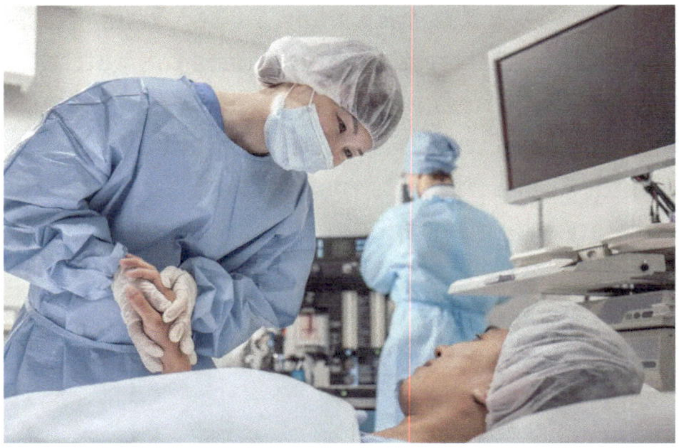

Figure 3.10. Moderate sedation.

Source: https://ysm-res.cloudinary.com/image/upload/c_limit,f_auto,h_630,q_auto,w_1200/v1/yms/prod/e9c456e7-1f49-4d6f-a3d3-18fd92932e6e.

Thus, moderation in the practice of moderate sedation is essential to create a balance between provision for patient comfort and safety. Furthermore, integration of moderate sedation increases patient comfort during the experience and streamlines procedural workflow efficiency. Reduced anxiety typically corresponds with shorter recovery periods, leading to faster discharges and more efficient use of healthcare resources (Mitchell, 2003). Patients receiving procedures with moderate sedation often experience higher satisfaction rates, which is paramount in the value-based care era. Clinically, this satisfaction is seen as improved adherence to post-procedure instructions and fewer complications, hence lower overall healthcare system burden. Hence, moderate sedation stands as a critical patient preparation and sedation approach with a wide range of benefits impacting from the patient level to healthcare as a whole (Figure 3.10).

3.2.3. Deep Sedation and Its Risks

Optimal patient preparation for deep sedation is crucial in minimizing procedural hazards and enhancing patient safety. Deep sedation entails a controlled state of unconsciousness with patients being unresponsive but spontaneously breathing. Although this approach is useful to control pain and anxiety during invasive interventions, it poses an array of risks that need to be thoughtfully weighed. Risks , such as respiratory depression, cardiovascular instability, and lengthened sedation can occur, requiring an advanced level of understanding about the drugs employed and the patient's baseline state of health.

Monitoring of vital signs and maintenance of a clear airway are absolutely essential components of patient care during deep sedation, as even minor deviation can result in disastrous consequences. Thus, stringent pre-procedure assessment and patient-specific sedation protocols are vital elements in preventing the risks involved in deep sedation. In addition to patient factors, the procedural environment plays a crucial role in deciding what risks accompany deep sedation. The intricacy of the process, duration, and use of adjunct drugs can all cause side effects. For instance, for patients who are undergoing painful procedures that are involved in cancer therapy, deep sedation may enable analgesia required, but can inhibit a child's autonomic feedback to unpleasant stimuli, thereby complicating their care. There is research to indicate that the use of adequate pain management strategies, both pharmacological and psychological, can improve patient outcomes for deep sedation. Preoperative counseling and the application of cognitive-behavioral therapies have been discovered to enhance a child's coping strategies, thereby diminishing the psychological disturbance commonly associated with sedation and procedure pain in pediatric cancer patients (Liossi, 1999). Furthermore, discussion of quality measures related to endoscopic procedures highlights the critical nexus between sedation practices and patient outcomes. Studies contrasting variations in the performance of colonoscopy, that is, in organized colorectal cancer screening programs, have established that the regular use of sedation impacts adenoma detection rate (ADR) as well as overall success of the procedure.

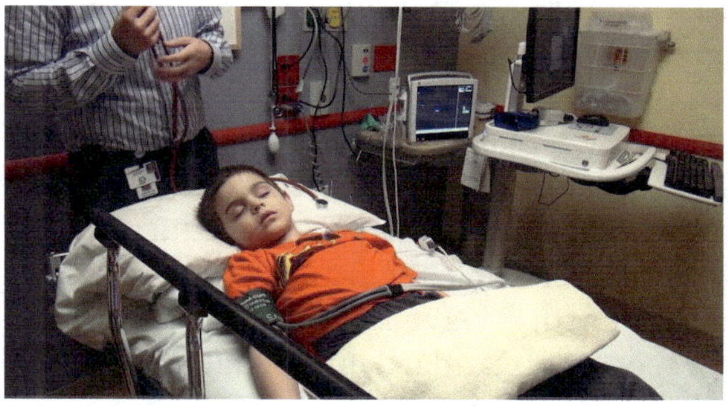

Figure 3.11. Pediatric deep sedation.

Source: https://i.ytimg.com/vi/74GocsLGMvo/maxresdefault.jpg.

Higher levels of sedation correspond to lower ADR, and that means that while sedation may more likely ensure patient comfort, it may inadvertently compromise procedural efficiency (Barca et al., 2014). That necessitates that the professionals balance the need for deep sedation against the issues of complications, being cautious that practices of sedation would not compromise the quality of diagnostic tests. Lastly, knowledge of these dynamics is necessary to optimize patient preparation, optimize procedural safety, and minimize the risks of deep sedation (Figure 3.11).

3.3. Pre-Sedation Protocols

Effective pre-sedation protocols are essential in preparing the safety and psychological readiness of patients for procedures under sedation. There should be an accurate assessment of the patient's medical history, especially past reactions to anesthetic agents or sedation. This will help determine the potential risks associated with sedation, which can vary significantly among individuals, especially in the vulnerable population , such as children or persons with underlying conditions. Furthermore, comprehensive knowledge of the proffered procedures allows medical practitioners to personalize their sedative approach, incorporating pharmacologic methods and psychological comfort measures. The combination of care is critical for anxiety relief, as it can enhance pain perception and overall distress involved in medical procedures (Liossi, 1999). Other than medical history surveying, implementing psychological interventions represents a standard pre-sedation protocol. Techniques , such as cognitive-behavioral therapy or hypnosis have gained popularity in reducing anxiety levels and enhancing patient compliance during medical procedures. Clinical evidence supports hypnosis's efficacy, having been shown to decrease acute procedural pain significantly and enhance overall outcomes when applied within pre-sedation regimens. Specifically, hypnosis has been found to be of great utility in minor surgical procedures, where patients are more apt to exhibit increased anxiety related to pain (Kendrick et al., 2016). Training of medical staff on the application of such techniques alongside traditional sedation methodologies can create a comprehensive approach to patient treatment, satisfying both physical and psychological requirements within one unified process. Last but not least, patient education is essential to the success of pre-sedation protocols. Providing clear, concise information regarding the sedation process, potential results, and recovery will help to demystify the experience for patients, allowing them to feel empowered and confident in the medical team. Well-informed patients are more likely to express their concerns and desires, allowing for more tailored care. Part of a successful pre-sedation strategy is that informed consent not only be ethically obtained but also understood by the patient. This discussion is not only limited to the procedural routine but also encompasses the anticipated effect of sedation and associated risks (Liossi, 1999). At some point, an integrated pre-sedation protocol that involves assessment, psychological intervention, and education fares well in promoting patient outcomes and satisfaction with medical procedures.

3.3.1. Fasting Guidelines Before Sedation

Pre-sedation fasting guidelines are critical components of patient preparation with an immediate bearing on the safety and efficacy of anesthesia. They are designed to minimize the risk of aspiration and consequent complications during sedation procedures. Patients have previously been requested to avoid solid food for at least six hours before sedation, while clear fluids are generally permitted up to two hours prior. These restrictions not only lower the risk of regurgitation but also ensure clear airways during intubation, if intubation is required. Compliance with such fasting guidelines can significantly reduce the occurrence of procedure-related complications, resulting in a smoother anesthetic experience for both patients and clinicians. Strong clinical evidence supporting their use highlights the importance of how they are woven into patient safety. Studies demonstrate that adherence to prescribed fasting periods is positively correlated with reduced rates of postoperative nausea and vomiting and shorter recovery times following sedation. For example, even though intravenous sedation has been employed effectively for a variety of outpatient procedures, including carpal tunnel releases, compliance with appropriate fasting guidelines plays a key role in minimizing the duration of postanesthesia care unit stays. While no significant differences in total operative time between techniques of sedation existed, the better perioperative outcomes that ensue from adequate fasting highlight the importance of such recommendations to overall patient comfort and safety under procedure under sedation (Youha et al., 2018). Also, there cannot be an overestimation of the importance of individualized fasting recommendations because patient-specific factors , such as age, medical status, and type of anesthetic method may influence fasting requirements. Particularly, vulnerable populations, such as the elderly, can be assisted using adjusted fasting protocols that take into account their physiological changes and risk, as confirmed in anesthetic regimens studies. For instance, it has been established that a combination of sedative agents , such as propofol and etomidate, is amenable to hemodynamic stability, but the effectiveness of the regimens is subject to proper patient preparation, for instance, compliance with fasting instructions. The use of individualized testing along with evidence-based fasting regimens will enhance safety and efficacy under sedation, ultimately developing an environment where patients would feel safe and cared for (Meng et al., 2016).

3.3.2. Medication Review and Adjustments

Patient preparation and sedation are mostly dependent on comprehensive reviews and modifications of medications before any procedure. This procedure includes evaluating a patient's existing medications, such as over-the-counter medications, supplements, and any past treatments that may interact negatively with anesthetic agents. By thoroughly examining this drug profile, clinicians can recognize potential contraindications and fine-tune the pharmacological strategy for sedation. For example, some drugs may enhance the effects of sedation or lead to cardiovascular instability. In this context, medication reviews are a crucial part of informing sedation protocols to enhance patient comfort and safety, ultimately leading to smoother procedural outcomes. Moreover, medication changes are often important factors in prepping patients for sedation. These include adjusting dosages or even the timing of administering medications based on individual patients' needs, patients' own medical conditions, or the specific needs of an individual surgical procedure. At this level, pharmacotherapy ability is paramount. Take patient management with chronic pain syndromes, for example: Practitioners must ensure that acute pain management is compatible with their ongoing treatment regimens so as not to detract from sedation results. Incorporating evidence-based practices in medication adjustment, practitioners can actually improve the effectiveness of sedation and mitigate possible harmful side effects of polypharmacy, outlining a profound appreciation for the pharmacological climate with regard to patient preparation. Second, individualized medication review and adjustment are in keeping with the most current models of education in healthcare. Through illustration in the form of educational programs to enhance students' clinical reasoning, a structured process of reviewing patient medications allows for enhanced learning and competency. Outcomes of such education demonstrate that students who engage in rigorous case analysis develop more effective skills in pain and symptom control, crucial in sedation settings. This pedagogical approach corroborates the significance of evidence-based clinical practice, preparing healthcare professionals adequately to handle the complexities of medication regimens among patients in practice settings. Secondly, optimal drug selection before procedure enhances patient safety but also guarantees therapeutic responses post-sedation, hence furthering ongoing clinical excellence within the healthcare system (Juba et al., 2014; Pandurangi et al., 2017) (Figure 3.12).

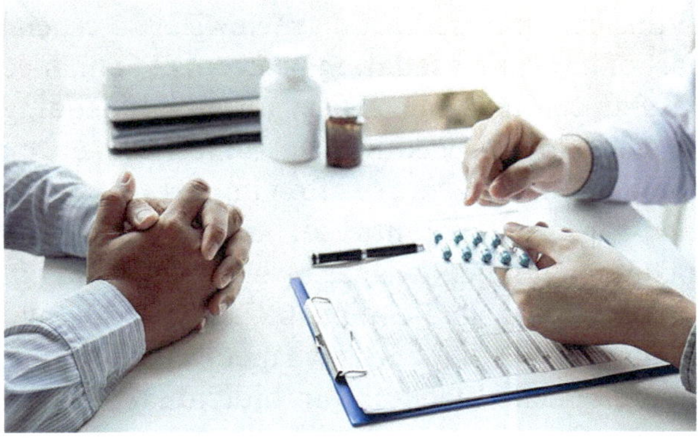

Figure 3.12. Conducting a medication review.

Source: https://ausmed-images.s3-ap-southeast-2.amazonaws.com/ausmed.com/ausmed-articles/20200915_body_3.jpg.

3.3.3. Informed Consent Process

The informed consent process is one of the central aspects of patient preparation, particularly with regard to sedation treatments. This process informs patients about the benefits, risks, and alternatives of their treatment. Informed consent is not just having a signature in writing; it brings healthcare professionals into serious conversation with patients, allowing them to ask questions and raise concerns. This is important, as it facilitates trust and informs patients to make decisions about their care. The complexities of sedation bring about the necessity for substantive informed consent, as patients are typically anxious and less resilient. Hence, a complete understanding of the informed consent process not only optimizes patient autonomy but also goes a long way in helping ensure patient safety as a whole when receiving sedation. Moreover, legal as well as moral implications of informed consent have evolved in tandem with advances in medical procedures. Medical practitioners are tasked with working within these sophisticated systems and maintaining information flow with patients. For instance, standards for informed consent of outpatient procedures, such as sedation procedures, typically demand evidence-based guidelines. A comparison of standards across various medical specialties reveals that, unlike highly politicized areas , such as abortion, outpatient procedures typically conform to set professional protocols designed by specialty groups (Berglas & Roberts, 2018). These systematic approaches promote consistency in informed consent practices, thereby guaranteeing that patients are informed to promote their well-being and safety. Further, research into the process of informed consent indicates its relevance to patient outcomes in sedation cases. The success of tracking pain following sedation, as done through studies that employ new pain measurement tools, supports the contribution of informed consent towards the safeguard of patient interests (Copot et al., 2020). Aspects , such as an appreciation of potential pain grade, sedation side effects, and postoperative care responsibility are crucial aspects to be addressed during the process of obtaining consent. Developing a robust informed consent process not only safeguards patient autonomy, but it also makes medical interventions meaningful to patient values and preferences. Generally speaking, the informed consent process is a cornerstone of sedation preparation of patients, enhancing both the ethical practice of medicine and patient care quality.

3.4. Monitoring During Sedation

Monitoring sedation represents a crucial element of patient safety and procedural success. By monitoring physiological parameters closely, healthcare providers can recognize any adverse reactions or deviations from the expected levels of sedation in a timely fashion. This continuous monitoring is particularly important in vulnerable populations, such as the elderly, who can react unpredictably to sedative medications. There are recent publications reporting alarming trends in the overuse of benzodiazepines and opiates in GI endoscopy in elderly patients and ensuing unnecessary complications. Guidelines requesting appropriate dosing of sedation are intended to outweigh these hazards and promote overall patient care, referencing the aggressive importance of monitoring in sedation practice (Lord et al., 2006). To better reach optimal levels of sedation, practitioners must possess both the data and technology required for adequate monitoring during treatment. In pediatrics, the complexity of monitoring in sedation is even higher. Procedures are a common source of distress among children undergoing them, and they associate with high levels of pain and discomfort. As indicated, cancer procedures often involve repeated painful interventions that interfere with the onset and resolution of distress if not properly managed. Physical safety and psychological well-being during the procedure require age-appropriate monitoring techniques to be utilized. Pediatric sedation demands greater vigilance for physiological indicators and the potential need for tailored pharmacologic interventions to adequately mitigate pain related to procedures (Liossi, 1999). It demands a multidisciplinary intervention incorporating both pharmacologic and psychological approaches to assessment and management of pain, with special emphasis placed on close observation during sedation procedures. Also, the use of technology in sedation monitoring protocols can be used to enhance patient safety and procedural efficiencies. More advanced monitoring equipment has the capacity to monitor heart rate, oxygen saturation, and respiratory rates in real time, allowing rapid intervention should any anomalies be found. Such equipment can be useful where procedures are of a high risk and patient response to sedation may vary significantly. With advancing healthcare, the demand for strong monitoring guidelines, with support from sophisticated technologies, will enable better patient outcomes and minimize occurrences of sedation-related complications. Training healthcare practitioners to effectively interpret data from such monitoring systems is essential so that they can act fast and efficiently in response to sedation (Liossi, 1999; Lord et al., 2006). Hence, the commitment to improved monitoring habits is crucial to the future of patient-directed sedation guidelines (Figure 3.13).

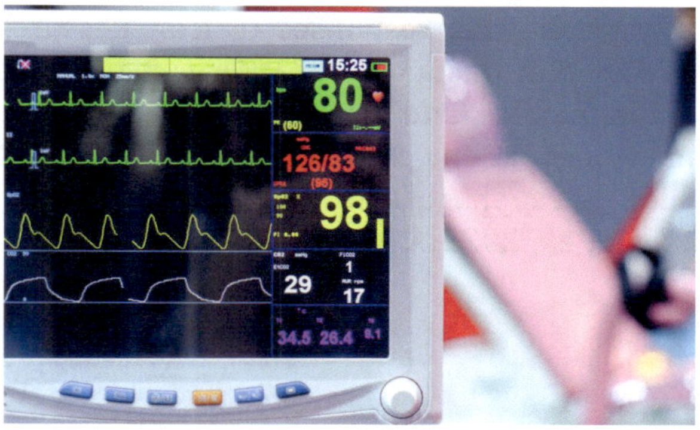

Figure 3.13. Monitoring during anesthesia.

Source: https://radiusga.com/wp-content/uploads/2022/11/endtidalCO2anesthesia.jpeg.

3.4.1. Vital Signs and Their Significance

In the preparation of patients and sedation, the monitoring of vital signs is a core aspect of safety and efficacy in medical procedures. Vital signs like heart rate, blood pressure, respiratory rate, and body temperature are the markers of a patient's body physiological condition and help healthcare professionals detect any deviation from the normal. This active monitoring is particularly important during sedation, when the likelihood of cardiovascular instability and respiratory depression is presumably higher. Systematic assessment of these parameters allows healthcare teams to make logical decisions about the depth of sedation and to intervene immediately if there is any sign of distress or instability in the vital signs, thus eliminating the risk of adverse events. Along with the immediate physiological monitoring, the significance of vital signs extends beyond the immediate; they can also provide valuable information on a patients psychological status. Patients tend to go into procedures with an element of anxiety, which tends to alter their vital signs greatly, particularly heart rate and blood pressure. Awareness of this psychological effect allows doctors to tailor their sedation techniques to each patient. For example, sedation not only aims for the alleviation of bodily pain but also for psychological responses to fear. Research clarifies that adequate sedation can preserve hemodynamics and decrease anxiety levels, improving patient experiences in procedures , such as esophagogastroduodenoscopy (EGD) (Izaki et al., 2022).

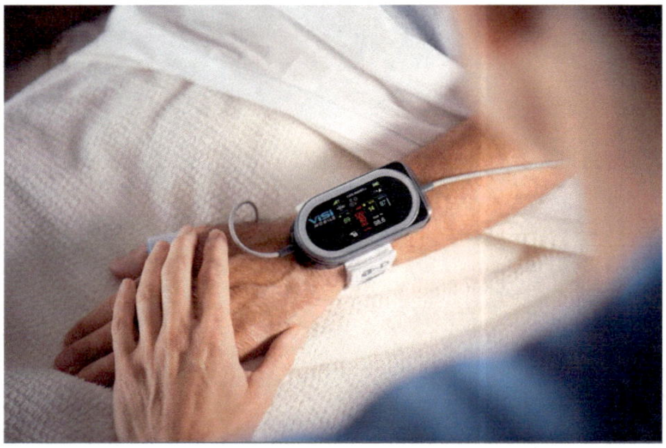

Figure 3.14. Continuous vital signs monitoring.

Source: https://soteradigitalhealth.com/hs-fs/hubfs/Sotera%20Digital%20Health%20-%20Continuous%20Vital%20Signs%20Monitoring%20%7C%20Effectiveness%20of%20CVM%20on%20General%20Wards.png?width=992&height=656&name=Sotera%20Digital%20Health%20-%20Continuous%20Vital%20Signs%20Monitoring%20%7C%20Effectiveness%20of%20CVM%20on%20General%20Wards.png.

Monitoring vital signs thus becomes critical not only for procedure safety but for providing comprehensive patient management. Also, present guidelines emphasize strongly the vigilant observation of vital signs with reference to sedation guidelines, particularly within psychiatric settings where immediate tranquillization may become a priority. The NICE guideline for managing violent or aggressive behavior states that an organised system for monitoring vital signs can significantly enhance patient safety when sedatives are being given (Branford et al., 2008). The absence of an accepted, universal regimen of medications for rapid tranquillization underscores the importance for clinicians to prioritize assessment of vital signs when determining the appropriateness of offered sedation options. By establishing a solid platform that integrates vital signs into sedation planning, healthcare professionals can encourage safer, more efficient treatment plans, ultimately resulting in enhanced patient outcomes in numerous clinical contexts (Figure 3.14).

3.4.2. Use of Monitoring Equipment

Monitoring device utilization in patient preparation and sedation is an essential component in the provision of safe and good-quality care. Continuous monitoring modalities, such as electrocardiography (ECG), pulse oximetry, and capnography, allow clinicians to detect physiological changes in real time. For instance, ECG can help identify arrhythmias that may occur during sedation, and pulse oximetry can readily show any changes in oxygen saturation levels. Such real-time monitoring, apart from bringing to the clinician's notice the patient's immediate response to sedation, also enables intervention in a timely fashion in the event of any complications developing. The inclusion of sophisticated monitoring techniques is a reflection of improved patient outcomes with procedural sedation, including the central role of monitoring in contemporary medical practice. The challenges posed by patients with special needs, particularly in pediatric patients, also underscore the value of customized monitoring strategies. Pediatric patients with procedures are at greater risk for anxiety and distress related to the invasive nature of medical interventions. In pediatric malignancy, for instance, fear of painful procedures may significantly enhance the procedural process, compromising compliance and overall outcome. Thus, through the employment of effective monitoring equipment, not only will the physiological integrity of these frail children be protected, but, perhaps more importantly, a feeling of security imparted. Better monitoring approaches may be integrated with psychological treatments to prepare children for procedures and, in the long run, reduce their pre-procedure anxiety and improve their overall experience in healthcare settings, as proposed in procedure-related pain management research (Liossi, 1999).

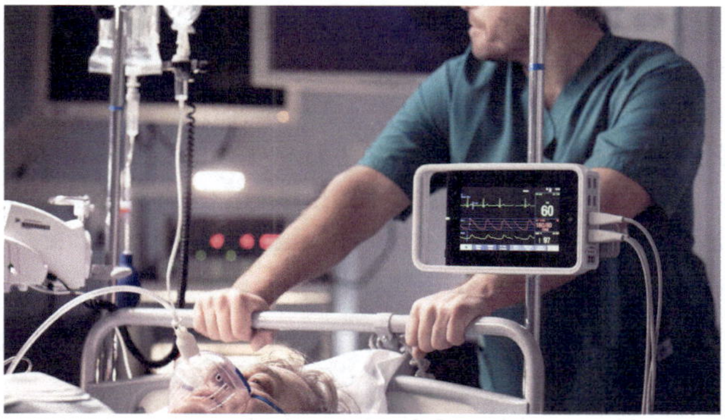

Figure 3.15. Patient monitoring.

Source: https://www.gehealthcare.com/-/jssmedia/be144729bab44bd7afa65f18b093ac5b.jpg?h=1080&la=en-US&w=1920&rev=661cd591032849cda2004b9f6bcc56d4&hash=9B8B25FE37B04DA2B0B2EDF7705BE30E.

Additionally, there are specific difficulties in monitoring the use of equipment when patients have developmental disorders, such as ASD. The behaviors of the child with ASD—, such as defensiveness and non-compliance to sensory input—can make monitoring vital signs when a child is sedated challenging. Special monitoring devices can eliminate some of these challenges by giving more precise measurements while accommodating the special needs of such children. Collaborating with the parents to understand the triggers and wants of the child is essential in a way that the environment is well adapted for effective monitoring. This comprehensive strategy not only delineates the significance of monitoring in the protection of vulnerable groups but also emphasizes the need for a compassionate healthcare plan that is patient-focused, centered on comfort and safety (Johnson & Rodriguez, 2013) (Figure 3.15).

3.4.3. Role of Healthcare Professionals in Monitoring

In patient preparation and sedation, the role of the healthcare professionals in monitoring is integral to patient safety and optimal outcomes. An effective monitoring strategy includes close observation of vital signs, including heart rate, blood pressure, and oxygen saturation, which provide the basis for observing any drift away from baseline status. This is particularly crucial in pediatric populations, where anatomical and physiological heterogeneity make the process of sedation challenging. Clinicians must receive training to identify respiratory distress and hemodynamic instability, which, if not treated, can lead to serious complications. Therefore, their function is not ancillary but critical in the pre- and post-sedation monitoring processes to permit timely intervention in the event of issues, thereby enhancing recovery outcomes and patient safety. Also, integration of multidisciplinary teams spotlights the complexity of monitoring sedation. Professionals like anesthesiologists, pediatricians, and nurses collaborate to create an atmosphere that guarantees patient safety through combined expertise and efficient communication. The necessity of round-the-clock monitoring, especially in complicated cases , such as handling difficult airways, cannot be overstressed, as noted by Czajka et al. (2024). This reference highlights the sophisticated steps to minimize the hazards presented by sedation, including advanced monitoring technology and protocols. Cooperation not only advances the direct safety of patients receiving sedation but also permits longitudinal observation with the ability to predict future health consequences, provide input for further progress in practices of patient care. Educating health workers in the principles of good monitoring further sets the foundation of secure sedation practices. Continual learning and training on new best practices, technology integration, and the ethical concerns in sedation are essential for achieving high-quality care. Case studies of healthcare organizations illustrate successful innovations that can be replicated to enhance patient safety in sedation, as discussed by McCarthy & Blumenthal (2006). By analyzing the actions implemented and results achieved in these instances, medical professionals can utilize evidence-based practice that improves monitoring protocols and patient interaction. This commitment to continuing education and adjustment is essential because it enables the professional not only to react to clinical problems effectively but also to anticipate potential complications, thereby developing an ethos of active care within the sedation process.

3.5. Post-Sedation Care

Post-sedation care is a critical phase in the continuum of patient care that ensures patients' safety and comfort upon regaining full consciousness from a state of sedation. Under this phase, patient care attendants must be observant while observing vital signs , such as heart rate, blood pressure, and respiratory status to identify any developing complications , such as hypoxia or hypotension. Efficacy of sedation is very sensitive to dosage and the agent being used, so recovery parameters must be carefully monitored. In addition, proper recovery can avert the development of postoperative complications like pain or anxiety, which have also been reported to disproportionately affect vulnerable groups, e.g., pediatric patients, for invasive interventions. Specific post-sedation assessments are particularly relevant in these populations, as shown by studies reporting that children recognize painful procedures as the most challenging aspect of hospitalization (Liossi, 1999). Pharmacological interventions may also be applied to post-sedation care in an attempt to mitigate discomfort or anxiety experienced by patients. The use of analgesics, for instance, has been revealed to reduce postoperative pain as well as improve recovery results. In the area of post-sedation care, psychological and pharmacological interventions are central to addressing potential distress. An example is the use of local anesthetics in procedural interventions, which has been seen to have a positive effect on postoperative pain perceptions, although results are found to vary with patient uniqueness (Kass et al., 2014). Besides, the inclusion of psychological care, including reassurance and emotional counseling, can ensure increased compliance by patients and lower levels of anxiety, making recovery less difficult. These multi-disciplinary approaches underscore the importance of holistic post-sedation care addressing individual needs of patients. Finally, effective post-sedation care includes educating patients, and their families on what to expect during recovery. Effective communication will alleviate fears and prepare them for any potential distress or side effects of sedation. The patients must be informed about common symptoms, such as drowsiness or confusion, which may be present even after recovery of consciousness. Instructions for postoperative care, including complications requiring immediate health care, are essential in creating a supportive environment for recovery. By educating and empowering patients and families, healthcare clinicians can enhance compliance and patient satisfaction with the sedation process. Ultimately, an adequately crafted post-sedation care plan not only ensures safety but also supports a positive therapeutic relationship among clinicians and patients, affirming the commitment to quality care throughout the sedation continuum (Figure 3.16).

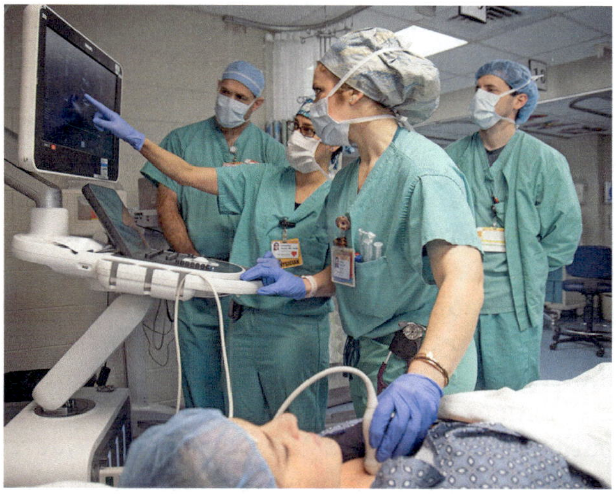

Figure 3.16. Post anesthesia care.

Source: https://cdn.atriumhealth.org/-/media/wakeforest/school/images/page-content/education-and-training/residencies-and-fellowships/anesthesiology-residency/anes-res-curr-pacu.jpg?h=666&w=800&rev=b88717c1c42b44b8a51afb0dbfeab78a&hash=2BE2CEC8F20B832BD015BE380ACAB6FD.

3.5.1. Recovery Room Protocols

The use of recovery room protocols is a significant aspect of the continuum of patient care, particularly after surgeries using sedation. This phase is crucial for monitoring patients emerging from anesthesia, making them comfortable and safe while their vital signs become normal. Health professionals in recovery rooms typically adhere to standardized protocols for assessing patients' respiratory and cardiovascular status, thus minimizing post-anesthetic complications. Nurses' attention during this interval can profoundly influence patient outcomes, since early detection of complications enables immediate intervention and reduction in morbidity. Effective recovery room regimens therefore, not only enhance patient safety but also foster a reassuring environment that supports uneventful recovery from operating room to outpatient status. The addition of guidelines to recovery room procedures also highlights the significance of personal care for patients. Each patient's reaction to anesthesia can be dramatically different as a function of age, state of health, and procedure type performed. Personalized recovery methods are therefore required in addressing individual needs and solving potential complications. Comorbid patients, say, may require special monitoring in contrast to relatively healthy patients, and thus personalized measures and assessment criteria must be followed. This strategy is aligned with modern healthcare models, which emphasize per-patient strategies to the detriment of generalized, all-encompassing protocols. Utilizing targeted assessment and individualized care plans, health practitioners are able to maximize the overall efficacy of the recovery process, highlighting the significance of patient-centered practices that ultimately enhance satisfaction and health outcomes. Furthermore, takeaways from emergent situations , such as the COVID-19 pandemic underscore the significance of robust recovery room protocols with emphasis on safety for high-risk patients. Amidst waves of patients requiring airway and respiratory complication management, healthcare systems inspected practices and enhanced safety guidelines to protect both patients and healthcare workers. These protocols include the wear of personal protective equipment (PPE) and heightened hygiene levels in recovery settings, which lower the likelihood of transmission of airborne pathogens. The learning from different medical circles reminds us that diligent adherence to recovery protocols can greatly enhance the level of safety and quality of care, keeping staff safe while ensuring that care offered to patients is of high quality. Hence, routine review and revision of recovery room procedures guarantee that they remain beneficial and relevant in the presence of new medical settings, contributing to the general patient preparation and safety of sedation.

3.5.2. Assessing Patient Readiness for Discharge

The process of patient readiness for discharge determination is a significant area of patient preparation, particularly for the example of sedation. Good discharge planning needs to be initiated early in the patients hospital stay so that they learn everything and are able to achieve everything they require before going home. Nurses play a critical role in this teaching process, delivering individualized discharge education on medication management, activity restrictions, and signs and symptoms to observe upon discharge. This quality of teaching has a significant influence on parental readiness, as revealed in research in which improved nurses' abilities to give information are connected with fewer parental coping issues and decreased use of post-hospitalization care (Jerofke et al., 2008). The more information the patients have regarding their postoperative treatment, the more they are prepared to manage by themselves once they are home. Another significant criterion of discharge readiness evaluation is evaluating the physical and emotional status of patients. Before discharge, health practitioners need to ascertain whether patients can carry out common self-care activities and recognize any complications of their surgery or sedation. Checking patients' cognitive function, pain, and overall stability of health is part of this evaluation. Of significance also to be considered is the environment in which patients are being discharged. For instance, patients who are transferring from an inpatient setting to home or a rehabilitation facility must be given special attention so support systems can be implemented. If knowledge deficits or inadequate home support are observed by the health care provider, additional resources or follow-up appointments may be arranged. Implementing current nursing practice into routine discharge procedures continues to be essential to enhance patient outcomes (Mitchell, 2003). Finally, facilitating effective communication among healthcare professionals and patients or their relatives is included in the discharge readiness assessment. Encouraging patients to participate in discussions about their treatment processes and recovery expectations is a major factor in minimizing discharge-related anxiety. When empowered and informed, patients have a high rate of overall satisfaction regarding discharge. Furthermore, collaborative communication can also determine any outstanding questions or concerns related to postoperative care and thus facilitate individualized teaching and reinforcement of instruction. Through attention to efficient nurse-patient relationships, healthcare providers can create a comprehensive grasp of patient needs and possible setbacks toward successful recuperation. In the end, these processes equate to an improved discharge process and increased long-term health outcomes for home-recuperating patients (Jerofke et al., 2008).

3.5.3. Instructions for Post-Procedure Care

It is imperative that after a procedure where sedation is used, clear instructions for patients must be provided and in detail. These are necessary to ensure smooth recovery with the minimum number of complications. Patients must first be monitored for adverse effects of sedation, which may be in the form of drowsiness, nausea, or confusion. Caregivers should closely monitor vital signs, particularly respiratory function, because sedation impacts respiratory drive. Provision of clear verbal and written instructions regarding the limitations imposed on activity—e.g., driving, machinery operation, or the making of significant decisions—can also be a safeguard against potential harm due to residual sedation effects. Also, the role of hydration and proper nutrition post-procedure cannot be overstated because such factors contribute significantly to recovery and overall patient comfort. Moreover, effective pain control following procedural procedures is vital to the process of successful recovery. The patients typically report various degrees of pain or discomfort based on the procedure that is being undertaken. Prevention of this pain should be patient-specific, including pharmacological as well as non-pharmacological interventions. Proper monitoring of analgesic consumption should be performed, and patients should be educated to adhere to dosing regimens and understand when to take medication. Non-pharmacological pain control approaches , such as relaxation or distraction, may reinforce pharmacologic approaches and enhance patient satisfaction. Cognitive-behavioral therapy, among psychological treatments, can further enhance the patient experience after recovery from a post-procedure by facilitating enhanced emotional coping with pain and thereby enhancing compliance with care instructions, as suggested by Liossi (1999). Finally, follow-up care is part of the ongoing continuum of patient preparation and success with sedation. Patients should be given clear instructions regarding when to come in for medical treatment if they experience complications , such as heavy bleeding, infection symptoms, or unforeseen changes in their condition. Remembering follow-up visit appointments ensures timely and effective treatment of resultant problems. Active engagement of patients with healthcare professionals fosters a situation under which all can collaborate to enhance patient care as a comprehensive entity. Utilizing evidence-based practice, as in Meng et al. (2019), will assist in guiding healthcare professionals to develop comprehensive post-procedure care guidelines focusing on addressing pain, psychological support, and proper communication. Thus, robust post-procedure care not only results in improved recovery but also ensures active participation by patients in their care, eventually leading to increased satisfaction and outcomes (Figure 3.17).

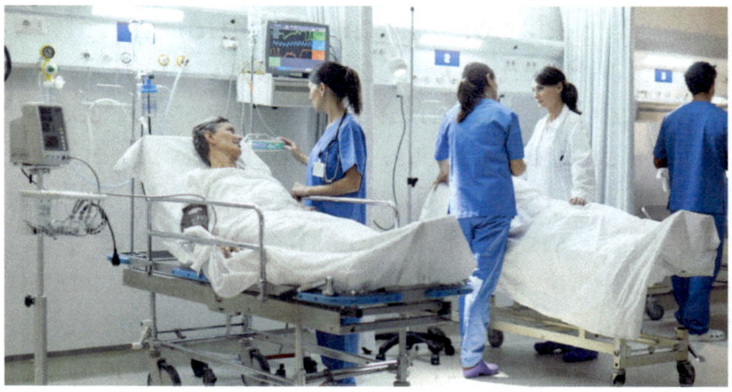

Figure 3.17. Post-operative care.

Source: https://veritascare.co.uk/wp-content/uploads/2022/08/Featured-image1200-%C3%97-628px-1-1030x539.png.

3.6. Complications and Risks

Sedation in medical and dental procedures has major issues regarding complications and risks that may arise during treatment. As sedation is administered by healthcare professionals, they need to be constantly sensitive to possible side effects like respiratory depression, hypotension, or even cardiac arrest. Such risks are amplified in patients with pre-existing health ailments, which becomes a pressing concern since most patients for whom sedation is needed may be presenting with physical, mental, or medically compromising illness, thereby risking complications. For instance, the patients are unlikely to yield to behavioral modification plans, and a careful sedation management strategy should be adopted to ensure their safety and well-being (Al-hidabi et al., 2009). Thus, before a sedation procedure, there is a requirement to thoroughly screen the patient for any underlying condition that would escalate the risks of the procedure. Moreover, the impact of pain caused by the procedure cannot be overstated, particularly for susceptible populations , such as children. Children who have conditions like cancer often receive multiple, painful procedures, which are a major cause of distress, making sedation in these children rather difficult. Painful procedures have been found to be rated by children as the most distressing aspect of their illness, as repetitive repetition are not as desensitizing (Liossi, 1999). Thus, the management plan for these patients must extend beyond sedation only; it must blend both pharmacological and psychological approaches to ensure proper care. This will enable healthcare providers to minimize procedural pain and anxiety, thereby enhancing the overall experience of the patients as well as curtailing the dangers of sedation procedures. When the risk of sedation and pain due to the procedure is appreciated, there is a need to employ effective preparation tactics to prevent complications. Effective patient preparation should involve effective communication, addressing concerns of patients, and setting realistic expectations for the procedure of sedation and what can be anticipated. Additionally, treatments , such as cognitive-behavioral therapy and hypnosis can be utilized to reduce anxiety before the procedure, thus minimizing the incidence of side effects during sedation (Liossi, 1999). Overall, an integrated patient preparation and sedation procedure dealing with both the physical and emotional realities of care will not only protect patients from potential harm but also optimize the effectiveness of utilized therapies. The complexity of sedation management stresses the importance of a cautious preemptive strategy, in turn raising the demand for prudent planning in clinical settings.

3.6.1. Common Complications Associated with Sedation

Sedation is typically employed to facilitate various medical interventions, yet the therapy has its complications. Common complications include respiratory depression, cardiovascular instability, and over-sedation. The most frequent cause of respiratory depression is the sedative drugs themselves, which can produce suppression of the central nervous system and respiratory drive. Such a state needs to be monitored closely for patients' oxygen saturation and respiratory effort because failure to recognize and reverse respiratory issues in a timely fashion may result in major morbidity or death. Cardiovascular instability, including hypotension or bradycardia, can also occur and particularly in patients with pre-existing cardiovascular disease. These cases typically require immediate intervention, like fluid resuscitation or pharmacologic intervention, requiring vigilant monitoring of the patient during the sedation process. Another serious complication of sedation is the potential for aspiration in patients with impaired gag reflexes or those with altered mental status. Aspiration can occur when the patient's airway is inadequately protected, resulting in pulmonary complications in the form of aspiration pneumonia. This is especially true in sedation cases among patients undergoing gastrointestinal procedures or pre-existing esophageal illness. To prevent aspiration, the guidelines propose fasting before sedation procedures and the utilization of appropriate airway management protocols. Besides, communication and patient preparation are of utmost importance. Through education of the patient about risks and cooperation throughout the process, providers can enhance patient adherence and potentially prevent these complications during sedation. Last but not least, the psychological impacts of sedation, even though they are sometimes overlooked, should be noted. Sedation patients usually worry about the procedure itself, which not only increases their perception of pain and discomfort but also plays a role in patient agitation and aggression. Complications involving psychological distress can include postoperative pain, duration of recovery period, and enhanced sedation-related anxiety on future medical procedures. Psychological intervention can be introduced to minimize these problems through preparatory interventions and cognitive-behavioral therapies. Not only do interventions here condition the patient mentally and psychologically for the procedure, but they also serve to improve overall outcomes. Patient safety and comfort thus necessitate attention to both the physiological and psychological determinants of sedation, encapsulating the holistic thinking involved in patient preparation and sedation (Liossi, 1999; Beard et al., 2019).

3.6.2. Risk Factors That Increase Complications

Complications from sedation in medical procedures can often be explained by various risk factors that may cause potential danger to the patient. One primary one among them is the age and overall health of the patient. Older patients, for instance, tend to have more comorbidities, making the process of sedation very complicated. It has been proven that sedative overdoses, particularly benzodiazepines and opioids, are prevalent in such groups and lead to adverse consequences , such as respiratory depression as well as prolonged recovery times. Also, lack of monitoring of patients who undergo procedures adds to such risks, necessitating the highest priority for adhering to available guidelines for sedation to avoid such complications. The choice of sedation agent and method can significantly impact the risk of complications during procedures. In particular, over-administration of sedatives to patients without adequate evaluation leads to severe side effects, most notably in gastroenterology procedures. UK reports indicate that improper application of high dosages to old patients for gastrointestinal endoscopy has resulted in excessive morbidity and even fatality. Such alarming findings underscore the imperative for personalized sedation protocols based on patient-specific factors and adverse reaction history to sedatives. Vigilant compliance with revised guidelines, which stress conservative titration and dose adjustment, is essential to patient safety and best procedural outcomes. Furthermore, the organizational environment of the healthcare setting can also impact complication rates in sedated patients. Factors , such as the type of endoscopy center, endoscopist experience, and availability of dedicated screening sessions may be involved in variation in the quality of care. For instance, centers with high rates of sedation use and dealing with screening dedicated sessions have reported improved quality indicators, with significant impact on ADR and caecal intubation rate (CIR). Consequently, policy making and implementation focusing on these organizational variables can potentially enhance patient outcomes as well as reduce the incidence of complications of sedation. The focus on systemic changes, coupled with patient-related as well as endoscopist-related parameters, is an important aspect in addressing challenges regarding complication in sedation practice (Lord et al., 2006; Barca et al., 2014).

3.6.3. Strategies for Minimizing Risks

Successful patient preparation is most important in reducing sedation risks, especially in susceptible groups like children. Development of detailed protocols covering psychological and physical elements of patient preparation can improve outcomes remarkably. As an example, careful pre-sedation evaluation is critical in recognizing any covert or overt health condition or special patient factor that could predispose patients to increased risks from sedation, including age, medical history, and anxiety score. Infants less than three years old, as noted in past studies, regularly need anesthesia/ sedation (A/S) for medical procedures, while the demand decreases with age, which requires differentiated strategies based on stages of development. In addition, involving parents or guardians during the preparation phase can allay their fears and foster cooperation and resulting in fewer opportunities for complications during and after sedation as outlined in the institutional sedation requirements study among pediatric patients (Bratton et al., 2015). Another important prevention measure for risks of sedation is through the cautious use and application of sedation techniques tailored to individual patients. In endoscopic procedures like colonoscopy, patient factors—female gender, older age, and certain medical histories—can hinder the success of sedation, causing complications. Endoscopists should enhance their technical skills using varying techniques in the management of difficulties, e.g., in terms of taking up water-aided techniques, changing the position of patients, and utilizing abdominal pressure (Bayupurnama et al., 2013). Additionally, utilizing appropriate sedation protocols that take into account the requirements of patients—choosing agents with rapid onset and short durations—reduces the time patients are under sedation, ultimately limiting the risk of prolonged recovery and adverse effects to minimal levels. These protocols enable a safer sedation process by factoring in each patient's individual factors affecting their response to sedation. Finally, ongoing monitoring during the process of sedation is essential in detecting and rectifying any complications arising immediately. Real-time monitoring of patients' vital signs and comfort allows clinicians to respond rapidly to changes, thus reducing the risk for adverse events. Training staff to detect respiratory depression or hypotension in high-risk patient populations is essential to enable timely intervention. The addition of advanced monitoring technologies can provide additional levels of safety with alerts that enable clinicians to intervene in a timely fashion. In pediatric patients, monitoring must be done not only during the procedure but also during the recovery phase, so that patients are returned to baseline function in the absence of unnecessary delay or complication. By harmonious blending of patient-focused preparation with appropriate technique choice and vigilant monitoring, healthcare providers are able to ameliorate risks associated with sedation, delivering successful and safe results to all involved patients.

SUMMARY

Overall, patient preparation for sedation is a process with various facets that requires careful planning and execution to ensure safety and effectiveness. Effective patient preparation not only enhances the experience of the sedated patient but also avoids complications. The importance of in-depth assessments, medical histories, as well as psychological testing cannot be overemphasized because these are important in determining appropriate sedation protocols. Besides, patient preparation through informing them of the sedation process lowers their anxiety and fosters the team atmosphere of interdisciplinary care providers and patients. Lastly, the incorporation of the best practices in the preparation of patients is critical for optimal outcomes in sedation. The literature verifies that there exist significant variances in sedation- and patient preparation-related practices, which necessitate standard procedures across all environments. Poor guidance can lead to inconsistent practice, which can have effects on patient safety and patient satisfaction. Perhaps none is as important as the NICE guideline on rapid tranquillization, which identifies the importance of establishing a framework for effective sedation practice in psychiatric and emergency settings. By adhering to evidence-based advice and drawing together the findings of systematic reviews like that of NICE, clinicians can enhance the quality of care received by patients requiring sedation. Lack of consensus regarding first-line sedative medications points toward ongoing research that seeks to standardize safe and efficacious processes, as a response to the unique requirements of patients and environments (Branford et al., 2008). Furthermore, the need for targeted interventions in managing undesirable behavior, particularly in special groups , such as children with ASD, becomes apparent under sedation conditions. Health care practitioners must contend with complex behaviors that render sedative delivery a potentially arduous process. Identification of the exact categories of behavior and how they must be treated comes to reveals the necessity of an individualized method of sedation. Engaging parents and caregivers to develop individualized strategies is not only proving to establish improved compliance but also a more secure care setting for these vulnerable populations. With further development of medicine, the interaction between some behavioral control methods and sedation protocols will play a crucial role in better patient outcomes overall, particularly in challenging cases (Johnson & Rodriguez, 2013).

Patient preparation before surgery plays a significant role in the success of sedation protocols. Sensitivity to the psychological and physiological responses inherent in surgery can provide hints for improved patient outcomes. For instance, studies show that ideal patient preparation can include the application of hypnosis as an adjunct therapy. Hypnosis has been found to reduce levels of perceived pain during minor surgery more than conventional care approaches. As seen in randomized controlled trials, hypnosis not only leads to reduced pain but also encourages patients to be constructively proactive toward the procedural process. Therefore, integrative approaches incorporating preoperative hypnotic sessions can contribute to overall patient satisfaction and procedural sedation-related outcomes (Kendrick et al., 2016). Anxiety tends to emerge as a universal factor affecting patients scheduled for surgical operations, particularly gynecologic surgeries. Clinical practice experience indicates that anxiety tends to grow when the surgery date is approached, peaking on the eve of anesthesia induction. Increased anxiety is also linked with higher levels of postoperative pain, creating a combined effect that complicates recovery. Qualitative assessment through interviews shows that patients report consistently anxiety driven by inadequate information and preparation regarding the process of surgery. These findings underscore the necessity for adequate preoperative counseling and education, through which patient anxiety can be addressed and ultimately lead to improved surgical results. Health professionals should recognize that part of addressing both psychological and physical aspects of patient well-being should be included in their preparatory planning (Carr et al., 2006). Ultimately, a combination of psychological methods , such as hypnosis, and robust educational frameworks, acts to optimize the sedation experience and positively influence patient outcomes. Enhanced preoperative preparation can potentially lead to reduced levels of anxiety, having a secondary effect on pain control following surgery in a positive manner. With the strong interrelationships among preoperative anxiety, procedural information adequacy, and post-surgery recovery, health professionals have the responsibility of ascertaining that the measures of the reduction of anxiety are prioritized. There must be evidence for the efficacy of interventions , such as hypnosis and thorough preoperative education to be utilized in the development of the best practices within operating rooms. By securing patient mental health alongside intact physiological safety, healthcare professionals can facilitate a more complete and effective process of patient preparation and sedation, with improved overall experiences and results for surgical care (Carr et al., 2006; Kendrick et al., 2016).

CLOSER LOOK

PATIENT-SPECIFIC SEDATION:

Patient-specific sedation refers to the individualized selection and administration of sedatives tailored to a patient's unique medical profile, procedural needs, and safety considerations. Unlike standardized sedation protocols, a patient-specific approach emphasizes personalization—accounting for factors such as age, weight, medical history, anxiety level, comorbidities, and the anticipated complexity of the procedure. This individualized strategy improves patient comfort while maintaining the highest standards of safety and clinical effectiveness. A central principle of patient-specific sedation is risk assessment. Before any sedative is administered, clinicians evaluate the patient's cardiovascular and respiratory status, allergies, prior reactions to anesthesia, and current medications. Special attention is given to populations with heightened vulnerability, such as pediatric patients, older adults, individuals with obstructive sleep apnea, or those with chronic respiratory disease. These assessments influence the choice of sedative agents, dosing strategies, and required monitoring intensity.

Another key element is the selection of the sedation level. Depending on the patient's needs and the procedure being performed, clinicians may choose minimal, moderate, deep sedation, or general anesthesia. For example, a patient with high anxiety undergoing a lengthy dental or endoscopic procedure may benefit from deeper sedation, while someone with significant medical risks might be better suited for a lighter, more controlled approach. Tailoring the sedation depth helps balance comfort with physiological stability. Pharmacologic choices also reflect individualized planning. Different drugs—such as benzodiazepines, propofol, or nitrous oxide—vary in onset, duration, and side-effect profiles. Combining agents may allow for lower doses of each, reducing risk. Adjustments based on patient metabolism, liver and kidney function, and potential interactions further ensure precise dosing. Pharmacogenomic insights, although still emerging in routine practice, offer additional avenues for optimizing drug response.

Monitoring and recovery are equally critical to patient-specific sedation. Continuous assessment of oxygenation, ventilation, cardiac status, and level of consciousness ensures early detection of adverse events. Post-procedure, clinicians consider the patient's baseline health and response to sedation to determine recovery time and discharge readiness. Clear communication with caregivers and tailored post-sedation instructions support safe recovery at home.

Overall, patient-specific sedation enhances patient-centered care by aligning sedation choices with individual characteristics and clinical realities. As healthcare increasingly values personalization, this approach promotes comfort, minimizes complications, and supports positive procedural experiences. It reflects the broader shift toward precision medicine—one in which every sedation plan is crafted not just for a procedure, but for the person undergoing it.

REFERENCES

1. Carr, E., Brockbank, K., Allen, S., & Strike, P. (2006). Patterns and frequency of anxiety in women undergoing gynaecological surgery. *Journal of clinical nursing, 15*(3), 341–352. https://doi.org/10.1111/j.1365-2702.2006.01285.x(accessed on 15th July 2025).
2. Al Youha, S., Apfel, A., Carroll, D., Codding, J., Davison, C., Hill, M., Ketonis, C., et al. (2018). *A cost analysis of carpal tunnel release surgery performed wide awake versus under sedation.* https://core.ac.uk/download/213444643.pdf (accessed on 15th July 2025).
3. Bray, L., Snodin, J., & Carter, B. (2015). Holding and restraining children for clinical procedures within an acute care setting: an ethical consideration of the evidence. *Nursing inquiry, 22*(2), 157–167. https://doi.org/10.1111/nin.12074(accessed on 15th July 2025).
4. Al-hidabi, D., & Fatima. (2009). *Usage of dental general anesthesia and assessment of fear among special needs and non-special needs children in Kota Bharu, Kelantan.* https://core.ac.uk/download/32600639.pdf (accessed on 15th July 2025).
5. Barca, A., Naldoni, C., Senore, C., Hassan, C., Rex, D., Di Giulio, E., Da Re, F., et al. (2014). *Quality of colonoscopy in an organized colorectal cancer screening program with immunochemical fecal occult blood test. The EQuIPE study (Evaluating Quality Indicators of the Performance of Endoscopy).* https://core.ac.uk/download/80311410.pdf (accessed on 15th July 2025).
6. Bayupurnama, P. (P.), & Cahyono, S. B. (S.). (2013). *How to negotiate difficult colonoscopy to optimize cecal intubation rate.* https://media.neliti.com/media/publications/63912-EN-how-to-negotiate-difficult-colonoscopy-t.pdf (accessed on 15th July 2025).
7. Beard, T. L., Bergese, S. D., Berkowitz, R. D., Brzezinski, M., et al. (2019). *ATHENA: A phase 3, open-label study of the safety and effectiveness of oliceridine (TRV130), a G-protein selective agonist at the μ-opioid receptor, in patients with moderate to severe acute pain requiring parenteral opioid therapy.* https://core.ac.uk/download/323063237.pdf (accessed on 15th July 2025).
8. DA, Lord & Bell, Geoffrey & A, Gray & A, Quine & J, Bowles & A, Reynolds. (2006). Sedation for Gastrointestinal Endoscopic Procedures in the Elderly: Getting Safer but Still Not Nearly Safe Enough. Br Soc Gastroenterol. (accessed on 15th July 2025).
9. Berglas, N. F., & Roberts, S. C. M. (2018). *The development of facility standards for common outpatient procedures and implications for the context of abortion.* https://core.ac.uk/download/323063555.pdf (accessed on 15th July 2025).
10. McCarthy, D. , & Blumenthal, D (2006). *Committed to safety: Ten case studies on reducing harm to patients.* https://core.ac.uk/download/71350251.pdf (accessed on 15th July 2025).
11. Branford, D., Chandler-Oatts, J., Johnston, S., Nelstrop, L., et al. (2008). *Establishing gold standard approaches to rapid tranquillization: A review and discussion of the evidence on the safety and efficacy of medications currently used.* https://core.ac.uk/download/48632.pdf (accessed on 15th July 2025).
12. Bratton, J., McMullen, K. P., Johnstone, P. A. S., & Hanson, T. (2015). *Parameters of anesthesia/sedation in children receiving radiotherapy.* https://core.ac.uk/download/pdf/81874376.pdf (accessed on 15th July 2025).
13. Meng, Q. T., Cao, C., Liu, H. M., Xia, Z. Y., Li, W., Tang, L. H., Chen, R., Jiang, M., Wu, Y., Leng, Y., & Lee, C. C. (2016). Safety and efficacy of etomidate and propofol anesthesia in elderly

patients undergoing gastroscopy: A double-blind randomized clinical study. *Experimental and therapeutic medicine, 12*(3), 1515–1524. https://doi.org/10.3892/etm.2016.3475(accessed on 15th July 2025).

14. Carella, S., Fino, P., Fioramonti, P., Marchese, C., et al. (2016). *Improvement of mouth functional disability in systemic sclerosis patients over one year in a trial of fat transplantation versus adipose-derived stromal cells.* https://core.ac.uk/download/54526751.pdf (accessed on 15th July 2025).
15. Chinn, S. B., Clayburgh, D., Davies, L., Givi, B., et al. (2020). *Safety recommendations for evaluation and surgery of the head and neck during the COVID-19 pandemic.* https://core.ac.uk/download/322846968.pdf (accessed on 15th July 2025).
16. Coghill, E., Crow, W., Richardson, A., Turnock, C., et al. (2007). *A comparison of sleep assessment tools by nurses and patients in critical care.* https://core.ac.uk/download/4146365.pdf (accessed on 15th July 2025).
17. Copot, D., Ghita, M., Ghita, M., Ionescu, C., et al. (2020). *Pain detection with bioimpedance methodology from 3-dimensional exploration of nociception in a postoperative observational trial.* https://core.ac.uk/download/322827629.pdf (accessed on 15th July 2025).
18. Czajka, A., Piaszczyński, S., Płeska, K., Reguła, J., et al. (2024). *Difficult pediatric airway in anesthesia practice and future sport performance.* https://core.ac.uk/download/613192436.pdf (accessed on 15th July 2025).
19. Kendrick, C., Sliwinski, J., Yu, Y., Johnson, A., Fisher, W., Kekecs, Z., & Elkins, G. (2016). Hypnosis for Acute Procedural Pain: A Critical Review. *The International journal of clinical and experimental hypnosis, 64*(1), 75–115. https://doi.org/10.1080/00207144.2015.1099405(accessed on 15th July 2025).
20. Euliano, T. Y., Lee, A. I., Melker, M., et al. (2003). *Development and evaluation of an internet-based airway evaluation tutorial.* https://core.ac.uk/download/pdf/85715.pdf (accessed on 15th July 2025).
21. Hamilton, J. M. (2015). *An evidence-based approach to prepare interdisciplinary team members for implementation of the ABCDE bundle.* https://core.ac.uk/download/217685663.pdf (accessed on 15th July 2025).
22. Izaki, Y., Okahisa, T., Sogabe, M., Takayama, T., et al. (2022). *Acceptability in Subjects Undergoing EGD.* https://core.ac.uk/download/521170943.pdf (accessed on 15th July 2025).
23. Jerofke, T. A., Johnson, N. L., Lang, C., Malin, S., et al. (2008). *Readiness for discharge in parents of hospitalized children.* https://core.ac.uk/download/213078372.pdf (accessed on 15th July 2025).
24. Johnson, N. L., & Rodriguez, D. (2013). *Children with autism spectrum disorder at a pediatric hospital: A systematic review of the literature.* https://core.ac.uk/download/213081757.pdf (accessed on 15th July 2025).
25. Juba, K., & Ricca, B. P. (2014). *Design of a problem-based learning pain and palliative care elective course.* https://core.ac.uk/download/48616928.pdf (accessed on 15th July 2025).
26. Kass, P. H., Lascelles, B. D. X., McKune, C. M., Pascoe, P. J., et al. (2014). *The challenge of evaluating pain and a pre-incisional local anesthetic block.* https://core.ac.uk/download/323070364.pdf (accessed on 15th July 2025).

27. Liossi, C. (1999). *Management of Pediatric Procedure-Related Cancer Pain.*

28. Mitchell, M. J. (2003). *Patient anxiety and modern elective surgery: A literature review.* https://core.ac.uk/download/104290.pdf (accessed on 15th July 2025).

29. Pandurangi, A., Snyder, A. D., & Venkatachalam, V. (2017). *Electroconvulsive therapy in geriatric patients: A literature review and program report from Virginia Commonwealth University, Richmond, Virginia, USA.* https://core.ac.uk/download/215482217.pdf (accessed on 15th July 2025).

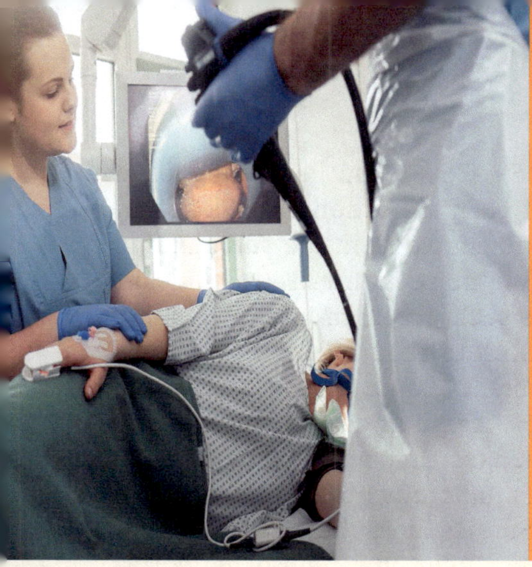

Chapter 4

UPPER GASTROINTESTINAL ENDOSCOPY (ESOPHAGOGASTRODUODEN-OSCOPY – EGD)

Contents

Introduction 95
4.1. Indications for Esophagogastroduodenoscopy (EGD) 99
4.2. Preparation for Esophagogastroduodenoscopy (EGD) 103
4.3. The Esophagogastroduodenoscopy (EGD) Procedure 106
4.4. Risks and Complications 109
4.5. Post-Procedure Care 112
4.6. Advances in Esophagogastroduodenoscopy (EGD) Technology 116
Summary 120
References 123

Introduction

Upper gastrointestinal endoscopy, or esophagogastroduodenoscopy (EGD), is an essential procedure in modern gastroenterology with the advantage of both diagnostic and therapeutic maneuvers. The EGD is performed to enable visualization of the esophagus, stomach, and duodenum to enable clinicians to obtain useful information on various types of gastrointestinal disorders. The procedure has gained significance with the advent of diagnosing conditions , such as gastrointestinal bleeding, dysphagia, and neoplasms. The utility of EGD transcends diagnostic purposes and can also encompass therapeutic purposes , such as biopsies, foreign body removal, and stricture treatment. Thus, EGD is a multifunctional tool in the clinician's arsenal with the capability to view and intervene simultaneously to optimize patient outcomes in upper gastrointestinal wellness. Despite all its advantages, the efficiency of EGD has some limitations. Early detection of malignant lesions, particularly gastric cancer, remains a challenge within the medical world. Gastric cancer is the fifth most common malignancy worldwide, and survival rates plummet to as little as 5%-25% upon being diagnosed at late stages. The cold, harsh reality is that the technologies of early detection are needed in the field of EGD because early lesions become essentially indistinguishable from the surrounding normal tissue. Second, the risk of missing injured areas through the inspection raises significant questions concerning the validity and completeness of the test. As such, research into developing diagnostic technology, such as artificial intelligence, is being explored to ensure EGD findings are more complete and valid and therefore enhance patient management (Lopes, 2021). Lastly, the diagnostic and therapeutic function of EGD in managing diseases of the upper gastrointestinal tract becomes increasingly critical but is also fraught with challenges that necessitate ongoing innovation. Integration of new technologies into EGD procedures is imperative to further improve diagnostic accuracy and overcome the dangers of missed lesions. Studies have shown that the use of machine learning methodologies, and specifically the use of convolutional neural networks, can present promising avenues through which to overcome these issues by allowing for better image analysis and identification of more subtle lesions that could be missed under conventional methods of examination. As the gastroenterological landscape moves forward, it is essential that physicians remain informed of developments and how they can implement them in their practice to maximize patient outcomes. The future of EGD may well lie at the crossroads of traditional diagnostic methods and emerging technologies (Tringali et al., 2017) (Figure 4.1).

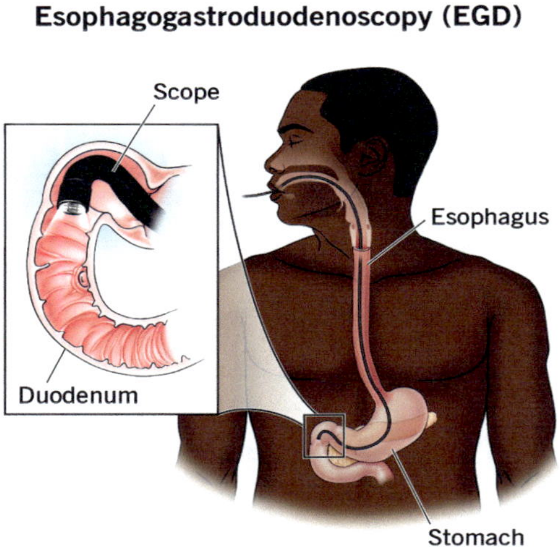

Figure 4.1. Esophagogastroduodenoscopy (EGD) procedure (Upper endoscopy).

Source: https://my.clevelandclinic.org/-/scassets/images/org/health/articles/22549-esophagogastroduodenoscopy.

Definition of Upper Gastrointestinal Endoscopy

Upper gastrointestinal endoscopy (EGD) is a therapeutic and diagnostic tool that enables direct visualization of the duodenum, stomach, and esophagus. This procedure uses a flexible endoscope, a very thin tube that has a light and a camera within it, which allows physicians to examine these upper GI structures in detail. The indications for EGD range from the evaluation of gastrointestinal symptoms , such as dysphagia (swallowing difficulty), gastrointestinal bleeding, and persistent abdominal pain, to the establishment of diseases , such as inflammation, ulcers, and cancers. Consequently, EGD is commonly indispensable in the diagnosis and treatment of many gastrointestinal disorders, thus leaving a final mark on the decision of therapy and the result for the patients. The results of EGD can be greatly influenced by the skill of the endoscopists, particularly as indicated by the endoscopist biopsy rate (EBR). The EBR, as the proportion of procedures in which biopsies are taken, is a critical quality measurement of the overall efficacy of the procedures. Research has confirmed that an increased EBR is correlated with improved detection rates of gastric premalignant conditions (GPCs) and the decreased missed rate of gastric cancers (GCs) (Bialek et al., 2019).

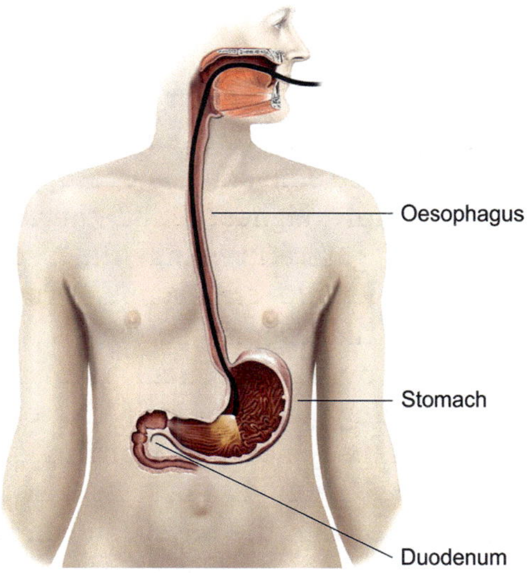

Figure 4.2. Upper gastrointestinal endoscopy.

Source: https://media.healthdirect.org.au/images/inline/original/upper-gi-endoscopy-illustration-2679eb.png.

Specifically, endoscopists who have a higher EBR have a superior ability to detect significant pathologies, supporting the contribution of skill and experience towards EGD procedures. Thus, as a measure of quality and competence, the EBR not only establishes clinical expertise but also carries the stakes of patient safety and care. The diagnostic function, upper gastrointestinal endoscopy plays a central role in therapeutic interventions too. Therapeutic maneuvers in the course of EGD can include stricture dilation, extraction of foreign bodies, and biopsy for histopathological examination. Furthermore, EGD is applied in the management of patients with specific clinical conditions , such as gastrointestinal bleeding and corrosive ingestions, thereby acting as a significant resource in pediatric and adult gastrointestinal care (Tringali et al., 2017). The fact that EGD has the capacity to diagnose and treat simultaneously testifies to its usefulness in modern gastrointestinal medicine. As endoscopic technology evolves, the future of EGD is anticipated to be broader as it becomes increasingly able to treat an increasingly broad range of gastrointestinal diseases more efficiently (Figure 4.2).

Esophagogastroduodenoscopy (EGD) Significance in Medical Diagnosis

Upper gastrointestinal endoscopy (EGD) is closely involved in diagnosing gastrointestinal illness. By direct visualization of the esophagus, stomach, and duodenum, EGD can diagnose a variety of conditions , including ulcers, tumors, and bleeding. The ability to take biopsies during the procedure enhances the diagnostic clarity of the procedure, enabling healthcare practitioners to decide on care for patients based on evidence. It is particularly vital in the case of risk groups, such as patients aged more than 50, because they are likely to exhibit symptoms typical of serious diseases, for example, esophageal cancer or advanced gastritis. Early detection and treatment, particularly for these people, are best, and therefore, it is essential that EGD be incorporated in regular medical checkups and preventive healthcare practices. Extensive guidelines affirm that EGD remains the most effective diagnostic procedure when upper digestive tract symptoms show up, cementing its position as a cornerstone in traditional medicine. The efficacy of EGD also relies on adherence and the cooperation of the patient to have it conducted. A study indicates that there is a huge gap between the awareness of the necessity of EGD among patients, particularly those with less severe symptoms. For instance, a study from Greece found that a high number of dyspeptic patients refused endoscopic examination and listed fears, pain myths, and logistical challenges as their explanations (Tringali et al., 2017). Such barriers are a critical shortfall in patient management, as refusal or delay of EGD can be linked to worsening outcomes. For this purpose, soothing patient anxiety and educating them on the benefits and safety of EGD are crucial to ensuring optimal compliance. Understanding these dynamics is necessary to enable healthcare providers to maximize diagnosis strategies and enhance patient participation in their own health care management.

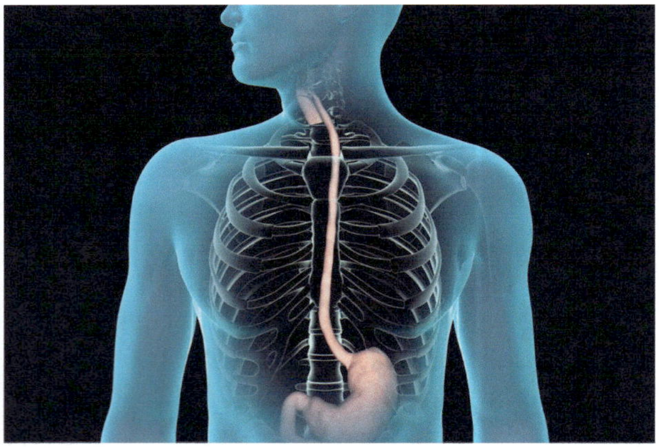

Figure 4.3. Esophagogastroduodenoscopy (EGD) procedure for diagnosis.

Source: https://mss-p-057-delivery.stylelabs.cloud/api/public/content/c8f2530301834d679dd4710f942d73bc?v=25fa5062.

Beyond mere diagnostics, the effects of EGD are profound and manifest within a broader paradigm of directed therapeutic intervention. EGD is not just limited to the identification of gastrointestinal conditions, but it also finds application in procedures , such as dilating strictures, removal of foreign bodies, and biopsies. The dual use of EGD in diagnosis and treatment increases the importance of the procedure in gastroenterology. Professional guidelines state the application of EGD in the treatment of various pathological conditions like corrosive injuries and upper GI bleeding that require immediate medical attention and intervention (Tringali et al., 2017). Thus, integration of EGD in routine medical practice not only makes early diagnosis possible but also aids in the mitigation of complications due to untreated gastrointestinal diseases. Lastly, the numerous benefits of EGD reflect its imperative role in contemporary medical diagnosis and treatment (Figure 4.3).

Overview of the Procedure

Esophageal, gastric, and duodenal visualization through upper gastrointestinal endoscopy (EGD) is a fundamental diagnostic and therapeutic tool for many gastrointestinal illnesses. By employing a flexible endoscope, providers may visualize the esophagus, stomach, and duodenum, providing critical information about underlying pathology of the organs. The procedure is typically performed on the patient under sedation to ensure that he/she is comfortable so that the physician can insert the endoscope softly into the mouth and pass it into the upper digestive system. The area of the body visualized using visualization may reveal diseases , such as ulcers, erosive disease, strictures, polyps and tumors, hence allowing timely and proper clinical management. The endoscope also possesses the ability to perform biopsies, polypectomies and cauterizations, thereby broadening its role from simple looking in managing conditions , such as upper GI bleeding or potential lesions as explained by Tringali et al. (2017). Furthermore, EGD performs a critical role in the management of the majority of gastrointestinal emergencies. For instance, when there is massive gastrointestinal bleeding, the endoscopic approach allows for timely therapeutic interventions , such as banding or clipping, to halt hemorrhage. This efficiency is exemplified by its application in the treatment of corrosive ingestion or foreign body trauma complications, where visual control can be potentially crucial to effect removal or management of damaged tissue safely.

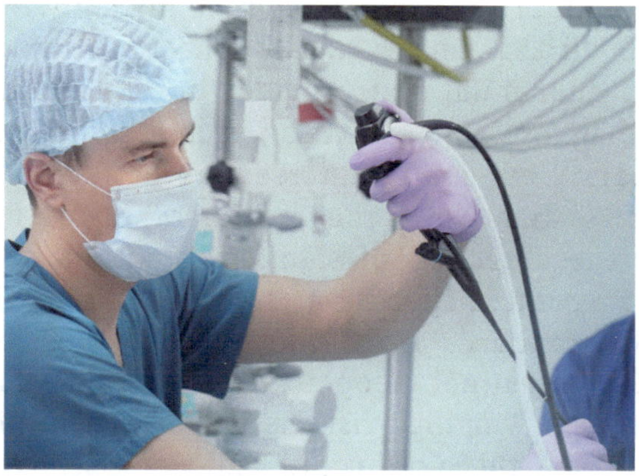

Figure 4.4. Upper endoscopy procedure.

Source: https://medlineplus.gov/images/Endoscopy_share.jpg.

The technique also serves as a valuable diagnostic aid for more long-term conditions like motility disorders and malignancies. For instance, evaluation of a patient with previous iron deficiency anemia and occult GI blood loss can necessitate a combination of diagnostic procedures like EGD, as indicated under duodenal adenocarcinoma management discussion in Berger et al. (2010). Preparation and follow-up that accompany EGD are also essential in ensuring optimal benefits. Patients typically have a pre-procedure workup, including fasting and the stopping of some medications that will compromise the procedure or recovery post-procedure. Post-EGDEX, patients are monitored while the anesthesia wears off, typically requiring education in diet habits and identification of signs of complications, including infection and bleeding. The technological progress of endoscopic techniques not only enhanced diagnostic accuracy but also reduced procedural morbidity and recovery times, to showcase the overall safety of EGD as a procedure. The interdisciplinarity of patient care—integrating pre-procedure management, procedure execution, and post-procedure care—demonstrates the wholistic approach of EGD in upper GI well-being as sworn by widespread inclusion in recent guidelines (Tringali et al., 2017) (Figure 4.4).

4.1. Indications for Esophagogastroduodenoscopy (EGD)

Upper GI endoscopy (EGD) possesses a varied set of diagnostic and therapeutic indications, reflecting its essential role in modern gastroenterology. In practice, the most significant indications for EGD are symptom evaluation , such as dysphagia, chronic gastrointestinal bleed, or recurrent abdominal pain or vomiting. Dysphagia or swallowing difficulty may be indicative of structural disease like stricture or malignancy and warrants visualization of the esophagus. Similarly, chronic gastrointestinal bleeding is caused by pathologies like peptic ulcers or variceal bleeding and therefore needs immediate evaluation and possibly therapeutic intervention. With direct visualization, EGD not only allows doctors to diagnose but even treat various lesions, highlighting its significance not merely as a diagnostic tool but also as a therapeutic option. Beyond the accepted clinical indications, EGD is also important in the management of more exotic gastrointestinal complications. For instance, guidelines state that EGD is indicated in patients with conditions , such as Barrett's esophagus, where surveillance is necessary to prevent the development of esophageal cancer. The test is relatively safe and can identify precancerous lesions that may otherwise not be detected (Gross et al., 2017). EGD is also indicated in foreign body ingestions and corrosive injury, where early intervention may be required to prevent further complications. Identification of these specific signs demonstrates the extent of EGD applications, beyond straightforward diagnosis to various therapeutic roles. For youngsters, utilization of EGD may bear minor variation from its usage in adults, in light of the unique challenges that come with pediatric patients. Indications for EGD in children include chronic gastrointestinal symptoms, foreign body ingestion, and evaluation of inflammatory bowel diseases. A guideline for these pediatric applications is directed to the significance of proper training and updating of skill in practitioners performing such processes (Tringali et al., 2017). EGD also can enable interventions , such as balloon dilatation for strictures in esophageal atresia or inflammatory disorders. By tailoring the use of EGD to the specific requirements of various age groups, clinicians can deliver optimal care to all the groups, further justifying the application of this endoscopic technique in diagnosis and therapy (Figure 4.5).

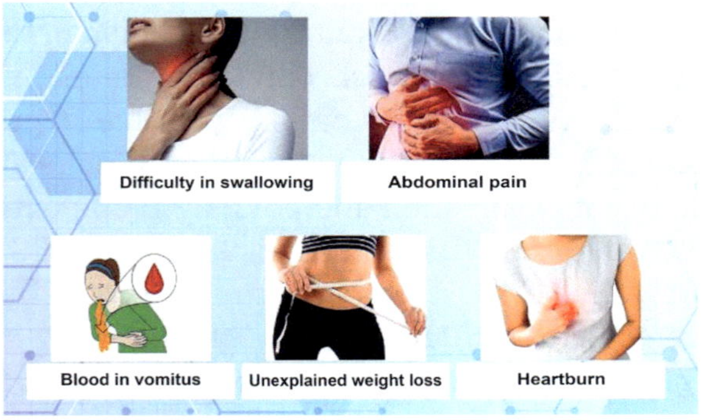

Figure 4.5. Upper Gi endoscopy indications types.

Source: https://healthsoul.s3.amazonaws.com/uploads/ec9ea02f-ef57-4856-afe4-f057e96b3c2a.jpg.

4.1.1. Evaluation of Gastrointestinal Symptoms

The evaluation of gastrointestinal symptoms is critical in making underlying conditions that will necessitate subsequent diagnostic procedures , such as upper gastrointestinal endoscopy (EGD). The three most frequent presenting symptoms are dysphagia, gastrointestinal bleeding, and persistent abdominal pain, prompting clinicians to think of EGD as a diagnostic modality. The EGD directly images the esophagus, stomach, and duodenum and provides an opportunity to diagnose abnormalities , such as strictures, ulcers, or malignancies. Evidence also shows that while the revival of endoscopy for the detection of significant pathology is often context-specific, it remains one of the gold standards in the detection of possible gastrointestinal neoplasia or inflammation, particularly in high-risk individuals. The utility of EGD is therefore contingent upon sensitive symptom evaluation, which can help clinicians make informed decisions regarding procedural necessity (Gross et al., 2017). In addition, in children, evaluation of gastrointestinal symptoms generally necessitates an adapted strategy due to variations in gastrointestinal disorders between children and adults. Symptoms that suggest EGD in children cover a range of diseases, including dysphagia, vomiting, and abdominal pain, and can be manifestations of severe underlying pathology, for example, inflammatory bowel disease or foreign body ingestion. As highlighted in national guidelines for pediatric endoscopy, identification of the special indications can maximize the minimization of inappropriate procedures while allowing timely intervention in the at-risk group. These assessments should be determined by clinicians carefully, maximizing diagnostic accuracy versus the accompanying risks of endoscopic procedures (Tringali et al., 2017). These efforts ultimately maximize patient safety and maximize gastrointestinal symptom management overall. Moreover, an effective evaluation is important in separating benign from potentially malignant gastrointestinal illnesses, especially in patients with alarming features , such as weight loss or anemia. The presence of such symptoms will encourage a more aggressive diagnostic approach, including the use of EGD in establishing potential malignancies or other serious gastrointestinal diseases. Findings on EGD have been meaningful in the management of conditions like Barrett's esophagus, a risk factor for esophageal cancer. Studies indicate decreased yield of malignancy in certain patient populations, and therefore symptom evaluation should guide selective application of EGD to enhance patient benefit. By the integration of clinical evaluations, the effectiveness of procedures, and the related risk factors, the assessment of gastrointestinal symptoms continues to evolve, so interventions like EGD continue to be relevant and clinically effective (Gross et al., 2017) (Figure 4.6).

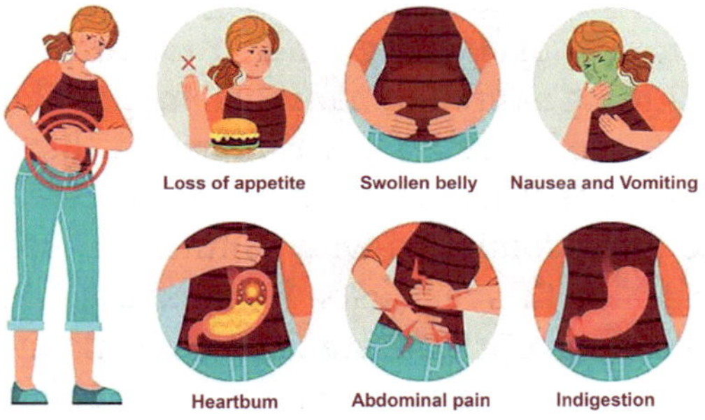

Figure 4.6. These are the symptoms of gastrointestinal syndrome.

Source: https://cdn.medizzy.com/XMvWXN4zZ4iACGtYHoVJynit5lI=/680x453/img/posts/91d4fbd2-3cac-41a7-94fb-d23caca1a789.

4.1.2. Diagnosis of Esophageal Disorders

The multifaceted diagnostic processes of the determination of esophageal disorders are focal, particularly in the application of upper gastrointestinal endoscopy or EGD. This minimally intrusive procedure allows direct endoscopic visualization of the esophagus, enabling visual detection of varied conditions , such as strictures, lesions, and inflammation. Among the common indications for EGD is dysphagia, which may result from mechanical obstruction or inflammatory diseases , such as eosinophilic esophagitis. Accurate diagnosis necessitates awareness of the potential underlying etiologies, including gastroesophageal reflux disease (GERD) and viral or fungal esophagitis, which are known to present with similar clinical features. In addition, growing appreciation of conditions like rumination syndrome highlights the importance of precise evaluations to differentiate them from more common esophageal illnesses (Tringali et al., 2017). Ultimately, precise and timely diagnosis with EGD can significantly improve patient management and outcome. In esophageal disease diagnosis, the role of EGD is greater than mere visualization. The procedure permits therapeutic maneuvers of a different sort, such that it gains added diagnostic significance. EGD, for example, can be utilized to obtain a biopsy from suspect lesions, with histological diagnosis afterward identifying malignancies or inflammation. Besides, endoscopic assessment is particularly valuable in bleeding of the esophagus, where EGD is not just diagnostic of etiology but therapeutic as well, for example, cauterization or varices banding. The guidelines to EGD underscore its application in a number of clinical scenarios, such as foreign body removal and corrosive injury treatment, wherein immediate intervention can prevent further complications (Tringali et al., 2017). From these multiple uses, EGD is a crucial part of the overall process of diagnosing and managing esophageal diseases. Result interpretation during EGD plays a critical role in accurate diagnosis and in planning the management plan. Heterogeneity of clinical presentation and symptoms, particularly in esophageal diseases, demands careful consideration while evaluating. For instance, erosive esophagitis and eosinophilic esophagitis may present with dysphagia or chest pain, posing a challenge to the clinical decision-making process. Research has shown that a full upper gastrointestinal workup, for instance, EGD, can uncover unorthodox presentations of common diseases. Patients in some cases may present with symptomatology common in rumination syndrome in addition to severe esophageal lesions that require treatment (Sidhu & Rick, 2009). This helps in emphasizing the necessity for incorporating a broad differential diagnosis in addition to the endoscopic presentation. As clinical knowledge of disorder advances, so must the practices adopted in treatment and diagnosis, affirming the vital place of EGD in the overall care of the esophagus (Figure 4.7).

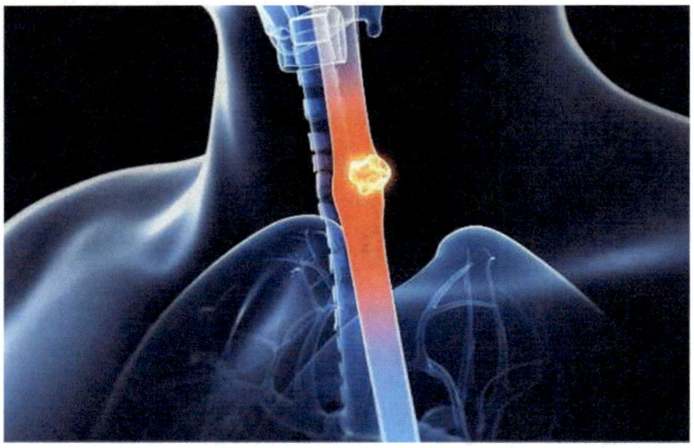

Figure 4.7. Esophageal disorders.

Source: https://www.dradityagastro.com/images/understanding-esophageal-disorders-symptoms-types-and-treatment-options.jpg.

4.1.3. Assessment of Gastric and Duodenal Conditions

Assessment of gastric and duodenal conditions through upper gastrointestinal endoscopy, that is, EGD, plays a pivotal role in the clinical management of symptomatic patients of the gastrointestinal tract. This procedure permits visualization of the esophagus, stomach, and duodenum directly and facilitates accurate inspection and diagnosis of several pathologies , such as peptic ulcers, erosive gastritis, and neoplastic lesions. The advantage of EGD extends beyond mere diagnosis since it also permits therapeutic interventions , such as biopsies, stricture dilatation, and foreign body removal. The use of EGD in younger populations, namely children with idiopathic gastrointestinal symptoms, necessitates the use of specific guidelines addressing the unique challenges encountered in this age group. As quoted in the guidelines, indications for EGD encompass a wide range of diagnostic indications aimed at optimizing patient care (Tringali et al., 2017). Technical advancements in endoscopy have similarly enhanced the efficiency of tests performed during EGD. The incorporation of endoscopic ultrasonography (EUS) has greatly enhanced the assessment of subepithelial lesions and deeper tissues surrounding the gastrointestinal tract by giving the clinician valuable information that standard EGD might miss. Consequently, application of adjunctive techniques , such as wireless capsule endoscopy and double balloon enteroscopy has expanded the range of gastric and duodenal tests, constituting a three-dimensional method for the diagnosis of obscure gastrointestinal bleeding and other disorders. The consistent evolution of these tests, combined with continuous training courses for GI specialists, remains essential in maintaining optimal standards in diagnostic accuracy and patient safety (Nguyen et al., 2010). Considering the above advancements, assessment of gastric and duodenal conditions during EGD not only meets the prescribed guideline but also emphasizes the importance of patient-based care strategies. Physicians must keep themselves updated with the dynamic landscape of endoscopic practices so that the most recent recommendations and guidelines are integrated into daily practice. The ability to rapidly and accurately diagnose life-threatening disease can significantly influence the success of treatment and quality of life for patients, thereby underlining the crucial role that EGD plays as a cornerstone of gastrointestinal medicine. As suggested by recent guidelines, correct utilization of EGD can lead to significant improvement in both treatment and diagnosis management, particularly relevant to chronic gastrointestinal disease and complication management due to illnesses , such as inflammatory bowel disease (Tringali et al., 2017).

4.2. Preparation for Esophagogastroduodenoscopy (EGD)

Preparation for an upper GI endoscopy (EGD) is a critically important process that has a significant bearing on the success of the procedure and patient safety. Patients are typically requested to undergo extensive pre-procedure work-ups before the endoscopy which may include physical examinations and health histories. Having an understanding of the patient's history of allergic reactions, current medication regimen, and previous medical illnesses is important because it may dictate the preparatory steps involved in the safe delivery of sedation as well as prepare the endoscopist to treat any potential complications. Additionally, patients are typically ordered to fast for a period of time, typically 6–8 hours, to reduce the risk of aspiration and improve visualization during the procedure. This period of fasting is critical, and one needs to adhere to this advice to prepare themselves effectively for a successful EGD so that the procedure can be carried out in the best possible conditions without interruption or delay. Medication management is also an important aspect of EGD preparation that requires special consideration. Some medications may be requested to be stopped by the patient before the procedure, especially anticoagulants and NSAIDs, as they predispose to bleeding during and after endoscopy. This management is particularly applicable for those with chronic illness, whose drug regimens must be harmonized while keeping procedural risk to a minimum, which necessitates the use of clear communication between the healthcare provider and the patient. The healthcare team should provide clear guidance regarding which medications may be continued and which must be held temporarily. The patient education function in this case cannot be overstated, as accurate counseling works to eradicate fear of drug manipulation by patients and overall procedure anticipation, alongside facilitating drug preparation adherence vital to safety guarantee during EGD (Tringali et al., 2017). In addition to fasting and drug manipulation, psychosocial factors also play a very significant role in the overall preparation for EGD.

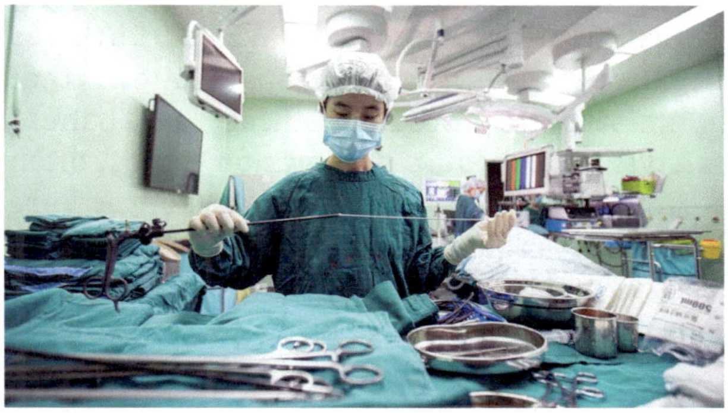

Figure 4.8. Esophagogastroduodenoscopy (EGD) procedure.

Source: https://i0.wp.com/post.medicalnewstoday.com/wp-content/uploads/sites/3/2022/08/what_esophagogastroduodenoscopy_GettyImages1232843685_Header-1024x575.jpg?w=1155&h=1528.

Anxiety and fear of the diagnostic procedure can overwhelm many patients, potentially affecting their adherence to pre-procedure protocols. For this reason, incorporating measures to reduce anxiety and improve patient comfort is an optimal practice for medical staff. It could involve preparing patients for what to expect from endoscopy and providing them with information regarding sedation and its impact, and reminding them of the skill and qualifications of the endoscopy team. Educative sessions and counseling may also serve to demystify fears regarding potential outcomes, thus making the patient better equipped for the procedure. Furthermore, as highlighted in such guidelines, collaboration among healthcare workers and patients provides a platform where questions can freely be answered, resulting in making patients feel consulted and informed in their preparation period for an EGD (Tringali et al., 2017) (Figure 4.8).

4.2.1. Pre-procedure Instructions for Patients

Preparation of a patient for an upper gastrointestinal endoscopy (EGD) involves significant pre-procedure instructions that optimize both procedure efficacy and patient safety. Pre-procedure preparation is most often attained through diet modification, where patients are required to refrain from eating for at least six to eight hours before the examination. This fasting time is required to ensure that the stomach is free from food particles so that the upper gastrointestinal tract can be better visualized. Patients are also typically cautioned against taking certain medications , such as blood thinners or nonsteroidal anti-inflammatory drugs, that have the risk of causing bleeding complications during the procedure. By adhering to these guidelines, patients are themselves a significant contributor to their safety, minimizing any risk of complications and ensuring the endoscopic experience is as efficient as possible. In addition to diet limits, adherence also a significant influenced by patient education. Anxiety and nervousness regarding the procedure are the primary obstacles noted by many patients, which can deter them from undergoing an EGD. It is necessary that the healthcare providers correctly explain the rationale for the pre-procedure preparations. Knowledge of the reason for fasting and stopping medications can demystify patients' fears. This is necessary considering the fact that studies, such as the ones reported in Lionis et al. (2011), indicate that a significant percentage of patients may refuse to go through the procedure due to ignorance or misinformation about endoscopy. Therefore, informed discussions that demystify the importance of pre-procedure instructions can lead to improved compliance and patient outcomes. Management of psychosocial issues is also an important aspect of preparing a patient for EGD. Anxiety, health literacy, and socio-demographics can have a significant impact on adherence to pre-procedure instructions. Family and friend social support and reassurance from healthcare professionals can have a positive influence on patient attitudes about the procedure. Research highlighted in Abdelmohsen et al. (2018) has proven that endoscopy processes' routine auditing can improve procedural performance indirectly, portraying the importance of proper patient education. As patients are assisted and properly educated, it enhances their overall experience as well as allows the timely completion of the procedure. Thus, there is a need for health care providers to make pre-procedure instructions clear, supportive, and individualized to meet the diverse needs of their patient populations (Figure 4.9).

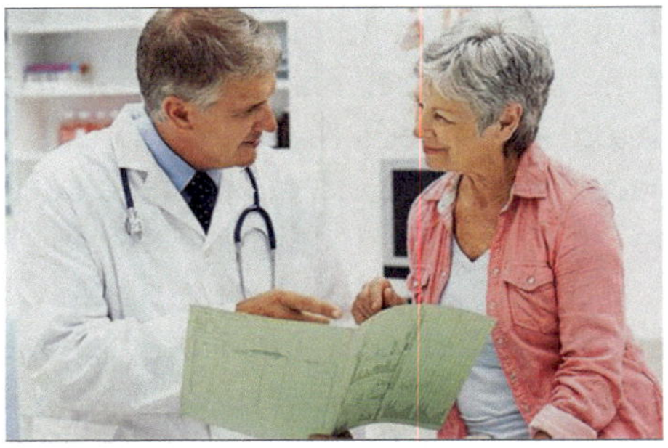

Figure 4.9. Pre-procedure instructions.

Source: https://external-content.duckduckgo.com/iu/?u=https%3A%2F%2Ftse3.mm.bing.net%2Fth%3Fid%3DOIP.MC8aVFux7FNmEKu0IJwfLgHaE8%26pid%3DApi&f=1&ipt=80a47b65d63535faed847885ccfb4441f3d2e6f7721430ade62844239079a9b1.

4.2.2. Dietary Restrictions Before the Procedure

Preparation for an upper gastrointestinal endoscopy (EGD) is made up of certain dietary restrictions that are of paramount importance in aiding to provide optimal visualization and evaluation during the procedure. The patients are typically asked to remain on a clear liquid diet for at least 24 hours before EGD. This dietary limitation decreases the quantity of solid food in the stomach and lowers the risk of aspiration due to sedation, thereby maintaining patient safety. Clear liquids , such as water, broth, and certain juices, are preferred, while beverages that leave residues, such as milk or alcohol, should be avoided. By adhering to these guidelines, not only is imaging clearer, but it also facilitates the taking of precise histological examination in case biopsies are needed intra-procedure. Patients undergoing an EGD also usually get advice they refrain from any solid foods and usually beginning the evening before their visit. This restriction is especially significant for individuals with pre-existing gastrointestinal pathology, such as GERD, because it allows more selective examination of the esophagus, stomach, and duodenum. The preparation instructions for diets are designed to avoid interference with diagnostic findings by food particles and thus maximize endoscopists' ability to detect abnormalities , such as esophagitis or gastric ulcers. Adherence to pre-procedure dietary limitations significantly impacts the quality of the endoscopic procedure and the reliability of the resultant findings, especially where biopsy is being performed to rule out conditions like eosinophilic esophagitis or gastric cancer. Beyond avoiding solid foods, patients also need to avoid some medications and supplements that will likely affect gastrointestinal function or bleeding risk before the EGD. They are normally advised to avoid anticoagulants and NSAIDs, as these can result in excessive bleeding both during and after the procedure. Drug and dietary restriction education is essential for patients, particularly vulnerable populations , such as children, as seen in a study that highlights the challenge of separating functional from organic gastrointestinal disorders (Helin et al., 2021). Particular dietary protocols, including avoidance of potentially offending foods and products, optimize the safety and efficacy of the EGD, ultimately enhancing patients' gastrointestinal care (Azueta et al., 2010).

4.2.3. Medications and Anesthesia Considerations

Inclusion of medications and anesthesia considerations in Upper Gastrointestinal Endoscopy (EGD) is critical to ensuring patients' safety and comfort. Procedural requirements demand the use of proper sedation methods for relief of pain that is associated with endoscopic examination. Moderate sedation, typically achieved with administration of a mixture of opioids and benzodiazepines, has been the dominant approach for EGD procedures. The need for quick recovery from sedation and efficient discharge processes has, however, created interest in alternative approaches to sedation. Particularly, sedation by anesthesiology staff with medications like propofol is emerging as a desirable consideration on the basis of its potential to cause greater patient comfort and shorter recovery times in the post-anesthesia care unit (PACU) (Tringali et al., 2017). Finally, it is important to consider certain patient factors when selecting appropriate sedation protocols for EGD. Factors , including patient age, history, and risk classification, all contribute to the optimal anesthetic approach. Because the population in question for EGD often includes both children and older adults, customized sedation regimens are most important. Children, for instance, may require individually tailored dosing protocols due to their pharmacokinetic differences. In addition, the administration of sedation in patients with chronic health conditions necessitates utmost caution to prevent side effects (Tringali et al., 2017).

An anesthesiology protocol for such patients calls for special emphasis on pre-procedure assessments to ensure that the chosen medications match the patient's individual health condition and procedural requirements. The selection of drugs and anesthetic forms to employ in EGD affects not only procedure duration but also broader implications for the success of healthcare. As the latest evidence has revealed, propofol administration for sedation has had significantly shorter discharge rates than traditional sedation, even though the cost could be heightened (Tringali et al., 2017). This reduction in the duration of recovery time can facilitate a higher turnover of patients, ultimately optimizing efficiency of operations in clinical settings. While increased speed of discharge is a desirable variable to take into consideration, cost considerations should not be overlooked; health care professionals must weigh the increased costs of propofol administration against possible returns on revenue from performing additional procedures (Mancini, 2017). Thus, a careful consideration of medication and anesthesia issues is essential in optimizing patient care in EGD surgery (Figure 4.10).

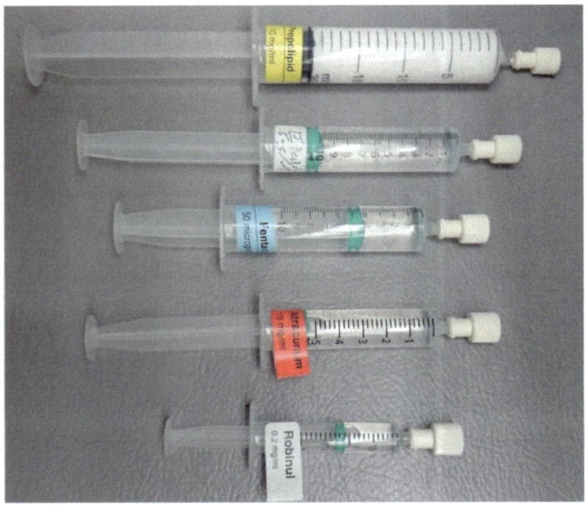

Figure 4.10. Anesthesia medications.

Source: https://upload.wikimedia.org/wikipedia/commons/thumb/e/ed/Anesthesia_medications.JPG/1200px-Anesthesia_medications.JPG.

4.3. The Esophago-gastroduodenoscopy (EGD) Procedure

The EGD procedure, clinically referred to as esophagogastroduodenoscopy, is a significant diagnostic and therapeutic tool for gastroenterology. This minimally invasive technique allows for direct visualization of the esophagus, stomach, and duodenum, thereby enabling the identification of many gastrointestinal disorders , such as inflammation, ulcers, and tumors. The technique is done through insertion of a flexible endoscope with an internal camera via the mouth and pressing it down into the gastrointestinal tract. Specific interventions , such as biopsies or polypectomies, can be made by practitioners to further enhance overall diagnostic yield and treatment efficiency. Therefore, the clinical usefulness of the EGD is more than mere observation; it promotes management of pathologies identified in real time, which will improve patient outcomes. The safety profile of EGD has been an area of emphasis, particularly in those patients with comorbidities that would potentially increase the difficulty of the procedure. For instance, patients with a history of myocardial infarction (MI) have an elevated risk of complications, like cardiopulmonary events, when undergoing endoscopic procedures. A retrospective cohort study demonstrated that MI patients tend to have a catalog of comorbid conditions, whose care process during EGD becomes more complicated (Al-Ebrahim et al., 2012). While the risk of complications is considerable, having the ability to diagnose and treat gastrointestinal bleeding in MI patients may outweigh potential negative effects. The outcomes underscore the need for accurate assessment and customized pre-procedure testing to ensure that the benefits of EGD are optimized and possible concomitant risks are prevented. Additionally, the EGD process is pivotal in diagnosing aggressive gastrointestinal neoplasias early, particularly in high-risk populations. A recent research estimated the impact of an endoscopic screening program in patients with neoplasms of the head and neck, where a high proportion of patients presented synchronous gastro-esophageal neoplasias (Luis, 2024). The ability to diagnose such lesions at an early stage permits immediate interventions, which play a central role in improving prognosis. Here, the use of systematic endoscopic screening can be life-saving in its intervention, cutting down on cases of advanced cancer. Thus, EGD not only enhances the accuracy of diagnosis but also forms a part of cancer preventive programs among high-risk populations (Figure 4.11).

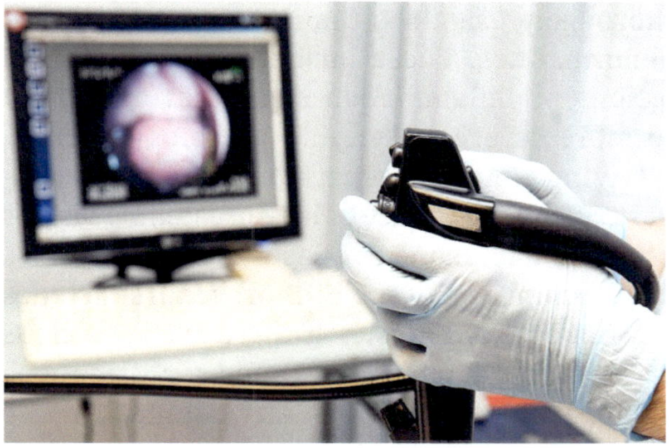

Figure 4.11. Esophagogastroduodenoscopy (EGD) procedure.

Source: https://www.verywellhealth.com/thmb/IzaXEulXhhFQvNQBkW8zWMZbbA8=/1024x683/filters:fill(87E3EF,1)/GettyImages-459771136-569755795f9b58eba49e59b2.jpg.

4.3.1. Description of the Equipment Used

Equipment utilized in upper gastrointestinal endoscopy, particularly in EGD, is a critical component of the success and comfort of the procedure. The primary instrument utilized is the flexible endoscope, a state-of-the-art device containing an embedded camera and light source that allows for high-definition visualization of the esophagus, stomach, and duodenum. These endoscopes have also made much advancement, with devices now available in various diameters to assist in comfort for patients and ease of entry. Miniature endoscopy, assisted by ultrathin endoscopes, has facilitated patient acceptability as well as discomfort relief, allowing easy observation of the gastrointestinal tract while maintaining instrument-related distress to a minimum. These advances are part of an overall trend to improve the efficacy and safety of gastrointestinal intervention in clinical practice (Ching et al., 2022). In addition, the performance of ancillary devices during EGD is the evolution of the examination procedure. Ancillary devices , such as biopsy forceps and snares, are employed for the excision of tissue and lesions with the maintenance of the integrity of adjacent structures. These instruments are made for exact maneuverability, using sophisticated engineering to handle the complex anatomy of the upper GI tract. Advances in instrumentation in recent studies show that changes to allow less patient discomfort during procedures play an important role in overall patient satisfaction. For instance, comparisons of traditional EGD and emerging technologies , such as magnet-controlled capsule endoscopy, have shown significant differences in patient tolerance, with patients describing less distress who are subjected to examinations that are less invasive (Ching et al., 2022). Miniaturization for endoscopic instruments is a watershed in technology and method. As noted in the literature, more compact equipment maximizes access to the alimentary tract, providing safer procedures and greater patient acceptability. The technology includes various technologies, including wireless and scanning fiber endoscopies, that maximize diagnostic capability while addressing past drawbacks with longer, more unmanageable scopes. Through the implementation of these newer technologies, medical professionals can offer more investigation and management of gastrointestinal disease. The ongoing process of designing and manufacturing endoscopic equipment not only ensure more accurate diagnosis but also aim to improve overall process experience for subjects undergoing EGD. (Haidry et al., 2019) (Figure 4.12).

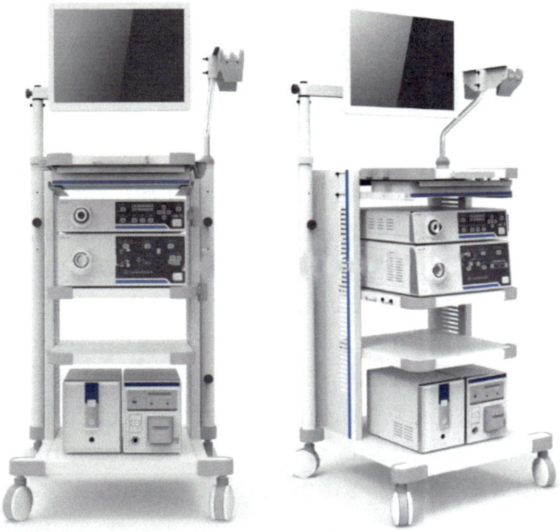

Figure 4.12. Profession medical equipment Aq-100 video endoscopy camera.

Source: https://sc01.alicdn.com/kf/Hc606711def784036952104fddff4791e6/227814542/Hc606711def784036952104fddff4791e6.jpg.

4.3.2. Step-by-Step Process of the Procedure

The step-by-step upper gastrointestinal endoscopy, or EGD, process begins with patient preparation. This step includes preparing patients who are about to undergo the procedure. Before the process, doctors ensure that the patient is well-informed about the process and why it is being done. Patients are usually advised against eating or drinking for at least six to eight hours before the test for an empty stomach, which is crucial to enable good imaging. Additionally, any medications that can affect blood clotting or stomach acid may need to be adjusted. Obtaining patient consent and assessing medical history, including any past gastrointestinal issues, allergies, or current medications, is important pre-procedure. This complete preparation is designed to maximize the safety and efficacy of the procedure as well as minimize potential complications that arise due to inadequate preparation. Once the preparations are completed, the EGD procedure starts with the administration of sedation or anesthesia to ensure patient comfort. This may involve intravenous sedation, so that there is a less tense state in which to carry out the test. The patient is then positioned comfortably, typically lying on his or her side, to enable easy access to the upper GI tract. The endoscope, a flexible tube with a camera and a light, is then passed through the mouth and guided down the esophagus, into the stomach, and into the duodenum. During this stage, the physician thoroughly examines the mucosal surfaces for abnormalities. These include the detection of lesions or inflammation signs that may point to more severe underlying pathology, thereby allowing immediate treatment if needed, particularly in the case of life-threatening lesions , such as malignancies (Rasul & Kandel, 2001). The termination of the EGD procedure includes the removal of biopsies if there are suspicious areas, and taking observations for diagnostic value. Following the visual examination, the endoscope is gradually withdrawn with a soft motion, allowing an exhaustive assessment of any potential complications arising from the procedure itself. Patients are monitored in a recovery room until the effects of sedation have dissipated, as well as their vital signs have normalized. Pre-discharge education regarding post-procedure care, resumption of normal activity and diet is provided. The importance of the outcome of the EGD can be significant, especially when pathological findings , such as gastritis or tumors are identified, influencing treatment and patient care in general (Arieira et al., 2019). Therefore, the EGD process not only assists in diagnosis but also plays a key role in guiding subsequent therapeutic interventions (Figure 4.13).

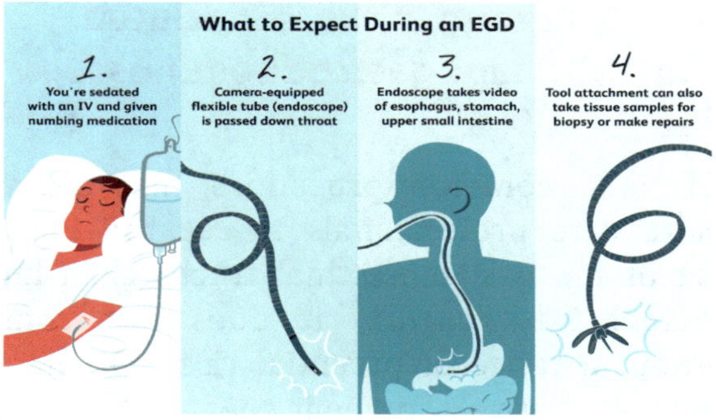

Figure 4.13. Esophagogastroduodenoscopy (EGD) procedure.

Source: https://www.verywellhealth.com/thmb/X-dYHwEMZldbqFuiHNZaYSTxJyI=/6000x4000/filters:no_upscale():max_bytes(150000):strip_icc()/1741797_color-5b9ab025c9e77c005088900b.png.

4.3.3. Duration and Setting of the Procedure

The duration and setting of an upper gastrointestinal endoscopy (EGD) are the determinants of both procedural success and patient experience. On average, the whole procedure may take 15–30 minutes, although this might be longer depending on the complexity of the case and the number of interventions that must be performed. Under ambulatory settings, such as endoscopy suites or specialized clinics, the procedure is often performed while under sedation to make the process more convenient to the patient. The procedural setting is optimized to be effective, with an emphasis on reducing waiting times and maximizing patient throughput safely and comfortably. Second, the handling of the patient position throughout the procedure is important, as ideal positioning can optimize visualization of the upper GI tract and, ultimately, procedural success. The foamy bubbles in the stomach and duodenum have a tendency to interfere with the visualization of the mucosal surface during EGD. Preemptive measures to decrease these phenomena have been observed to lower the incidence of these events considerably, thus reducing the procedure time by a notable extent. Research showed that administration of simethicone before EGD decreased the amount of gastric foam considerably and therefore facilitated easier visualization by endoscopists. This reduction not only improved imaging outcomes but also shortened the average duration of the endoscopy by around one minute to that of a placebo group. Such a finding points to the importance of considering pharmacological approaches that enhance clarity and make the procedure easier, ultimately benefiting both patients and physicians by making the endoscopy process more effective (Ahsan et al., 2011). The environment also plays an important role in the success of EGD as a whole. The use of dedicated endoscopic suites with advanced imaging technology can enhance the quality of the procedure and patient management. Compliance with indication guidelines for EGD is also important for optimizing procedure length. According to recommendations, correct patient selection based on their unique clinical conditions can lead to more focused examinations and interventions, reducing unnecessary procedure time. As the environment of gastrointestinal endoscopy evolves, with continuous advancements in environment, equipment, and pharmacologic support, these will remain centrally important to fine-tune the efficacy and effectiveness of EGDs (Tringali et al., 2017).

4.4. Risks and Complications

Upper GI endoscopy (EGD) is a valuable diagnostic tool, but it is not without risks and complications. Perhaps the most significant one is the risk for an adverse reaction to sedation or anesthesia during the procedure, leading to respiratory depression or cardiovascular instability. Patients with pre-existing medical conditions are potentially more prone to developing such complications. Furthermore, although rare, aspiration pneumonia secondary to sedation is a risk if the patient fails to adequately fast before the procedure. Knowledge of these risks is of significance to healthcare providers as well as patients as they weigh the benefits of EGD against possible adverse consequences. The other danger associated with EGD is the occurrence of procedural complications, albeit rare, with far-reaching implications. Please note that this answer doesn't fit well within any of the given categories. Perforation of the duodenum, esophagus, or stomach is a dangerous side effect that may occur during treatment, particularly if biopsies, polypectomies or therapeutic dilations are performed. The condition will result in life-threatening infections or peritonitis and will require surgical intervention. Bleeding within the biopsies or the treatments themselves is also possible, with a requirement for careful monitoring or specialized maneuvers to manage it.

Awareness of such risks allows medical practitioners to apply protective strategies and take immediate action i complications arise during the procedure. Besides physical risks, there are also psychosocial issues that can complicate the post-procedure scenario for patients. The psychological weight of having to undergo an invasive diagnostic test is significant and has the tendency to lead to elevated levels of anxiety or stress. Where findings from EGD point towards critical conditions, such as malignancies or chronic gastrointestinal illnesses, patients are more likely to be anxious about their health status. Besides, conditions , such as spontaneous bacterial infection or *Helicobacter pylori* status, while not necessarily connected with the procedure in itself, might also affect the patient's original diagnosis or treatment path, highlighting the correlation between body and mind in medical procedures (Nilsson, 2016; Tringali et al., 2017).

4.4.1. Common Risks Associated with Esophagogastroduodenoscopy (EGD)

EGD is a common procedure that allows health care professionals to see the upper part of the gastrointestinal tract. As in any medical intervention, it does not come without a range of potential risks. Of these, the most relatively frequent ones are bleeding, perforation, and infection. Bleeding tends to occur at the site of biopsy or the removal of polyps, particularly in patients with pre-existing coagulopathies or who are on anticoagulation therapy. Perforation is one of the potentially life-threatening complications that, although uncommon, will require an operation. Though infection is uncommon with the use of sterile precautions, it is still a possibility for some, i.e., immunocompromised patients. Allowing individuals to understand these complications is critical for those considering EGD because informed consent is essential in any procedure decision-making. Other than for direct risk from EGD, complications may occur in the longer term as well. Such patients with conditions , such as dermatomyositis may be particularly vulnerable to gastrointestinal neoplasia, as reported in studies on the incidence of upper endoscopic findings in such patients. Specifically, studies indicated that while the return of endoscopy in such patients is low, it does trigger awareness of the necessity for close follow-up for malignant changes (Gross et al., 2017). In patients undergoing EGD, close observation for long-term complications also assigns great importance to meticulous pre-procedure evaluation and ongoing post-procedure follow-up. This warning is particularly crucial not only to look after any urgent complications but also to manage any long-term or novel threats that will be made evident after the procedure. Furthermore, having pre-existing gastrointestinal conditions may complicate the threat of EGD. As an illustration, individuals with ulcerative colitis are particularly challenging, as investigations have reported a notable prevalence of upper gastrointestinal lesions in such individuals (Hiraoka et al., 2018). When they do occur, risks of the EGD can be heightened, namely the complication risk. These patients typically present with more severe disease and high comorbidities, necessitating a tailored course of management. Providers must weigh the necessity for performance of the EGD against the higher risk of adverse outcomes in such groups. Last but not least, meticulous patient planning and education are most significant to optimally achieve the potential benefits of EGD. This will allow the optimal optimization of patient outcomes and care.

4.4.2. Rare but Serious Complications

Though upper gastrointestinal endoscopy, or EGD, is widely regarded as safe and effective, the procedure is not exempt from the risk of rare but serious complications. Potential side effects can range from gastrointestinal tract perforation to massive bleeding, each with its unique challenges in the clinical setting. Perforation, occurring in about 1 in 1,000–2,000 cases, may lead to peritonitis if prompt treatment is not done, requiring surgery. Bleeding may also occur at the site of banding or biopsy, and this would require emergency endoscopic treatment or even hospital admission. Appreciation of these complications underscores the importance of operator skill and readiness for procedure, where proper training must be ensured to cope well in these rare occurrences. Furthermore, EGD complications may have more significant implications for patient populations who have special medical histories. Older patients, for instance, normally carry various comorbidities that complicate recovery from EGD complications. Research has pointed out that while the risk of complications can be viewed as greater in this age group, the therapeutic success of EGD still remains greater than the risks, even in patients older than 90 (Chang & Lei, 2007). Furthermore, additional precautions , such as monitoring of vital signs closely and pre-procedural testing, are critical in this age group to minimize complications. These figures and practices prove that, although EGD is relatively safe, caution in patient selection and procedure performance is necessary to limit risks. Finally, attention to rare complications must also include the late effects that can occur after an EGD procedure. Although immediate complications are usually foremost in our minds, the risk of post-endoscopic syndromes like post-ERCP pancreatitis reminds us to ensure complete follow-up care. The risk of pancreatitis after ERCP ranges from 3%–10%, and this is based on a number of variables , including the type of procedure and the patient's background (Tringali et al., 2017). This complication can lead to prolonged recovery, additional cost of care, and impaired quality of life, which necessitates a severe risk-benefit discussion before procedure of EGD. The study of such rare but severe complications again highlights the importance of informed consent and active patient involvement in planning their own care.

4.4.3. Management of Complications if They Occur

Complication management after upper gastrointestinal endoscopy (EGD) is critical to ensure patient safety and improve outcomes. Bleeding is one of the commonly seen complications and can occur at the polypectomy or biopsy site. In these cases, immediate control of hemorrhage is necessary. This can be done by endoscopic techniques , such as cauterization or clipping, which can cure the site of bleeding effectively. In addition to this, the hemodynamic status of the patients should be constantly monitored by the health care team since massive bleeding can lead to hypovolemic shock. Monitoring post-procedure for signs of continued bleeding is essential, particularly in the case of patients with coagulopathies or on anticoagulants. The practitioners need to be competent enough to detect and manage such a complication early to reduce EGD morbidity, according to guidelines suggested (Tringali et al., 2017). Perforation of the esophagus or the remaining gastrointestinal tract is another severe complication that occurs infrequently but needs urgent surgery. The presentation is typically severe abdominal pain, fever, and sepsis symptoms. Early identification and treatment are crucial; hence, close postoperative monitoring is appropriate to recognize potential symptoms. Perforation should be suspected early, and imaging of the abdomen , such as a CT scan, should be performed early to confirm the diagnosis. Surgical closure, frequently by laparotomy, may be necessary to successfully close the perforation. Moreover, active case-finding strategies , such as individual patient selection and algorithm-optimized procedural techniques, are crucial to decreasing the risk of perforation when undertaking EGD procedures. Awareness of the effects of perforation and the timing of intervention may affect the outcomes of patients after undergoing EGD procedures (Fuhs et al., 2016). Lastly, infection complications may ensue, particularly with invasive techniques , such as EGD. Even though the risk is low, transmission of the pathogens during instrumentation results in post-procedure infections , such as esophagitis or pneumonia. Precautions , such as instrument sterilization and strict infection control procedures during the procedure are necessary in avoiding these complications. When infection does take place, early detection and implementation of appropriate antibiotic therapy are crucial to the treatment of the condition of patients optimally. Regular training and retraining courses in infection prevention procedures among endoscopy staff also ensure heightened patient safety. Overall, the ability to anticipate complications through adequate control measures ensures better patient outcomes following EGD and proves the merit of rigid compliance with suggested clinical guidelines (Tringali et al., 2017) (Figure 4.14).

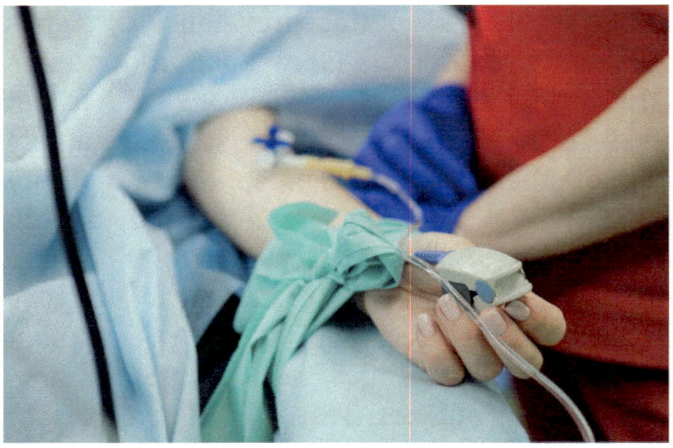

Figure 4.14. Medical complications.

Source: https://healthscopemag.com/wp-content/uploads/2021/05/olga-kononenko-98_MsKaUsI-unsplash-2048x1365.jpg.

4.5. Post-Procedure Care

Once an upper gastrointestinal endoscopy (EGD) has been performed, post-procedure care is necessary to avoid injuring the patient and assist with recovery. Afterward, patients are usually monitored for any sign of adverse reaction to sedation, including over-sedation or respiratory depression. Due to possible risk from sedation, especially in vulnerable patients , such as the elderly, precautions must be exercised to prevent complications. Evidence indicates that excessive doses of sedation drugs are responsible for unnecessary morbidity and mortality, particularly in the elderly population, thus highlighting the significance of following established guidelines for sedation dosing during procedures (Lord et al., 2006). Informing a person of how they feel post-procedure and monitoring for any potential side effects facilitates effective recovery and reassures patients throughout this process. Following the procedure, patients are normally instructed not to eat and drink for a while, allowing any residual anesthesia to dissipate.

This fasting from food and liquid is crucial in preventing complications , such as aspiration, especially since the gag reflex may temporarily be depressed. Following the initial postoperative healing time has passed, a gradual resumption of oral intake is usually advised, starting with clear liquids and gradually advancing to a solid diet. Patient teaching regarding recognizing signs that necessitate immediate medical care, such as abdominal distress or fever, is also an essential aspect of care. This education facilitates empowering the patient, in that they are made aware of potential complications that can arise after an EGD and can intervene accordingly when necessary.

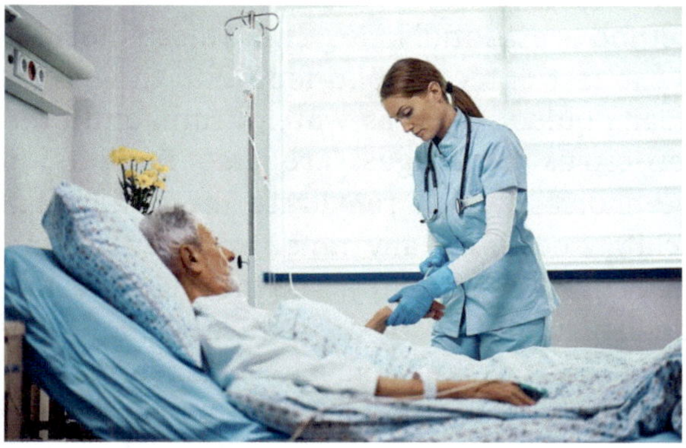

Figure 4.15. Post-operative care.

Source: https://sukinohealthcare.com/wp-content/uploads/2023/06/Post-operative-cares-1024x683.jpg.

Also, the follow-up visit and further diagnostic testing can be warranted based on what is discovered by endoscopy. If biopsies had been taken or lesions identified, the post-procedure course will often include a follow-up visit at a specified time to receive pathology reports and potential interventions. These follow-up appointments not only offer a forum for the discussion of outcomes, but also as an opportunity to plan further screening or surveillance modalities, especially given in the situation of gastrointestinal neoplasms (Gerada, 2012). Reassuring patients that they understand the importance of these follow-ups can have a dramatic impact on their overall long-term health outcomes, particularly in at-risk populations for conditions diagnosed by endoscopic evaluation. Generally speaking, intensive post-procedure care plays a significant role in facilitating maximum patient outcomes during the process of performing an EGD (Figure 4.15).

4.5.1. Recovery Process and Monitoring

Recovery from an upper gastrointestinal endoscopy (EGD) is of great importance to facilitate patient safety and comfort. Monitoring after the procedure is normally conducted in the recovery room, where patients are observed for any emergent complications , such as bleeding or perforation. Nursing staff assesses vital signs, level of consciousness, and any sign of distress, ensuring that the patient is returning to the baseline state. This is important because the action of sedative medication administered during the procedure can last long, and that needs careful surveillance. Patient teaching during this period is extremely important; patients are taught how to monitor themselves when they return home, which helps to detect early possible complications. Such rigorous post-procedure follow-up not only enhances outcomes but also reinforces faith in the healthcare system, gaining adherence to follow-up care protocols. The presence of quality monitoring in the recovery process can play a significant role in greatly impacting the effectiveness of EGD procedures greatly impact. Regular audits and assessments have been found to enhance performance metrics in endoscopy practice. For example, a yearly review conducted over the course of 10 years revealed notable improvements in completion rates and successful initial hemostasis in EGDs, as indicated in results where the completion rate improved to an average of 99% during the last five years of the study (Abdelmohsen et al., 2018). This information demonstrates the positive correlation between meticulous performance monitoring and procedure outcomes. These audits provide a forum for the determination of areas to change, ultimately leading to better patient care. By continually refining their practices based on audit feedback, healthcare professionals ensure a culture of learning and improvement, which is central to the effective recovery and follow-up of patients after EGDS. Continuous evaluation of the recovery of patients is also pivotal towards enhancing procedural protocols and the patient's experience.

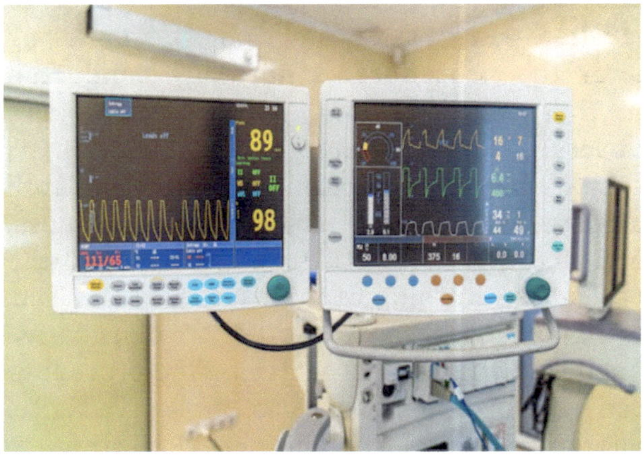

Figure 4.16. Recovery monitoring.

Source: https://img.freepik.com/premium-photo/hospital-recovery-monitoring-check-up-emergency-technologies_116317-21167.jpg.

Follow-up also does not cease when the patient leaves the recovery room; follow-up visits play a crucial role in measuring the success of the EGD and addressing persisting symptoms. Procedures for endoscopy in designated populations , such as pediatric patients, call for continued upkeep of healthcare provider technique and proficiency to render high-quality services (Tringali et al., 2017). These guidelines are crucial to the proceduralists as well as to the people who oversee recovery because they ensure all staff are in a position to detect early complications. Through an emphasis on such protocols and constant refinement, healthcare workers have the ability to significantly enhance the safety and efficacy of recovery following an EGD, lowering complications and maintaining favorable patient outcomes (Figure 4.16).

4.5.2. Dietary Recommendations After Esophagogastroduodenoscopy (EGD)

Dietary guidance after an EGD is necessary for smooth recovery and to prevent complications. Patients are advised to start with liquids to allow the stomach and esophagus to resume normal function after the procedure. This gradual method is essential in lessening discomfort due to the fast entry of solid food into the system. Clear liquids , such as water, broth, and other non-citrus beverages, are also included in the choices, which rehydrate the patient and facilitate healing of any minor irritation that may occur due to endoscopy. The process of feeding can be simplified by introducing bland, soft foods , such as applesauce or mashed potatoes progressively within the next 24 hours. One should also monitor for any sign of dysphagia or discomfort upon eating when the patient is on the way to a more consistent diet, which would be an indication of a complication or issue that needs to be addressed. This phase should include low-fat and low-fiber food and a ban on spicy, acidic, or extremely hot foods that may irritate the gastrointestinal tract. The recommendations emphasize the consumption of easily digestible and nutritious foods that do not strain the healing tissue. Patients are also advised to drink plenty of fluids, as appropriate fluid consumption is fundamental to ideal recovery. By a conservative strategy of food consumption after EGD, patients can significantly enhance their comfort level and overall recovery process. In some situations, such as eosinophilic esophagitis or food intolerance, the diet may also need to be further specified. For instance, for those patients with a history of presentation symptoms of food intolerance, an elimination diet following EGD to determine specific allergens responsible for their clinical presentation can be beneficial. Research has indicated that patients with certain esophageal histologic pathology, in some cases identified on EGD, may have their dietary restrictions clearly spelled out to them to reduce the risk of exacerbating their condition (Barfjani et al., 2016). Patient demographics and symptomatology and tolerance levels need to be carefully evaluated in formulating individualized diets. Having these recommendations followed up on not only allows for physical healing but also benefits patients' long-term well-being through better control of any underlying gastrointestinal conditions (Figure 4.17).

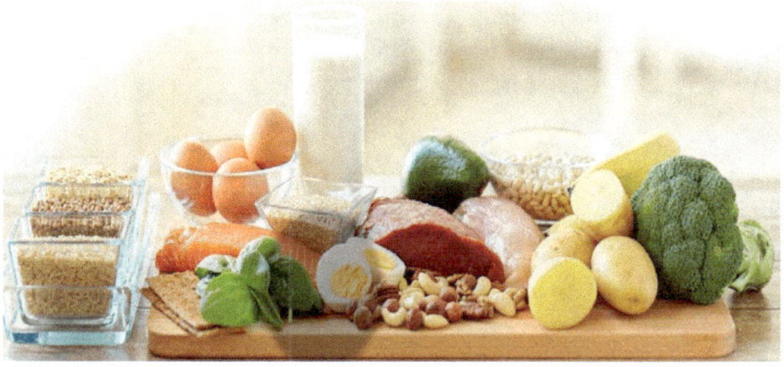

Figure 4.17. Post-surgery diet plan: How to get on the fastest road to recovery.

Source: https://www.indiahomehealthcare.com/wp-content/uploads/2019/06/IHHC-Blog-01.png.

4.5.3. Follow-Up Appointments and Results Discussion

Post-EGD follow-up appointments are both beneficial for the patient and clinician because they provide time to discuss the findings with any appropriate treatment plan. After an EGD, clinicians will typically sit down with patients and provide a complete overview of any abnormal or normal results obtained during the procedure. This consultation can improve patient concern over symptoms, particularly where results indicate GERD or minimal histological alterations to be assessed further. Knowledges regarding the meaning of results facilitate better patient involvement in their own care, facilitating compliance with follow-up treatment regimens or lifestyle adjustments. Moreover, reporting of outcomes is important to setting realistic recovery expectations and long-term prognosis, as noted by the little influence many results of EGD place on treatment plans overall (Helin et al., 2021). Furthermore, follow-up visits are an important check-in for monitoring patients' recovery and symptom resolution following an EGD. As longitudinal studies show, about 83% of children who take the test for suspected GERD have normal findings, and this calls for a reassessment of management strategies for symptoms (Helin et al., 2021). The visits also give medical practitioners a chance to determine the effectiveness of prescribed medications, such as proton pump inhibitors or dietary modification. It is at these follow-ups that patients are able to reveal any existing problems or new symptoms as they arise. This provides an ongoing feedback that contributes to improved clinical decision-making. Regular follow-ups enable identification of possibly missed conditions as well as enhance patient care through the provision of adequate adjustments in treatment regimens that are relevant based on the changing health status of the patients. Furthermore, discussions during follow-up consultations can alter subsequent medical evaluations and general treatment of gastrointestinal wellness. Clinicians are able to recommend additional testing, such as 24-hour pH monitoring, when symptoms fail to resolve after a normal EGD, illustrating an important factor in complete gastroenterological management. By critical analysis of the results gained from the EGD and follow-up testing, health care providers can aid in distinguishing between functional and more intense-intervention gastrointestinal illness. This is used to maintain both the provider and patient active within an ongoing discussion of the condition of gastrointestinal health, ultimately maximizing patient satisfaction and results. With this in mind, repeat consultations enhance personal treatment and also inform broader knowledge regarding child gastrointestinal disorders, emphasizing the need for meticulous clinical practice informed by patient history and shifting evidence (Helin et al., 2021).

4.6. Advances in Esophagogastroduodenoscopy (EGD) Technology

Technological advances in EGD have significantly enhanced diagnostic and therapeutic options for gastrointestinal (GI) disease. Historical techniques were successful but often lack scope and specificity. Technological advancements , such as high-definition imaging and chromoendoscopy, however, have provided GI specialists with tools to see mucosal details and detect abnormalities that escaped diagnosis in the past. High-definition EGD employs better resolution to detect lesions, polyps, and cancer at an early stage, which is essential for timely intervention. This increased visibility has led to a notable increase in the detection rates of diseases like Barrett's esophagus and early gastric carcinoma, bringing to the fore the revolutionary potential of such technological achievements in maximizing patient outcomes in upper GI tract evaluation and therapy. A second important advancement in EGD technology involves the integration of EUS, where the virtues of endoscopy are augmented with ultrasound imaging. EUS allows for high-resolution visualization of the layers of the gastrointestinal wall and adjacent structures, allowing accurate tumor staging and nodal involvement. This ability is most critical in complex cases , such as pancreatic and esophageal cancer, where accurate measurements can guide surgical as well as non-surgical treatment planning. New EUS techniques, including fine-needle aspiration, have established new avenues for biopsies, making them minimally invasive and more effective. Therefore, the addition of EUS into EGD planning not only maximizes diagnostic procedures but also radically improves the overall therapeutic paradigm for patients, enabling a more personalized and efficient management approach for upper GI cancers and other pathologies. Technological developments have also moved in favor of minimally invasive approaches, such as wireless capsule endoscopy and double balloon enteroscopy, that expand the boundaries of traditional EGD.

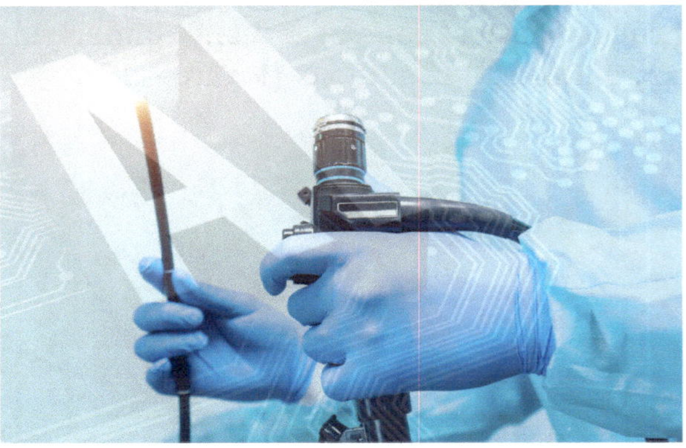

Figure 4.18. Artificial intelligence (AI) in endoscopy.

Source: https://miracleadvance.com/wp-content/uploads/2023/11/AI-in-Endoscopy-IT.png.

While dual balloon enteroscopy is able to penetrate the small intestine more deeply, wireless capsule endoscopy offers an unobtrusive window into seeing the entire GI tract, including typically inaccessible areas by means of traditional endoscopy. These advancements have proved extremely useful in the diagnosis of diseases like Crohn's disease or small bowel tumors, as demonstrated by case studies documenting the efficacy of these new diagnostic tools. The continued progress in these technologies points towards a commitment to optimizing patient care, enabling early diagnosis, and providing detailed examination of the complexities of gastrointestinal health, and thus making the importance of integrating advanced techniques into practice (Berger et al., 2010; Nguyen et al., 2010) (Figure 4.18).

4.6.1. Innovations in Endoscopic Equipment

The practice of upper gastrointestinal endoscopy, in particular EGD, has seen significant transformations with technological advancements in endoscopic equipment. Some of the advances have enabled a transition from traditional diagnostic methods to sophisticated interventional treatments. State-of-the-art endoscopes come equipped with high-definition cameras and sophisticated imaging technologies, which better visualize mucosal architecture and allow for more accurate diagnosis of gastrointestinal illness. The integration of digital technologies, such as computer-aided imaging, has enabled real-time analysis and improved outcomes in various interventions. Sophisticated instrument design possibilities, such as the application of thinner endoscopes, enable access to complex anatomical areas, enhancing the procedural efficacy and safety profile of EGD procedures (Tringali et al., 2017). Beyond direct visualization, developments in endoscopic instruments have expanded the therapeutic modalities available for application during EGD. Traditional practices have been complemented by innovative tools , such as the over-the-scope clip and hemostatic powder, which offer endoscopists successful means of managing complications , such as acute non-variceal upper GI bleeding (ANVUGIB). The existence of these sophisticated tools allows endoscopists to intervene directly and minimize the complications of this frequent medical emergency. Based on recent research findings, emerging treatment modalities enhance the ability to achieve hemostasis in difficult cases, thereby reducing morbidity and potentially decreasing mortality rates among patients, particularly in elderly patients, in whom comorbidities complicate treatment (Alali & Barkun, 2023). The path of innovation within endoscopy technology also encompasses progress in ancillary technologies. As an example, the development of artificial intelligence (AI) image analysis programs brings the potential for improved diagnostic accuracy through facilitating detection by healthcare professionals of lesions or abnormalities that the unaided eye may not be able to detect. Furthermore, optimization of methods of sedation and monitoring devices has assisted in improving the patient's comfort and safety throughout the course of EGD procedures, smoothing the examination process. With each advance in technology, the synergistic relationship between human experience and machine learning will bring even more dramatic improvements in the efficiency of endoscopic procedures. The promise of these innovations predicts a new era of gastrointestinal health, with quick, accurate interventions the norm and not the exception, leading to better patient outcomes in EGD practice (Tringali et al., 2017).

4.6.2. Development of Minimally Invasive Techniques

The evolution of minimally invasive techniques has revolutionized the landscape of medical diagnosis and intervention, particularly in upper GI procedures , such as EGD. Upper GI patients were traditionally subjected to more invasive surgical procedures with larger incisions and longer hospital stays. As technology evolved, the introduction of endoscopic techniques revolutionized the approach by which clinicians treat the diagnosis and management of a vast array of GI conditions. Refinements in instrument and technique have made possible visualization and intervention in the esophagus, stomach, and duodenum with less traumatic, smaller incisions, with less distress to the patient and faster recovery. This emphasis on less invasive techniques reflects the healthcare sector's ongoing preoccupation with improving patient outcomes and maximizing procedural efficacy. The invention of flexible endoscopes has also acted as a driving force for the spread of minimally invasive techniques. Compared to the rigid traditional instruments, the flexible endoscope provides greater maneuverability that enables complete visualization of the gastrointestinal tract without the need for large incisions. Not only does this transform diagnostic capability, but it also enables therapeutic procedures , such as biopsies and foreign body removal in real time, resulting in better integrated care for the patient. Patients treated with endoscopic procedures tend to perceive less pain compared to patients treated with standard surgery and might only require conscious sedation, which makes the experience more pleasant and secure.

The minimally invasive nature of endoscopy corrects not only the treatment approach but also the overall patient experience, leading to increased satisfaction and reduced recovery periods. The consequences of these advances extend beyond the procedural scope of EGD to encompass any more general effects on patient care and healthcare delivery. As highlighted in current guidelines, indications for endoscopy, either for diagnosis or treatment, continue to expand to cover all kinds of diseases from gastrointestinal bleeding to foreign body ingestion (Tringali et al., 2017). The need for ongoing training of practitioners to excel in such skills cannot be overemphasized, given that skill maintenance affects the care quality delivered. Development of minimally invasive methods, as with EGD, points towards the need for innovation in medical practice underpinned by measures responding to patient safety and comfort and enhancing the efficiency of gastrointestinal diagnostics and interventions (Perumal, 2012).

4.6.3. Future Trends in Gastrointestinal Endoscopy

As endoscopy of the gastrointestinal tract evolves, the future directions lean towards further inclusion of newer technology in EGD and so forth. The use of AI is particularly fascinating because it has the potential to enhance diagnostic yield through assisting clinicians in identifying irregularities in the gastrointestinal tract. Real-time processing AI that works on endoscopic images can virtually remove a lot of the human element of error, enabling detection of a condition , such as esophageal cancer at an early stage. Moreover, simulation-based learning technologies are becoming ever more mandatory for boosting procedural competency among medical professionals. Current reviews suggest that training methods involving robotics and virtual reality can shorten the learning curve for new practitioners, thereby enhancing patient safety and quality of care (Hernansanz et al., 2021). These technologies not only prepare clinicians for complex procedures but also meet the increasing demand for high-performance endoscopic procedures. The demand for standardized endoscopy training emphasizes the need for ongoing training and support for registered nurses (RNs) conducting gastrointestinal procedures. The technical nature of endoscopic procedures has risen in recent years and requires RNs to have a solid foundation in gastrointestinal anatomy, pathophysiology, and procedural knowledge. The development of detailed orientation documents, such as Endoscopy Intraprocedural Orientation Manuals (EIOM), may neutralize education gaps ascertained from stakeholder meetings and review of literature (Rose et al., 2020). By the implementation of formal education materials, healthcare centers can ensure that RNs have necessary skills to manage complex endoscopic procedures efficiently. This added focus on nursing education not only elevates the quality of care provided but also prepares the healthcare provider for evolving demands on gastrointestinal endoscopy. Lastly, the future of gastrointestinal endoscopy will include new approaches to patient interaction and follow-up after the procedure. As telemedicine continues to advance, providers will utilize more remote monitoring and consultation to follow up on patients post-EGD procedures. This enables medical practitioners to assess recovery, manage complications, and reinforce prevention care protocols remotely. Further, engagement of patients through digital interfaces can enable them to learn and adhere to post-procedure care better. Technology adoption in patient care, including educational resources and interactive learning tools, will be instrumental in debugging endoscopic procedures among patients, finally reducing anxiety and improving overall outcomes. As these trends materialize, focus will not only be given to technical expertise in endoscopy but also to maximizing patient experience and satisfaction throughout the healthcare journey (Figure 4.19).

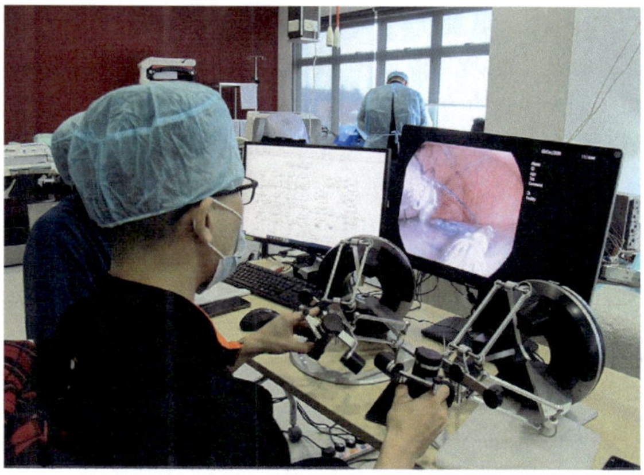

Figure 4.19. Using robotic endoscopic platforms to perform gastric endoscopic.

Source: https://els-jbs-prod-cdn.jbs.elsevierhealth.com/cms/attachment/b5ab5609-3a1b-4e78-b1aa-142f2041a6e7/gr1_lrg.jpg.

SUMMARY

In conclusion, EGD is a useful diagnostic and therapeutic modality for the evaluation of the upper gastrointestinal tract. This technique not only allows visualization of mucosal lesions but also facilitates intervention , such as biopsy and polypectomy. Performance and outcomes associated with EGD can be significantly improved with repeated measures of quality over time through systematic audits, as demonstrated. For example, research brought to light the fact that completion rates and procedure effectiveness increased substantially within a decade, reflecting the significance of frequent quality audits in refining clinical practice. In particular, adjusted completion rates increased from 80% 95%, which reflects a strong strategy in developing endoscopic procedures (Abdelmohsen et al., 2018). This evidence reaffirms that organized improvement efforts are imperative for maximizing patient care in gastrointestinal health. Furthermore, the foreign evidence of gastric cancer screening portrays the success of EGD as a population-based screening, particularly in high-risk regions. Japan and Korea are good examples of countries that have successfully rolled out systematic EGD screening protocols, whose results show high proportions of early diagnosis for gastric cancer. The aggressive approach not only increases the likelihood of early diagnosis but also lowers mortality from this neoplasm, perhaps. Research has proven that endoscopy-based screening is better compared to the standard approaches, with improved adherence and detection in diverse populations (Faria, 2020). Therefore, its encouragement in clinical guidelines around the world is justified, in consideration of its advantage towards early diagnosis and therapeutic potential. Finally, the implications of more EGD use extend past mere diagnostics; they involve trained personnel and resource planning to address mounting requirements. Instituting effective screening programs will take a dedication to enhancing endoscopic care and making it universally available to various populations. As the enhanced results in those regions with intensive endoscopic practice show, there is an excellent argument to be made for , including EGD as part of routine screening for gastrointestinal disease. The future will hold continuous research and innovation to enhance EGD techniques and create standardized protocols that can be uniformly applied to all patients. Lastly, the prioritization of EGD within healthcare systems is a well-informed step toward improving gastrointestinal healthcare outcomes globally and should be embraced as a foundation for contemporary medical practice.

Upper endoscopy or EGD is a significant diagnostic and therapeutic intervention in the field of gastroenterology. It is largely aimed at visualizing the esophagus, stomach, and duodenum to facilitate doctors in the assessment of chronic dysphagia, nausea, or unexplained loss of weight. Significantly, EGD enables interventions , such as biopsy sampling, polyp resection, and treatment of bleeding lesions. The requirement for accurate and less invasive procedures highlights the importance of technological developments in endoscopy, enhancing visibility and therapeutic capabilities and leading to improved patient outcomes. Moreover, newer research emphasizes the utility of upper gastrointestinal endoscopy across a range of patient groups, including the aged. Research has established that EGD can be safely and effectively performed even in patients aged 90 years and above, dispelling concerns of age-related risks. The decision to have EGD largely remains dependent on clinical need rather than age itself and represents a maturity in patient-led care. This finding aligns with the broader discussions in the literature regarding the importance of critical evidence-based practices to informing interventions for gastrointestinal disease. The dynamic nature of diagnostic and therapeutic criteria for gastrointestinal illness also highlights the worth of endoscopic procedures. Revised diagnostic criteria amendments for pediatric-onset inflammatory bowel disease (IBD), such as advanced biomarker and imaging technology, demonstrate greater recognition of EGD worth. As these standards are centered on aggressive diagnostic systems , such as the Paris classification, endoscopy is today at the forefront of defining and treating conditions , such as ulcerative colitis and Crohn's disease. Thus, the application of endoscopic technology not only improves diagnostic precision but also allows for customized treatment regimens, an overall strategy in gastrointestinal well-being centered on patient health and safety.

CLOSER LOOK

POST-ENDOSCOPIC SYNDROMES:

Post-endoscopic syndromes refer to a group of symptoms or clinical conditions that arise after gastrointestinal endoscopic procedures, such as colonoscopy, upper endoscopy, or endoscopic therapeutic interventions. While most endoscopies are safe and well tolerated, the mechanical manipulation of the GI tract, the use of insufflation, and occasional therapeutic maneuvers can lead to transient or, less commonly, clinically significant symptoms. Understanding these syndromes helps clinicians distinguish expected postoperative effects from complications that require intervention. One of the most recognized conditions is post-polypectomy syndrome, also known as post-electrocautery syndrome. It occurs when thermal injury from polyp removal causes localized inflammation of the bowel wall without full-thickness perforation. Patients may experience abdominal pain, fever, or leukocytosis, often mimicking perforation, though imaging typically shows only localized wall thickening. Management is usually conservative, focusing on rest, hydration, and clinical observation.

Another frequent complaint after endoscopy is post-procedural bloating and discomfort. This often results from residual air or carbon dioxide used to distend the GI lumen for visualization. While CO_2 insufflation reduces lingering gas more quickly than room air, some patients still report cramping, gas retention, or mild abdominal fullness for several hours. These symptoms typically resolve spontaneously.

Patients may also experience post-endoscopy sore throat, hoarseness, or mild dysphagia after upper GI endoscopy due to transient irritation from the endoscope passing through the oropharynx and esophagus. These symptoms are usually short-lived and respond to hydration and throat lozenges.

In more interventional procedures—such as endoscopic mucosal resection, ERCP, or dilation—post-endoscopic syndromes may present differently. Post-ERCP pancreatitis is a well-known complication characterized by abdominal pain and elevated pancreatic enzymes. Although not universally categorized under "syndromes," it remains an important post-endoscopic condition requiring medical evaluation. Similarly, patients undergoing dilation or stent placement may experience chest discomfort or transient dysphagia related to esophageal stretching.

Psychological and physiological factors can also contribute to post-procedure fatigue, nausea, or dizziness, often related to sedation rather than the endoscopy itself. Tailoring sedation to patient needs and ensuring adequate recovery time can help minimize these effects.

Overall, post-endoscopic syndromes span a wide spectrum—from benign, self-limiting symptoms to clinical conditions requiring careful assessment. Increased awareness and timely recognition allow clinicians to reassure patients when symptoms are expected and intervene promptly when signs suggest a more serious underlying issue. As endoscopic techniques evolve, continued monitoring and research help refine prevention and management strategies for these post-procedure experiences.

REFERENCES

1. Tringali, A., Thomson, M., Dumonceau, J. M., Tavares, M., Tabbers, M. M., Furlano, R., Spaander, M., Hassan, C., Tzvinikos, C., Ijsselstijn, H., Viala, J., Dall'Oglio, L., Benninga, M., Orel, R., Vandenplas, Y., Keil, R., Romano, C., Brownstone, E., Hlava, Š., Gerner, P., ... Zambelli, A. (2017). Pediatric gastrointestinal endoscopy: European Society of Gastrointestinal Endoscopy (ESGE) and European Society for Paediatric Gastroenterology Hepatology and Nutrition (ESPGHAN) Guideline Executive summary. *Endoscopy*, *49*(1), 83–91. https://doi.org/10.1055/s-0042-111002(accessed on 15th July 2025).
2. Abdelmohsen, A., Axon, A., Ebeid, B., Gado, A., et al. (2018). *Endoscopy audit over 10 years in a community hospital in Egypt.* https://core.ac.uk/download/478436806.pdf (accessed on 15th July 2025).
3. Ahsan, M., Babaei, L., Emami, M. H., Gholamrezaei, A., et al. (2011). *Simethicone for the preparation before esophagogastroduodenoscopy.* https://core.ac.uk/download/pdf/8603302.pdf (accessed on 15th July 2025).
4. Al-Ebrahim, F., Alhazzani, W., Alnemer, A., Alzahrani, A., et al. (2012). *Safety of esophagogastroduodenoscopy within 30 days of myocardial infarction: A retrospective cohort study from a Canadian tertiary center.* https://core.ac.uk/download/194194737.pdf (accessed on 15th July 2025).
5. Alexander, J., Ashorn, M., Barth, C., Bartunkova, J., Bernstein, C., Bousvaros, A., Boyce, E., et al. (2013). *ESPGHAN revised Porto criteria for the diagnosis of inflammatory bowel disease in children and adolescents.* https://core.ac.uk/download/83095760.pdf (accessed on 15th July 2025).
6. Arieira, C., Carvalho, P. B., Castro, F. D., Cotter, J., et al. (2019). *Esophagogastroduodenoscopy findings in patients on the waiting list for bariatric surgery.* https://core.ac.uk/download/344901430.pdf (accessed on 15th July 2025).
7. Azueta, A., Batheja, M., Heigh, R., Leighton, J., et al. (2010). *The Face of Tropical Sprue in 2010.* https://core.ac.uk/download/pdf/8445775.pdf (accessed on 15th July 2025).
8. DA, Lord & Bell, Geoffrey & A, Gray & A, Quine & J, Bowles & A, Reynolds. (2006). Sedation for Gastrointestinal Endoscopic Procedures in the Elderly: Getting Safer but Still Not Nearly Safe Enough. Br Soc Gastroenterol. (accessed on 15th July 2025).
9. Berger, A., May, A., Moglia, A., Postgate, A., Ross, A., Tocchi, A., Neugut, A. I., et al. (2010). *Duodenal carcinoma at the ligament of Treitz: A molecular and clinical perspective.* https://core.ac.uk/download/78918848.pdf (accessed on 15th July 2025).
10. Bialek, A., Januszewicz, W., Kaminski, M. F., Karpinska, A., et al. (2019). *Endoscopist biopsy rate as a quality indicator for outpatient gastroscopy: A multicenter cohort study with validation.* https://core.ac.uk/download/237712914.pdf (accessed on 15th July 2025).
11. Chang, W. H., & Lei, W. Y. (2007). *Endoscopic retrograde cholangiopancreatography in elderly patients.* https://core.ac.uk/download/pdf/82371991.pdf (accessed on 15th July 2025).
12. Ching, H. L., McAlindon, M., Sidhu, R., Sloan, J., et al. (2022). *Comparison of patient tolerance and acceptability of magnet-controlled capsule endoscopy and flexible endoscopy in the investigation of dyspepsia.* https://core.ac.uk/download/542497334.pdf (accessed on 15th July 2025).

13. Dellon, E. S., Gebhart, J. H., Hathorn, K. E., Higgins, L., et al. (2016). *The esophageal biopsy "pull" sign: A highly specific and treatment-responsive endoscopic finding in eosinophilic esophagitis (with video).* https://core.ac.uk/download/304663540.pdf (accessed on 15th July 2025).
14. Faria, L. M. A. (2020). *Gastric Cancer Screening: A Systematic Review.* https://core.ac.uk/download/334528648.pdf (accessed on 15th July 2025).
15. Fuhs, A. K., & Prahlow, J. A. (2016). *Death resulting from pneumocephalus complicating endoscopic food bolus retrieval in a patient with eosinophilic esophagitis.* https://core.ac.uk/download/228066076.pdf (accessed on 15th July 2025).
16. Gerada, J. (2012). *Gastrointestinal cancer screening and surveillance programs: A worldwide perspective – Part 2.* https://core.ac.uk/download/46604359.pdf (accessed on 15th July 2025).
17. Gross, A. J., Kidambi, T. D., Lee, J. K., Ostroff, J., et al. (2017). *Endoscopy is of low yield in the identification of gastrointestinal neoplasia in patients with dermatomyositis: A cross-sectional study.* https://core.ac.uk/download/323074387.pdf (accessed on 15th July 2025).
18. Haidry, R., Iyer, P. G., Lovat, L. B., McAlindon, M., et al. (2019). *Miniature gastrointestinal endoscopy: Now and the future.* https://core.ac.uk/download/227338082.pdf (accessed on 15th July 2025).
19. Hajizadeh Barfjani, S. (2016). *The utility of esophagogastroduodenoscopy with biopsy in diagnosis and treatment of children presenting with failure to thrive.* https://open.bu.edu/bitstream/2144/17007/1/HajizadehBarfjani_bu_0017N_11991.pdf (accessed on 15th July 2025).
20. Helin, N. (2021). *Outcomes of early childhood non-specific gastrointestinal symptoms: From diagnosis to long-term follow-up.* https://core.ac.uk/download/401693725.pdf (accessed on 15th July 2025).
21. Hernansanz, A., Casals, A., Koulaouzidis, A., Menciassi, A., Amram, D., Ciuti, G., Finocchiaro, M., et al. (2021). *Training simulators for gastrointestinal endoscopy: Current and future perspectives.* https://core.ac.uk/download/534195207.pdf (accessed on 15th July 2025).
22. Hiraoka, S., Inokuchi, T., Iwamuro, M., Kato, M., et al. (2018). *Evaluation of the upper gastrointestinal tract in ulcerative colitis patients.* https://core.ac.uk/download/156900873.pdf (accessed on 15th July 2025).
23. Rasul, I., & Kandel, G. P. (2001). An approach to iron-deficiency anemia. *Canadian journal of gastroenterology = Journal canadien de gastroenterologie, 15*(11), 739–747. https://doi.org/10.1155/2001/202035
24. Le Nguyen, V. T., Nguyen, C. C., & Nguyen, V. X. (2010). *Appropriate use of endoscopy in the diagnosis and treatment of gastrointestinal diseases: Up-to-date indications for primary care providers.* https://core.ac.uk/download/pdf/8490315.pdf (accessed on 15th July 2025).
25. Lionis, C., Oikonomidou, E., Kouroumalis, E., Anastasiou, F., Pilpilidis, I., & Null, N. (2011). *Upper gastrointestinal endoscopy for dyspepsia: Exploratory study of factors influencing patient compliance in Greece.* https://core.ac.uk/download/pdf/81191860.pdf (accessed on 15th July 2025).
26. Lopes, I. F. F. V. (2021). *Redes neurais convolucionais para deteção de landmarks gástricas.* https://core.ac.uk/download/492992973.pdf (accessed on 15th July 2025).

27. Mancini, C. B. (2017). *Decreasing cost in the GI endoscopy suite by utilizing best sedation practices.* https://core.ac.uk/download/301289065.pdf (accessed on 15th July 2025).

28. Marinho Luis, B. V. V. (2024). *Endoscopic screening of the upper digestive tract in patients with head and neck neoplasms.* https://core.ac.uk/download/619522256.pdf (accessed on 15th July 2025).

29. Alali, A. A., & Barkun, A. N. (2023). An update on the management of non-variceal upper gastrointestinal bleeding. *Gastroenterology report, 11*, goad011. https://doi.org/10.1093/gastro/goad011(accessed on 15th July 2025).

30. Nilsson, F. (2016). *Association between Helicobacter pylori status and self-rated health: A population based cross-sectional study.* https://core.ac.uk/download/75913305.pdf (accessed on 15th July 2025).

31. Perumal, P. (2012). *Endoscopy.* https://core.ac.uk/download/pdf/1570017.pdf (accessed on 15th July 2025).

32. Sidhu, S. S. ., & Rick, J. R (2009). *Erosive eosinophilic esophagitis in rumination syndrome.* https://core.ac.uk/download/46969151.pdf (accessed on 15th July 2025).

33. Rose, S. (2020). *Endoscopy intraprocedural orientation manual for registered nurses.* https://core.ac.uk/download/478634902.pdf (accessed on 15th July 2025).

34. シマダ, セイタロウ., 島田, 清太郎. (2023). *Endoscopic causes and characteristics of missed gastric cancers after endoscopic submucosal dissection.* https://core.ac.uk/download/636993660.pdf (accessed on 15th July 2025).

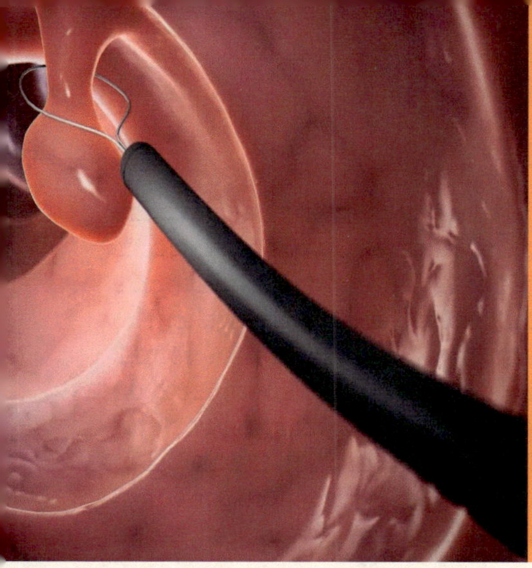

Chapter 5
COLONOSCOPY

Contents

Introduction..127
5.1. Purpose of Colonoscopy 130
5.2. The Colonoscopy Procedure...133
5.3. Risks and Complications..137
5.4. Benefits of Colonoscopy 140
5.5. Patient Experience..144
5.6. Alternatives to Colonoscopy 147
Summary 151
References 154

Introduction

Colonoscopy, a valuable tool in the prevention and diagnosis of colorectal cancer, is a procedure that allows for direct visualization of the colon and rectum. To understand the significance of this intervention, one must have a background about its primary functions, such as screening, surveillance, and therapeutic treatment of gastrointestinal disease. The process allows practitioners to detect abnormalities , such as polyps, tumors, and inflammatory disease, which play a critical role in clinical decision-making. As the evidence on specialized health centers has demonstrated, there is growing awareness that interventions like colonoscopy are essential to the achievement of patient-centered care. Such observations support the emphasis on having services for colonoscopy not only available but effective in addressing the diverse needs of the patient population. Given the increasing prevalence of colorectal cancer, thorough examination of colonoscopy is essential to enhance patient outcomes and healthcare. The history of change in colonoscopy practice has also followed technological advancement, which maximizes the efficiency and comfort of the procedure for the patient. Technologies , such as high-definition imaging and the development of subspecialty instruments have enhanced the process to be safer and more accurate, enabling lesions that could otherwise go unnoticed to be identified. Moreover, comparing the impacts of colonoscopy procedures on whole healthcare systems emphasizes the fine balance between subspecialty centers and overall general hospitals. The controversy surrounding the design and configuration of these institutions, as studies have found, is that while specialized settings can optimize provision of care for patients, expected impacts on hospital networks overall must be considered with great caution, as expounded in current reviews synthesizing these dynamic interactions (De Regge et al., 2013). Thus, the introduction of this essay speaks of the extent to which procedures of colonoscopy not only signify developments in medical practice but also must look to their broader implications carefully. Since health systems battle on with issues concerning access as well as the quality of care, colonoscopy is still at the forefront. The significance of early detection through screening has the potential to reduce mortality rates associated with colorectal cancer substantially, pointing towards a public health drive towards taking up screening programs. Furthermore, the intricacy of conditions regarding colorectal issues that may involve procedures , such as colonoscopy necessitates an in-depth understanding of clinical guidelines and evidence-based practice. Similarly, the necessity to assess the implications of ancillary findings , such as gastrointestinal cytomegalovirus infection, highlights the importance of ongoing clinical research and debate (Goodman et al., 2015). The introduction of the essay seeks to situate colonoscopy not simply as a procedural intervention, but as an integral part in the complex dance of patient care, diagnostic innovation, and advocacy for community health (Figure 5.1).

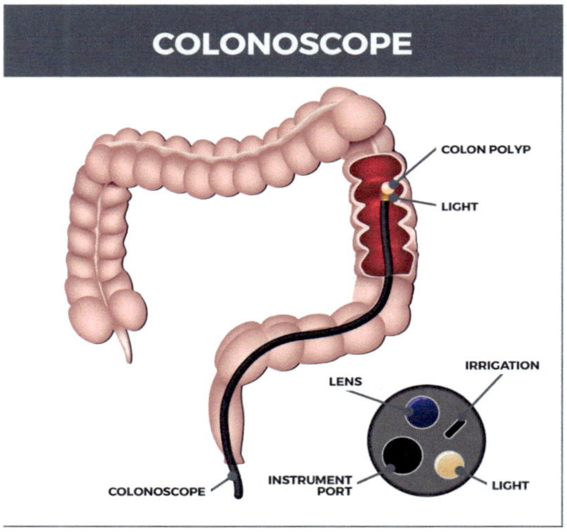

Figure 5.1. Colonoscopy.

Source: https://gastro-md.com/wp-content/uploads/2022/10/Colonoscopy3-1-scaled.jpg.

Definition of Colonoscopy

Colonoscopy is a vital medical examination that allows the interior of the colon, rectum and up to the terminal ileum to be viewed using a flexible tube with a camera known as a colonoscope. The diagnostic tool has several key functions, such as the determination of any abnormalities like inflammation, polyps, and tumors, which can detect a variety of gastrointestinal diseases. The importance of colonoscopy is reaffirmed by its role in colorectal cancer screening, where it has been shown to reduce disease-related mortality to a significant degree. Colonoscopy allows for the visualization of the mucosal surface directly, thereby enabling diagnosis as well as therapeutic interventions , such as biopsy or polypectomy, hence inclusion in a full care and management of the patient. The procedure is typically done under sedation, thereby making the patient comfortable and allowing doctors to examine the colon very carefully. Preparations for a colonoscopy entail cleansing of the bowel, via dietary modification and laxative use, to create clear visibility during the exam. Moreover, information about a person's GI health could be highly important following colonoscopy findings. Invasive, the process is done by skilled gastroenterologists or colorectal specialists in a contained health setting. Such skill is necessary, particularly in interpreting outcomes that indicate precursors to colorectal cancer, including Aberrant Crypt Foci (ACF), which are pre-detectable cellular anomalies on colonoscopy images, according to the literature (Engquist et al., 2016). Throughout recent decades, the landscape of colonoscopy has evolved with emerging technology and techniques in imaging and methodologies for enhancing diagnostic quality while improving patient comfort. Studies into the effectiveness of specialty centers, including ambulatory surgery facilities for endoscopic colonoscopy, have brought quality and access debate into the discussion (De Regge et al., 2013). Monitoring and evaluation of such facilities must continue to further develop the field. With the medical community increasingly aware of colorectal cancer's origin and pathogenesis, the role of colonoscopy remains paramount. The information that is extrapolated from this procedure not only contributes to early detection but also is significantly involved with demystifying the underlying pathobiology of colorectal cancers, emphasizing the procedure's relevance in modern medicine.

Importance of Colon Health

Colon health is most critical to overall well-being because the colon plays a central role in the gastrointestinal system, nutrient absorption, and elimination of waste. Sustaining body homeostasis and modulating immune function, a healthy colon is crucial. Colorectal cancer, inflammatory bowel disease, and diverticulitis are some of the conditions that can significantly impair colon function, causing morbidity and excessive healthcare costs. Regular screening, in particular colonoscopy tests, facilitates early detection and prevention of chronic diseases. Not only are healthy lifestyle and dietary habits important factors in keeping the colon healthy, but also preventive health practices that can cut down on the risk of chronic diseases of colorectal health. The relationship between microbiota composition and colon health has been the subject of much interest in recent times, recognizing the capacity of probiotics to enhance gut integrity. Studies have demonstrated that consumption of probiotics, or Lactobacillus rhamnosus GG (LGG), can strengthen mucosal adhesion as well as exert anti-inflammatory effects in the colonic environment. LGG, according to Corleto et al. (2018), has been established to adhere very well to colonic mucosa and reduce the levels of inflammatory markers , such as tumor necrosis factor alpha (TNFα) and interleukin (IL)-17. This also shows that probiotics can be employed as an adjunct treatment in colon health, controlling inflammation, and even averting conditions , such as ulcerative colitis and colorectal cancer. Thus, the addition of probiotics to dietary interventions holds promise for enhancing colon health. Demographics also have significant effects on colon health consequences, which serves to emphasize the importance of direct public health interventions. Health disparities among women in cities point toward race, level of income, and accessibility of care as affecting health outcomes relative to colorectal disease. New York City studies have determined that some subgroups are at higher risk for colon health problems, and targeted policies for health must be implemented to attend to disparities (De Regge et al., 2013). Colon health should be improved through education about screening and preventive services, especially in healthcare disadvantaged communities. Through bringing awareness and raising access to information about colon health, we can together enhance the efficiency of preventives, ultimately leading to greater health outcomes and reduced incidence of colorectal disease (Figure 5.2).

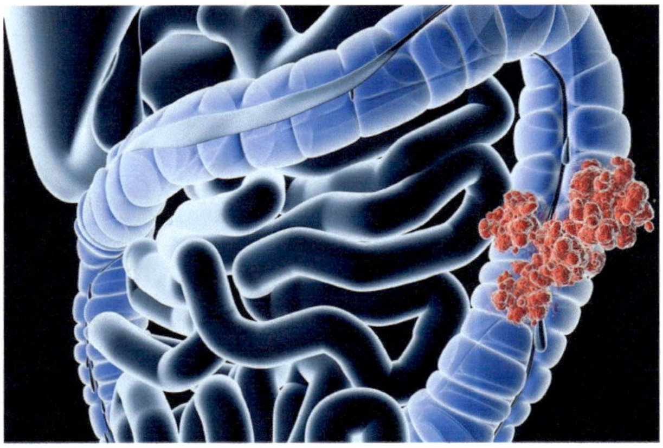

Figure 5.2. Colon health.

Source: https://www.healthspectra.com/wp-content/uploads/2017/02/Healthy-Colon02.jpg.

5.1. Purpose of Colonoscopy

The primary goal of a colonoscopy is to serve as a critical screening test for colorectal cancer (CRC) and other gastrointestinal disease. Because CRC is the third most common cancer to be diagnosed in the United States, early identification through screening is critical in improving patient outcomes. The procedure allows for direct viewing of the colon, which enables healthcare practitioners to identify abnormalities , such as polyps and lesions that could develop into cancer if left untreated. However, colonoscopy success also relies on adequate bowel preparation, which is necessary for proper visibility and examination. Notably, studies indicate that inadequate bowel preparation significantly lowers polyp detection rates as well as necessitates repeat procedures, emphasizing the importance of optimizing preparation protocols to ensure effective screening (Kastenberg et al., 2018). Moreover, colonoscopy also plays a crucial role in preventive care, particularly among high-risk populations. The procedure not only allows for early diagnosis of cancer but also allows for polyp removal on the same day, thus reducing the incidence of CRC. Despite its advantages, inequalities exist in screening rates between groups. African Americans, for instance, experience greater mortality due to CRC, yet have concomitant reduced access to screening than among their Whites. Educational interventions focusing on targeted groups are vital to developing knowledge and promoting anticipatory health behaviors for CRC screening. Through the identification and removal of barriers , such as medical mistrust and anxiety, these interventions can encourage greater colonoscopy screening uptake in the underserved (DuHamel et al., 2012). In addition to its diagnostic and prophylactic applications, colonoscopy has a therapeutic function through the opportunity for intervention during the procedure itself. Not only can doctors excise polyps, but they can also treat other gastrointestinal ailments, such as bleeding or strictures, thereby avoiding complications of these issues. This dual ability emphasizes the importance of colonoscopy not just as a screening test but as a therapeutic intervention as well. A shift in attitudes toward this procedure and emphasis on its proactive nature can result in greater acceptance and induction into screening programs. Subsequently, promoting awareness of the multitude of benefits of colonoscopy is to reinforce its status as a cornerstone of colorectal prevention and healthcare (Kastenberg et al., 2018) (Figure 5.3).

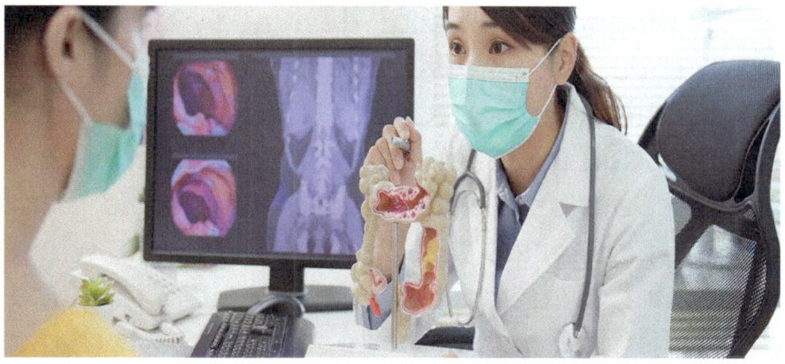

Figure 5.3. Colonoscopy: Purpose.

Source: https://ckbh.ckbirlahospitals.com/storage/rbh/uploadedfiles/gallery/1648987638_Colonoscopy.jpg.

5.1.1. Screening for Colorectal Cancer (CRC)

Screening for CRC is a key element of preventive medicine, particularly as the incidence of the disease continues to rise in various populations. The United States Preventive Services Task Force (USPSTF) advises that colorectal cancer screening should start at the age of 50 years and go up to age 75, stressing the need for detection at an early stage to minimize mortality related to this condition. Colorectal cancer tends to develop silently, and the majority of patients stay asymptomatic until the disease has progressed significantly. In such a case, adherence to screening guidelines, like the utilization of colonoscopy as an effective alternative, is obligatory if early treatment is to be obtained. CRC screening, in addition to allowing for early detection of cancer, also allows for the identification and removal of precancerous polyps, therefore significantly lowering the risk of colorectal cancer as well as related deaths among screened subjects (Schmidt, 2017). Screening barriers persist in most communities, however, leaving a significant majority of the eligible population unscreened. Lack of education, cultural attitudes about medical procedures, and socioeconomic disparities are typical root causes for lower screening rates. Research at Stowe Family Practice and Community Health Services of Lamoille Valley provides some insight into these barriers. By reviewing charts and interviews assessing patient compliance with screening guidelines, the research tries to establish some barriers that restrict frequent engagement in screening programs. Additionally, testing provider-patient shared decision-support instruments and educational tools as approaches to augment screening levels is also essential. These interventions can lead to improved communication, ultimately expanding patients' willingness to participate in preventive efforts against colorectal cancer (Schmidt et al., 2017). Further, educational outreach also plays a crucial role in increasing screening rates and educating patients on the importance of routine colorectal cancer screening.

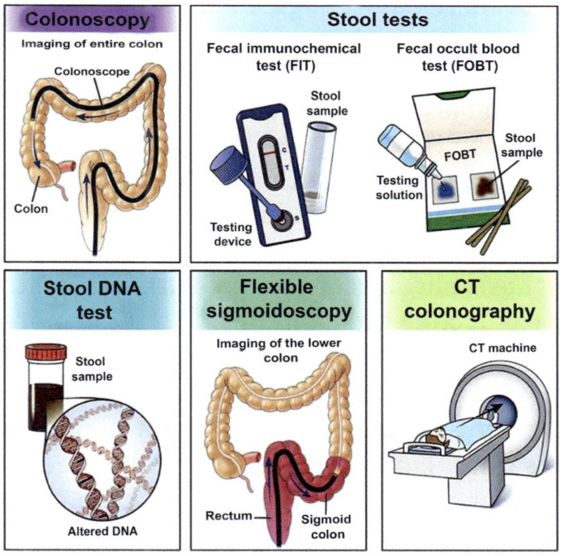

Figure 5.4. Colorectal cancer screening options.

Source: https://els-jbs-prod-cdn.jbs.elsevierhealth.com/cms/attachment/a5a960eb-5bb7-44ab-906c-99043ae300dc/gr1_lrg.jpg.

Effective communication efforts have the potential to dispel myths surrounding colonoscopy and associated risks. Healthcare professionals not only have the duty of prescribing screenings but also of giving patients information that will allow them to make informed decisions. Besides, in reaching out to include the particular needs of diverse populations, including minority populations and rural dwellers, there lies a potential in narrowing the gap in screening disparities. By establishing an enabling environment that sees patients empowered and motivated to pose queries and inquire about concerns in their well-being, healthcare systems can play a great role in adherence to screening recommendations, thereby resulting in a measurable decline in the occurrence and mortality of colorectal cancer (Figure 5.4).

5.1.2. Diagnosing Gastrointestinal Disorders

The complex nature of gastrointestinal disorders means that a variety of diagnostic techniques are needed, and colonoscopy is a leading tool. This enables direct visualization of the rectum and colon, allowing for the identification of abnormal growths , such as polyps and tumors, as well as signs of inflammatory bowel disease. Furthermore, colonoscopy serves not only for diagnosis but also for therapy, with the capacity for conducting interventions , including biopsy, polypectomy, and the management of bleeding lesions. Apart from colonoscopy, there are other diagnostic modalities in the form of imaging tests and laboratory assessment used for obtaining an overall picture of gastrointestinal illnesses. Each of these methods, from serologic testing to advanced imaging tests, complements colonoscopy's advantages as well as makes up for its deficiencies, enabling a thorough diagnosis of the condition of the patient. Beyond colonoscopy, the role of advanced imaging tests is paramount in gastrointestinal disease diagnosis. Methods , such as magnetic resonance enterography and computed tomography scans provide information regarding small bowel conditions, particularly in cases of suspected Crohn's disease. Small bowel endoscopy, like capsule endoscopy, has been an added dimension to the diagnostic arsenal, designed particularly for the ability to visualize areas that cannot be visualized using regular endoscopy. With a combination of imaging technology, doctors are able to develop an integrated diagnostic plan. Evidence suggests that these techniques, when combined, enhance diagnostic yield and guide subsequent management approaches toward the utilitarian value of a diverse diagnostic toolset for the detection of gastrointestinal disease.

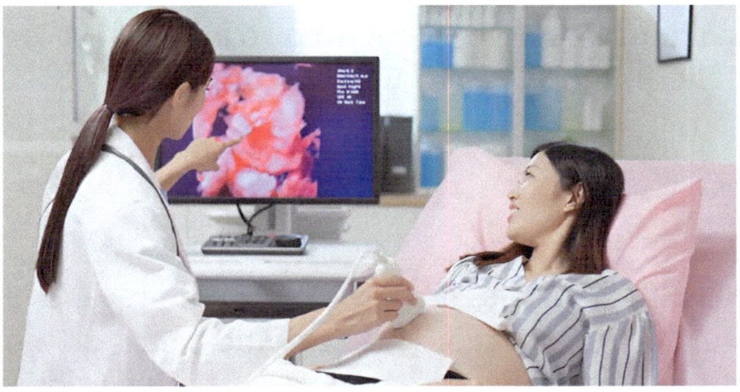

Figure 5.5. Ultrasound in diagnosing gastrointestinal disorders.

Source: https://ehealthcommunity.org/wp-content/uploads/2025/03/ultrasound-in-diagnosing-gastrointestinal-disorders.webp.

These techniques' ability to visualize the entire gastrointestinal tract makes them highly valuable in contemporary medical practice. Economic implications of detecting gastrointestinal disease, specifically Crohn's disease, are only becoming increasingly powerful as healthcare determinants. The application of wireless capsule endoscopy (WCE) has been in the limelight because it can accomplish more diagnostic yield than traditional diagnosis like colonoscopy and small bowel follow-through. Not only is WCE superior in presenting clear pictures, but also it reduces repeat testing, which is costly and burdensome to patients. Evidence more recently available indicates that using WCE as a first-line diagnostic agent has the potential to result in significant cost savings for payors. And, beyond financials, the implications are further that early and accurate diagnosis will lead to improved treatment outcomes, enhancing patients quality of life and productivity level. Lastly, effective use of diagnostic tools like WCE aligns with the overall objective of facilitating the provision of healthcare in gastrointestinal disorders (Goldfarb et al., 2004; Hausmann & Albert, 2011) (Figure 5.5).

5.1.3. Monitoring Inflammatory Bowel Diseases (IBD)

IBD care must be followed up carefully to monitor disease activity and the response to treatments. Colonoscopy is a valuable tool for this surveillance process because it can directly visualize the gastrointestinal mucosa and quantify the severity of inflammation. Colonoscopy is particularly useful since it can potentially enable biopsy collection, which can be used for histological analysis in an attempt to identify active inflammation or dysplasia. Colonoscopy has also been made more useful by recent advances in imaging technology. The integration of other diagnostic imaging modalities, such as scintigraphy, contributes to the utility of colonoscopy by providing additional insight into disease behavior, enabling prediction of relapses and enhancing optimal treatment planning. Utilization of a multidimensional approach involving colonoscopy and ancillary imaging techniques enables clinicians to attain precise monitoring of IBD, finally improving patient outcome and quality of life. Despite the supremacy of colonoscopy in IBD monitoring, challenges persist in the accurate reporting of endoscopic activity. Scoring methods have been proposed to introduce mucosal healing assessment into standardization in the case of diseases like ulcerative colitis (UC) and Crohn's disease (CD). The majority of these tools are badly validated, and therefore, the tools have failed to be well accepted in clinical practice. As research emphasizes the importance of mucosal healing as a treatment endpoint, improved methodologies in the definition of endoscopic activity are increasingly needed. Furthermore, the suboptimal application of endoscopic scores typically reduces their use in routine monitoring and therefore their capacity to quantify treatment effectiveness. These barriers are relevant to overcome during the advancement of IBD management and highlight the necessity for ongoing study to optimize endoscopic evaluation approaches. According to these aspects, it is presumed that the future of the surveillance of IBD may rely on the development and application of more sophisticated strategies centered on mucosal healing. Current literature suggests that biomarkers, in conjunction with colonoscopy, may provide an improved level of understanding of disease activity. For instance, adopting the mucosal healing paradigm as a primary outcome measure can revolutionize treatment by encouraging widespread adoption of sustained remission as a therapeutic goal over symptom management. In addition, the introduction of technologies , such as point-of-care imaging and digital surveillance may support the role of colonoscopy by decreasing patient burden and improving monitoring compliance. The ongoing evolution of IBD monitoring techniques is a new frontier in gastroenterology, with enhanced health care and more efficient management in terms of unique patient needs. Therefore, the union of colonoscopy with innovations in diagnostics and biomarkers will play a vital role in further elevating the efficacy of IBD treatments in the future.

5.2. The Colonoscopy Procedure

The colonoscopy procedure is a crucial diagnostic tool in the diagnosis and early prevention of CRC, a highly prevalent yet largely preventable disease. Through viewing the inside of the colon and rectum via a flexible tube with a camera on the end, physicians can identify any irregularities , such as polyps or tumors. These precursors to cancer highlight the importance of regular screening, particularly in individuals 50 years and older, according to national guidelines. An effectively planned communication strategy with patients will promote a significant uptake of screening. For instance, adding multi-modal interventions , such as mailed information letters and pre-colonoscopy counseling has reflected dramatic rate increases of screening uptake from 65.1%–76.6% in managed care populations, as shown by recent evidence (Yu et al., 2018). This illustrates a causal relationship between knowledge and the use of preventive healthcare. Colonoscopy preparation is required to facilitate the optimization of procedures accuracy and effectiveness. Patients typically have a bowel-cleansing protocol to clear any residual stool from the colon that hinders visualization. Preparatory steps include dietary restriction and administration of aggressive laxatives, highlighting the importance of adequate patient education about expectations and possible discomfort during the same. Proper preparation is not only important for procedure success but also for the prevention of the risks of complications. As it is estimated that 5.5% of screening patients will be positive on a fecal immunochemical test requiring follow-up testing with colonoscopy, the need for a process that has a well-defined and effective procedure, as well as appropriate patient communication, cannot be overstated. It follows that the application of navigators and facilitated scheduling is critical in enhancing the quality of the process and outcomes for the patients (Yu et al., 2018). In real colonoscopy practice, physicians utilize state-of-the-art imaging technology both for therapeutic and diagnostic purposes. The integration of machine learning into endoscopic procedures is a breakthrough for polyp detection, and tools , such as the Faster R-CNN are making encouraging breakthroughs. The ability to automate and enhance polyp detection can potentially reduce the "miss rate" secondary to variable experience of physicians, thereby improving diagnostic accuracy and patient outcomes. As early diagnosis of precursors of colorectal cancer is of utmost importance, these technological advancements in the detection of polyps can go a long way in early intervention. Therefore, the supplementary use of modern thoughts to traditional practice provides an environment in which preventive therapy becomes increasingly beneficial in the long term, eventually serving the general purpose of reducing morbidity and mortality of colorectal cancer. Through continuous learning, preparedness, and application of technology advancements, the colonoscopy process not only functions as a diagnostic procedure but as a core strategy against colorectal cancer (Figure 5.6).

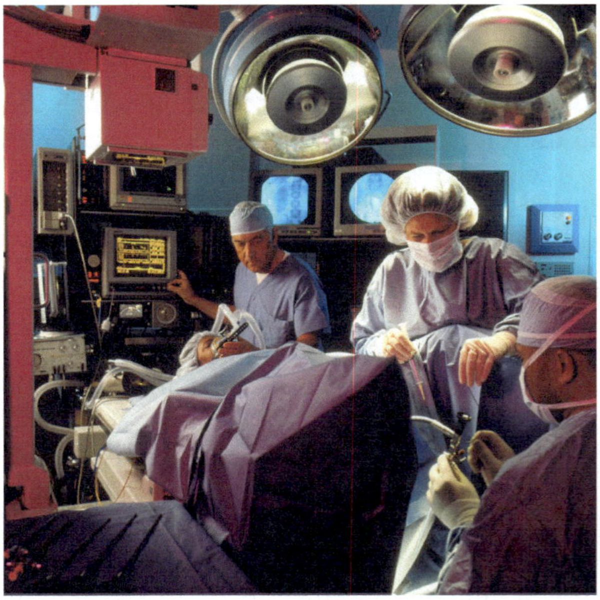

Figure 5.6. Colonoscopy procedure.

Source: https://images.fineartamerica.com/images-medium-large-5/colonoscopy-surgical-procedure-on-a-patient-ed-youngscience-photo-library.jpg.

5.2.1. Preparation for the Procedure

Preparation of a colonoscopy is a sensitive process that significantly affects the quality and reliability of the examination. Proper bowel preparation is required to ensure that the colon is adequately cleansed of fecal matter, so that visualization during the procedure can be optimal. Poor preparation will render potential polyps and lesions unseen, leading to a false-negative diagnosis or spurious results. There is evidence to indicate that up to one-quarter of colonoscopy procedures can be attributed to suboptimal bowel preparation, calling for patients to adhere rigidly to the rigorous preparatory regimens provided by clinicians. Thus, uniform bowel preparation protocols have become a necessity in enhancing the diagnostic efficacy of colonoscopy (Kastenberg et al., 2018). Patients typically have a full pre-procedural education process, such as an explanation of the bowel prep protocol and the importance of dietary restrictions in the run-up to the exam. The routine is normally a clear liquid diet 24 hours before the procedure and the consumption of a laxative that has been prescribed for the purpose of bowel cleansing. Adherence to these standards not only improves the quality of the colonoscopy but also minimizes patient anxiety regarding the procedure. Moreover, the relationship between the preparation period and conducting colonoscopy in general is that high-volume centers and specialist procedures have been shown to be linked with higher detection rates of pertinent lesions. Therefore, emphasis on adequate preparation is key to the success of the colonoscopy and overall health outcomes of the patients (Holly et al., 2025). In light of the numerous factors that ascertain the success of colonoscopy performances, it's understood that systematic improvements in bowel preparation protocols can reduce variations in outcome. For instance, the application of validated scales for bowel preparation quality would enhance consistency and clarity in preparation, eventually having a positive impact on the diagnostic yield. The scales would provide a framework for measuring the quality of bowel preparation across different clinical settings, reducing the inconsistency that occurs with non-validated measures. As healthcare systems strive to enhance patient care, the establishment of specialized units for colonoscopy, coupled with stringent but uncomplicated preparation procedures, is imperative. Such actions would not only enhance patient cooperation but also lead to enhanced detection and diagnosis, achieving the primary objective of this life-saving gastrointestinal procedure (Kastenberg et al., 2018) (Figure 5.7).

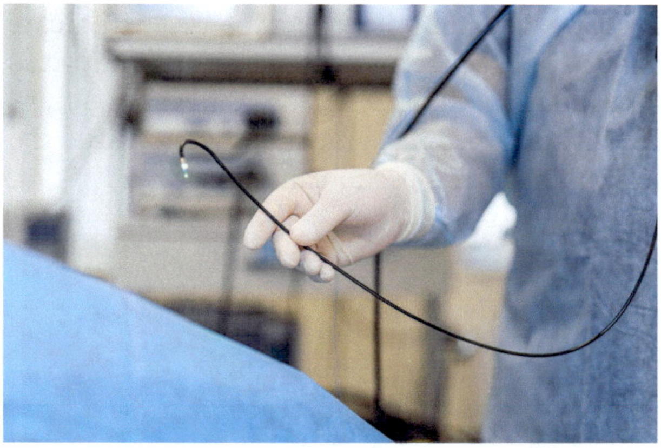

Figure 5.7. Colonoscopy preparation.

Source: https://www.jeffersonhealth.org/content/dam/health2021/images/photos/photo-shoots/people/clinical/colonoscopy-preparation-and-procedure.jpg.

5.2.2. The Actual Procedure Process

The procedure itself for a colonoscopy is a component of colorectal cancer screening, with distinct steps that collectively ensure patient safety and diagnostic yield. Before the process, prolonged preparation is needed; this includes dietary modifications and administration of a bowel lavage solution to clear the colon of any obstructive material. This preparation aids in enhancing the visualization of the gastrointestinal tract during testing. When the patient arrives at the facility, there will be a rapid assessment for readiness, typically with sedation to facilitate ease of comfort during the procedure. Sedation serves to emphasize one of the distinctive aspects of colonoscopy that differentiates it from other screening tests, which are otherwise conducted by the patient without such interventions (Yu et al., 2018). When the actual procedure is performed, the physician takes a flexible tube with a camera attached to it—a colonoscope—to view and examine the lining of the rectum and colon. As the slow passage of the colonoscope takes place within the GI tract, the physician can identify and perhaps cut away polyps or biopsy suspicious lesions that could indicate cancer. This process is not only diagnostic; it is therapeutic in tone, with the removal of polyps serving as a prophylactic measure towards the formation of colorectal cancer.

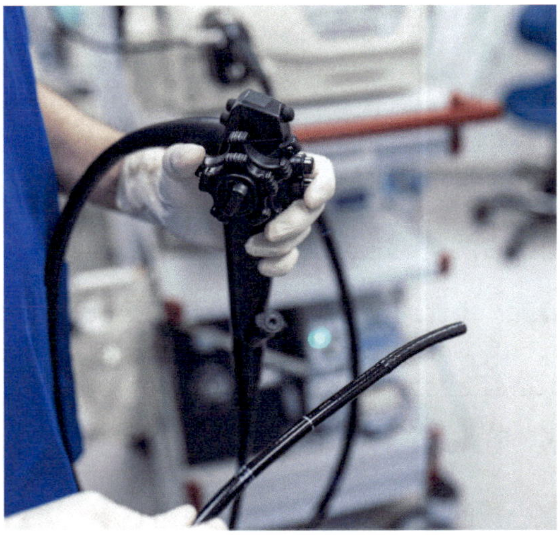

Figure 5.8. Preventing colorectal cancer: The vital role of colonoscopy screening.

Source: https://merusgastro.com/wp-content/uploads/2024/05/The-Vital-Role-of-Colonoscopy-Screening-1.png.

The activity of performing colonoscopies has seen remarkable results in the detection of precancerous conditions through routine screenings, thereby emphasizing the importance of such an activity in population health policy towards colorectal cancer (Yu et al., 2018). Post-procedure, the patients are monitored as the sedation wears off and given information on recovery and follow-up. Since sedation is frequently used being the case, post-procedure journeys need consideration, involving the presence of an escort person for safety reasons. This is consistent with greater logistical issues associated with the process; research has indicated that social and pragmatic barriers to patients—e.g., acquiring a driver—can influence whether they can complete screenings (Curbow et al., 2019). Thus, healthcare providers are encouraged to implement measures of support in addressing the barriers, thereby improving overall screening rates and ensuring that patients utilize the preventive potential of colonoscopy, especially since the incidence of colorectal cancer remains a significant health concern (Figure 5.8).

5.2.3. Post-Procedure Care and Recovery

Post-procedure after colonoscopy is a critical phase that guarantees patient safety and successful recovery. Patients are typically observed in a recovery room post-procedure to assess vital signs and improve any resulting discomfort. The effects of sedatives administered during colonoscopy can last for several hours, and observation is required to establish that the patient regains sufficient awareness before discharge. Health care professionals will typically provide both oral and written instructions for post-procedure care, including such things as dietary modifications, activity restrictions, and potential complications to be monitored, e.g., uncontrolled bleeding or sudden sharp pain in the abdomen. These precautions show how important it is that communication between the health care professionals and the patient must be effective because it significantly assists them in understanding and adhering to care instructions given (NDe Regge et al., 2013). Other than follow-up observation in the early post-procedure course, patients are instructed on measures of self-care to enhance recovery.

Cramping and bloating after a colonoscopy are not uncommon; therefore, gradual reintroduction of a normal diet, beginning with clear liquids, is recommended. This allows the gastrointestinal system to adjust and minimizes gastrointestinal discomfort. Patients are also asked to drink sufficiently, as this aids in bowel function restitution. Additionally, individuals are generally discouraged from heavy activity for a day or two in an effort to provide their bodies with the time to recover.

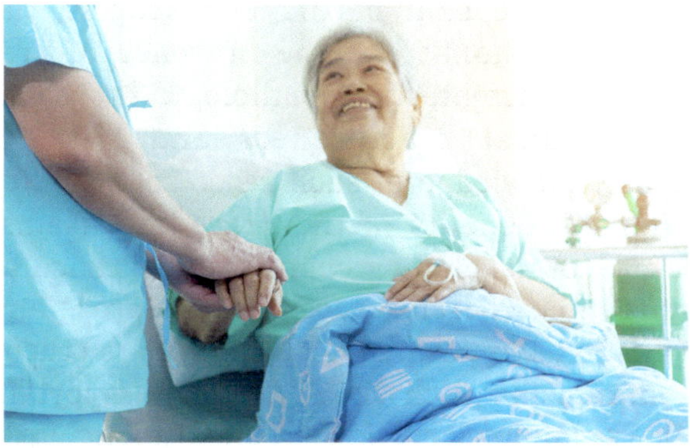

Figure 5.9. Post-operative care.

Source: https://uesrnc.com/wp-content/uploads/2019/03/post-operative-care.jpg.

By practicing such measures, patients can significantly minimize risks and enhance their general recovery process following colonoscopy (De Regge et al., 2013). The psychological care of post-procedure care also needs to be mentioned, in that most patients are able to feel anxious or fearful following a colonoscopy. Education on the reason and possible outcomes of the procedure can calm fears and improve recovery experiences. Health care professionals have an important role to de-escalate fears through empathetic interaction and affirmation of the benefits of the procedure. Furthermore, making appointments for follow-up serves to create a continuity of care, where any remaining questions or issues are addressed in depth. Leaving the facility with a full grasp of their post-colonoscopy care plan not only improves patient recovery but also fosters compliance in follow-up screening or treatments if necessary, ultimately leading to better health outcomes (De Regge et al., 2013) (Figure 5.9).

5.3. Risks and Complications

When contemplating the colonoscopy process, one should also have in mind the risks and complications which may happen. Although the procedure is generally secure in a majority of instances, it is not free of certain potential adverse outcomes. Among the most significant risks are colon perforation, which might happen seldom during polyp removal or aggressive manipulation. The risk for perforation is 0.1%–0.3% in the average patient, but it can be elevated with pre-existing gastrointestinal disease. Bleeding risk, particularly with biopsies taken out or polyps excised, is another side effect. This bleeding can be managed in most cases, but in some instances, it will require additional control measures , such as blood transfusions or additional procedures to stabilize the bleeding, thus demonstrating the importance of a comprehensive pre-procedure review of patient history and health. Another concern of interest with colonoscopy is the detection of conditions present that would complicate the procedure outcomes. For instance, as described in recent studies, acromegalic patients had an appreciable rate of colorectal polyps. Of 21 patients with acromegaly surveyed, 88% of the patients were identified by colonoscopy examination to have detectable polyps, thus establishing the significant contribution of widespread screening in patients with some risk factors. The study highlights that despite the potential for complications from colonoscopy, such as incomplete procedures and unnecessary testing, the benefit from the detection of colorectal lesions in high-risk populations cannot be ignored. Thus, judicious screening algorithms based on individual patient needs must be advocated by practitioners, particularly in symptomatic or high-risk patients for advanced neoplasia. Also, the patient's gender and age can become a deciding factor influencing the risks and complications associated with colonoscopy. Clinical trials have indicated that men are at higher risk of having advanced neoplasia at younger ages compared to women. In a mass screening of outpatient colonoscopies, 8.6% of men and 4.6% of women were found to have advanced neoplasia, which justified the suggestion for screening at an earlier age in men. This disparity extends to the number of colonoscopies required to uncover such conditions, with men often requiring fewer tests to diagnose advanced adenomas. As a result, the risk of complications must be weighed against the benefit of early treatment, particularly in high-risk groups. Hence, an enhanced understanding of these factors is essential to optimize colonoscopy practices and outcomes of patients in the early prevention and detection of colorectal cancer (Figure 5.10).

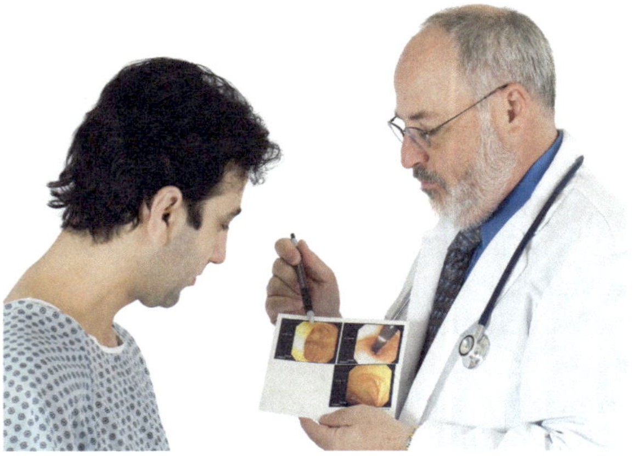

Figure 5.10. Colonoscopy risks and complications.

Source: https://www.verywellhealth.com/thmb/upg4zqbTTe1M69dvIzWtjx1e5-A=/1500x1000/filters:fill(87E3EF,1)/colonoscopy-56a8ec5c3df78cf772a1f28c.jpg.

5.3.1. Common Risks Associated with Colonoscopy

Colonoscopy is a routine procedure for cancer screening and diagnosis of gastrointestinal conditions; however, it also has some associated risks. Bowel perforation, one of the serious complications, occurs in approximately 1 in 1,000 procedures. This type of injury can cause fatal infections, requiring surgery and hospitalization for several days. The perforation risk can be established by multiple factors, including the skill of the endoscopist, the patient's anatomy, and the presence of pre-existing gastrointestinal pathology. Therefore, both medical practitioners and patients require knowledge of such risks, so that they weigh the benefits of the procedure against the risk of developing complications , such as perforation. Therefore, accurate pre-procedure evaluation and scrupulous technique are crucial in minimizing such risks. Another important risk of colonoscopy is bleeding, particularly if polyps are removed. There can be a small amount of bleeding following polypectomy that resolves without treatment. Severe bleeding is a possible complication that can cause the need for hospitalization or even emergency surgery. Bleeding related to polypectomy has been reported at rates of 0.3%–6%. Variables , such as polyp size and type, as well as anticoagulant therapy, may affect the risk of complications of bleeding. Patients with a history of coagulopathy or on anticoagulant therapy must be carefully monitored and, possibly, alternative treatment options considered to avoid this. To this end, an awareness of the risk of bleeding is necessary to help decide whether or not to proceed with the procedure. Besides physical diseases, colonoscopy also carries the risk of sedation and anesthetic side effects, which induce respiratory depression or side effects, especially among patients with comorbidities. Sedatives or anesthetics cannot be helped to render the patient comfortable during the procedure, but pose potential harm to the patient as well.

According to research, major adverse events from sedation are noted in approximately 1 in 2,000 procedures. Furthermore, strict stratification of patients based on their overall health conditions can help address such risks. In conclusion, although colonoscopy is useful in the early detection of colorectal cancer and other gastrointestinal ailments, patients must be well-educated about the current risks of the procedure, such as those associated with sedation, to make well-informed decisions regarding their healthcare options (De Regge et al., 2013; Garcia et al., 2019).

5.3.2. Rare But Serious Compli cations

The colonoscopy procedure, while generally regarded as safe, carries with it the potential for rare but serious complications that should be considered very seriously. Some of them include the most significant risk being perforation of the colon, which occurs in approximately 0.1%–0.5% of procedures. This kind of complication can lead to serious morbidity as it necessitates surgery and a prolonged hospital stay. If the bowel is perforated, contents can spill into the peritoneal cavity and peritonitis will occur, which is an acute and potentially fatal condition. Also, there is an increased risk of perforation in patients with a pre-existing condition, such as advanced diverticular disease or IBD. Thus, awareness of the risks of colonoscopy becomes important in patient selection and pre-procedure counseling. Another rare but serious complication of colonoscopy is post-polypectomy bleeding, which occurs in up to 1% of procedures. The bleeding is typically from where the resections of the polyps were performed and is either immediate or days following the procedure. The majority of instances are minor and can be managed conservatively, yet heavy bleeding may require surgical or endoscopic intervention to achieve hemostasis. Further, the severity of bleeding can be enhanced in patients with anticoagulant therapy or coagulopathies. Therefore, clinicians take utmost care to assess the patient's risk of bleeding before the procedure as well as keep them closely observed following the procedure for any evidence of complications. These potential risks, when effectively communicated, can alleviate patient anxiety as well as enhance informed consent. Lastly, complications associated with sedation employed in colonoscopy can also be developed by patients, such as respiratory depression and cardiovascular complications, although these are not common. Sedative agents must be given cautiously, and despite the risk for severe adverse effects being unlikely, they may occur in susceptible patients, such as the elderly or those with underlying conditions. Obstructive sleep apnea or significant cardiac history patients can also have special risks when given sedation.

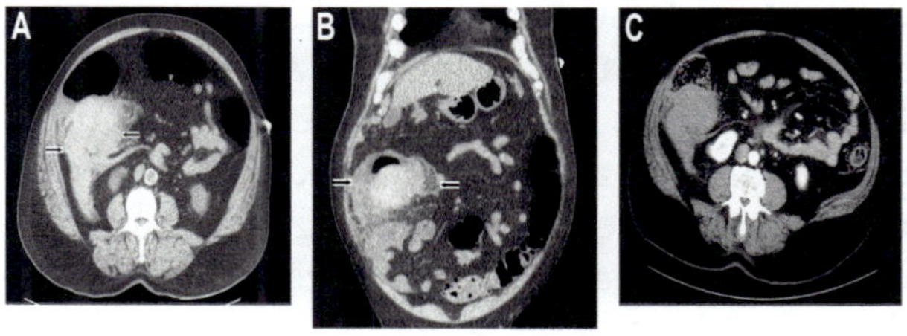

Figure 5.11. Intramural cecal hematoma: A rare complication after colonoscopy.

Source: https://els-jbs-prod-cdn.jbs.elsevierhealth.com/cms/attachment/1e28daa4-de76-4633-912b-c0cded6e78aa/gr1_lrg.jpg.

Awareness of these potential complications underscores the importance of comprehensive pre-procedure assessment, a tailored sedation method, and continuous monitoring during the procedure. With technological and technical innovation continuing to increase, proactive management of such rare complications remains key to further ensuring patient safety during colonoscopies, maintaining their status as a critical diagnostic and therapeutic tool in gastrointestinal health, as highlighted by the association with serious conditions like gastrointestinal disease and adenomatous polyps reported in Khare et al. (2015) and Moldovan et al. (2017) (Figure 5.11).

5.3.3. Factors That Increase Risk

An understanding of the diverse risk-increasing factors that predispose to colorectal cancer is important in maximizing the efficacy of colonoscopy as a screening method. All studies have established that age is one of the most significant risk factors, with individuals over the age of 50 having a significantly heightened risk of developing colorectal abnormalities , such as adenomas or cancers. Moreover, gender also plays a crucial role in the evaluation of the risk; studies have found that males are more likely to develop advanced neoplasia compared to women, and more regular screening to detect precancerous lesions is normally needed. This differential prevalence suggests that younger screening initiation among men will predict better outcomes through the detection of asymptomatic advanced adenomas, showing the importance of age and gender as risk determinants of tailored screening advice. Beyond demographic factors, individual clinical history has a significant influence on one's risk profile for colorectal disease. Patients with a history of polyps or colorectal cancer, for example, are at heightened risk that require careful follow-up with periodic surveillance colonoscopies. Evidence points to surveillance of patients with a history of polypectomy as underused, a prime example of an important gap in care. Expansion of Medicare coverage for screening has attempted to address this, but bureaucratic barriers reign in practice, resulting in inappropriate surveillance behavior. Hence, medical history is an important determinant to determine patients at high risk, thereby enabling healthcare providers to design proactive screening plans to address colorectal cancer risks effectively (Fedewa et al., 2014). Genetic conditions and family history are the important determinants that can greatly raise the chances of getting colorectal cancer. Genetic syndromes , such as Lynch syndrome and familial adenomatous polyposis significantly raise the risk of developing polyps and cancer at an earlier age, necessitating the need for earlier and more frequent screening treatments. The information shows that individuals with a history of colorectal cancer in the family should already be having consultations with their health care providers in their 20s, emphasizing early awareness. Besides, lifestyle determinants , such as diet, physical activity, and smoking contribute to the risk profile. A low fiber intake diet with excess red and processed meat consumption, combined with physical inactivity, is associated with increased risks, and this is a demonstration of the complexity of factors influencing colorectal health (Crispin et al., 2011) (Figure 5.12).

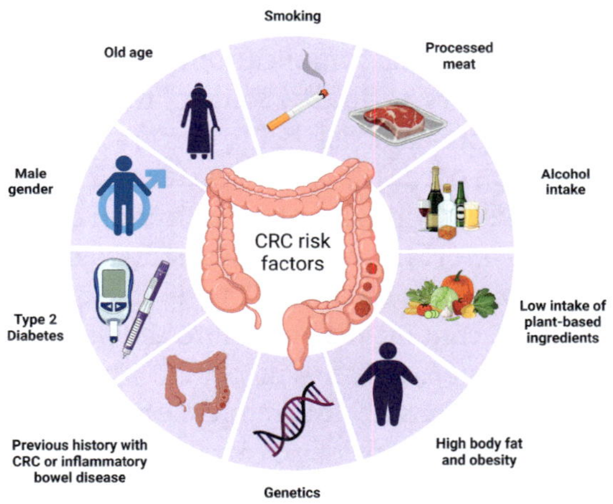

Figure 5.12. Risk factors of colorectal cancer.

Source: https://cdn.prod.website-files.com/621e95f9ac30687a56e4297e/65dfaaa6deeb44de8d1472a1_V2_1680184064635_c1f0aa25-6168-47f6-80a5-0f40a1904162_HIGH_RES.png.

5.4. Benefits of Colonoscopy

Colonoscopy advantages extend far more than mere screening, making the procedure an essential tool in proactive colorectal disease treatment. Arguably, the most critical advantage of colonoscopy is that it can detect cancer of the colon in its early stages, which is paramount since cancer identified at an early stage is often more curable. Statistically, individuals with an early diagnosis of colorectal cancer have an extremely good prognosis, with survival rates much better than those who are diagnosed later. Moreover, colonoscopy is a preventive; during the procedure, polyps can be identified and removed before they become malignant cells, thereby reducing the incidence of colorectal cancer and, in fact, mortality due to the disease. As health education programs confirm, a better-educated population is more likely to take advantage of this preventive potential, and thereby have improved outcomes in the management of colorectal health (Gipsh et al., 2004). Furthermore, a significant gap in the use and acceptance of colonoscopy screening exists among varied populations, and most significantly among African Americans, who are disproportionately affected by colorectal cancer. Cultural perceptions and beliefs play a significant role in influencing screening behavior within this population. An understanding of these factors enables healthcare practitioners to develop successful education interventions that promote screening program participation. Literally, for instance, which is culturally tailored, can debunk widespread myths , such as pain during procedures and medical mistrust, which are generally barriers to screening (DuHamel et al., 2012). Resolution of these problems with specially devised communication plans provides a positive environment, encouraging people to place preventative exams like colonoscopy on their agenda. Ultimately, through increased awareness and accessibility, colonoscopy use can result in decreased death rates and overall improved public health. Furthermore, the psychological benefits of a colonoscopy cannot be overlooked. All patients report feeling empowered and relieved after the procedure, particularly when given a clean bill of health. Even if the prospect of a colonoscopy initially causes anxiety, reassurance that comes with regular screenings can cut down on fears of colorectal cancer. This is in accordance with findings that successful health education can create people's willingness to undergo such screenings by confirming the importance of prevention as well as early detection. Though public awareness of colorectal cancer is the intent of community health programs, the promotion of colonoscopy as a fundamental aspect of health maintenance becomes increasingly important. Ultimately, promoting an understanding of the benefits of the procedures can promote society toward prioritizing preventative measures of care to advance population health outcomes (Gipsh et al., 2004) (Figure 5.13).

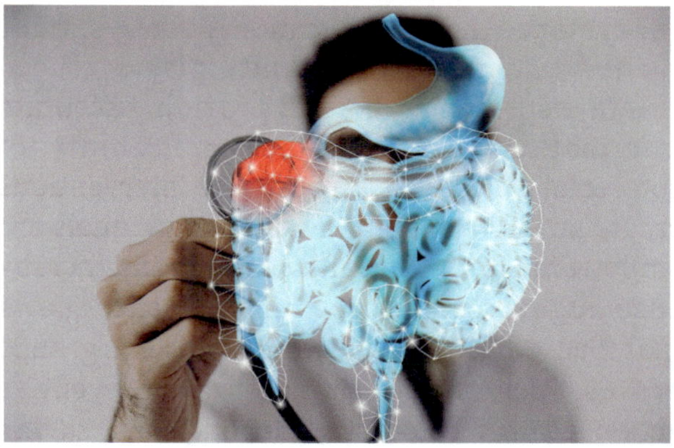

Figure 5.13. Benefits of a colonoscopy.

Source: https://virginiacolonoscopy.com/wp-content/uploads/2023/01/2150942845-min.jpg.

5.4.1. Early Detection of Cancer

Early detection of cancer, particularly CRC, is a milestone in patient care with significant implications on treatment and survival. Colonoscopy plays a central role within this early detection system with the capability for direct visualization and intervention within the colon. Through the identification of precancerous polyps and removal before malignancy develops, colonoscopy not only reduces rates of incidence but also promotes an active colorectal health management. The effectiveness of this therapy is dependent on mass screening protocols, particularly among the 50-and-older group known to have higher risks of colorectal cancer. Since public health programs encourage screening on a regular basis, there is a need to understand what underlies beliefs and behaviors toward influencing health decisions for having a colonoscopy since these are critical in enhancing early detection and decreasing morbidity and mortality due to cancer among the population (Gipsh et al., 2004). Increasing awareness regarding health beliefs is critical to enhancing early detection of cancer through colonoscopy. Evidence indicates that knowledge about the benefits of screening in childhood can be a contribution to patient behavioral change. For instance, health educational interventions carried out in the community play a crucial role in dispelling myths and providing accurate information regarding the applicability of colorectal cancer screening. These interventions create an environment in which individuals are empowered to make healthy choices and thereby encourage screening programs. Evidence shows that focused health education in specific groups proves to be a good initiator for preventive action against colorectal cancer, hence saving lives and slowing the economic burden of treating advanced cases of cancer (Gipsh et al., 2004). Moreover, the interaction between education and the quality of information provided has a high effect on early detection rates. Evidence indicates that individuals with higher education tend to adopt screening interventions like colonoscopy. The correlation posits the importance of a healthy relationship between patients and health care providers concerning the complexity of cancer risk and prevention measures. When well-educated patients receive high-quality advice from their providers, they are better able to process and react to information about their health, with a notable increase in their willingness to accept screening advice. Thus, by raising patient education and offering higher-quality primary care, healthcare systems are better able to increase early detection rates and facilitate an improved public health response to colorectal cancer.

5.4.2. Prevention of Colorectal Cancer (CRC)

Prevention of CRC has a close association with effective screening methods, and colonoscopy has emerged as a vital tool. As most health authorities, including the U.S. Preventive Services Task Force, recommended, routine screening initiated at age 50 continues until age 75; this program has shown a notable decrease in incidence and mortality due to colorectal cancer. Colonoscopy not only allows for the detection of precancerous polyps but also allows for their removal at the same time, further inhibiting cancer development. With late detection significantly decreasing survival rates, preventive screening through colonoscopy is seen to be a significant measure towards avoiding cancer by not only taking into consideration early intervention but also informing patients about regular screening. Despite the proven efficacy of colonoscopies in preventing colorectal cancer, participation rates have often fallen short of public health expectations. A study in Germany highlighted that only 26% of non-screened individuals had received recommendations for screening, indicating a substantial gap in provider-patient communication. This lack of engagement may stem from misconceptions surrounding the necessity and safety of colonoscopies. Most people wrongly assume that such screenings have to be done only in case of prevalent symptoms, which directly discourages compliance with preventive health measures. Demystifying these myths by conducting targeted education programs is necessary. By raising awareness among the public regarding the dangers of colorectal cancer and the importance of screenings, health professionals can substantially enhance the usage rate of such critical preventive services, which will eventually translate into improved health outcomes. Besides increasing worry about low screening rates, psychosocial concerns about the procedure itself are a significant contributor to discouraging individuals from undergoing colonoscopy. Anxiety about the experience of colonoscopy and general knowledge deficit regarding colorectal cancer emerge as determinants for not complying with screening recommendations, as evidenced by multivariate analysis. Thus, it is essential to develop shared decision-making tools and overall educational materials as part of the process to enhance patient readiness for screenings. Through patient participation in decision-making, health care providers can alleviate fear and misinformation regarding colonoscopy, creating an active public approach to colorectal cancer prevention. As work to enhance patient engagement advances, promise of transforming screening compliance and, in turn, rates of prevention of colorectal cancer increases significantly, demonstrating the central intersection of education, communication, and preventive health (Figure 5.14).

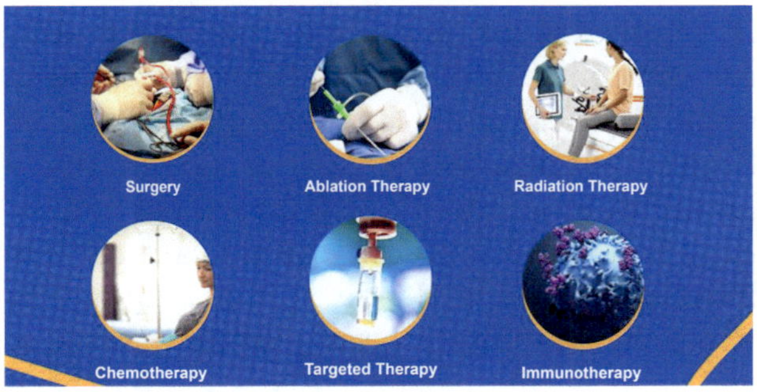

Figure 5.14. Colorectal cancer.

Source: https://actchealth.com/images/treatment/colo-treat.png.

5.4.3. Improved Management of Gastrointestinal Conditions

Advances in diagnostic techniques and technology have significantly enhanced the care of gastrointestinal diseases, particularly those needing colonoscopy. Colonoscopy is not only an extremely useful diagnostic tool but also for intervention , such as polypectomy and control of gastrointestinal hemorrhage. The precision made possible by high-definition imaging and chromoendoscopy allows gastroenterologists to visualize lesions that might otherwise have been missed. Also, integration of artificial intelligence and machine learning into colonoscopy image interpretation represents a milestone development in boosting the precision of diagnoses for colorectal disease. Focusing on readiness and response, the streamlined process of obtaining timely colonoscopic evaluation ensures that patients receive instant and effective intervention, thus avoiding potential morbidity that can accumulate from delays in care. Effective treatment of gastrointestinal disease via colonoscopy is also risk-stratified and tailored to individual patients. Personalized scheduling of colonoscopy based on individual risk factors, such as family history and genetic susceptibility, offers the prospect of surveillance and preclinical detection of colorectal cancer. For instance, suggestions have been given regarding varying screening intervals depending on a patient's initial result and risk factors; patients with a family history of colorectal cancer are most likely to require more frequent testing than the general-risk population. In addition, sedation care and analgesia innovations in colonoscopies minimize pain and anxiety, thereby dispelling patient fear of the procedure. More education on colon health, as well as increased public awareness, achieves a cultural shift towards anticipatory gastrointestinal care, which empowers individuals to access necessary screenings without apprehension. Moreover, care for gastrointestinal disease involves not only immediate intervention by colonoscopy but also holistic treatment of gastrointestinal well-being. Coupling the multidisciplinary nature with the addition of dietary modifications, lifestyle modifications, and continued medical intervention helps improve outcomes. For example, with the condition being soil-transmitted helminths, which infects a substantial percentage of the population, public education and early detection with colonoscopy can help in intervention at an appropriate time and limit complications (Addiss et al., 2018). The multidisciplinary approach is most evident in the management of conditions , such as IBD, when serial endoscopic follow-up has a central role to play in the evaluation of disease activity and also the response to therapy. As healthcare systems seek tighter control of gastrointestinal illness, the central contribution that colonoscopy makes as a diagnostic, as well as a therapeutic modality, will remain within a holistic patient care model (Figure 5.15).

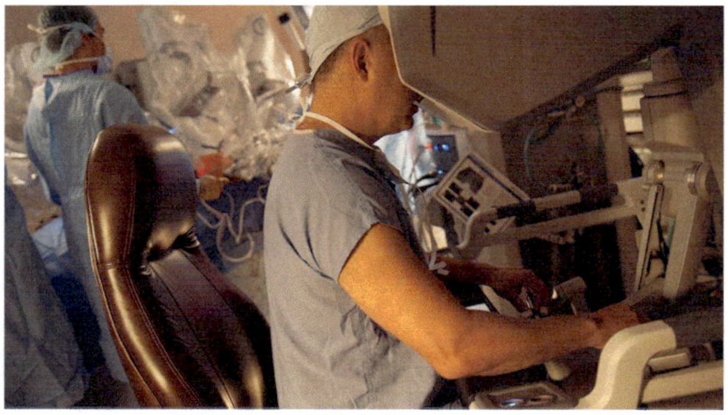

Figure 5.15. Robotic surgery for digestive & gastrointestinal conditions.

Source: https://nyulangone.org/files/surgeon-and-robotic-technology.jpg.

5.5. Patient Experience

Patient experience with a colonoscopy is a significant factor that can influence both immediate and long-term outcomes of this common diagnostic test. The quality of communication, the amount of support from health care professionals, and the overall ambiance of the site are all significant variables in what produces patient perceptions. This experience is particularly important, as most individuals feel uncomfortable and apprehensive when exposed to a colonoscopy. Research has established that specialized centers have the tendency to enhance patient care through encouraging innovation in service provision by taking care of the medical needs while offering a patient-centered service. By dealing with these issues initially, clinicians can relieve patient fear, increase levels of satisfaction, and therefore encourage a more favorable association with the health-care system, an essential foundation for follow-up and compliance with future screening advice (De Regge et al., 2013). Moreover, the conditions of the colonoscopy procedure itself—pre-procedure instructions, sedation options, and follow-ups after the procedure—can have a significant impact on the patient experience. High-deductible health plans (HDHPs) are increasingly prevalent, affecting patient attitudes and behavior towards the healthcare system. The financial burden of HDHPs places patients at a disadvantage in making well-informed decisions, particularly for preventive services like colonoscopies that may be viewed as both critical and costly. This stress could lead to the delay or avoidance of screening tests, with adverse effects on their health. Resolution of these fiscal concerns in the patient pathway is significant to healthcare providers, who are confronted with balancing best treatment opportunities with the evolving nature of health coverage and cost-sparing initiatives (Fendrick et al., 2014). To improve the patient experience of colonoscopy, healthcare centers must include a multi-disciplinary approach based on supportive care, patient education, and patient compassion. Facilitating feedback loops where patients can offer concerns and share experiences allows healthcare providers to continually adjust the quality of service. Expanding pre- and post-procedure education provided can also enable patients, making them feel in charge of their treatment. Having gastroenterologists, nurses, and administrators collaborate to offer congruent information and care to patients throughout the process makes this possible. While undergoing the process, not only do healthcare organizations enhance the immediate patient experience, but also promote adherence to preventative care practice, which ultimately results in improved public health outcomes (De Regge et al., 2013).

5.5.1. Emotional and Psychological Aspects

The psychological and emotional factors involved with colonoscopy procedures are normally overlooked but largely impact the overall experiences of patients and subsequent health outcomes. Levels of anxiety can also be critical in a patient's adherence to the procedure, as well as in their memory and compliance with post-procedure care. For many individuals, fear of discomfort, embarrassment, or the outcome of colorectal cancer creates an invisible mental block that could deter them from undergoing recommended screening programs. The Halton report discusses that the quality of perceived care manifests so that patients feel more comfortable and secure in accepting colonoscopy when they experience empathetic and caring care subjectively, and this establishes the need for health professionals to enhance emotional support systems throughout the screening process (Kirby et al., 2003). Moreover, ethnic and cultural heritage make these kinds of emotional challenges worse. Studies have indicated that ethnic minority groups have extremely low screening rates due to complex reasons, including past mistrust of the healthcare establishment, fear of discrimination, and a lack of culturally appropriate care. The emotional burden of dealing with these disparities is likely to create isolation and hopelessness among these populations, leading to missed opportunities for early detection and colorectal cancer prevention. Through the identification of the psychological barriers that different groups face, healthcare providers are able to modify communication and support, hence improving levels of participation and completion for colonoscopy screenings (Szczepura et al., 2003). This is an important step in ensuring equitable healthcare as well as building a safer, more inclusive healthcare environment for patients. Dealing with the emotional and psychological components of colonoscopy is not only crucial for the patient but also for enhancing the overall effectiveness of public health interventions that seek to improve screening rates. Interventions that aim to raise awareness regarding the need to be screened and those that provide counseling for the psychological impact have shown potential results. Such programs can alleviate anxiety, create a sense of mastery, and encourage patients to resist any threats of both procedure and potential diagnoses. Moreover, an environment in which disclosure of colorectal health is fostered can empower, especially among the underrepresented ethnic populations, patients to be proactive in seeking care. These pre-emptive measures are required for the success of national colorectal cancer screening initiatives, with all patients' psychological well-being taking precedence over clinical care (Clay et al., 2025).

5.5.2. Patient Testimonials and Perspectives

Comments from patients play a crucial role in shaping public views and opinions regarding colonoscopy. Patients who undergo the procedure usually offer feedback, highlighting both the physical and emotional aspects of the process. Many of the testimonials emphasize the anxiety that accompanies waiting for the colonoscopy, mentioning initial fear about the pain entailed in undergoing it as well as the intrusiveness of the process. However, many testimonials reflect a change of heart after experiencing the procedure, with patients tending to express relief and appreciation for the preventive value it offers against colorectal cancer. By sharing their experiences, patients not only demystify the procedure itself but also encourage others to place importance on their gastrointestinal health, which in turn leads to higher screening rates within communities. Patient comments about colonoscopy also provide useful information concerning areas where healthcare providers can do better. Patient testimonials tend to make observations on the need for good communication between provider and patient, with emphasis on the preparation process and what one experiences during the procedure. Patients have indicated that clear descriptions and empathetic communication significantly alleviate pre-procedure anxiety. These results can serve as valuable resources for physicians who are striving to provide a welcoming environment for open communication.

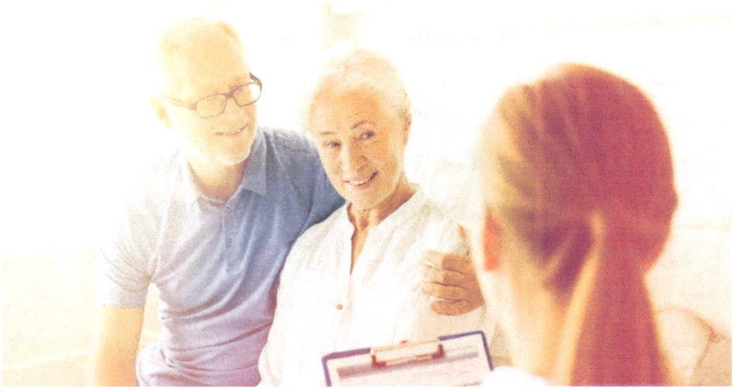

Figure 5.16. Patient perspectives.

Source: https://www.hccnthecharity.org/wp-content/uploads/2021/11/Patients-perspectives-1280x640.jpg.

Moreover, the communication of positive testimonials will deconstruct myths and stigma surrounding colonoscopy, allowing for a better-informed patient population that is more willing to engage in required screenings for their health. In addition to patient testimonies, patient feedback can also highlight the inherent benefit of employing complementary means of mitigating pain from colonoscopy. For instance, patients have expressed satisfaction upon integrating back-up modes of pain control, such as music therapy or mindfulness meditation, within their pre-and post-procedure protocols. Such modes, beyond alleviating pain, provide patients with empowerment by allowing them to feel they are in control of their healthcare process. This reflects a growing trend in medicine, where patient-centered care includes exploring various methods to enhance comfort and satisfaction during medical procedures. As seen in projects aimed at increasing healthcare provider awareness of such modalities, patient testimonials can drive the adoption of these innovative methods, ultimately improving overall patient outcomes in colonoscopy procedures (Boyles, 2021) (Figure 5.16).

5.5.3. Addressing Common Fears and Misconceptions

Colonoscopy, much feared, is accompanied by an array of fears and myths that have a very strong influence on people's decisions in relation to this crucial screening test. Patients usually fear the pain or embarrassment caused by the passage of the colonoscope. Medical science has made advancements to turn colonoscopy into a relatively smooth procedure, particularly with sedation techniques available for patient comfort during the procedure. Research has indicated that a majority of patients experience minimal pain rather than severe pain, thus making it important to eliminate such myths and educate worthy candidates on how others actually feel. Eliciting emotion-based fears, e.g., fear about the outcome, is also essential; articulating the argument for colonoscopy's central role in early detection of colorectal cancer can diminish this fear and enable informed participation in screening programs (Szczepura et al., 2003). Further, inaccuracy regarding age and family history is usually the source of misinformation regarding the need for a colonoscopy. The overall perception is that screening is only for those who are known to have a history of colorectal cancer in their families, and as such, most disregard their own health. In actuality, routine screenings are recommended by medical professionals to be conducted on everyone starting at age 45, irrespective of personal or family medical history. This eligibility expansion is key in mirroring the rising rate of colorectal cancer among youths, wherein education and preemptive screening lag behind. In eliminating such myths and reasserting that colonoscopy as a preventive measure can be applied to a wider population, medical practitioners can be in a position to increase participation rates in regular screenings, thus optimizing early detection procedures (Andrew et al., 2023). Finally, the taboo on bowel health adds to the complexity of attitudes towards colonoscopy. Patients feel shy bringing up gastrointestinal problems, which results in decreased interaction with healthcare professionals. The silence reinforces bad myths, such as that only very bad symptoms need to be felt before consultation. There is a need to create a setting that normalizes talking about bowel health, with its importance to overall well-being. Screening programs that introduce personal narratives of the colonoscopy-done individuals can make the process more personal, with relatable stories that alleviate anxiety and shame. Education campaigns to both the public and the health care providers on the significance of maintaining colon health may lead to a change in attitude, eventually translating into increased screening rates as well as improved outcomes for at-risk populations (Andrew et al., 2023).

5.6. Alternatives to Colonoscopy

Even though colonoscopy has been considered the "gold standard" for the screening and diagnosis of colorectal cancer, all the while, over time, other techniques were created that give patients less invasive options without compromising diagnostic accuracy. Stool-based testing is one of the primary alternatives, i.e., the Fecal Immunochemical Test (FIT) and the Multi-Target Stool DNA test (MT-sDNA). These tests operate on the basis of finding residual blood or DNA markers in the stool that validate the presence of colorectal abnormalities. The non-invasive nature of these tests is a big draw for most patients who otherwise would be nervous about the preparation and procedure of a standard colonoscopy. By providing an accessible alternative for people who might refuse screening due to fear or discomfort, stool-based tests are a key element in raising overall rates of screening and early diagnosis of colorectal cancer. Another useful alternative to colonoscopy is CT colonography, or virtual colonoscopy. This imaging technique uses computed tomography to produce high-resolution images of the rectum and colon. Like standard colonoscopy, CT colonography attempts to visualize polyps and other diseases but does so noninvasively. Although direct intervention during CT colonography, such as polyp removal or biopsy, cannot be performed, the sensitivity for the detection of large lesions is as good as with standard colonoscopy. Importantly, the absence of sedation and smaller amounts of bowel preparation make it more attractive to patients. Nevertheless, the health workers need to weigh the benefit against the risk for radiation exposure as well as follow-up testing on confirmed cases, hence placing into context the requirement for judicious patient selection and informed decision in choosing screening options. Recent technologies , such as capsule endoscopy, are also gaining popularity as alternatives to the conventional colonoscopy. This test employs a tiny, swallowable capsule that holds a camera to photograph the gastrointestinal tract, including the colon. The chief advantage of capsule endoscopy is that it does not involve a break in the skin and is not painful, which could be more inviting for potential patients than other colonoscopy methods. However, there is a necessity to recognize that while capsule endoscopy is most effective in small bowel examination, one of its limitations is that it cannot perform biopsies or even remove polyps. The evolving profile of colorectal cancer screening makes the imperative for continuous investment in and research on these newer modalities, as each has its own relative strengths and limitations that must be addressed to optimize patient care and outcomes in screening modalities (Lam et al., 2016; Aas, 2025) (Figure 5.17).

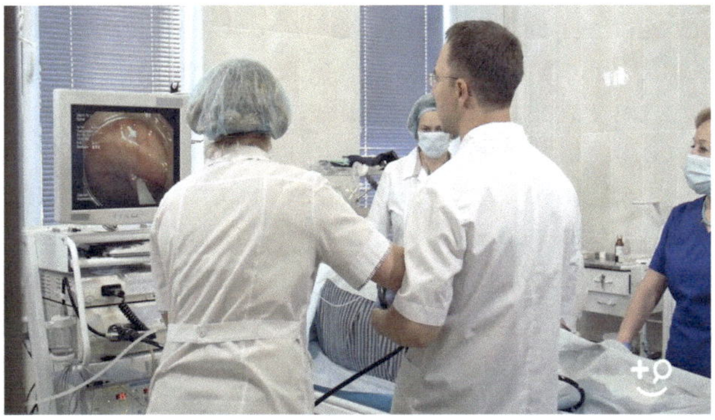

Figure 5.17. Colon cancer – Alternatives to colonoscopy.

Source: https://doctorpedia-dev.s3.us-east-2.amazonaws.com/wp-content/uploads/2021/08/19085728/Colon-Cancer-Colonoscopy.jpg.

5.6.1. Other Screening Methods

The function of alternative screening tests to colonoscopy has now emerged for the early detection of CRC. A prominent alternative is FIT, which detects occult blood in stool samples, an early indicator of potential neoplastic change. It has been found that FIT sensitivity for advanced adenomas is as good as that of colonoscopy, with sufficient yield in asymptomatic individuals at average risk. Additionally, the fact that FIT is non-invasive renders it a favored option among those who are reluctant to undergo a colonoscopy, thereby potentially raising overall screening levels. Specifically, efficacy is assured by regular annual screening, as studies have shown that such interventions provide early interventions and reduce mortality from CRC, thus firmly establishing FIT as an effective adjunct to conventional colonoscopic screening, particularly among populations who may avoid invasive testing (Crispin et al., 2011). Emerging technologies also provide promising alternatives for CRC screening. Such is the case with the Cologuard test, a multi-target stool DNA test that analyzes stool samples for DNA and hemoglobin biomarkers for CRC and advanced adenomas. This non-surgical method is particularly valuable for those patients who are not yet candidates for routine colonoscopy, since it carries both sensitivity and specificity combined, creating high detection rates for precursors and cancerous lesions alike. The convenience of conducting the test at home, combined with superb patient compliance, sets it apart as a choice for complementing screening practices. It is vital, however, that education on the different screening modalities available be promoted, since varied options offered will ensure that broader participation is drawn from the heterogeneous population bases and eventually translate to lowered CRC incidence and mortality (Boggi et al., 2017). Another important screening process involves the utilization of advanced imaging technologies , such as virtual colonoscopy, also referred to as CT colonography.

It employs computed tomography to create high-quality images of the rectum and colon and has increasingly been valued for its ability to detect large polyps without necessarily utilizing the invasive method of traditional colonoscopy. Although virtual colonoscopy is not as painful and does not involve sedation, it should be noted that a positive result would also require a follow-up colonoscopy to validate the diagnosis and removal of detected lesions. The presence and creation of such alternatives highlight an evolving paradigm in the screening for colorectal cancer, emphasizing the value of individualized modes of healthcare provision. As these methods evolve and improve, they form a critical component of the broader spectrum of options for CRC prevention alongside colonoscopy (Crispin et al., 2011).

5.6.2. Pros and Cons of Alternatives

The controversy over alternative alternatives to colonoscopy generally revolves around the effectiveness and accessibility of such procedures to identify colorectal issues. FIT and stool DNA tests are useful substitutes, primarily due to their non-invasive nature and reduced levels of distress compared to standard colonoscopy. However, even with their potential to provide initial screening, their sensitivity will be less than that of colonoscopy, particularly for polyps or early cancer. The challenge remains how to recommend using them as single screening tests without the verification from colonoscopy. With increasingly sophisticated genetic and epidemiological risk evaluation, the potential for these alternatives to complement or even partially replace colonoscopy may increase, although current constraints render one vulnerable to careful consideration of the trade-offs in abandoning further diagnostic follow-up upon receiving positive results on such non-invasive studies (Allegretti et al., 2017). Further, the limitations of only doing non-invasive screening tests highlight a significant deficit in patient management. Whereas others like FIT or stool DNA tests can identify abnormalities but not direct visualization and polypectomy, real-time diagnostic capabilities like colonoscopy, their efficiency in elderly populations also needs to be compared against individual health status, given special attention to comprehensive geriatric assessments for screening regimens (Balducci et al., 2017). Health care providers are confronted with a multifaceted setting in which the potential benefits of these options, e.g., increased patient convenience and comfort, are contrasted with the potential harms of possibly avoided diagnosis or delay in treatment. Options are thus understandably attractive, yet must be considered within the context of a comprehensive strategy that is based on best practices in colorectal health. The integration of alternative screening processes into the conversation for the prevention of colorectal cancer opens up differential views for patient participation and compliance. Most patients would likely be more inclined to undergo non-invasive screening owing to their ease and comfort, with a possible increase in overall screening rates among populations who are reluctant to conventional colonoscopy. However, medical clinicians must address the educational aspect of such options, reiterating that follow-up intervention will be necessary in an attempt to decrease the chances of the development of advanced disease." Moreover, as outlined in current literature, decision-making regarding screening for older individuals can be enhanced through a focus on the measurement of physiologic versus chronologic age alone, thereby allowing for more tailored care. By increasing awareness of the strengths and weaknesses of alternatives, healthcare providers can improve informed decision-making by patients in terms of their colorectal health and screening (Balducci et al., 2017).

5.6.3. Recommendations for Different Patient Needs

The disparities in CRC screening rates necessitate patient-specific recommendations that meet differential patient needs. Results from a UK pilot study identify a serious gap in the uptake of colonoscopy among ethnic minorities, despite otherwise positive attitudes in regular screening programs. What such findings suggest is that programs must be adapted to the particular situation and barriers faced by such groups, emphasizing the need for culturally appropriate outreach. Active engagement with local community organizations and with the use of local knowledge can promote awareness and improve take-up rates for screening programs. With the knowledge that a generic solution will only strengthen disparities, it is crucial to define particular interventions according to socio-economic, cultural, and linguistic differences between potential participants (Szczepura et al., 2003). Clinicians must also consider the specific demands of minority groups when responding to CRC screening. Research within the United States indicates that screening rates can be profoundly impacted by healthcare systems through effective intervention programs tailored to their patient population. Implementation of a systematic approach that utilizes a learning community strategy can make it feasible to establish best practices to improve screening in underserved populations. By assembling interprofessional teams with stakeholders and community representatives, health systems can pilot and refine evidence-based interventions in an effort to improve accessibility, raise awareness, and ultimately improve outcomes in various patient populations. Such modifications can incorporate outreach activities or educational campaigns that speak to the concerns and values of ethnic minorities, thus building a trust relationship that can increase participation in screening programs (DiCarlo et al., 2018). Finally, continuous evaluation and revision of CRC screening guidelines are crucial to ensure that they continue to be effective and relevant to the populations targeted. As uncovered in the UK pilot study, low take-up rates for screening in certain groups impose a necessity for active intervention to break down access barriers. Health policy-makers need to practice strategic planning to tackle the intricate challenges ethnic minorities face in accessing colonoscopy programs. Having evidence-based recommendations from data collected through ongoing surveillance allows the construction of sustainable interventions that can be replicated in most health systems. Prioritizing equity and inclusivity in CRC screening programs allows the authorities to try and reduce health disparities and ensure every patient is provided with the care they are entitled to in a timely and respectful manner (Szczepura et al., 2003).

SUMMARY

In concluding the subject of colonoscopy, it must be stressed that it is a powerful tool for the prevention and early detection of colorectal cancer. Although shown to be effective, there are issues with interpreting data from various practices, in particular, those billing screening exams through billing codes. As indicated by analysis of medical billing data, while a 61% screening rate conforms to national norms, on closer inspection through manual audit, inconsistencies that significantly influence the accuracy of such statistics are discovered, leading to a revised rate of screening at 85%. This demonstrates the intricacies involved in the utilization of billing information for the evaluation of health quality, indicating that prudence is advisable when making assumptions regarding population-level screening efficacy using such measures (Avila et al., 2020). Additionally, the significance of compliance with the best practices in procedural guidelines cannot be emphasized enough. The Italian Society of Colorectal Surgery (SICCR) emphasizes the use of evidence-based recommendations for the diagnosis and treatment of diseases of the colon and rectum, including those managed through colonoscopy. The SICCR tries to maximize patient care and equip health care providers with the information they need to conduct screening effectively by presenting full guidelines. This is particularly pertinent given that the quality of colonoscopy care can vary based on procedural ability and strict adherence to standard protocol. Towards this end, the use of standardized procedures based on thoroughly investigated guidelines can take on a central role in improving health outcomes for screening patients (Annibale et al., 2015). Finally, increasing awareness and education on colonoscopy is crucial to increasing screening rates and increasing patient compliance. Public health intervention programs must clear some myths and misconceptions related to the procedure so that more individuals are encouraged to undergo recommended screening. Integrating patient education into the healthcare system also demystifies the procedure and underlines its preventive role in colorectal cancer. Given that discrepancies in screening data indicate, elevating the systematic process to practice and patient participation is critical. Colonoscopy is not merely the technical performance; it involves the broader goal of establishing a society that is health-conscious and encourages prevention, to eventually achieve improved public health outcomes (Annibale et al., 2015).

Colonoscopy is a vital screening method in modern medicine, routinely used to detect CRC and its precursors, such as adenomatous polyps. Colonoscopy-based early diagnosis has been proven to significantly enhance the prognosis and reduce mortality rates of CRC. Colonoscopy offers a direct visual inspection of the colon and rectum, and clinicians can identify abnormalities and utilize interventions accordingly. With the development of technology over the past decades, computer-aided detection (CAD) system integration has enhanced polyp detection during colonoscopy. As discussed in the literature, CAD-CTC systems offer high sensitivity rates for polyps of varying sizes, and hence screening findings can be potentially improved with reduced missed diagnoses and less radiologists' manual analysis time (Chowdhury et al., 2008). In addition, the effectiveness of colonoscopy as a screening procedure hinges on a wide range of factors , including physician incentives and health policies. Research indicates that when primary care physicians are incentivized through bonus eligibility, the rate of their patients being screened for CRC substantially increases. More specifically, research has shown that patients whose doctors were eligible for bonuses saw their screening rates increase by 3% points (Armour et al., 2025). This linkage points to the importance of coordinating incentives for doctors and public health objectives, in that organizational encouragement can lead to improved screening outcomes and, consequently, improved patient treatment. Therefore, reform of healthcare policy must examine how best to optimize physician involvement in screening programs to extend CRC detection in a productive way. In conclusion, the importance of colonoscopy as a preventive intervention for preventing colorectal cancer cannot be overstated. Its role in detection early on, along with the technological progress achieved using CAD systems and the role played by physician incentives, turns out to be an interdisciplinary approach in maximizing screening efficiency. As medicine evolves, a focus on improving the optimization of screening practice through innovative technology and good policy solutions will be essential in resolving the burden of CRC. The inclusion of these factors not only leads to better patient outcomes but also fosters an aggressive approach to cancer prevention that can ultimately save lives and more effectively utilize resources in healthcare systems.

CLOSER LOOK

HIGH-DEDUCTIBLE HEALTH PLANS (HDHPS):

High-deductible health plans (HDHPs) are insurance plans characterized by lower monthly premiums paired with higher out-of-pocket costs before coverage begins. Designed to encourage cost-conscious healthcare decisions, HDHPs have become increasingly common among employers and individuals seeking more affordable premiums. Understanding how these plans function—and how they affect patient behavior, financial risk, and access to care—is essential for assessing their role in today's healthcare landscape.

A defining feature of HDHPs is the large annual deductible, which patients must pay before most insurance benefits take effect. Preventive services are typically covered regardless of deductible status, but diagnostic tests, specialist visits, and non-emergency care often remain fully out-of-pocket until the threshold is met. For healthier individuals or those who use services sparingly, the monthly savings can outweigh these higher deductibles, making the plan financially attractive. However, for people with chronic conditions or unpredictable medical needs, HDHPs can result in substantial upfront expenses. To offset some of these burdens, HDHPs are frequently paired with Health Savings Accounts (HSAs). HSAs allow patients to set aside pre-tax funds that can be used to pay for qualified medical expenses, effectively offering a built-in financial buffer. Contributions grow tax-free, and unused balances roll over from year to year, encouraging long-term savings. For individuals who can afford to contribute regularly, HSAs can provide both flexibility and significant tax advantages.

Despite their potential benefits, HDHPs raise important questions about healthcare access and decision-making. Research consistently shows that when faced with high out-of-pocket costs, patients may delay or skip care—sometimes even essential or chronic-disease management services. This response is not always linked to improved cost-conscious behavior but rather to financial pressure. Delayed care can lead to more severe health issues, ultimately increasing long-term costs for both patients and the healthcare system.

HDHPs can also disproportionately impact low-income individuals and families. While they may benefit from lower premiums, the high deductible can be a significant barrier. Even with HSAs available, many households lack the disposable income needed to contribute meaningfully, widening health and financial disparities.

In the broader healthcare ecosystem, HDHPs reflect a shift toward consumer-directed care, where individuals shoulder more responsibility for navigating costs and treatment choices. Whether HDHPs ultimately improve affordability or exacerbate inequity depends on plan design, patient education, and ongoing policy development. As healthcare costs continue to rise, HDHPs will remain a topic of debate, balancing financial incentives with patients' ability to access timely, essential care.

REFERENCES

1. Aas, E. (2025). *The effect of screening on treatment cost: The case of colorectal cancer.* https://core.ac.uk/download/pdf/7107393.pdf (accessed on 15th July 2025).
2. Abedi, J., Amiriani, T., Assadi, M., Besharat, M., et al. (2013). *Scintigraphy with 99mTc(V)-DMSA in monitoring patients with inflammatory bowel disease.* https://core.ac.uk/download/52204679.pdf (accessed on 15th July 2025).
3. Addiss, D. G., Fenwick, A., Jourdan, P. M., Lamberton, P. H. L., et al. (2018). *Soil-Transmitted Helminth Infections.* https://core.ac.uk/download/96884381.pdf (accessed on 15th July 2025).
4. Hausmann J, Albert JG (2011) Detecting and Managing Small Bowel Crohn's Disease – Capsule Endoscopy Becoming a First Line Diagnostic Method? J Gastroint Dig Syst S1:002. doi:10.4172/2161-069X.S1-002(accessed on 15th July 2025).
5. Allegretti, J. R., Budree, S., Fischer, M., Kassam, Z., et al. (2017). *The 5D framework: A clinical primer for fecal microbiota transplantation to treat Clostridium difficile infection.* https://core.ac.uk/download/129148516.pdf (accessed on 15th July 2025).
6. Andrew, L., Kirk, D., & Szmaglinska, M. (2023). *Reporting and mapping research evidence on perceptions of clinical hypnosis among the general population and patients receiving health care , including cancer care: A scoping review.* https://core.ac.uk/download/613952299.pdf (accessed on 15th July 2025).
7. Melissa De Regge, Jeroen Trybou, Paul Gemmel, Philippe Duyck, and Lieven Annemans, 2013: Physician-Owned Specialized Facilities: Focused Factories or Destructive Competition?. *Proceedings,* **2013**, https://doi.org/10.5465/ambpp.2013.13667abstract(accessed on 15th July 2025).
8. Annibale, B., Bellini, D., Binda, G. A., Cuomo, R., et al. (2015). *Practice parameters for the treatment of colonic diverticular disease: Italian Society of Colon and Rectal Surgery (SICCR) guidelines.* https://core.ac.uk/download/54522076.pdf (accessed on 15th July 2025).
9. Armour, B. S., Friedman, C., Etchason, J., Wike, J., Alley, L., & Pitts, M. M. (2025). *The influence of year-end bonuses on colorectal cancer screening.* https://core.ac.uk/download/pdf/6924530.pdf (accessed on 15th July 2025).
10. Avila, P., Butte, A. J., Glicksberg, B. S., Harding-Theobald, E., et al. (2020). *Accuracy of medical billing data against the electronic health record in the measurement of colorectal cancer screening rates.* https://core.ac.uk/download/323062526.pdf (accessed on 15th July 2025).
11. Avitabile, C., Jappelli, T., & Padula, M. (2008). *Screening tests, information, and the health-education gradient.* https://core.ac.uk/download/1687675.pdf (accessed on 15th July 2025).
12. Balducci, L., Carrato, A., Manzano García, M., Ortiz Romero, M., et al. (2017). *Secondary prevention of cancer in the older individual.* https://core.ac.uk/download/83599302.pdf (accessed on 15th July 2025).
13. Kastenberg, D., Bertiger, G., & Brogadir, S. (2018). Bowel preparation quality scales for colonoscopy. *World journal of gastroenterology, 24*(26), 2833–2843. https://doi.org/10.3748/wjg.v24.i26.2833(accessed on 15th July 2025).
14. Yu, C., Skootsky, S., Grossman, M., Garner, O. B., Betlachin, A., Esrailian, E., Hommes, D. W., & May, F. P. (2018). A Multi-Level Fit-Based Quality Improvement Initiative to Improve Colorectal Cancer

Screening in a Managed Care Population. *Clinical and translational gastroenterology, 9*(8), 177. https://doi.org/10.1038/s41424-018-0046-z(accessed on 15th July 2025).

15. Boeving, A., Parolim, B., Cé, J., Jú, J., João, O. R., De Bem, R., et al. (2008). *First reports of computed tomographic colonography for the screening of colorectal polyps in acromegalic patients.* https://core.ac.uk/download/pdf/288056.pdf (accessed on 15th July 2025).
16. Boggi, R., Hassan, C., Lorenzetti, R., Morini, S., et al. (2017). *Association between diverticulosis and colonic neoplastic lesions in individuals with a positive fecal immunochemical test.* https://core.ac.uk/download/231748785.pdf (accessed on 15th July 2025).
17. Boyles, H. (2021). *Increasing healthcare providers' intent to utilize alternative and complementary pain management with their patients.* https://core.ac.uk/download/519918332.pdf (accessed on 15th July 2025).
18. Bühner, M., Kolligs, F. T., Schubring-Giese, B., Ziegler, D., et al. (2010). *Attitude to secondary prevention and concerns about colonoscopy are independent predictors of acceptance of screening colonoscopy.* https://core.ac.uk/download/16432735.pdf (accessed on 15th July 2025).
19. Chowdhury, T. A., Ghita, O., & Whelan, P. F. (2008). *A fully automatic CAD-CTC system based on curvature analysis for standard and low-dose CT data.* https://core.ac.uk/download/11308846.pdf (accessed on 15th July 2025).
20. The UK CRC Screening Pilot Evaluation (Ethnicity) Team (Including: Szczepura, Ala, Johnson, Mark R. D., Orbell, Sheina, Gumber, Anil, O'Sullivan, I., Clay, Diane and Owen, David). (2003) Ethnicity : UK colorectal cancer screening pilot : final report. [London]: [Department of Health]. (Final report).(accessed on 15th July 2025).
21. Corleto, V. D., D'Ambra, G., Di Giulio, E., Fave, G., et al. (2018). *Mucosal adhesion and anti-inflammatory effects of Lactobacillus rhamnosus GG in the human colonic mucosa: A proof-of-concept study.* https://core.ac.uk/download/195777522.pdf (accessed on 15th July 2025).
22. Corleto, V. D., Delle Fave, G., Desideri, F., Di Giulio, E., et al. (2016). *Endoscopic scores for inflammatory bowel disease in the era of 'mucosal healing': Old problem, new perspectives.* https://core.ac.uk/download/74319420.pdf (accessed on 15th July 2025).
23. Crispin, A., Göke, B., Kolligs, F. T., Mansmann, U., et al. (2011). *Risk of advanced colorectal neoplasia according to age and gender.* https://core.ac.uk/download/12175588.pdf (accessed on 15th July 2025).
24. Curbow, B. A., George, T. J., Jr., Hyams, T., et al. (2019). *Social vs. practical problems in attaining a colonoscopy: Different patient profiles?* https://digitalscholarship.unlv.edu/cgi/viewcontent.cgi?article=1851&context=jhdrp (accessed on 15th July 2025).
25. DiCarlo, M., Fleisher, L., Lambert, E., Man, M., et al. (2018). *A learning community approach to identifying interventions in health systems to reduce colorectal cancer screening disparities.* https://core.ac.uk/download/213444218.pdf (accessed on 15th July 2025).
26. DuHamel, K. N., Freeman, K. L., Jandorf, L., Thompson, H. S., et al. (2012). *Colorectal cancer brochure development for African Americans.* https://digitalscholarship.unlv.edu/cgi/viewcontent.cgi?article=1042&context=jhdrp (accessed on 15th July 2025).
27. Engquist, B., Figueiredo, I. N., Leal, C., Romanazzi, V., et al. (2016). *Homogenization model for aberrant crypt foci.* https://core.ac.uk/download/pdf/151539069.pdf (accessed on 15th July 2025).

28. Fedewa, S., Jemal, A., Lansdorp-Vogelaar, I., Lin, C. C., et al. (2014). *Utilization of surveillance after polypectomy in the Medicare population.* https://core.ac.uk/download/43314758.pdf (accessed on 15th July 2025).

29. Fendrick, A. M., Cliff, E. Q., Milkovich, K., Spangler, K., McKellar, M. R., Chernew, M., & Parents, S. (2014). *Health savings account-eligible high-deductible health plans: Updating the definition of prevention.* https://core.ac.uk/download/75777849.pdf (accessed on 15th July 2025).

30. Goldfarb, N. I., Pizzi, L. T., Fuhr, J. P., Jr, Salvador, C., Sikirica, V., Kornbluth, A., & Lewis, B. (2004). Diagnosing Crohn's disease: an economic analysis comparing wireless capsule endoscopy with traditional diagnostic procedures. *Disease management : DM, 7*(4), 292–304. https://doi.org/10.1089/dis.2004.7.292(accessed on 15th July 2025).

31. Garcia, J., Gross, S. A., Lahr, R., Rex, D. K., et al. (2019). *Endocuff Vision reduces inspection time without decreasing lesion detection in a randomized colonoscopy trial.* https://core.ac.uk/download/187423803.pdf (accessed on 15th July 2025).

32. Gipsh, K. (2004). *Assessing health beliefs about colonoscopy.* https://core.ac.uk/download/223074300.pdf (accessed on 15th July 2025).

33. Goodman, A. L., Griffiths, P. D., Murray, C. D., Watkins, P. J., et al. (2015). *CMV in the gut: A critical review of CMV detection in the immunocompetent host with colitis.* https://core.ac.uk/download/29414101.pdf (accessed on 15th July 2025).

34. Holly, A., Burnand, B., Froehlich, F., Gonvers, J. J., Vader, J. P., Lamiraud, K., Juillerat, P., et al. (2025). *The effect of non-medical factors on variations in the performance of colonoscopy among different health care settings.* https://core.ac.uk/download/pdf/6617669.pdf (accessed on 15th July 2025).

35. Khare, P., Saraswat, P., & Tiwari, R. (2015). *Recent Advancement in Diagnosis of Gastrointestinal Diseases.* https://core.ac.uk/download/328159812.pdf (accessed on 15th July 2025).

36. Kirby, K., Perry, C., & Thurston, M. (2003). *Exploring Colorectal Cancer Patients' Perceptions of the Quality of Their Care.* https://core.ac.uk/download/364086.pdf (accessed on 15th July 2025).

37. Lam, A. H. K., Cheung, C. C. L., Foo, D. C. C., Chan, H. H. W., Chiang, M. F., Null, N., Chan, T. T., et al. (2016). *Alternatives to colonoscopy for population-wide colorectal cancer screening.* https://core.ac.uk/download/95552954.pdf (accessed on 15th July 2025).

38. Mo, X., Tao, K., Wang, G., Wang, J., et al. (2018). *An efficient approach for polyps detection in endoscopic videos based on Faster R-CNN.* http://arxiv.org/abs/1809.01263 (accessed on 15th July 2025).

39. Moldovan, C. A., Alexandru, S. C., & Ungureanu, F. D. (2017). *The prevalence of high dysplastic colonic adenomatous polyps in a 3-year endoscopic retrospective study from a single clinical center.* https://core.ac.uk/download/144553184.pdf (accessed on 15th July 2025).

40. Platell, C., Preen, D. B., Cenin, D. R., Ee, H. C., Lansdorp-Vogelaar, I., Troeung, L., et al. (2017). *Optimizing patient risk stratification for colonoscopy screening and surveillance of colorectal cancer: The role for linked data.* https://core.ac.uk/download/213607291.pdf (accessed on 15th July 2025).

41. Schmidt, E. (2017). *Colorectal Cancer Screening.* https://core.ac.uk/download/79664966.pdf (accessed on 15th July 2025).

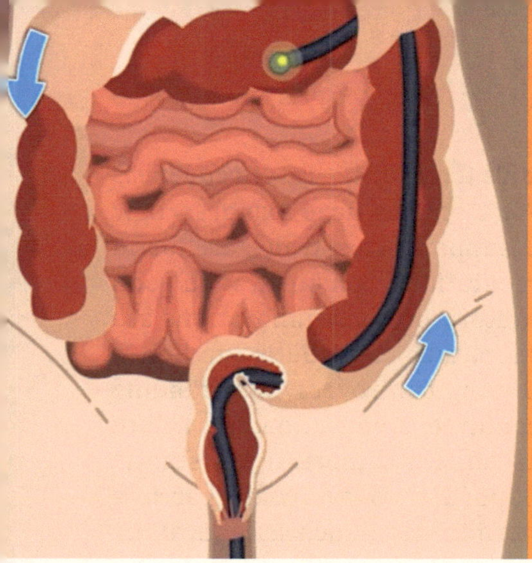

Chapter 6

SIGMOIDOSCOPY AND PROCTOSCOPY

Contents

Introduction 157
6.1. Historical Background 160
6.2. Indications for Procedures 163
6.3. Procedure Overview 167
6.4. Risks and Complications 170
6.5. Patient Experience 173
6.6. Comparison of Sigmoidoscopy and Proctoscopy 177
Summary 181
References 184

Introduction

The necessity of colorectal screenings, particularly sigmoidoscopy and proctoscopy, has been more apparent in the public health arena. Sigmoidoscopy and proctoscopy are screening procedures that serve as integral parts of early detection and treatment of colorectal cancer (CRC), a leading cause of morbidity and mortality from cancer in the United States. In spite of increased screening rates among different groups, there remain disparities, underscoring the need for targeted education and outreach to underserved populations. For instance, research indicates that in Tennessee state, percentages of those people who were up to date on CRC screening increased from 49% in 2002 to 55% in 2006 before declining to 46% by 2008, demonstrating the volatility of knowledge and access to such essential screenings, particularly by individuals lacking health-care coverage or education (Veeranki & Zheng, 2014). In the area of gastrointestinal diagnosis, sigmoidoscopy and proctoscopy give practitioners more advanced information about the colorectal system so that interventions can pre-empt the malignancies. Both procedures involve minimally invasive techniques, but effectiveness depends greatly on the quality of pre-exam bowel preparation. New studies have explored new approaches to bowel preparation, such as the use of free fatty acid suppositories, which are found to be very effective in terms of efficacy comparable to standard preparations, combined with good tolerance among patients (Asgrimsdottir et al., 2016). Such preparatory protocol innovations are essential in the quest to increase patient compliance and satisfaction, thus contributing to better diagnostic outcomes in the fight against colorectal cancer. The ongoing controversy surrounding sigmoidoscopy and proctoscopy is underscored by the need for continuous education and health awareness campaigns among healthcare providers and patients alike. As there is constantly evolving technology in colorectal cancer screening, it is most important to overcome barriers that limit people from accessing these lifesaving screenings. Determinants , such as education, socioeconomic status, and availability of healthcare have a significant influence on screening rates, making universal approaches responsive to populations inevitable. The evolving methods and findings highlight the necessity to remain vigilant in screening practice to foster an enhanced degree of knowledge about colorectal health and promote timely intervention where indicated, as the foundation for the better-informed process of prevention and management of colorectal cancer (Veeranki & Zheng, 2014) (Figure 6.1).

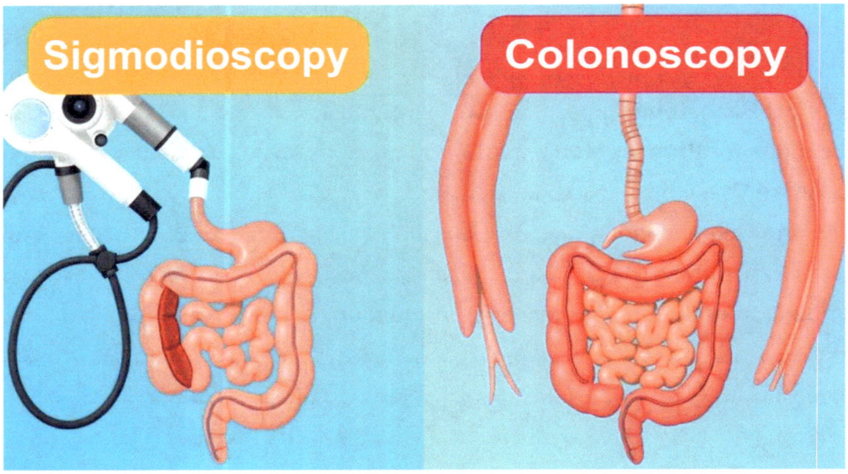

Figure 6.1. Sigmoidoscopy vs. colonoscopy.

Source: https://drniveditapandey.com/wp-content/uploads/2024/10/sigmoidoscopy-vs-colonoscopy-differences-1024x585.jpg.

Definition of Sigmoidoscopy and Proctoscopy

To understand the significance of sigmoidoscopy and proctoscopy, one should first describe the two similar yet distinct tests. Sigmoidoscopy is the investigation by a flexible or rigid endoscope of the rectum lining and the lower colon, otherwise known as the sigmoid colon. This diagnostic modality is held accountable for the identification of abnormalities like polyps, tumors, and inflammation that can be harbingers of more severe illnesses like colorectal cancer or inflammatory bowel disease. As a minimally invasive test, it allows clinicians to extract valuable diagnostic data with consideration for patient comfort. Proctoscopy, which is similar in nature, focuses particularly on the examination of the rectum and lower anal canal, thus enabling practitioners to conduct more focused tests when necessary, enhancing overall efficiency in gastrointestinal diagnoses. Proctoscopy and sigmoidoscopy are practiced primarily in outpatient units and are characterized by their lack of invasiveness. Conscious sedation can be given to patients who are undergoing these procedures, which aids in alleviating any pain felt during the procedure. It is this ease that is so crucial in convincing patients to undergo these important diagnostic tests, particularly when presenting with bleeding per rectum or other alarming symptoms. With the flexibility of instruments used being so superior, there is not only visual examination feasible but also procedures , such as biopsies, thereby providing diagnosis and treatment at the same time.

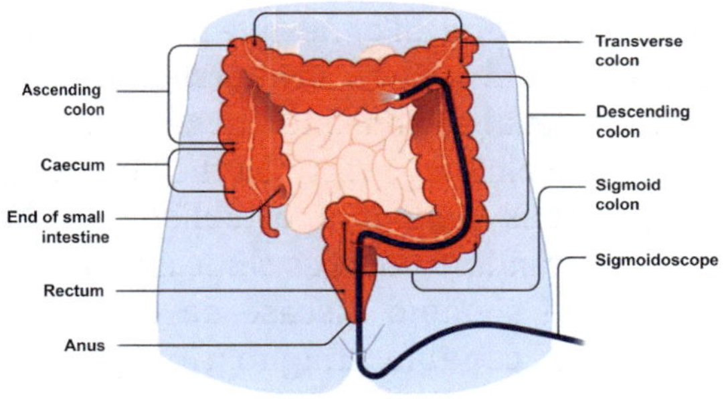

Figure 6.2. Sigmoidoscopy.

Source: https://post.medicalnewstoday.com/wp-content/uploads/sites/3/2022/07/2005311-Sigmoidoscopy_1296x975-body-1-1024x771.png.

As stated, endoscopy is the cornerstone of minimally invasive surgery, highlighting the essential role of such interventions in modern medical practice and patient management (Perumal, 2012). The application of sigmoidoscopy and proctoscopy extends beyond diagnosis, encompassing the recent patterns of malpractice suits for gastrointestinal endoscopic procedures. One analysis of closed claims from 1985–2008 identified colonoscopy as the most common procedure with claims, closely associated with sigmoidoscopy, emphasizing the necessity of procedural hazard awareness in gastroenterology. Proctoscopy and sigmoidoscopy are both components of routine screening and follow-up in patients at risk of colorectal disease, emphasizing the necessity for constant practitioner training on complications and optimal practice. These innovations are imperative in preventing risks of malpractice while affirming the incorporation of procedural efficiency and the safety of the patient as a top priority in the clinical agenda (Hernandez et al., 2013) (Figure 6.2).

Significance of These Procedures in Gut Health

The significance of sigmoidoscopy and proctoscopy is that they are key diagnostic tools for ensuring gastrointestinal health. Endoscopic tests allow medical personnel to visualize the lower gastrointestinal tract, allowing them to identify pathological states early, such as polyps, inflammatory bowel disease, and colorectal cancer. These must be detected early because they have the potential to develop into more serious complications unless they are treated. For instance, clinical research has proven that screening tests—encompassing these endoscopic tests—are essential in reducing mortality rates of colorectal cancer through facilitating timely interventions. The ability to detect abnormalities early in the course of these diseases further confirms the worth of incorporating these procedures into routine gastrointestinal health screening, thereby lending itself to preventative healthcare modalities. In addition to their diagnostic value, sigmoidoscopy and proctoscopy also have significant roles to play in guiding therapy. Both tests allow for not only visualization but also therapeutic maneuvers, such as polypectomy or biopsy. Their dual function adds to their worth in managing gastrointestinal health, as it minimizes the need for more invasive interventions that would be required later if conditions are not addressed early. Further, the findings of these evaluations can also be utilized to inform treatment approaches, thus maximizing patient outcomes and facilitating a customized model of care. Procedural effectiveness demonstrated in studies emphasizes the need for prudent evaluation of colorectal pathology, which indicates that such kinds of interventions may lead to fewer levels of complications like anastomotic leaks and infections, particularly if results in relation to rigid proctosigmoidoscopy versus flexible sigmoidoscopy are taken into consideration (Carmichael & Mills, 2023).

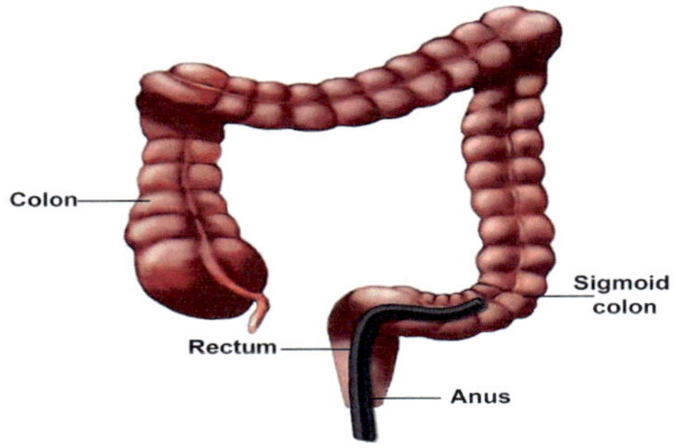

Figure 6.3. Flexible sigmoidoscopy.

Source: https://i.ytimg.com/vi/ffWViNy-q_k/maxresdefault.jpg.

Sigmoidoscopy and proctoscopy have a broad influence beyond caring for individual patients; these procedures lie at the heart of the advancement of public health goals. Globally, the increasing prevalence of colorectal cancer necessitates awareness of risk factors and symptomology via such endoscopic tests. Systematic symptom detection and risk predictors can easily influence early detection, as seen in various predictive models that integrate multiple risk factors associated with colorectal cancer (Williams et al., 2016). Such models can simplify screening processes and ensure that individuals at higher risk receive priority for testing, thereby optimizing resource utilization by health systems. Subsequently, through promotion of routine use of sigmoidoscopy and proctoscopy within screening investigations, health authorities can manage to reduce the public health burden of gastrointestinal diseases and maximize population-level health benefits (Figure 6.3).

6.1. Historical Background

The history of sigmoidoscopy and proctoscopy can be traced back to the end of the 19th century, which was a time of major advances in techniques and technology in medicine. Early exploration of the lower gastrointestinal tract was primitive and depended on the use of mere instruments, which did not always offer a significant understanding of mucosal conditions present in patients. The arrival of flexible instruments in the mid-20th century was a watershed, allowing improved visualization and diagnosis. These advances in technology rectified the deficiencies of the previous technique, establishing a new procedural standard. Also, as clinical knowledge of rectal and sigmoid disease developed, the demand for capable diagnostic apparatus grew. Consequently, the use of combined visual modalities during medical procedures emphasized patient comfort and accessibility, paving the way for contemporary sigmoidoscopy and proctoscopy techniques, which concentrate on extensive examinations of the rectosigmoid area. Advances in surgical processes have also influenced the historical background of sigmoidoscopy and proctoscopy. As surgical methods improved, the merging of diagnostic tools became the order of the day in evaluating conditions , such as total rectal prolapse. Historically, various techniques of surgery were employed, ranging from full abdominal surgery to simpler perineal operations, with widely varying success and complications. Abdominal rectopexy emerged as an evolved choice among surgeons, particularly in patients with rectal prolapse, with low rates of recurrence and successful achievement of continence (Jinreeve

2015). These technological advances in surgery necessitated proper diagnostic equipment that would study not only the physical anatomy of the rectum but also its surgical function outcomes, thus the role of sigmoidoscopy and proctoscopy in the process of surgery. The development of these medical devices has significantly enhanced diagnostic effectiveness and patient care. As detailed in recent evaluations, modern proctosigmoidoscopes are designed to provide improved visibility and accurate visual accounts of the rectosigmoid mucosa in real-time, enhancing a more satisfactory diagnostic outcome (Anselm et al., 2025). The ongoing inquiry into technology development and the use of such in clinical settings validates the importance of continuous innovation in improving patient outcomes. Moreover, the growing knowledge of colorectal illnesses has created a greater focus on minimally invasive techniques, which could be supplemented by the precise vision provided through sigmoidoscopy and proctoscopy. The above history highlights not only the technology evolved within these disciplines but also their irreplaceable role in today's gastroenterological practice and procedures.

6.1.1. Development of Sigmoidoscopy and Proctoscopy Techniques

The establishment of sigmoidoscopy and proctoscopy procedures has been a great advancement in gastrointestinal diagnostics history. It was originally developed during the early 20th century, and it employed rudimentary tools that limited visualization and diagnostic capability. Over time and with innovations in technology, endoscopic devices have been evolving. Flexible endoscopes revolutionized these procedures, enabling improved maneuverability and the visualization of lesions and abnormalities more clearly. This shift provided the way for higher patient comfort and lower procedural risks, making sigmoidoscopy and proctoscopy gold standards for diagnostic examinations of the lower gastrointestinal tract. The continuous improvement of these instruments underlines the necessary role they play in contemporary medicine. The function of sigmoidoscopy and proctoscopy is not visualization alone; they are also essential diagnostic instruments employed in the detection of other colorectal pathology, including cancer and inflammatory bowel disease. Adapations , such as transanal endoscopic microsurgery (TEM) have emerged in the current literature, an indication of a trend towards local treatment of early rectal cancer. Techniques like TEM and TAMIS have advantages over the traditional methods in the sense that they allow safe resection with minimal complications and satisfactory oncological outcomes.

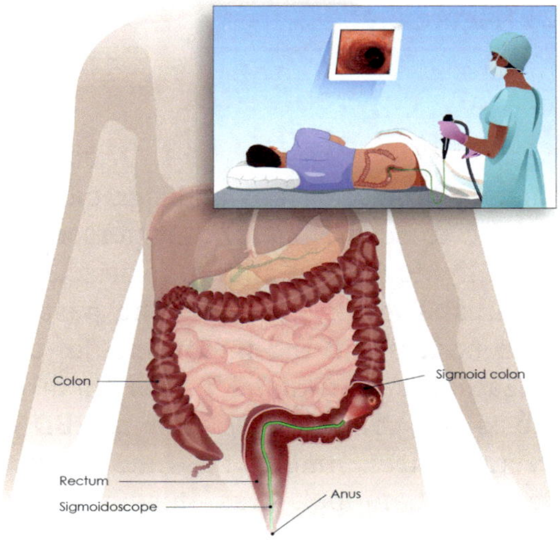

Figure 6.4. Sigmoidoscopy procedure.

Source: https://digestivecancers.eu/wp-content/uploads/2021/05/3.Sigmoidoscopy_withlegend.jpg.

From the literature presented in recent studies, the innovations are not only advancements but a shift in paradigm in how surgeons approach surgical treatment for rectal pathologies and thus improve the prognosis of and management options for patients (Ahmed et al., 2020). Furthermore, the application of such endoscopic techniques to practice demonstrates their vital role in prevention. Despite the historic initial emphasis of sigmoidoscopy and proctoscopy as diagnostic tools, they also provide therapeutic potential. For instance, while examining, practitioners are not only able to visualize abnormalities but can also biopsy or remove polyps, preventing the cancer from developing. This two-in-one feature extends the collective competence of colorectal screening programs, thereby allowing doctors to tackle colorectal disease at an earlier level. As studies continue to indicate the safety and effectiveness of these newer endoscopic methods, their arrival is a reflection of the ongoing pursuit of better patient care in gastroenterology (Perumal, 2012) (Figure 6.4).

6.1.2. Key Figures in the Advancement of These Procedures

The history of proctoscopy and sigmoidoscopy is credited to several significant persons who significantly developed and popularized these procedures. The physicians of the past have come to understand the importance of direct visualization of the distal bowel in disease diagnosis for conditions , such as IBD and colorectal cancer. Among the innovators, Dr. William W. Campbell was instrumental in defining the diagnostic possibilities of flexible sigmoidoscopy in the mid-20th century. His work laid the basis for procedural protocols and validated the essence of proper examinations, which would later guide subsequent iterations of the procedure. These advances are a continuation of the push toward improved patient outcomes, evidenced in the intentions of most early adopters, who focused on optimizing diagnostic quality with lesser patient discomfort. The addition of technological innovation has also played a major role in the development of sigmoidoscopy and proctoscopy. Professionals like Dr. J. Bruce M. Smith advocated for the integration of video technology into endoscopic procedures. Not only did this innovation enhance visual quality in testing, but it also allowed results to be recorded for research and educational use. By pushing the need for proper visualization, Dr. Smith's efforts helped to standardize higher-quality tests for colonoscopies. Also, this quality focus has further been recognized as crucial in the context of screening programs to detect colorectal cancer earlier to prevent disease mortality (Meester, 2017).

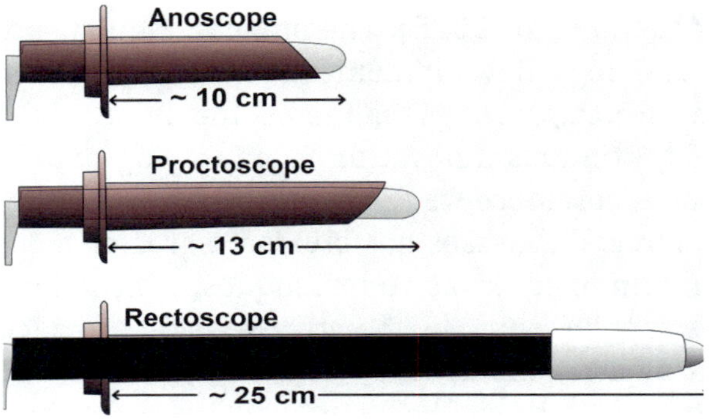

Figure 6.5. Proctoscopy.

Source: https://upload.wikimedia.org/wikipedia/commons/b/be/Anoscope%2C_proctoscope_and_rectoscope.png.

Along with technological innovation, the incentive for preventive treatment and early detection has been reinforced by leading physicians pointing towards the significance of sigmoidoscopy and proctoscopy. Their comments have supported the integration of these processes into routine screening programs, and it has been central to effective colorectal cancer screening practice. Knowledge of the diagnostic delay contribution in IBD, as mapped in patient experience studies, shows how crucial early diagnosis is. Physicians in the medical profession continue to point to the correlation between appropriate diagnoses and favorable patient outcomes, reaffirming the necessity for ongoing education of clinicians incorporating the current research findings (Cross, 2019). The cumulative impact of these individuals points to a broader trend towards preventive medicine in the diagnosis and treatment of colorectal disease (Figure 6.5).

6.1.3. Evolution of Medical Instruments Used

The evolution of medical instruments has significantly enhanced the practice of sigmoidoscopy and proctoscopy, transforming diagnostic capabilities and patient care. Early instruments used for examining the rectum and sigmoid colon were rudimentary and often limited in their effectiveness. However, the introduction of more sophisticated endoscopes in the late 19th and early 20th centuries marked a pivotal moment in the modernization of these procedures. Advances in optics and the creation of flexible endoscopes enabled enhanced visualization of the lower gastrointestinal tract, giving medical professionals the capability to detect abnormalities with increased accuracy. The tremendous progress in materials and design methodologies has enabled these instruments to become less invasive and more patient-friendly, which has also improved their acceptability and application in medical practice. In the 20th century, there has been a focus on developing effective and user-friendly medical instruments. Moving away from stiff metal scopes to flexible fiber-optic instruments was a landmark in accomplishment, allowing effortless maneuverability inside the colon. With advancements in the instruments themselves, the application of video technology has also improved the procedures of sigmoidoscopy and proctoscopy, providing real-time images and better diagnostic results. Techniques , such as narrow-band imaging have emerged, whereby the detection of polyps and lesions that are otherwise unseen is facilitated. These advances not only maximize detection rates but also minimize the risk of complications during intervention, ultimately leading to improved patient outcomes and a greater understanding of colorectal disorders. The growing awareness of colorectal cancer as a significant health hazard and leading cause of morbidity and mortality has also been the impetus for research and development and the utilization of diagnostic modalities. Screening tests, including the faecal occult blood test (FOBT) and subsequent sigmoidoscopy, have been critical instruments in the early detection of this disease, as has been seen in studies documenting their importance in clinical practice (Raj et al., 2015). Importantly, while these tests have proved to be useful in isolating cases for intervention, they work best when used alongside follow-up diagnostic tests. In spite of certain flaws in sensitivity and specificity, the ongoing development of clinical guidelines and equipment continues to enhance these screening tests. In addition, as the healthcare environment moves toward evidence-based practice, the incorporation of sophisticated medical devices into standard screening and diagnostic workups will continue to play an important role in the battle against colorectal cancer (Figure 6.6).

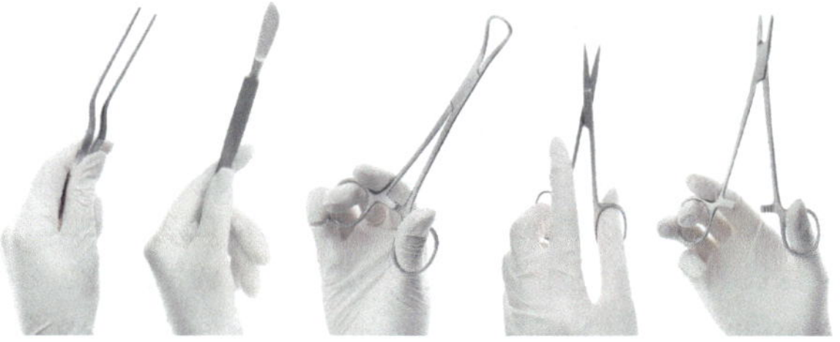

Figure 6.6. Evaluation of surgical instruments.

Source: https://myronmeditech.com/wp-content/uploads/2020/09/Surgical-Instrument-scaled.jpeg.

6.2. Indications for Procedures

Use of proctoscopy and sigmoidoscopy is heavily reliant on the existence of clinical indications that justify their utilization in evaluation of colorectal health. Both are frequently used as diagnostic measures to identify the occurrence of abnormalities , such as polyps, tumors, and inflammatory bowel disease. Referrals for these procedures are usually made for patients with symptoms of rectal bleeding, chronic abdominal pain, or a change in bowel habits. Such symptomatic presentations are close enough to warrant investigation, as they could be warning signs of serious pathologies, like colorectal cancer or diverticulitis. Close surveillance for these pathologies to be identified early will improve patient outcomes significantly, since numerous studies have shown the need for timely screening of persons at risk, particularly those 50 years and older (Asgrimsdottir et al., 2016). Along with symptomatic examinations, these methods play an important preventative function in colorectal cancer screening regimens. Practice guidelines suggest repeated sigmoidoscopy regularly for individuals within certain age groups, generally starting at 45 years of age, to support early diagnosis. The information indicates a parallel relationship between screening rates and outcomes of colorectal cancer, underscoring the need to target screening inequalities between population groups. On the basis of evidence, access to healthcare has a critical role in determining whether patients are screened on time, leading to late diagnosis among people who are not covered or are not informed. Additionally, application of new preparation methods, such as suppositories like free fatty acids, has been investigated for their efficacy in bowel preparation before such procedures, and they have demonstrated commitment to enhancing patient comfort while maintaining diagnostic integrity (Asgrimsdottir et al., 2016). In addition, the role of sigmoidoscopy and proctoscopy as a sign for its performance goes beyond the diagnosis to include therapeutic intervention. Both procedures can allow for polyp removal, treatment of localized bleeding, and relief of obstructing strictures. For example, the ability of sigmoidoscopy to carry out polypectomies makes it a diagnostic and therapeutic aid in the care of the colon and rectum. As proof mounts regarding the effectiveness of these interventions in cancer prevention, the procedures are increasingly becoming integral components of colorectal management as a whole. The ongoing optimization of techniques, such as improved bowel preparation protocols, contributes not only to their efficacy but to their safety and patient satisfaction in these invasive exams, thereby making them entirely worth implementing across clinical environments (Veeranki & Zheng, 2014).

6.2.1. Diagnostic Purposes for Gastrointestinal Disorders

The diagnostic setting for gastrointestinal disease has grown much more sophisticated, including advanced modalities like sigmoidoscopy and proctoscopy. These examinations serve an important role for the direct visualization of the colon and rectum and allow practitioners to identify abnormalities that produce gastrointestinal symptoms. Not only do these endoscopic techniques enable assessment of mucosal inflammation, polyps, and lesions, but also therapeutic intervention in the form of biopsies. This twofold utility serves to point out the worth of such interventions in diagnostic indications, particularly when standard imaging techniques are non-specific. As described in recent clinical practice guidelines, the benefit of collecting tissue specimens during the time of endoscopy is crucial for accurate diagnoses of illnesses like inflammatory bowel disease and colon cancer, and therefore these procedures are precious tools in modern gastroenterology (Perumal, 2012). Moreover, the utility of sigmoidoscopy and proctoscopy extends beyond mere visual diagnosis; they have an important role to play in patient outcomes by offering early detection of gastrointestinal disease. Evidence points to the fact that timely detection and follow-up treatment of neoplasia or dysplasia, for instance, can lead to improved survival among patients with colorectal cancer. By offering a minimally invasive option for screening, such procedures not only reduce the need for more invasive surgical techniques but also encourage patient compliance with screening programs to the fullest extent. Further, guidelines from organizations , such as the International Urogynecological Association (IUGA) and International Continence Society (ICS) point to the importance of uniform vocabulary to improve clinical dialogue regarding anorectal dysfunction, further reinforcing the importance of precise diagnosis via modalities , such as sigmoidoscopy and proctoscopy (Sultan et al., 2016). Moreover, the integration of endoscopic techniques into the diagnostic armamentarium of gastrointestinal illness demonstrates a broader shift toward individualized medicine. As diagnostic criteria become more sophisticated, patient tailoring becomes most crucial. Sigmoidoscopy and proctoscopy support the diagnosis of recognized disorders and direct preparation of treatment plans tailored to the individual patient, with ongoing monitoring and follow-up a requirement. These procedures are particularly valuable in the assessment of chronic gastrointestinal disorders that frequently affect the quality of life in the patient. Accordingly, by joining together advanced imaging techniques and an understanding of underpinning pathophysiological processes, clinicians can embrace a more integrated approach to diagnosing and managing gastrointestinal disease, ultimately resulting in enhanced patient satisfaction and outcomes (Perumal, 2012).

6.2.2. Screening for Colorectal Cancer

Screening for colorectal cancer is an important population-based initiative that significantly reduces mortality from this neoplasm. There are various screening methods, some of which include sigmoidoscopy and proctoscopy, that play a vital role in the early detection process. Both procedures enable visualization of the lower gastrointestinal tract, enabling the clinician to identify polyps or abnormal growths that could be an indication of cancer. Of importance, research has established that systematic screening through interventions , such as client reminders and education is associated with increased test uptake among tests like FOBT and sigmoidoscopy. By increasing awareness and access, these interventions are able to reach population groups with historically low screening rates effectively, promoting a shift towards more engagement in preventive health behaviors (Sabatino et al., 2012). Colorectal cancer screening rates, as witnessed in Tennessee from 2002 through 2008, indicate improvement and struggle in achieving optimal screening levels. Trends indicate that the proportion of adults receiving the recommended screenings rose from 49% in 2002 to 55% in 2006, then declined to 46% in 2008. Variations demonstrate the necessity for ongoing surveillance and modulation of screening behaviors. Age, education level, income, and access to health care are the primary determinants of these proportions. Adults aged 65–74 years had the greatest compliance rates, while those with no health insurance were much less likely to adhere to screening recommendations. This places a demand for special intervention among low-income populations to ensure equal access to screening for colorectal cancer (Veeranki & Zheng, 2014). In the changing landscape of colorectal cancer screening, the inclusion of technologies , such as sigmoidoscopy and proctoscopy is still crucial. Such procedures not only provide diagnostic function but also therapeutic intervention platforms, potentially eliminating the need for more invasive surgery. Ongoing education of healthcare providers as well as patients about the importance of regular screening, along with a program aimed at reducing structural barriers, can optimize rates of participation and ultimately reduce cancer-related mortality. Besides, ramping up outreach efforts to educate target populations about the importance of early detection can spur a more active role for health. By offering comprehensive screening programs and making them accessible, the fight against colorectal cancer can make significant strides toward better community health outcomes and patient survival (Sabatino et al., 2012) (Figure 6.7).

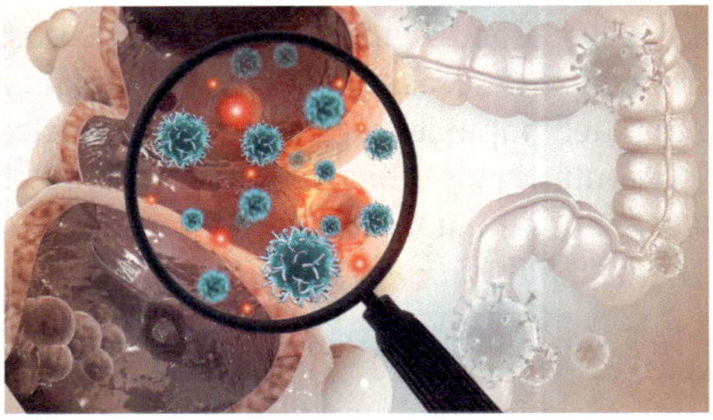

Figure 6.7. Colorectal cancer screening options.

Source: https://res.cloudinary.com/broadcastmed/image/fetch/ar_16:9,c_fill,g_auto,f_auto,q_auto,w_1300/https://55933-bcmed.s3.amazonaws.com/bcp/images/dmImage/SourceImage/study_gettyimages-13914246925.jpg.

6.2.3. Evaluation of Inflammatory Bowel Diseases (IBD)

IBD assessment is also crucial in clinical care, as early and accurate diagnosis significantly affects patient management and prognosis. Devices , such as sigmoidoscopy and proctoscopy play a critical role in investigating the lower GI tract, particularly to detect pathological alterations due to diseases , such as ulcerative colitis and Crohn's disease. These endoscopic processes allow direct visualization of the colonic mucosa, making it possible for the clinician to see inflammation, ulceration, and bleeding and take biopsy samples for histopathological examination. Targeted biopsies can be done to enhance diagnostic accuracy to differentiate between IBD subtypes, complications, and associated diseases. The inclusion of sigmoidoscopy and proctoscopy in routine evaluation thus provides relevant information that guides therapeutic maneuvers and follows up on disease progression. Furthermore, new evidence has defined the efficacy of most endoscopic modalities for assessing IBD. For instance, there exists a relative advantage of flexible sigmoidoscopy compared to rigid proctosigmoidoscopy in terms of reduced anastomotic leaks and organ space infections during colorectal evaluations. Specifically, data show that patients examined with flexible sigmoidoscopy reveal lower complication rates, such as organ space infection (3.8% vs. 4.8%) and anastomotic leak (2.9% vs. 3.8%) compared to rigid procedures. These findings highlight the importance of selecting appropriate endoscopic techniques based on clinical conditions and patient considerations to facilitate maximal management options in accordance with individual needs.

Effective evaluation methods are not only crucial for diagnosis but also for therapeutic efficacy assessment and making the necessary therapeutic regimen adjustments. Outside of endoscopic evaluation, comprehensive management of IBD involves an understanding of the underlying pathophysiology of these diseases and complications involved.

Those presenting with lower GI bleeding typically need to be assessed urgently through tests , such as colonoscopy or flexible sigmoidoscopy to identify the site of the bleeding and to implement appropriate treatment. A systematic review found early intervention with colonoscopy to have higher diagnostic and therapeutic yields compared to postponed procedures. These are of particular significance in the case of sigmoidoscopy and proctoscopy, indicating the necessity for early evaluations in acute cases to prevent adverse outcomes. Therefore, the addition of advanced endoscopic techniques to routine evaluations for IBD not only enhances the diagnostic accuracy but also plays a vital role in optimizing patient outcomes and minimizing complications of the chronic diseases (Figure 6.8).

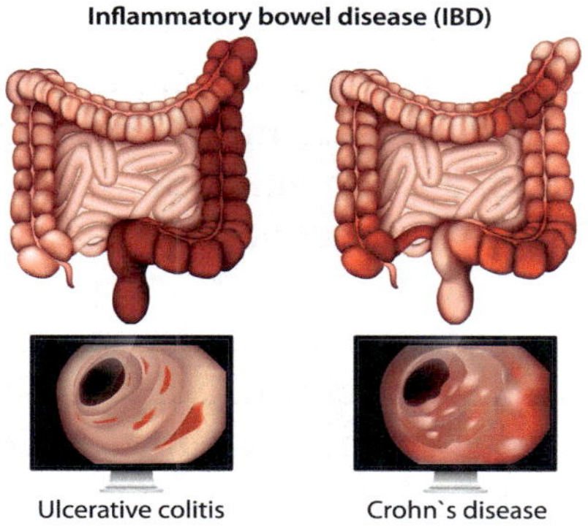

Figure 6.8. Inflammatory bowel disease (IBD).

Source: https://sanmateorheumatology.com/wp-content/uploads/2019/06/shutterstock_1307614990-1.jpg.

6.3. Procedure Overview

The procedural setting of sigmoidoscopy and proctoscopy is of critical importance in the diagnosis and treatment of several colorectal disorders. Sigmoidoscopy, which is a non-surgical procedure, allows for examination of the rectum and the descending part of the colon, providing valuable information on pathologic details , such as polyps, inflammation, and cancer. Proctoscopy, however, is specific to the examination of the rectum and anal canal. Sigmoidoscopy and proctoscopy are both outpatient procedures, typically performed with the patient under local anesthesia or conscious sedation to ensure comfort. In addition, as suggested by current practices, sigmoidoscopy is not only used for diagnostic purposes but also forms an integral part of therapeutic procedures, such as polypectomy and biopsy, which can be crucial in the early diagnosis and treatment of colorectal cancer, thereby pointing to its clinical relevance in current gastroenterology. Besides their diagnostic purposes, the choice of doing a proctoscopy or a sigmoidoscopy may rely on the clinical presentation and presentation at examination. For instance, with suspicion of rectal cancer, practitioners may use more sophisticated techniques , such as TEM or transanal minimal invasive surgery (TAMIS). These techniques can be utilized to obtain local tumor resection with acceptable recurrence rates based on recent literature. The capacity to treat early rectal cancer, particularly stages TiS and T1, by local excision methods determines the procedural significance of sigmoidoscopy in colorectal oncology. Consequently, the findings from these processes that are informative not only allow for accurate staging of cancer but also present a framework for making future therapeutic treatment decisions, further demonstrating that they aid in advocating patient care and outcomes, as the local excision techniques literature review discusses (Ahmed et al., 2020). Additionally, the acknowledgment of the practical use and outcome of sigmoidoscopy and proctoscopy enhances the management of conditions like rectal prolapse. Recently, a paper reported findings on patients who were submitted to surgical operations for rectal prolapse and observed that a majority had returned to normal sigmoidoscopy results with significant symptoms , such as mass per rectum and discharge of mucus (Aravind, 2013). The findings highlight the importance of these procedures in both therapeutic and diagnostic settings, where accurate procedure selection can have a notable influence on recurrence rates and recovery courses. As highlighted, perineal procedures are associated with lower morbidity and decreased hospital stays when compared to abdominal procedures, thereby signaling the importance of tailoring interventions in relation to the outcomes and patient conditions. Lastly, the incorporation of these processes into a general management plan lays a good platform for enhanced quality of life and treatment outcomes for patients with colorectal pathology (Figure 6.9).

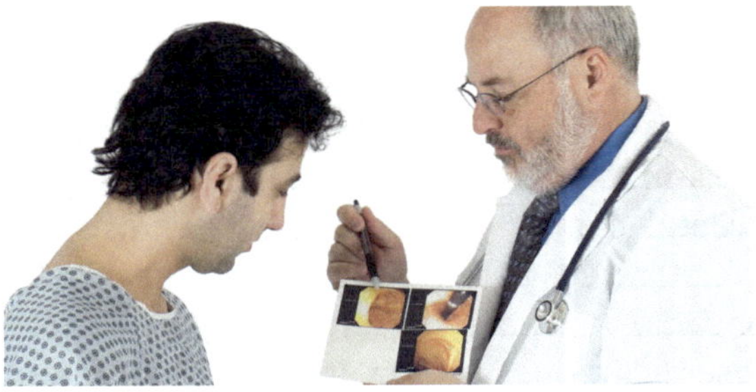

Figure 6.9. Sigmoidoscopy and proctoscopy.

Source: https://hips.hearstapps.com/netdoctor.cdnds.net/15/45/4000x2000/landscape-1446741703-g-sigmoidoscopy-and-proctoscopy-172874238.jpg?resize=1200:*.

6.3.1. Preparation Required for Patients

Patients need to be prepared if they are going to undergo sigmoidoscopy or proctoscopy, since this does a lot to enhance the diagnostic yield and the overall procedural experience. Preparation is usually begun with changes in diet, whereby a clear liquid diet for 24 hours preceding the test is employed. This should be supported by oral laxatives or enemas, such that the bowel is cleaned adequately. Ideal bowel preparation allows visualization of the rectosigmoid mucosa so that clinicians can detect abnormalities like lesions or polyps efficiently. Effective preparation, as per studies, can lead to more favorable outcomes in diagnostic yield and potential therapeutic interventions in endoscopic procedures, highlighting the importance of adhering to preparatory guidelines (Colman et al., 2017). In addition to dietary preparation, effective communication among healthcare workers and patients is necessary for ensuring the patients understand and follow the prescribed regimen. Healthcare workers must ensure that patients understand the need to strictly adhere to bowel preparation processes since variation may inhibit the effectiveness of diagnostic tests. Providing clear instructions about the timing and mode of administration of medication, along with the avoidance of solid food, assists in the enhancement of patient compliance. Moreover, talking to patients about concerns related to the preparation process reduces anxiety and hence enhances the overall patient experience before the procedure. One cannot overestimate the significance of open communication since it is at the core of the readiness of patients to prepare for sigmoidoscopy or proctoscopy (Anselm et al., 2025). Last but not least, psychological readiness is another essential aspect that cannot be disregarded in the preparation process by healthcare providers. Patients may experience anxiety owing to the invasiveness of these tests, and this can be alleviated through education-based interventions. Giving clear explanations regarding what the procedures are, such as the length, feelings, and possible discomforts, can strengthen patients and minimize anticipatory anxiety. In addition, visual aids or pre-procedure counseling sessions can enable patients to see the process, thus making their experience more routine-like and facilitating a sense of control. In summary, physical and mental preparation equally contribute a significant influence on patient outcomes, and, hence, emphatic importance should be given to intensive and patient-centered approaches in the case of sigmoidoscopy and proctoscopy (Colman et al., 2017).

6.3.2. Step-by-Step Process of Sigmoidoscopy

The step-by-step procedure of sigmoidoscopy begins with patient preparation, which is greatly essential to achieve accurate results. Doctors typically order patients to follow a special diet before the procedure and prescribe laxatives to cleanse the bowel. Preparation is needed to provide clear observation of the rectal and sigmoid areas during testing. Patients may also be instructed not to eat solid foods for a certain period and transition gradually to a clear liquid diet to cleanse the bowel. These pre-procedure measures reduce the chance of complications and can maximize the effectiveness of the procedure, ultimately resulting in better diagnostic outcomes. Educating the patient regarding what to expect during the sigmoidoscopy process is often emphasized as well, which allays fear and promotes cooperation, thereby leading to smoother overall experience. The sigmoidoscopy procedure really begins with the patient being in a comfortable position, usually on their side. The physician then gradually passes a lubricated sigmoidoscope – a flexible, soft tube with a camera and light – into the rectum. The instrument allows direct visualization of the sigmoid colon and areas of the rectum. While advancing the sigmoidoscope, air is introduced into the colon to distend it, allowing one to obtain an entire view of the mucosal lining. The physician carefully examines for abnormally appearing features , such as polyps, inflammation, or signs of cancer. In some cases, tissue samples are taken for biopsy, and the procedure can be the key to the diagnosis of numerous disorders. The doctor can also make critical decisions during the procedure based on the images provided by the sigmoidoscope in real-time, which enhances diagnostic outcomes. After finishing the sigmoidoscopy, the doctor slowly withdraws the sigmoidoscope while monitoring the patient's comfort throughout the procedure. Afterwards, patients are typically monitored for a period of time to avoid any emergent complication, for instance, bleeding or pain in the abdomen. Patients may experience mild cramping or discomfort from the air introduced, but otherwise tend to resume normal activities shortly afterwards. Follow-up includes relating findings to the patient and possibly ordering additional diagnostic studies, depending on what is observed. The information obtained through sigmoidoscopy is invaluable since it may inform further screening or treatment strategies, particularly in the context of outcomes related to colorectal cancer risks and control, as discussed in more recent research studies on the impact of screening processes like the fecal immunochemical tests for hemoglobin (Ahlquist et al., 2014) and socioeconomic disparities in cancer survival (Barbiere et al., 2011) (Figure 6.10).

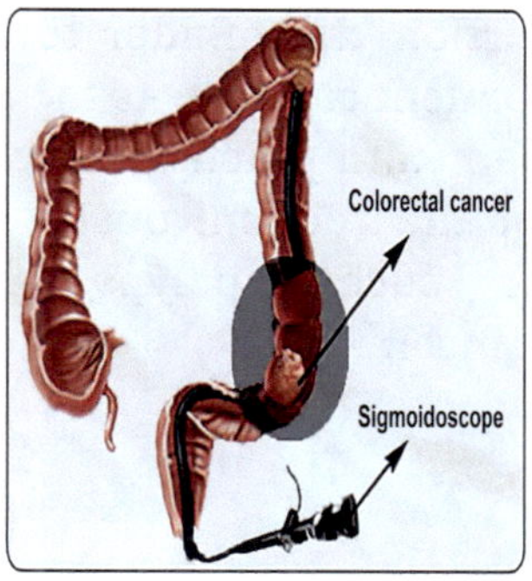

Figure 6.10. Sigmoidoscopy procedure.

Source: https://images.medindia.net/amp-images/patientinfo/Colorectal-cancer-screening.jpg.

6.3.3. Step-by-Step Process of Proctoscopy

The step-by-step procedure of proctoscopy begins with preparations to keep the patient safe and comfortable. Initially, the physician reviews the patient's history, focusing on gastrointestinal symptoms or prior procedures that can influence the exam. Next, the patient is informed about the procedure, its indication, risks, and what he or she can expect during the procedure. This communication is necessary because awareness of the procedure can alleviate patient fear and ensure cooperation. The correct position on an examining table—usually the left lateral position—is then achieved, which offers greater access to the rectum. This preparation time not only optimizes patient comfort but also makes the clinician ready to examine with precision and minimal complications, forming the basis for further invasive procedures where needed, particularly in light of mounting evidence suggesting screening effectiveness in reducing mortality rates from colorectal cancers (Sabatino et al., 2012). Proctoscope insertion constitutes the next critical step after preparations are complete. The tool, typically a rigid tube with a light source and an optical system, is gently introduced into the rectum. The health practitioner applies a lubricant to decrease pain on insertion, a reminder to be cautious to maintain patient comfort. As the proctoscope advances, the health practitioner can visualize the lining of the rectum, observing for any irregularities , such as polyps, inflammation, or signs of cancer.

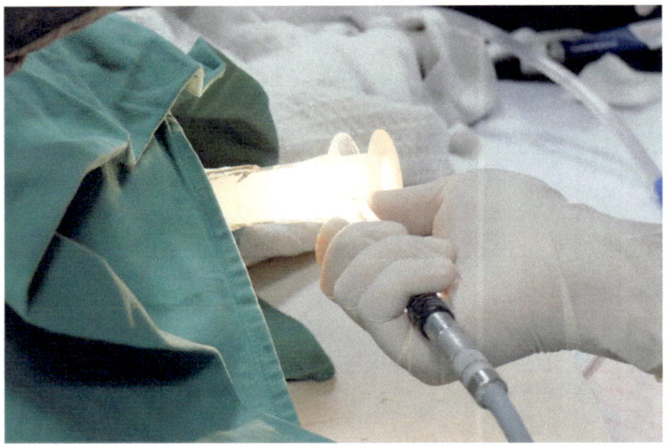

Figure 6.11. Proctoscopy.

Source: https://eremedium.in/wp-content/uploads/2024/06/proctoscopy-1200x800.jpg.

This is a key step since real-time visualization allows for immediate assessment of situations that require further intervention. Precise technique upon insertion is essential to preventing complications; therefore, clinicians are trained to be attentive while monitoring patient reactions during the procedure, which is supplemented by guidelines to ensure standardization and safety of anorectal emergency interventions (Abongwa et al., 2021). Finally, completion of the proctoscopy is required with a complete evaluation and follow-up regimen. After the examination, the findings must be well-documented to inform patient care decisions and subsequent medical testing. In the event of abnormalities, such as polyps or lesions, the physician can order additional procedures, including biopsies or sigmoidoscopy for further testing. The importance of informing the patient of their findings cannot be overstated, as it induces understanding and adherence to any recommended treatment or follow-up therapy. Furthermore, the practitioner tends to discuss changes in lifestyle or additional screening based on results, which is in line with evidence supporting the promotion of preventive interventions to minimize future health risks, especially for colorectal cancer screening procedures, as quoted in current health literature (Sabatino et al., 2012) (Figure 6.11).

6.4. Risks and Complications

The sigmoidoscopy and proctoscopy procedure, though quite safe in general, is not risk-free with complications that should be carefully balanced. Among the risks of these procedures, one of the major ones is bowel perforation, which, though uncommon, may lead to dire consequences , such as peritonitis or sepsis. The risk of bowel perforation would typically be based on the nature of the procedure and patient features. Risk factors, including history of prior surgeries or inflammatory bowel disease, can increase the risk.

Furthermore, sedation performed during the procedure can also be a source of respiratory complications, particularly in individuals with underlying pulmonary issues. Therefore, the evaluation of patients before the procedure is necessary, helping healthcare providers weigh the benefit against potential adverse outcomes. Awareness of these hazards is important to the physician and patient alike to facilitate informed consent and preparation in the event of complications. Of note also is bleeding after a sigmoidoscopy or proctoscopy, particularly when biopsies are performed or polyps removed during the procedure. While most instances of bleeding are self-limited, it can become a medically challenging bleeding, such as transfusions or the necessity for repeat surgery. The occurrence of bleeding may be higher in patients who have coagulopathies or who are on anticoagulant therapy. Invariable follow-up of patients following the procedure is essential to identify any symptoms of abnormal distress or hemodynamic instability. As discussed in endoscopic procedure research, the probability of such complications proves the necessity for subspecialist training on the procedures done and competency in managing emergencies.

Patients should be educated regarding the signs of bleeding to facilitate early treatment if it occurs, thus minimizing risk and complications further. Finally, apart from bleeding, other complications of sigmoidoscopy and proctoscopy include infection and post-procedure pain. Infection may result from the entry of bacteria into the lumen of the bowel, particularly in individuals with compromised immune systems or underlying gastrointestinal diseases. The use of aseptic methods is of the highest significance in preventing such infections. Uncomfort during after the procedure, including bloating and cramping, is normal though typically transient. Such potential side effects ought to be appropriately explained to patients by healthcare professionals, encouraging open systems where patients are motivated to express their symptoms or concerns following the procedure. Historical data show a rising trend of malpractice cases in some endoscopic procedures, predominantly colonoscopy, supporting the necessity of careful follow-up treatment and vigilance in recognizing and treating such complications (Perumal, 2012; Hernandez et al., 2013). Both healthcare practitioners and patients may strive to ensure safer procedure outcomes through emphasis on awareness of risk.

6.4.1. Common Risks Associated with Both Procedures

Both sigmoidoscopy and proctoscopy are diagnostic examinations employed to view the rectum and descending colon, but carry risk. The risks of these examinations arise largely from the invasive nature of the examinations and potential complications of instrumentation within the gastrointestinal tract. Perforation of the intestinal wall is a common complication that can cause severe morbidity or necessitate emergency surgery. Furthermore, there is a risk factor for post-procedure bleeding in patients with pre-existing conditions that weaken the vascular integrity of the rectum. There is also a legitimate concern with anesthesia use; although generally mild, sedation carries side effects with it, adding one more risk factor to the procedures. Beyond the physical danger, the psychological impact of undergoing sigmoidoscopy and proctoscopy cannot be overlooked. They also experience anxiety or discomfort while undergoing and before such procedures, primarily because of the invasive nature of the tests. Such anxiety may lead to a delay in diagnosis or avoidance of needed evaluation. Lastly, the risk of complications like infection, though minimal, necessitates vigilant monitoring for signs of post-procedure adverse effects. Thus, health care providers must explain clearly the kind of risk involved in such procedures to patients and thus promote greater understanding and informed consent. Lastly, there are some instances that can increase the risk profile for such procedures, such as in pre-existing conditions , such as inflammatory bowel disease or in patients who have had previous surgeries of the gastrointestinal tract. Studies have indicated that procedures like sigmoidoscopy are capable of leading to high incidences of complications among patients suffering from conditions like sigmoid volvulus, which might entail a more complex surgical procedure (Assan & Slivanov, 2016). This is apart from potential complications arising from biopsies and polypectomies performed during the procedure. As procedures evolve, the understanding of associated risks must also progress, necessitating continuous education for practitioners to mitigate these risks effectively (Perumal, 2012). The overarching goal remains to balance diagnostic yield against potential harm for optimal patient outcomes.

6.4.2. Potential Complications During and After the Procedures

Sigmoidoscopy and proctoscopy, although fairly innocuous procedures, are not free from probable complications during or following their execution. The immediate complications of such procedures are bowel perforation, albeit rare, with grave intra-abdominal complications in the form of peritonitis. In addition, bleeding can occur, particularly if biopsies are taken or if there are pre-existing lesions along the lining of the intestine. The utilitarian advantage of these procedures, that is, obtaining diagnostic images and the capacity to intervene, requires that their risks be disclosed. Both patients who undergo sigmoidoscopy or proctoscopy must be properly informed about these risks as part of informed pre-procedure counseling. Safe practices and the use of endoscopic devices have reduced risks significantly, but personnel must be cautious since complications still arise in such settings (Perumal, 2012). Complications can also arise after the procedure, most often after the patient has been discharged. The patients might experience post-operative sensations of cramping or abdominal pain, which are a result of bowel manipulation during the procedure. Although mild discomfort is expected, pain accompanied by fever or heavy bleeding can be a sign of underlying complications. Transient bowel habit disturbances, including change of bowel habits or diarrhea, are also typical postoperative complications. Although these may resolve spontaneously, patients must be dutiful and maintain a line of communication with physicians to monitor and maintain these side effects in the best manner possible. Ergo, adequate post-procedure follow-up and education of patients regarding warning symptoms are vital in avoiding these risks and achieving the best patient outcomes (Perumal, 2012). In complicated conditions, particularly in rectal cancer, technical difficulty in sigmoidoscopy and proctoscopy procedures is added. After local excision techniques , such as TEM and TAMIS, patients may develop complications that are distinct from routine endoscopic procedures. Such advanced procedures yield recurrence rates that require close monitoring and perhaps adjuvant treatment based on tumor stage. Delayed early complications , such as local recurrence or anastomotic leaks, can significantly influence overall prognosis and quality of life for the patient. Multi-disciplinary input in the form of oncologists and experienced colorectal surgeons is therefore required in the management of complications. This collaborative strategy aims at enhancing patients' safety and clinical outcomes while capitalizing on the advancement of minimally invasive surgical techniques.

6.4.3. Strategies for Minimizing Risks

In diagnostic procedures, particularly sigmoidoscopy and proctoscopy, minimizing risks is crucial for patient safety and the efficacy of the procedure. One such effective strategy is the rigorous selection of candidates for these procedures. By deliberate analysis of patient history and current symptoms, clinicians can identify who will benefit most from the test and who may have risks that exceed potential benefits. For instance, patients with extreme underlying conditions or those on anticoagulant drugs may need alternative diagnostic tests to minimize the chances of side effects. Such prudent consideration is in line with evidence-based approaches to enhancing the quality of care, specifically for vulnerable groups , such as elderly patients who will tend to suffer more debilitating consequences due to invasive interventions, as reinforced in McCarthy & Leatherman (2005). Another significant factor in minimizing risks associated with sigmoidoscopy and proctoscopy is maintaining strict conformity with up-to-date technologies and techniques. Technological advances in endoscopic equipment have led to better visualization and diagnostic capability, which not only facilitate proper assessment but also minimize complications. For example, high-definition imaging can enhance the identification of lesions that would otherwise go undiagnosed.

Furthermore, the use of an individually prepared bowel protocol for the patient's overall health status can significantly enhance the efficacy of the procedure. As can be seen from studies, adequate patient preparation minimizes the chances of poorly conducted tests that may necessitate re-procedures and further add to patient distress and exposure to additional risks, pointing to the significance of optimizing preparatory procedures (Hemnath, 2014). Informed consent and patient education are key cornerstones in risk reduction associated with sigmoidoscopy and proctoscopy. Engaging patients in a process of explaining the procedure, its risks, and results creates a spirit of collaboration in which patients feel empowered and more active in their healthcare. Following adequate education, patients can more easily adhere to pre-procedure precautions and therefore lower the risk of complications due to inadequate preparation. Proper lines of communication should also be established with patients for receiving their worries both before, during, and after the procedure. This combined strategy not only raises patient satisfaction but also promotes a culture of safety, significantly lowering the incidence of adverse events associated with gastrointestinal endoscopic procedures (Hemnath, 2014).

6.5. Patient Experience

The patient experience of sigmoidoscopy and proctoscopy is critical in promoting early detection of colorectal disease and promoting widespread adherence to screening guidelines. An understanding of patients' short-term reactions may be a good predictor of the acceptability and effectiveness of the procedures. Based on research, patient-reported outcome measures (PROMs) have high satisfaction levels with sigmoidoscopy, as 87% of the participants in the research study indicated that the patient experienced no or very little pain during the procedure. This type of positive feedback is important as it counteracts fear that is commonly thought to be tied to colorectal screening, thus encouraging more individuals to get preventive medical care like flexible sigmoidoscopy. Such acceptability has a significant role in increasing screening rates and consequently improving health outcomes in risk groups for colorectal cancer (Atkin et al., 2012). Moreover, the psychological impact of sigmoidoscopy cannot be overemphasized; psychological comfort during such procedures is paramount to patient satisfaction. Evidence indicates that anxiety levels and self-assessed health did not actually change from pre-screening to follow-up, suggesting that the intervention per se does not have a detrimental effect on psychological status (Atkin et al., 2012). Furthermore, as the reported rate of colorectal symptoms declined after the procedure, patients feel that the screening is not only a necessary procedure for health but also a beneficial one for their good health. This finding indicates that good communication regarding the absence of physical distress and psychological neutrality of procedure can induce more patients to undergo screening, thus enhancing public health programs. In the broader context of screening for colorectal cancer, nevertheless, physicians' and incentive arrangements' functions can further shape patient experience to a significant degree. It has been discovered in studies that physician bonus eligibility could enhance screening adherence, with roughly 3% points more patients undergoing colorectal cancer screening when their physicians were eligible for bonuses. This correlation shows that motivation in healthcare practice can actually enhance patient outcomes, particularly in the context of prevention. Disparities in screening behavior across different populations still exist because the likelihood of screening also varies depending on gender and physician and patient income. Knowledge of such dynamics enables healthcare systems to better personalize approaches for optimal patient experience maximization and equitable access to necessary screenings (Figure 6.12).

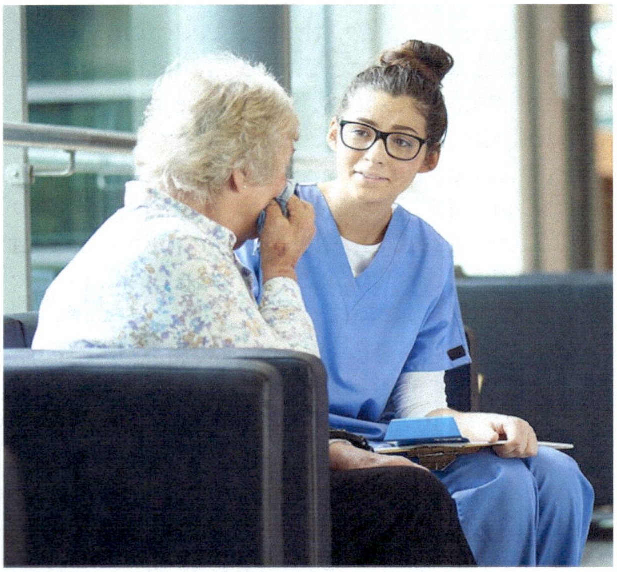

Figure 6.12. Value of patient experience.

Source: https://www.deloitte.com/content/dam/Deloitte/us/Images/promo_images/healthcare-medical/us-hospitals-patient-experience.jpg.

6.5.1. What Patients Can Expect During the Procedures

Patients undergoing sigmoidoscopy and proctoscopy can expect an efficient procedure with minimal discomfort to gather necessary diagnostic information. Before the procedure being performed, medical staff typically undertake a thorough explanation with patients, including steps to be followed, the reason for the test, and requirements for preparation. Pre-procedure discussion can assist in the alleviation of anxiety and allow patients to ask pertinent questions regarding treatment. The procedures are then likely to commence with the administration of a light sedative, whilst many patients remain awake and alert. It is important for patients to strictly follow pre-procedure directions, which might include diet restrictions or bowel prep to allow for adequate visualization of the intestinal mucosa. The preparations, aside from enhancing the accuracy of the test, also facilitate the process as a whole. Patients, in the process of sigmoidoscopy or proctoscopy, will be placed in a comfortable position while the health care provider inserts a flexible tube with an endoscope into the rectum. The procedure will typically last between 15–30 minutes, with some discomfort or pressure experienced by patients when the instrument is passed through the bowel. Providers normally employ lubrication and, in some instances, air insufflation in an effort to facilitate easier visualization. Patients are likely to expect to hear the sounds of the equipment or directions from the provider, but can generally remain engaged in small talk. Vital signs are taken routinely during the procedure to give safety to the patient. Patients also generally have expectations about what might be discovered, because they typically want to know about symptoms like rectal bleeding or bowel change, and thus expect a transparent explanation from the examining health care provider. Following the protocols, patients are usually monitored for a brief period of time to assess their recovery from sedation as well as to identify any side effects. Once cleared, patients may expect a customized plan of post-procedure care, such as review of results, potential follow-up appointments, and changes in lifestyle as may be needed. If there are abnormalities during the procedure, the provider can describe further diagnostic tests or treatments, highlighting the importance of this procedure in early disease diagnosis and preventative screening for conditions , such as colorectal cancer. Patients should also be taught how to recognize signs to watch out for after the procedure, such as uncontrolled bleeding or persistent pain, which ought to prompt medical assessment urgently. By and large, proper communication and full guidance throughout the process result in a more satisfactory and educational patient experience (Figure 6.13).

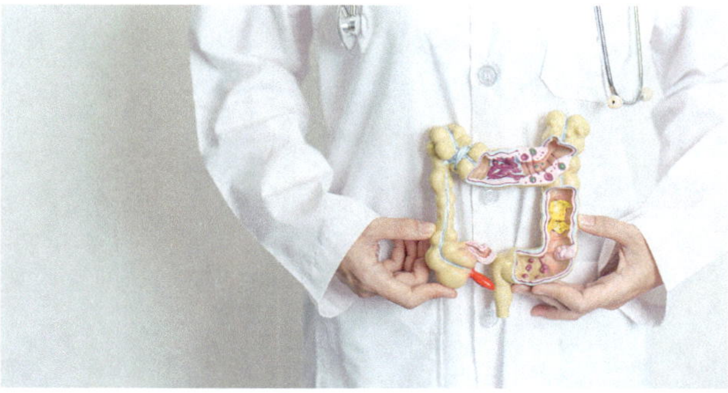

Figure 6.13. Sigmoidoscopy patient education.

Source: https://www.adlermicromed.com/wp-content/uploads/2024/06/Colorectal.jpg.

6.5.2. Pain Management and Sedation Options

Pain management and sedation are the indispensable components in the proper performance of sigmoidoscopy and proctoscopy. These examinations, designed for rectum and lower colon visualization, could cause significant pain based on their invasive nature. Hence, adequate pain relief and adequate use of sedation have a vital role to enhance patient experience and adherence. Sedation strategies can be of diverse choice, ranging from intravenous moderate sedation to deep sedation or general anesthesia, depending on patient need and procedure complexity. Adequate protocols of pain management not only decrease anxiety but also help in minimizing the physiological response of stress, potentially leading to an enhanced streamlined overall procedural outcome. This approach emphasizes the role of personalized sedation plans that are tailored to individual patient characteristics, history, and anticipated intensity of the procedure. More recently, the advances in sedation techniques have moved towards the restriction of deeper sedation and towards non-invasive methods that are more focused on comfort and quicker recovery. This evolution is especially seen in the handling of diseases like hemorrhoids, which, according to research, can be treated in different ways based on severity. For example, sclerotherapy has proved to be a successful and less agonizing first-line treatment for first-degree hemorrhoids, so that outpatient treatment could be achieved with minimal pain and no anesthesia (Kalpana, 2013). This reflects growing realization of the benefits of non-operative approaches, which can be added to pain control protocols in sigmoidoscopy and proctoscopy. These advances are particularly opportune because they lend themselves well to the prevailing pressures for patient-focused models of care that value both procedural efficacy and patient safety. Overall, the applicability of implementing thoroughly investigated sedation techniques cannot be overestimated. Pain control treatments, which are relevant to the specifics of sigmoidoscopy and proctoscopy, are far-reaching in guaranteeing patient satisfaction and compliance during the procedures. There is evidence that ineffective pain control can lead to poor patient outcomes, including delayed diagnosis and treatment complications (Abongwa et al., 2021). By establishing clearer clinical standards and using evidence-based care in sedation, there could be a better risk-benefit ratio during these diagnostic tests. As health care increases, emphasis on total pain management approaches will undoubtedly remain at the forefront of optimizing procedural success and quality of care for patients (Figure 6.14).

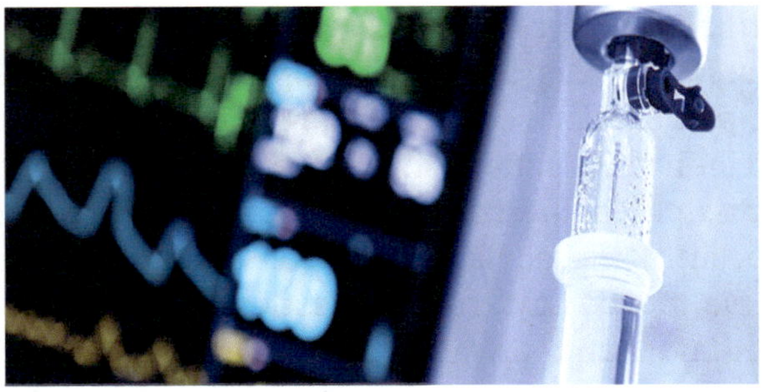

Figure 6.14. Sedation and pain management.

Source: https://www.thoracic.org/patients/patient-resources/managing-the-icu-experience/images/sedation.jpg.

6.5.3. Post-Procedure Care and Recovery

Post-procedure care and recovery from sigmoidoscopy and proctoscopy are necessary to ensure patient comfort and safety. Patients are typically monitored in a recovery area after the procedure to assess their vital signs and that they are stable. Since sedatives are often administered during the procedure, patients may be groggy, lightheaded, or mildly uncomfortable. It is important that they be taken home by a responsible adult because the effects of sedation can affect motor control and judgment. Good hydration is also important because patients are often told to start with clear liquids and gradually progress to a regular diet depending on how well they feel.

The systematic method benefits the recovery process through a quicker return to normal activity and minimizing complications of anesthesia. Once the patients are discharged home, some post-procedure instructions must be followed to ensure optimal recovery. Patients are usually recommended to check for any unexplained symptoms , such as heavy bleeding, stabbing pain in the abdomen, or fever, which may be indicative of complications. Pain relief may be prescribed with over-the-counter medication if needed, but generally, patients experience no more than mild pain. Avoidance of heavy activity for at least 24 hours after the procedure is also necessary, as it can prolong recovery and increase any pain. For patients undergoing procedures , such as local excision, for instance, in rectal adenocarcinomas, follow-up care guidelines become more critical, particularly in surveillance for possible recurrences, as noted by Glasgow et al. 2014). Adherence to such guidelines makes a significant difference in overall recovery and long-term outcomes.

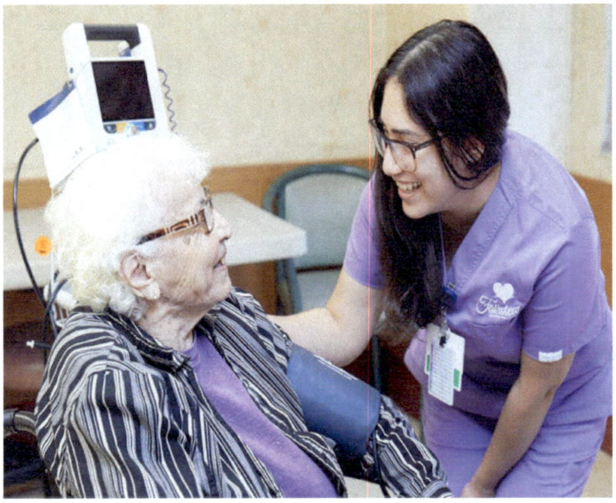

Figure 6.15. Post-operative care.

Source: https://www.fairviewrehab.com/wp-content/uploads/2022/08/post-operative-care-800x554.jpg.

Finally, healthcare providers have a tendency to emphasize the importance of follow-up visits in post-procedure care. On such visits, clinicians are able to evaluate the healing process, examine any biopsies taken during the procedure, and respond to concerns from patients regarding recovery. For the patients who received procedures with local excision or low anterior resection, post-operative follow-up is essential given the reported risk of anastomotic leak complications, as reported in Khan et al. (2014). Patients are encouraged to communicate freely with their care providers and report any suspicious signs immediately. Through the establishment of a relationship between patients and providers, the success potential for healing is realized, allowing individuals to enter their health positively and with confidence in their care processes (Figure 6.15).

6.6. Comparison of Sigmoidoscopy and Proctoscopy

Among the gastrointestinal diagnostic tests, sigmoidoscopy and proctoscopy have significant but distinct roles in their discovery. Sigmoidoscopy is designed primarily to look at the sigmoid colon and the rectum to establish symptoms like rectal bleeding or recurrent diarrhea. It has a flexible endoscope that is more flexible and offers a broader outlook than the rigid form of traditional proctoscopy. The flexibility of the tube makes it easier for the physician to follow the bends of the colon. This feature of sigmoidoscopy enhances its diagnostic potential significantly, and therefore, it is a method of choice for initial examinations of lower gastrointestinal disorders (Perumal, 2012). Proctoscopy is usually limited to the rectum alone and can be beneficial in the context of some rectal disorders, but is not helpful in the evaluation of more proximal lesions of the colon. It is more comfortable in terms of procedure comfort and invasiveness compared to some forms of proctoscopy. Usually, patients need only light sedation during sigmoidoscopy, and they can also be left awake and responsive, which is convenient for both the patient and the physician. It has fewer complications and faster recovery, and hence it is a good choice for diagnostic evaluation. Conversely, while relatively straightforward, proctoscopy may be a less comfortable experience due to its direct and stiff approach in examining the rectum. Hence, it is important to learn about the varying comfort of these procedures in the practice of patient care and satisfaction (del Governatore et al., 2024). Moreover, the choice between sigmoidoscopy and proctoscopy is significantly influenced by the clinical indication. Sigmoidoscopy is typically preferred in patients who have more generalized symptoms, particularly colonic-type symptoms, whereas proctoscopy can be utilized to the best advantage in more focal pathology of the rectum, i.e., hemorrhoids or prolapse of the rectum. Familiarity with the reason that one procedure is employed over the other ensures more precise management of the patient and can eventually enhance diagnostic yield. In regard to the capacities of both procedures, doctors must examine patient symptomatology and history to determine the best method to use. With increasing developments in diagnostic technology, additional research on comparisons between the methods will build a better image of their individual strengths and uses, resulting in optimal patient care in gastroenterology (del Governatore et al., 2024; Perumal, 2012).

6.6.1. Differences in Scope and Reach of Each Procedure

In evaluating sigmoidoscopy and proctoscopy, their differences in scope and scope of examination have profound implications for clinical practice and care of the patient. Sigmoidoscopy is a visual inspection of the rectum and the lower part of the colon, the sigmoid colon, and offers a wider view of potential abnormalities than proctoscopy. While proctoscopy limits its study to the rectum, sigmoidoscopy allows practitioners to recognize a wider range of conditions, including polyps and precancerous indicators of colorectal cancer. Since early detection is the point of improved patient outcomes, sigmoidoscopy thus has an obvious advantage where thorough investigation is required. Proctoscopy, while useful for focal application, is too limited for total cancer screening, which may lead to delayed diagnosis when clinicians miss distal colonic pathology. Procedural method and implications of every diagnostic method also further demarcate their scopes. Bowel cleansing is generally necessary for sigmoidoscopy, enhancing visualization of the lining of the colon, enabling accurate judgments of pathology. This preparatory element not only improves process quality but also allows for early treatment and diagnosis of colorectal disease. Proctoscopy, however, is typically performed without elaborate preparation and is therefore quicker and less invasive. This, however, is at the cost of reduced diagnostic capability, with frequent underdiagnosis of more complex disease beyond the rectum.

Thus, whereas proctoscopy may be chosen in certain localized assessment scenarios, sigmoidoscopy's increased usefulness maintains its essential role in the observation and screening of colorectal well-being. These differences become of particular importance in issues of healthcare delivery systems and their influence on outcomes of patients. Studies have established that referral patterns to specialty care can influence the detection stage of colorectal cancers, which calls for the utilization of appropriate procedures based on patient needs. As an example, in the Trust As healthcare model, the utilization of urgent referrals to specialty care has been associated with an increased detection rate of early-stage cancers, highlighting the effectiveness of sigmoidoscopy in early detection and intervention when utilized appropriately. On the other hand, the restricted field of proctoscopy can interfere with such avenues, possibly giving rise to lost opportunities for early diagnosis. Generally, recognition of the unique dissimilarities in the range and extent of each procedure is important for maximizing patient care and facilitating the ability of clinicians to make educated choices regarding methods of diagnosis.

6.6.2. Advantages and Disadvantages of Each Method

The methods of sigmoidoscopy and proctoscopy are valuable diagnostic tools for lower gastrointestinal disease, each with respective strengths to meet various clinical circumstances. Sigmoidoscopy, an examination in which a peek inside the sigmoid colon and rectum is taken, is typically praised as being minimally invasive and enabling direct visualization of abnormal lesions or pathology. This method not only allows physicians to diagnose conditions like polyps or colon cancer but also allows the conduct of targeted biopsies and therapy, thereby reducing the need for more invasive procedures. Perhaps most importantly, patients generally report minimal discomfort rather than pain, especially with conscious sedation, facilitating inspection to become more tolerable (Perumal, 2012). These characteristics make sigmoidoscopy a useful and cost-effective tool for early diagnosis in asymptomatic individuals undergoing routine screening or symptomatic patients with gastrointestinal symptoms. Proctoscopy, on the other hand, having access only to the rectal segment, offers some benefits in assessing rectal prolapse and other localized processes. As highlighted by studies, proctoscopy can help identify pathologies that have a direct impact on rectal function and health, for example, tumors of the rectum or hemorrhoids. Additionally, the procedure is typically quicker and performed on an outpatient basis, possibly leading to cost savings among patients and healthcare systems. In rectal prolapse, for instance, findings in the majority of the patients on proctoscopy were effective in guiding subsequent surgery (Aravind, 2013). However, though proctoscopy is a quick assessment of the rectal canal, its limitation is its limited coverage, not giving the entire perspective of the sigmoid colon and potentially missing proximal lesions that may require further investigation. Sigmoidoscopy and proctoscopy both have their drawback, which necessitate strictly balancing their limitations. One of the important limitations of sigmoidoscopy is the potential for incomplete evaluation of the entire colon in some patients, especially in those who are suspected to have extensive pathology. In some situations, physicians may need to ask the patient to undergo a complete colonoscopy, which adds further cost and inconvenience. On the other hand, although less invasive, proctoscopy sacrifices all-around evaluation to focally examine, a scenario that may lead to underdiagnosis of diseases outside the rectum. The two procedures also carry the risk of rectal perforation or bleeding, although these occurrences are relatively rare (Perumal, 2012). Therefore, the choice between these two should depend on the specific patient circumstances so that the benefits can outpace the inherent risk and limitations of each investigation method (Figure 6.16).

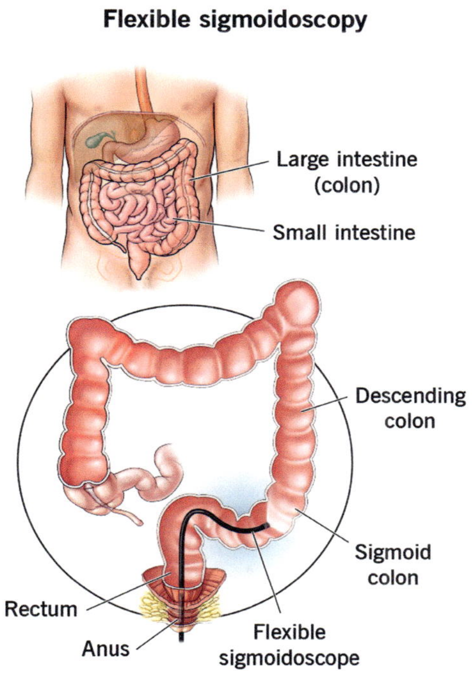

Figure 6.16. Flexible sigmoidoscopy.

Source: https://my.clevelandclinic.org/-/scassets/images/org/health/articles/4953-flexible-sigmoidoscopy.

6.6.3. Situational Appropriateness for Each Procedure

Situational appropriateness of sigmoidoscopy and proctoscopy resides largely in the individual clinical circumstances that demand these investigations. Sigmoidoscopy is most commonly employed as a diagnostic tool in patients who present with rectal bleeding, nonspecific abdominal discomfort, or alteration in bowel habit. Its applicability is also improved by the ability to perform tissue biopsies and administer therapeutic measures to local pathology. The direct assessment of the sigmoid colon is facilitated by this modality, thus giving valuable information regarding likely pathologies , such as polyps or inflammatory bowel disease. Conversely, proctoscopy is focused solely on the examination of the anal canal and lower rectum and would be indicated in patients presenting with local signs , such as anal fissures, hemorrhoids, or rectal prolapse. Definition of the specific clinical indications of each procedure enhances patient management and guides appropriate management strategies in colorectal practice. An understanding of the anatomical rationale of sigmoidoscopy and proctoscopy mostly informs their situational appropriateness. Each of these procedures requires a deep understanding of the anatomy involved, and this is essential for clinicians as they make diagnoses. The anal canal, pelvic floor, colon, and rectum involves problems that are not academically focused but of vital importance to be applied to patient care (Carmichael & Mills, 2021). This data enables clinicians and surgeons to quickly identify anatomical landmarks and potential pathological changes in the processes, facilitating accurate diagnoses and appropriate interventions. Furthermore, awareness of common conditions to arise in these anatomical sites enables clinicians to effectively report results to patients and other healthcare professionals. Thus, detailed anatomical understanding is behind the success of these procedures and modifies them to suit unique patient needs according to their own unique clinical presentations. Beyond anatomy awareness, patient-specific factors also play a role in determining situational appropriateness for sigmoidoscopy and proctoscopy. Patient history, age, and specific symptoms all factor into the decision-making process associated with selecting the appropriate examination. For instance, younger patients with rectal bleeding may be referred to sigmoidoscopy as a first-line procedure due to its minimal invasiveness and benign risk factor profile. Elderly patients with a history of inflammatory bowel disease may be diagnosed by proctoscopy to screen for complications. Having effective communication with patients regarding the purpose and expected outcomes of each procedure is likely to enhance their understanding and minimize fear (Keane, 2015). Lastly, a customized approach taking into account clinical as well as patient aspects ensures that the chosen diagnostic procedure optimally meets the needs of each individual and thereby contributes to better healthcare experiences.

SUMMARY

In short, sigmoidoscopy and proctoscopy are critical diagnostic and therapeutic instruments of gastroenterology. Their applications range from normal screening for colorectal cancer to finding reasons for gastrointestinal symptomatology , such as bleeding or pain. The procedure's success largely relies on the quality of bowel preparation, which has enormous effects on visibility during inspection. Research into newer bowel prep agents , such as free fatty acid suppositories, has provided encouraging results compared with traditional methods but with better patient tolerability. Innovations like these underscore the need for continued evaluation and refinement of preparation protocols to optimize procedure outcomes, hence enhancing patient experience with these procedures (Asgrimsdottir et al., 2016). In addition, the findings on patient outcomes and physician satisfaction endorse the importance of selecting proper methods for varied ailments. Studies have revealed that while traditional techniques of bowel preparation are predominantly effective, innovations can also achieve similar results with less patient discomfort and compliance. The success of local excision techniques in the management of early rectal cancers also gives significance to these diagnostic procedures, as these techniques are now of utmost significance in diminishing the rate of recurrence for some stages of tumors (Ahmed et al., 2020). Thus, the application of sigmoidoscopy and proctoscopy in routine clinical practice is significant for the early diagnosis and management of lower gastrointestinal disorders. The overall inference from sigmoidoscopy and proctoscopy findings is that not only are these methods crucial during early diagnosis, but even in therapeutic strategies employed in treating various proctological ailments. With technological growth in the area and practitioners getting greater training, the possibility of reduced morbidity and improved results of surgery materializes. New research into new modalities of bowel preparation and management of rectal cancer in early stages keeps refining the levels of clinical practice. Ultimately, combining new techniques with old practices allows for optimizing patient care in a manner that maintains sigmoidoscopy and proctoscopy as cornerstones of gastrointestinal health care in the future.

In exploring the application of sigmoidoscopy and proctoscopy in gastrointestinal diagnosis, it was discovered that there were certain points that were highlighted in their significance in the early detection of colorectal disease. These two procedures are necessary to visually examine the lower intestines for conditions , such as polyps, inflammation, and cancer. The significance of early detection was highlighted in most studies that indicated early referrals to specialist care significantly enhance patient outcomes. For instance, results from information accessed from Trust A and Trust B reveal that when general practitioners utilized urgent referral pathways, higher percentages of early-stage colorectal cancers were identified, highlighting the efficacy of systematized systems of referrals (Shah et al., 2012). It is hence essential to learn about procedural variations and patterns of referral for increasing diagnostic quality and treatment efficacy in the treatment of CRC. The history of colorectal cancer in the United States increases the need for such procedures even more. Colorectal cancer (CRC) remains a leading cause of cancer-related deaths and occurs among both men and women at alarming levels. The recent progress in screening procedures like sigmoidoscopy and proctoscopy plays a significant role in the decline in CRC incidence and mortality, reflecting increased improvements in early disease detection. Furthermore, the number of survivors with CRC increases over time, necessitating long-term management and follow-up measures. Where diagnostics blend into total patient care is most important, as survivors are not only at risk for recurrence but also for new cancers and late sequelae of treatment modalities. These intricacies necessitate an organized system of communication between oncologists and primary care physicians so that the greatest survivor benefit can be realized. Secondly, successful models of health care delivery are the determinants for the optimization of the utility of sigmoidoscopy and proctoscopy. The relative comparison of different systems of health care gives insight into how the structure affects the rate of cancer detection. While Trust A had a higher percentage of early detection using a streamlined system of referrals, it was found that both systems ultimately resulted in the same output in cancer diagnosis. Key conclusions highlight the importance of healthcare systems adopting best practice along referral pathways and specialist access for minimizing delay in diagnosis and treatment initiation (Shah et al., 2012). With an ever-changing healthcare setting, continued assessment of such diagnostic procedures will continue to be important in ameliorating approaches to colorectal health, enabling effective early diagnosis as well as best management of the patient in an era where increasing CRC incidence is more widespread.

CLOSER LOOK

PATIENT-REPORTED OUTCOME MEASURES (PROMS):

Patient-reported outcome measures (PROMs) are standardized tools used to capture patients' perspectives on their health, functioning, and quality of life without interpretation by clinicians or researchers. Unlike traditional clinical measures, which focus on objective indicators such as laboratory results or imaging findings, PROMs provide insight into how patients experience symptoms, treatment effects, and overall well-being. This patient-centered approach has become increasingly important in healthcare, particularly in chronic disease management, clinical trials, and quality improvement initiatives.

PROMs can be disease-specific or generic. Disease-specific PROMs target symptoms and functional limitations associated with a particular condition, such as the Asthma Control Test or the Western Ontario and McMaster Universities Osteoarthritis Index (WOMAC). Generic PROMs, like the Short Form-36 (SF-36) or EuroQol-5D (EQ-5D), assess broader aspects of health-related quality of life, allowing comparisons across different patient populations and conditions. Both types are essential for comprehensive evaluation, as they provide complementary perspectives on patient well-being. Administration of PROMs can be paper-based, digital, or via telephone interviews, with increasing adoption of electronic PROMs (ePROMs) due to their efficiency, real-time data capture, and integration with electronic health records. The frequency of PROM collection varies depending on the clinical context, ranging from single assessments in clinical trials to routine monitoring in chronic disease management programs.

The use of PROMs supports shared decision-making by highlighting patient priorities and facilitating individualized care plans. In clinical trials, PROMs serve as key endpoints, providing evidence on treatment impact from the patient perspective, which may not be fully captured by traditional clinical outcomes. Additionally, PROMs contribute to health system performance measurement, enabling benchmarking and evaluation of interventions based on patient-centered outcomes.

However, challenges remain. Ensuring the validity, reliability, and cultural appropriateness of PROMs is critical, as is minimizing patient burden during data collection. Interpretation of PROM data also requires careful consideration, as scores may be influenced by factors such as comorbidities, literacy, or socio-economic status. Despite these challenges, PROMs are increasingly recognized as essential tools in modern healthcare, offering a direct window into the patient experience and fostering a more holistic, person-centered approach to health assessment and care delivery.

REFERENCES

1. Abongwa, H., Abu-Zidan, F., Agnoletti, V., Ansaloni, L., et al. (2021). *Anorectal emergencies: WSES-AAST guidelines.* https://core.ac.uk/download/483745432.pdf (accessed on 15th July 2025).
2. Sultan, A. H., Monga, A., Lee, J., Emmanuel, A., Norton, C., Santoro, G., Hull, T., Berghmans, B., Brody, S., & Haylen, B. T. (2017). An International Urogynecological Association (IUGA)/ International Continence Society (ICS) joint report on the terminology for female anorectal dysfunction. *International urogynecology journal, 28*(1), 5–31. https://doi.org/10.1007/s00192-016-3140-3(accessed on 15th July 2025).
3. Ahlquist, D. A., Allison, J. E., Atkin, W. S., Barrows, G. H., et al. (2014). *Population screening for colorectal cancer means getting FIT: The past, present, and future of colorectal cancer screening using the fecal immunochemical test for hemoglobin (FIT).* https://core.ac.uk/download/30661134.pdf (accessed on 15th July 2025).
4. Ahmed, S., Mothe, B., & Zafar, H. (2020). *Management of Early Rectal Cancer: Current Practice and Future.* https://core.ac.uk/download/388606635.pdf (accessed on 15th July 2025).
5. Anselm, V. J., Frazer, R. E., Lecroisset, D. H., Roseboro, F. J., et al. (2025). *Feasibility study on the design of a probe for rectal cancer detection.* https://core.ac.uk/download/pdf/42877325.pdf (accessed on 15th July 2025).
6. Aravind, R. M. (2013). *A study on etiological factors and outcome of rectal prolapse.* https://core.ac.uk/download/235665817.pdf (accessed on 15th July 2025).
7. Armour, B. S., Friedman, C., Etchason, J., Wike, J., Alley, L., & Pitts, M. M. (2025). *The influence of year-end bonuses on colorectal cancer screening.* https://core.ac.uk/download/pdf/6924530.pdf (accessed on 15th July 2025).
8. Asgrimsdottir, G. M., Bjornsson, E. S., Kristinsson, J. O., Loftsson, T., et al. (2016). *Clinical trial: Free fatty acid suppositories compared with enema as bowel preparation for flexible sigmoidoscopy.* https://core.ac.uk/download/38283746.pdf (accessed on 15th July 2025).
9. Assan, A., & Slivanov, I. (2016). *Sigmoid volvulus: Management by resection and primary anastomosis.* https://core.ac.uk/download/478441261.pdf (accessed on 15th July 2025).
10. Atkin, W., Edwards, R., Kralj-Hans, I., Lo, A., et al. (2012). *Patient-reported outcomes following flexible sigmoidoscopy screening for colorectal cancer in a demonstration screening program in the UK.* https://core.ac.uk/download/16457880.pdf (accessed on 15th July 2025).
11. Barbiere, J. M., Baum, M., Coleman, M. P., Lyratzopoulos, G., et al. (2011). *Changes over time in socioeconomic inequalities in breast and rectal cancer survival in England and Wales during a 32-year period (1973–2004): The potential role of health care.* https://core.ac.uk/download/13093422.pdf (accessed on 15th July 2025).
12. Carmichael, J. C., & Mills, S. (2021). *Anatomy and embryology of the colon, rectum, and anus.* https://core.ac.uk/download/617035483.pdf (accessed on 15th July 2025).
13. Carmichael, J. C., Dekhordi-Vakil, F., Detweiler, K., Duong, A., et al. (2023). *Intraoperative anastomotic evaluation methods: Rigid proctoscopy versus flexible endoscopy.* https://core.ac.uk/download/614877242.pdf (accessed on 15th July 2025).

14. Colman, K. S., Desborough, M., East, J. E., Goldsmith, C., et al. (2017). *Diagnostic and therapeutic treatment modalities for acute lower gastrointestinal bleeding: A systematic review.* https://core.ac.uk/download/346536201.pdf (accessed on 15th July 2025).
15. Cross, E. L. (2019). *Understanding the extent of, and reasons for, diagnostic delay in inflammatory bowel disease.* https://core.ac.uk/download/333901336.pdf (accessed on 15th July 2025).
16. del Governatore, M., Ferla, S., Govoni, F., Guida, M., et al. (2024). *Feasibility of intraoperative proctosigmoidoscopy after discoid bowel resection for deep infiltrating endometriosis: A pilot multicenter study.* https://core.ac.uk/download/654521638.pdf (accessed on 15th July 2025).
17. Glasgow, S. C., & Heafner, T. A. (2014). *A critical review of the role of local excision in the treatment of early (T1 and T2) rectal tumors.* https://core.ac.uk/download/368707144.pdf (accessed on 15th July 2025).
18. Hemnath, U. A. (2014). *A prospective study on the diagnostic yield of lower gastrointestinal endoscopy for altered bowel habits, lower abdominal pain and rectal bleeding.* https://core.ac.uk/download/235668238.pdf (accessed on 15th July 2025).
19. Hernandez, L. V., Klyve, D., & Regenbogen, S. E. (2013). *Malpractice Claims for Endoscopy.* https://core.ac.uk/download/51141143.pdf (accessed on 15th July 2025).
20. Jena, A. B., Atkins, D., Baicker, K., Bovbjerg, R. R., Card, D., Centers for Medicare and Medicaid Services, et al. (2016). *Does medical malpractice law improve health care quality?* https://core.ac.uk/download/62571352.pdf (accessed on 15th July 2025).
21. Jinreeve, S. W. D. (2015). *Study of clinical and functional results of abdominal mesh rectopexy for complete rectal prolapse.* https://core.ac.uk/download/235667063.pdf (accessed on 15th July 2025).
22. Kalpana, R. (2013). *A comparative study on various treatment procedures in the management of hemorrhoids – Banding, sclerotherapy and hemorrhoidectomy.* https://core.ac.uk/download/235667805.pdf (accessed on 15th July 2025).
23. Kapil Raj, S. (2015). *Study on colonoscopic findings in positive fecal occult blood testing.* https://core.ac.uk/download/235667064.pdf (accessed on 15th July 2025).
24. Keane, D. J. (2015). *User-centered approach to the design, development and implementation of patient information.* https://core.ac.uk/download/42506661.pdf (accessed on 15th July 2025).
25. Khan, N., Mir, S. A., Parray, F. Q., Thoker, M., et al. (2014). *Role of diversion ileostomy in low rectal cancer: A randomized controlled trial.* https://core.ac.uk/download/pdf/82246232.pdf (accessed on 15th July 2025).
26. McCarthy, D., & Leatherman, S. (2005). *Quality of health care for Medicare beneficiaries: A chartbook.* https://core.ac.uk/download/71354155.pdf (accessed on 15th July 2025).
27. Meester, R. G. S. (2017). *Optimizing Outcomes of Colorectal Cancer Screening.* https://core.ac.uk/download/154416443.pdf (accessed on 15th July 2025).
28. Perumal, P. (2012). *Endoscopy.* https://core.ac.uk/download/pdf/1570017.pdf (accessed on 15th July 2025).
29. Sabatino, S. A., Lawrence, B., Elder, R., Mercer, S. L., Wilson, K. M., DeVinney, B., Melillo, S., Carvalho, M., Taplin, S., Bastani, R., Rimer, B. K., Vernon, S. W., Melvin, C. L., Taylor, V.,

Fernandez, M., Glanz, K., & Community Preventive Services Task Force (2012). Effectiveness of interventions to increase screening for breast, cervical, and colorectal cancers: nine updated systematic reviews for the guide to community preventive services. *American journal of preventive medicine*, *43*(1), 97–118. https://doi.org/10.1016/j.amepre.2012.04.009(accessed on 15th July 2025).

30. Shah, P. R. (2012). *Colorectal cancer: A comparative study of models of health care delivery in two adjacent trusts in South Wales.* https://core.ac.uk/download/pdf/6117433.pdf (accessed on 15th July 2025).

31. Veeranki, S. P., & Zheng, S. (2014). Trends and Determinants of Up-to-date Status with Colorectal Cancer Screening in Tennessee, 2002-2008. *International journal of preventive medicine*, *5*(7), 865–874. (accessed on 15th July 2025).

32. Williams, T. G. S., Cubiella, J., Griffin, S. J., Walter, F. M., et al. (2016). *Risk prediction models for colorectal cancer in people with symptoms: A systematic review.* https://core.ac.uk/download/83938441.pdf (accessed on 15th July 2025).

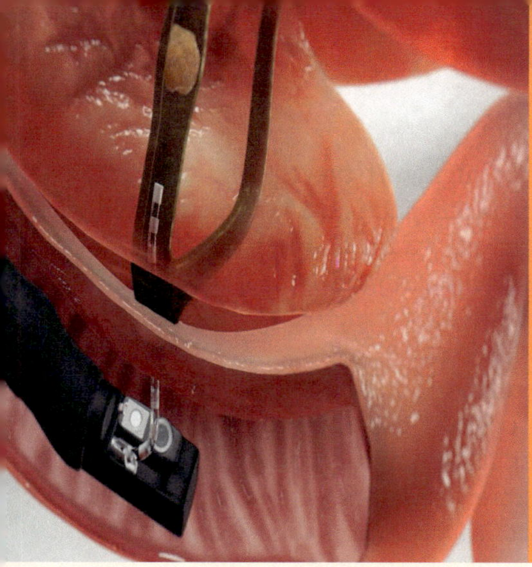

Chapter 7

ENDOSCOPIC RETROGRADE CHOLANGIOPANCREATOGRAPHY (ERCP)

Contents

Introduction 187
7.1. Indications for Endoscopic Retrograde Cholangiopancreatography (ERCP) 191
7.2. Procedure of Endoscopic Retrograde Cholangiopancreatography (ERCP) 195
7.3. Risks and Complications 198
7.4. Diagnostic Applications 201
7.5. Therapeutic Applications 204
7.6. Advances in Endoscopic Retrograde Cholangiopancreatography (ERCP) Technology 207
Summary 211
References 214

Introduction

The introduction of Endoscopic Retrograde Cholangiopancreatography (ERCP) has been a milestone in the history of gastrointestinal diagnosis and management. This innovative procedure allows visualization and intervention of the pancreatic and biliary ductal systems, thereby proving highly valuable for both therapeutic and diagnostic reasons. As a minimally invasive procedure, ERCP allows physicians not only to diagnose disorders , such as choledocholithiasis and obstruction of the pancreatic duct but also to perform interventions if necessary, thereby lowering the need for more invasive surgical procedures. Importantly, the safety and efficacy of ERCP have enhanced over time, with the procedure now being a widely used option in clinical practices. With anatomical complexity and potential complications, understanding indications for ERCP is most important to achieve maximum patient care and outcome in the management of complex gastrointestinal disease. In the evaluation of technicalities of ERCP procedures, it is also crucial that constant skill improvement among practitioners be maintained to achieve maximum safety and efficacy. Current recommendations highlight the significance of rigorous training and competence maintenance in endoscopic procedures, particularly in pediatric and adolescent patients, as noted by Tringali et al. (2017). This is actually a quite applicable focus given that younger patients' anatomy is quite different from adults,' requiring tailored approaches and treatments. Secondly, the procedural aspects of ERCP require ongoing practice maintenance to aid in risk minimization. Successful outcomes also depend not just on the technical proficiency of the endoscopist but on team-based care with multidisciplinary teams to address complications and post-procedure care in an optimal manner. Progress in the future will continue to be assured by emphasizing training that will maintain clinicians skilled at delivering high-quality care. Even repeat ERCP procedures have become a focus of ongoing research, namely, biliary stent management. Current studies have shown divergent requirements for therapeutic interventions following ERCP, with the suggestion that not all patients require follow-up ERCP for stent removal, such as in Ponugoti (2015). For example, uncomplicated bile leak patients showed a low requirement for follow-up procedures, which was in direct contrast to choledocholithiasis or stricture patients. Hence, protocols based on clinical presentation can optimize procedural efficiency with the least amount of unnecessary procedures. This criticism of follow-up requirements helps highlight the worth of individualized patient management plans, demonstrating along the way how ERCP can be streamlined for cost-saving strategies and increased patient comfort. Finally, these new observations regarding ERCP's procedural landscape help solidify ERCP's role as a cornerstone in the management of biliary and pancreatic disease (Figure 7.1).

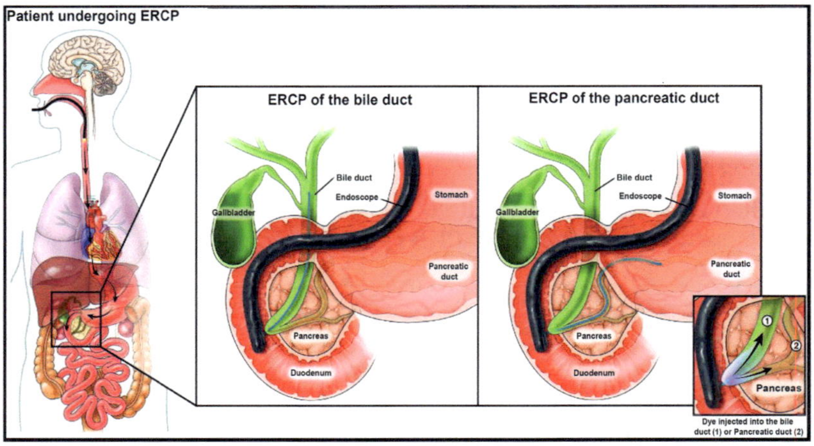

Figure 7.1. Endoscopic retrograde cholangiopancreatography (ERCP).

Source: https://www.regencymedicalcentre.com/wp-content/uploads/2021/03/ERCP-1536x1026.jpg.

Definition of Endoscopic Retrograde Cholangiopancreatography (ERCP)

ERCP is a valuable diagnostic and therapeutic instrument that is primarily utilized to manage diseases of the pancreatic and biliary ducts. ERCP integrates endoscopy and fluoroscopy to visualize the pancreatic duct and biliary tree. During the procedure, an endoscope, a long, flexible tube with a camera, is inserted through the mouth and advanced to the duodenum. Upon taking office, a contrast agent is injected into the bile duct, which allows precise imaging via X-ray.

The method has the potential to detect many conditions , such as biliary stones, strictures, and tumors. Procedural definition emphasizes the dual purpose of ERCP, both in diagnosis and management of the underlying pathology by facilitating the extraction of stones and stent placement, thereby improving outcomes in patients through less invasive interventions. Central to interpreting ERCP is its utility in the diagnosis and management of biliary strictures, which tend to present significant clinical problems. Biliary strictures, which involve narrowing of the bile ducts, can result from multiple benign or malignant causes and can cause serious complications if not treated. Proper diagnosis is necessary, as a number of the strictures have overlapping characteristics that make clinical management more difficult. ERCP is especially valuable in the diagnosis of benign and malignant types by direct visualization and possible tissue retrieval by brush biopsy or dilatation techniques. The integration of imaging methods along with ERCP, including MRCP and ultrasound, is intended to enhance diagnostic yield as a whole, indicating an integrative approach towards the evaluation of biliary illnesses and supplementing ERCP's capability for more drastic decision-making (Raza et al., 2025). In addition, the procedural efficiency and responsiveness of ERCP extend to its therapeutic applications, offering a range of interventions available in one session. These include clearance of obstructing biliary stones, biliary stenting, and dilation of stricture, which together underscore the procedure's application to gastrointestinal medicine. Such demands have created continuous advancements in technique and technology, leading to higher success rates and fewer procedure-related complications. Maintenance of proficiency and training in ERCP are necessary as the complexity and dynamic nature of the procedure necessitate continuous updates for physicians (Tringali et al., 2017). This dynamic ERCP environment not only reflects its critical significance to modern medicine but also suggests the necessity for harmonious interdisciplinary collaboration in the management of patients with any form of biliary disease, ultimately to the benefit of improved quality of care (Figure 7.2).

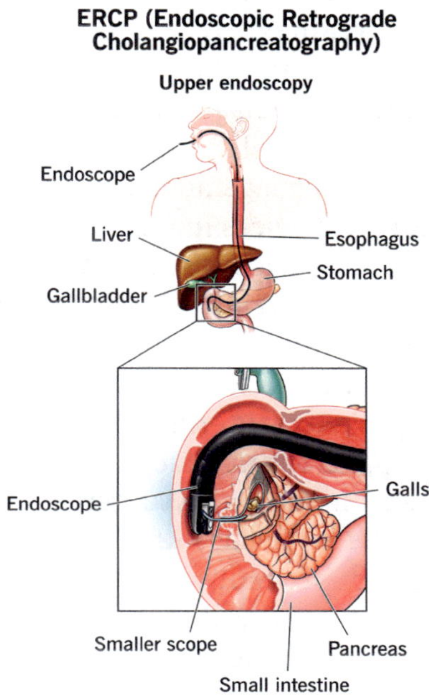

Figure 7.2. Endoscopic retrograde cholangiopancreatography (ERCP)

Source: https://my.clevelandclinic.org/-/scassets/images/org/health/articles/4951-ercp.

Historical Background and Development

The earliest historical origins of ERCP lie in the evolution of endoscopy from the mid-20th century. Initially, fiberoptic endoscopy formed the foundation for imaging the gastrointestinal tract as well as enabling physicians to diagnose a host of conditions of the digestive system. The work of pioneering physicians , such as Dr. Heinrich M. W. B. Kalloo during the 1960s and 1970s paved the way for the convergence of endoscopy with radiographic imaging, enabling targeted intervention within the biliary system. This period was marked by the development of duodenoscopy as a central procedure to access the ampulla of Vater, ultimately leading on to the revolutionary merging of endoscopy and retrograde techniques known as ERCP (Tringali et al., 2017). This revolution did not just enhance diagnostic capability but drove a trend towards less invasive treatment techniques, leading to progress in gastroenterology. By the 1980s, the function of ERCP as a diagnostic and therapeutic tool was increasingly valued, marking a watershed in the management of pancreatic and biliary disease. Advances in technology enabled the use of accessories , such as guidewires and balloons to provide improved precision in attempting to remove gallstones or place biliary stents. These developments brought a new era to patients suffering from obstructive jaundice or pancreatitis since ERCP was now less invasive than traditional surgery (Tomoda et al., 2020). While ERCP has hitherto been utilized for diagnostic procedures, its therapeutic applications have secured it as a treatment for various disorders of the biliary and pancreatic systems, further anchoring it to practice and improving patient care. Despite its progress, ERCP has not been complication-free, particularly acute pancreatitis, a procedure-related adverse event. While medical practitioners were making efforts to minimize such risks, research efforts were geared towards ascertaining preventive strategies. Medical Image Processing. Current evidence affirms that the prophylactic use of non-steroidal anti-inflammatory drugs (NSAIDs) , such as indomethacin may decrease the risk of post-ERCP pancreatitis, although the efficacy of such treatments is debated in clinical settings (Tomoda et al., 2020). Such ongoing research attests to the dynamic process of ERCP, whereby both its historical development and modern modifications continue to be led by improving scientific principles and concerns for patient safety. Appreciation for the universalizing role of ERCP in treating the gastrointestinal system is increased by this historical awareness, yet its continued necessity for research and protocol refinement.

Endoscopic Retrograde Cholangiopancreatography (ERCP) Relevance to Modern Medicine

ERCP is a valuable technology in modern medicine, particularly in the diagnosis and treatment of bile duct and pancreatic disease. ERCP is an intervention that is less invasive, allowing direct visualization, diagnosis, and treatment.

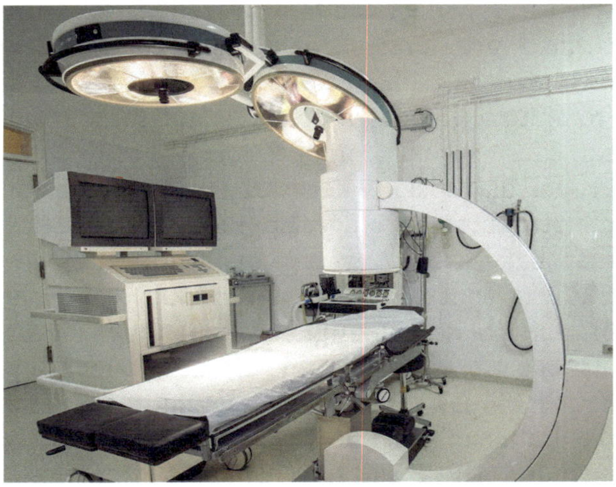

Figure 7.3. Endoscopic retrograde cholangiopancreatography (ERCP) machine.

Source: https://www.apsf.org/wp-content/uploads/newsletters/2020/3502/endoscopic-retrograde-cholangiopancreatography-ercp-featured.jpg.

This capability plays a critical role in the management of diseases , such as cholangitis, pancreaticobiliary malignancies, and bile duct gallstones, which can significantly influence patient morbidity and mortality.

The procedure not only provides valuable diagnostic insight but also allows for therapeutic interventions , such as sphincterotomy and stenting and therefore enhances patient outcomes. The ability to perform such advanced treatments endoscopically emphasizes ERCP's core role in contemporary hepatobiliary medicine, and as such, it is an essential competence for gastroenterologists and surgeons, as underlined in the profession-specific guidelines (Tringali et al., 2017). Beyond its therapeutic and diagnostic applications, ERCP is most significant in the management of chronic liver disease and complications. The advent of ERCP has transformed the treatment of conditions like recurrent pyogenic cholangitis, in which conventional surgical intervention is more hazardous. By means of real-time imaging of the biliary tract and its related pathology, ERCP provides for targeted intervention that can prevent further complications, i.e., infection and liver failure.

Also, the integration of advanced techniques, including endoscopic ultrasound with ERCP, has improved the staging accuracy of gastrointestinal cancer and assessment of vascular complications, significantly impacting management plans for patients (Lam et al., 1997). This demonstrates the versatility and effectiveness of ERCP in the treatment of complex gastrointestinal diseases in the contemporary clinic. While the effectiveness of ERCP is unquestioned, the value of procedures also exists in enhancing the efficiency of medical care. ERCP can reduce the need for more invasive surgeries in most situations, shortening hospital stays and healthcare costs.

Further, technology continues to enhance the safety and success rates of ERCP, solidifying its position in current medicine. Training and maintenance of competency are important components of delivering competence in ERCP, as outlined in several guidelines (Tringali et al., 2017). As the landscape of gastrointestinal disease evolves, ERCP remains an important part of clinical practice and study, proving its ongoing relevance and value in delivering comprehensive patient care in today's healthcare environment (Figure 7.3).

7.1. Indications for Endoscopic Retrograde Cholangiopancreatography (ERCP)

ERCP has a significant role to play in the treatment of various biliary and pancreatic illnesses, evidenced by the presentation of the diseases of choledocholithiasis, strictures, and pancreatitis. The most common indication of ERCP is choledocholithiasis or gallstones in the common bile duct. The procedure is both diagnostic and therapeutic, offering the potential for stone removal and the relief of obstruction. In biliary strictures, commonly caused by neoplasms or inflammatory conditions, ERCP is useful in diagnosis and may allow for stenting to preserve bile duct patency and avoid further complications.

Moreover, in acute pancreatitis, especially when obstruction of the bile duct is suspected, ERCP may be vital for diagnosis and possibly treatment, highlighting the diverse applications of ERCP in gut medicine. The worth of ERCP is also confirmed with the diagnosis and treatment of pancreatic ductal obstruction, including that due to pancreatic cancer and chronic pancreatitis. Visualization of the biliary tree in pancreatic cancer gives information regarding the extent of the disease and resectability. ERCP not only facilitates the procurement of tissue samples by brush cytology but is also therapeutic in relieving obstructive jaundice by drainage of the biliary tract. In the same way, in patients with chronic pancreatitis, where duct strictures may exacerbate symptoms, ERCP can both clarify the diagnosis and provide therapeutic intervention by way of balloon dilation or stenting. Its dual utility highlights the place of ERCP as a minimally invasive modality for addressing difficult pancreatic disease and makes it an essential procedure in gastrointestinal intervention. Lastly, there is abundant evidence at a large scale for the use of ERCP in jaundice patients with an unknown cause, particularly if differential diagnoses are choledocholithiasis or bile duct malignancies. It is routinely a first-line investigation because visualization and intervention can be done simultaneously, provided malignancy is not ruled out. ERCP process quality monitoring is crucial and can be performed through novel techniques , such as Natural Language Processing (NLP) and data mining, enabling enhanced provider accountability and adherence to established standards (Beesley et al., 2017).

In addition, guidelines strongly define the appropriate indications for ERCP, justify its application in children, as reflected in recent literature (Tringali et al., 2017). By emphasizing ERCP's indications, physicians can more appropriately place the procedure within the broader context of gastrointestinal treatment (Figure 7.4).

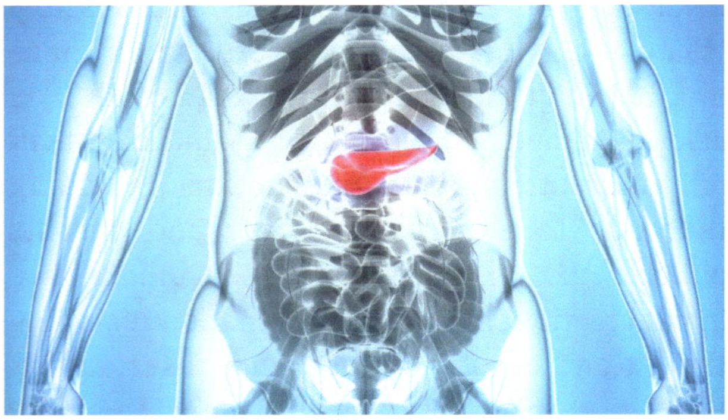

Figure 7.4. Endoscopic retrograde cholangiopancreatography (ERCP) indications.

Source: https://res.cloudinary.com/broadcastmed/image/fetch/q_auto,c_fill,w_1300,h_731,g_faces:center,f_auto/http://55933-bcmed.s3.amazonaws.com/bcp/images/orlVideoAssets/imgSource/istock-6720813881.jpg.

7.1.1. Diagnosis of Biliary Tract Disorders

In diagnosing biliary tract disorders, imaging modalities play an important role in determining underlying pathologies of bile ducts. Ultrasound (US) has been most frequently the first imaging modality used since it is noninvasive and can visualize biliary dilatation. Ultrasound was reported to be reliable in diagnosing conditions of the bile in one study with its high sensitivity, 100% in bile stone detection and 83.3% in bile duct system tumors. Moreover, the study found that in 92.5% of the cases, ultrasound was accurately diagnosed in relation to ERCP findings, indicating its possible value as a first-line diagnostic test. Early intervention becomes possible with this, particularly if experiencing acute cholecystitis or obstructive jaundice, and medical professionals are able to make patient management judgments. ERCP is now an integral diagnostic and therapeutic procedure in the management of biliary tract disease. ERCP allows for direct visualization of pancreatic and biliary ducts and hence for the diagnosis of a variety of conditions , such as choledocholithiasis and strictures. ERCP not only aids in diagnostic assessment but also therapeutic management, such as stone extraction and stenting. Integration of the therapeutic and diagnostic roles in one procedure optimizes its utility in day-to-day practice. Second, ERCP is also considered to be particularly valuable in patients with suspected neoplastic bile duct malignancies because it allows for the retrieval of cytological specimens that can establish the diagnosis of neoplastic changes (Tringali et al., 2017). These broad capabilities render ERCP an essential element in the diagnostic course of biliary tract disease, maximizing patient outcomes with targeted treatment protocols. While ERCP remains a cornerstone in the diagnosis and management of biliary tract disease, its success can be influenced by numerous variables, including the skill of the physician and the specific anatomical requirements of the patient. Complications, although rare, can arise with the procedure, such as pancreatitis, infection, or perforation, and need careful balancing of risk and benefit before attempting. The availability of advanced imaging modalities, such as magnetic resonance cholangiopancreatography (MRCP) and endoscopic ultrasonography (EUS), complements ERCP by providing diagnostic options through lesser invasiveness. These other modalities may also serve to provide further clarification of diagnosis in an inconclusive initial ultrasound or when ERCP is contraindicated due to patient problems (□□□□□□□ et al., 1391). A multidisciplinary approach that incorporates a variety of imaging modalities, therefore, provides comprehensive evaluation of biliary tract illnesses with the utmost patient management pathways and clinical results (Figure 7.5).

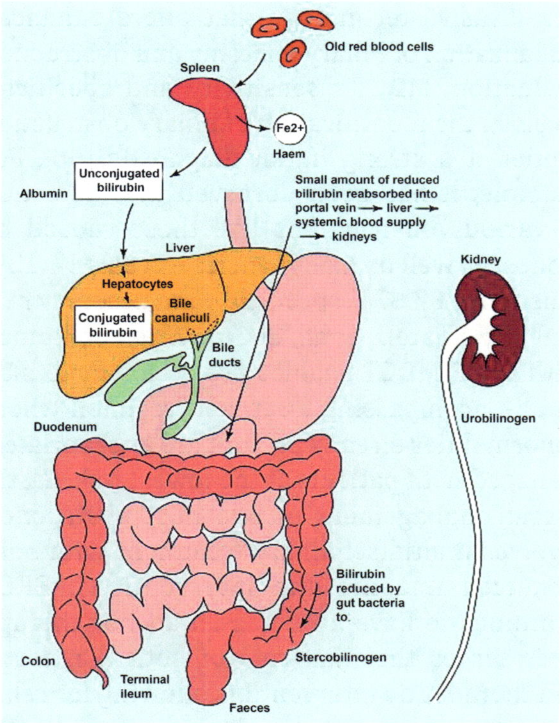

Figure 7.5. Biliary tract disorders.

Source: https://www.bmj.com/content/bmj/322/7277/33/F1.large.jpg?width=800&height=600.

7.1.2. Management of Pancreatic Diseases

The management of pancreatic diseases has seen drastic changes following the advent of endoscopic techniques , such as ERCP. The procedure is crucial for both diagnosing and treating pancreatic diseases , such as obstructive jaundice and pancreatitis. Effective management depends on awareness of complications associated with ERCP, notably post-endoscopic retrograde cholangiopancreatography pancreatitis (PEP). Preventive strategies for PEP risk include the use of prophylactic agents , such as rectal non-steroidal anti-inflammatory drugs (NSAIDs) and fluid regimens. The FLUYT trial highlights the significance of intravenous fluid therapy in patients who are already being given NSAIDs, meaning an integrated approach is able to reduce the incidence of severe PEP to improve patient outcome in treating pancreatic disease (Baak et al., 2018). Also not to be downplayed is the role of prophylactic antibiotics in ERCP, especially with the potential for complications following procedures , such as cholangitis and pancreatitis. Present guidelines from the main gastrointestinal societies advocate for antibiotic administration in the setting of obstructed biliary systems as a prophylactic measure. Efficacy of prophylactic antibiotics is substantiated by systematic review evidence that they can decrease bacteremia and cholangitis rates significantly following ERCP. However, the use of antibiotics must be individualized based on the patient's risk factors and procedure complexity (Brand, 2011). This quiet plan is aimed at balancing benefits with the risks of antibiotic resistance and making pancreatic disease management safe as well as effective. Pharmacological interventions are not the sole method of the management of ERCP-induced secondary pancreatic diseases; management of these diseases post-procedure is equally important in the overall treatment of diseases, however. Complication monitoring, symptom management, and imaging follow-up form major parts of post-ERCP management. Patients are assisted by education about signs that could indicate complications, such as fever or abdominal pain, so that they can report early to medical attention if necessary. A good aftercare program will provide for early intervention in the event of complications, therefore maximizing long-term prognosis. The intersection of endoscopic techniques with multidisciplinary care models points to the necessity of a collaborative approach in managing pancreatic diseases, ultimately for enabling patient-centered therapy and enhancing therapeutic intervention effectiveness related to ERCP (Figure 7.6).

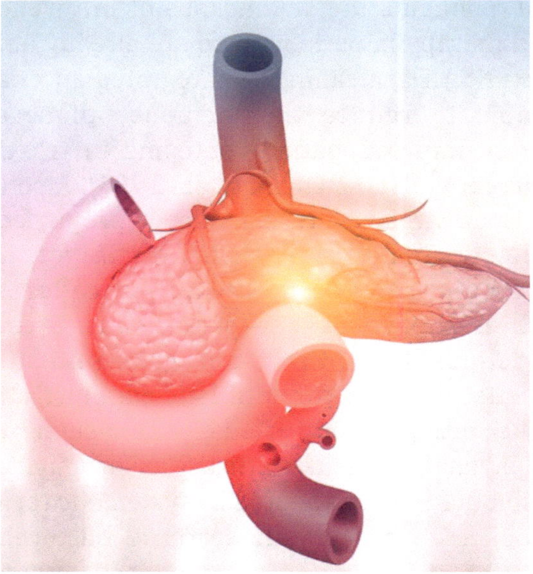

Figure 7.6. Pancreatic disease.

Source: https://www.uclahealth.org/sites/default/files/styles/portrait_3x4_024000_720x960/public/images/Pancreaticobiliary%20diseases%201200x1600.jpg?h=b69067a1&itok=PNFx5gX8.

7.1.3. Treatment of Bile Duct Obstructions

Treatment of bile duct obstruction typically involves a strategic plan with emphasis on both diagnosis and curative treatment. ERCP is today a critical procedure in the treatment of such disorders, both due to its diagnostic value as well as due to its scope of addressing underlying pathology. This is a minimally invasive technique that allows visualization of the bile ducts, along with the potential removal of the obstructions like stones, balloon dilatation, or stenting if required. With the rising incidence of bile duct stones and malignant illness, especially in the elderly, evaluation of the risks and benefits of ERCP is essential. There is current evidence that age alone should not be used as a contraindication for ERCP, especially if patients have an increased clinical need (Chang & Lei, 2007). Besides ERCP, other imaging modalities can be used in conjunction with bile duct obstruction assessment. Multidetector Computed Tomography (MDCT) is a useful non-invasive technology that offers enhanced visualization of biliary anatomy and obstruction evaluation. MDCT's sensitivity and specificity levels in the identification of biliary obstruction render it a strong initial diagnostic tool. For example, it has been observed that detection of various obstructions like those caused by stones, as well as malignancies, reveals 94.12% sensitivity, 87.87% specificity, and accuracy rate of 94.6% (Fatehi et al., 2016). When combined with ERCP, MDCT enables professionals to plan an all-encompassing treatment regimen where abnormalities already present are appropriately managed with patients at the lowest risk. Lastly, overall management of bile duct obstruction involves multidisciplinary treatment with both advanced imaging and interventions. ERCP continues to have a role as an anchor therapy as it serves the dual role of both diagnostic and therapeutic intervention, allowing for relief from obstructive symptomatology immediately, with the possibility of further assessment of malignancy in suspected cancer. The combination of MDCT as an auxiliary diagnostic agent allows for a more precise decision-making system, thereby reducing complications and enhancing patient outcomes. With the clinical community pushing these techniques forward and establishing their effectiveness in diverse populations, there is no question that age does not have to be the deciding factor in the choice of ERCP as a probable treatment method for bile duct obstructions (Chang & Lei, 2007) (Figure 7.7).

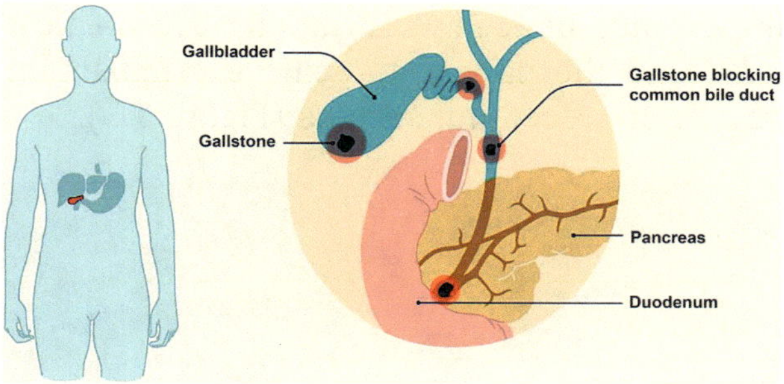

Figure 7.7. Bile duct obstruction.

Source: https://post.healthline.com/wp-content/uploads/2022/01/1827269-Biliary-Duct-Obstruction.png.

7.2. Procedure of Endoscopic Retrograde Cholangiopancreatography (ERCP)

The ERCP procedure is used to treat various biliary and pancreatic abnormalities. The patient receives sedation to be in a relaxed state during the procedure. An endoscope, a flexible catheter with a camera at the tip, is passed through the mouth and guided through the esophagus, stomach, and into the duodenum. This allows the physician to visualize the ampulla of Vater, where pancreatic and bile ducts drain into the intestine. The primary goal is cannulation of the bile duct to place contrast material, providing clarity on X-ray imaging. ERCP is particularly important in diagnosing disorders , such as choledocholithiasis, strictures, and pancreatitis-related disease and thus has a central role in therapeutic management (e.g., stone removal) (Tringali et al., 2017). During ERCP, meticulous attention to technique and equipment is important. After successful cannulation of the bile duct, a contrast agent is injected, and fluoroscopic images are obtained to assess ductal anatomy. These images not only reveal obstructions or abnormalities but also guide additional therapeutic interventions, such as sphincterotomy or balloon dilation. The procedure is all-embracing, uniting both diagnostic and interventional purposes, hence elevating its significance in treatment algorithms for conditions that require urgent intervention. As a reflection of the significance of the procedure, its use is linked to improvement in surgical practices. The spectrum of diseases treated with ERCP indicates its vital role in gastroenterology and emergency care (Tringali et al., 2017). Patient safety and procedure success are a priority during ERCP. Sedation alleviates discomfort, but the clinician must be attentive to potential complications , such as pancreatitis, infection, or perforation. Hence, a thorough pre-procedure evaluation is required to rule out any contraindications. Outcome and quality of procedure are a function of the experience and skill of the endoscopist, pointing to the requirement for training and continuous skill development in the field. Various resources, including clinical guidelines, recognize the importance of validating competence among endoscopists to optimize outcomes and minimize danger. With the development of ERCP, ongoing research and skill refinement are still the secrets to further advancing this basic diagnostic and therapeutic intervention for biliary and pancreatic disorders (Tringali et al., 2017).

7.2.1. Pre-Procedural Preparations

Effective pre-procedure preparations are required for risk mitigation and ERCP improvement. An extensive review of the patient's history and physical examination is critical to assess any underlying condition that may predispose an individual to complications. Nonetheless, pre-existing cardiac, pulmonary, or hematologic disease will significantly influence the risk profile both within and outside the procedure. Furthermore, the management of potential contraindications to anesthesia or sedation is important in a bid to ensure patient safety and comfort. Appropriate preparation not only serves to address risks but also assists clinicians in selecting an appropriate technique for biliary drainage. Such decisions to employ surgical or minimally invasive palliative therapies need to be made on a case-by-case basis, as nearly 80%–90% of malignant biliary obstruction is non-resectable and effective drainage methods are needed for symptom palliation (Hasan et al., 2001). Other pharmacologic interventions can be recommended to further reduce the frequency of complications related to ERCP. Pre-procedure measures , including intravenous fluid infusion or administration of certain medications , such as indomethacin can be a decisive factor to prevent post-ERCP pancreatitis, a known complication that arises in about 16% of patients (Abdullah et al., 2022). Administration of such drugs can help stabilize the functions of the pancreas and prevent ischemic damage to pancreatic tissue following the procedure. Moreover, educating the patient about the importance of adhering to pre-procedural dietary restrictions is also important. Patients typically are counseled to abstain from solid food intake for a few hours before the procedure so that the gastrointestinal tract can be well prepared, which is an important factor in optimizing the efficacy of the ERCP. Reassurance of the patient, appropriate education, and informed consent are also key components of pre-procedure preparation for ERCP. This phase provides an opportunity for the medical staff to explain the objectives, process of procedures, and potential complications of ERCP so that patients can possess informed expectations. Patient participation at the preparation phase is beneficial in facilitating trust and reducing anxiety that may otherwise complicate the procedure. Moreover, it is crucial to inform patients about post-procedure management and signs of complications, such as fever or abdominal distress, allowing for appropriate medical assessment if needed. Overall, a comprehensive pre-procedure plan makes ERCP more effective, emphasizing the importance of teamwork among the medical team and the patient to achieve a maximum degree of procedural success (Figure 7.8).

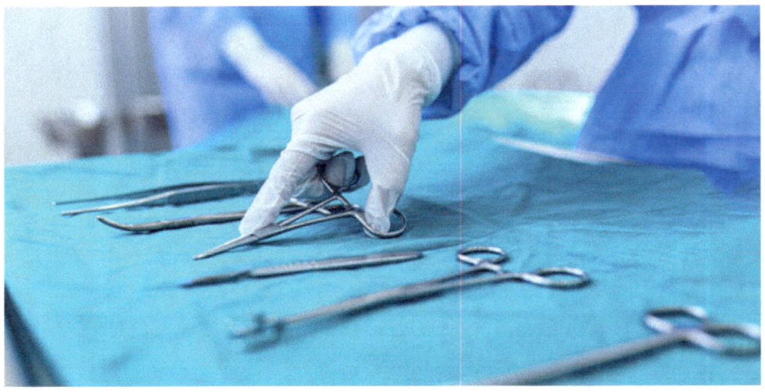

Figure 7.8. Pre-procedure preparation.

Source: https://aci.health.nsw.gov.au/__data/assets/image/0004/942673/Perioperative-Toolkit-digital-thumbnail.jpg.

7.2.2. Step-by-Step Process of the Procedure

The ERCP process is stepwise beginning from preparation of the patient, bringing the individual in the best state possible to undergo the procedure. Patient history is properly assessed before ERCP with focus on symptoms of jaundice or abdominal pain, which are the signs of choledocholithiasis. Patients can even be put through imaging studies like ultrasound or MRI to image the biliary system. In this initial phase, risk factors for the development of complications , such as a history of pancreatitis or coagulopathy, are addressed, making decision-making about the procedure easier. Balancing the possible benefit of ERCP in the removal of stones from bile ducts against the potential risk of complications, such as pancreatitis, in the appropriate ratio of harm and benefit is vital to ensure patient safety and technical success, as reported in predictive factors and pitfalls in the diagnosis of choledocholithiasis (Magalhães et al., 2015). The ERCP procedure starts after patient preparation with the induction of sedation. This is followed by the placement of the endoscope, which is a flexible tube that contains a camera, slowly into one of the patient's mouths, through the esophagus and into the duodenum. At the duodenum, the ampulla of Vater, where the bile duct opens up, is found. A cannula is then threaded through the endoscope into the ampulla so that contrast dye can be injected into the biliary tree. This decisive step enables fluoroscopic imaging, and hence it can visualize the bile ducts and identify any blockages, stones, or abnormalities. In case of detection of stones, the next step is to take endoscopic sphincterotomy, which enlarges the sphincter of Oddi to allow the effective removal of stones, as noted in studies that examine intraoperative modalities in addition to laparoscopic procedures (Magalhães et al., 2015). Following successful intervention and visualization, the second step is then the removal of stones using specialized equipment, such as balloons or retrieval baskets. Once the stones are out, the procedural team assesses for the presence of residual stones with additional fluoroscopic images. If necessary, balloon dilation of the biliary duct can be done to enable further manipulation and clearance. After the intervention, the endoscope is withdrawn, and the patient is monitored for early post-procedure complications , such as bleeding or perforation. The effectiveness of ERCP for the treatment of choledocholithiasis is typically measured in relation to the success rates of stone removal and the incidence of post-procedure complications and emphasizes the importance of maintaining strict operating procedures for better patient outcomes and minimizing concomitant risks (El-Bahrawy et al., 2009).

7.2.3. Post-Procedural Care and Monitoring

Monitoring and post-procedure care following ERCP are important aspects to ensuring patient safety and optimizing results. Since ERCP is an advanced technique used for diagnosing and treating pancreatic and biliary illness, special care must be taken during the recovery phase of the patients. Monitoring of vital signs, fluid status, and patient condition on a close basis is essential during the early recovery period. Post-anesthesia care should include monitoring for complications , such as bleeding, infection, or pancreatitis, which, though rare, require prompt treatment. Post-endoscopic retrograde cholangiopancreatography pancreatitis (PEP) has also been cited as the most common complication of ERCP. Supportive care and proper hydration may minimize this risk, emphasizing the need for a vigilant monitoring regime to address any emerging complications effectively (Chang & Lei, 2007). In addition to regular monitoring, clinicians must remain watchful for particular ERCP complications. In accordance with existing literature, the therapeutic efficacy of ERCP within geriatric cohorts suggests that the procedure is as safe for patients aged over 65 as it is for younger patients (Chang & Lei, 2007). Post-procedure care needs to be tailored to these at-risk patients, with ongoing monitoring to easily identify complications. For instance, comorbid patients, including respiratory or cardiovascular ones, may need extended monitoring to timely counterbalance expected complications. Furthermore, it is very important to have an established line of treatment for the management of adverse effects. Standardized rules on how to timely intervene should be available to medical staff, emphasizing the importance of cooperation and communication between carers in the post-procedure setting. Aside from reinforcing recovery, education on post-procedure self-care is also an essential element of post-ERCP monitoring. Patients and their families must be instructed on signs and symptoms of potential complications, such as abdominal pain, fever, or jaundice, and should be instructed when to report to the emergency department for treatment. Additionally, hydration recommendations, particularly for patients who are at moderate to high risk of PEP, should be clearly articulated and incorporated in discharge instructions. Recent studies, such as the FLUYT trial, point to a vital role for both hydration and prophylactic regimens like rectal NSAIDs in avoiding harmful consequences (Baak et al., 2018). Ultimately, a coordinated post-procedural care plan that combines meticulous clinical surveillance with patient education forms the basis of both safety and efficacy during the post-ERCP recovery process (Figure 7.9).

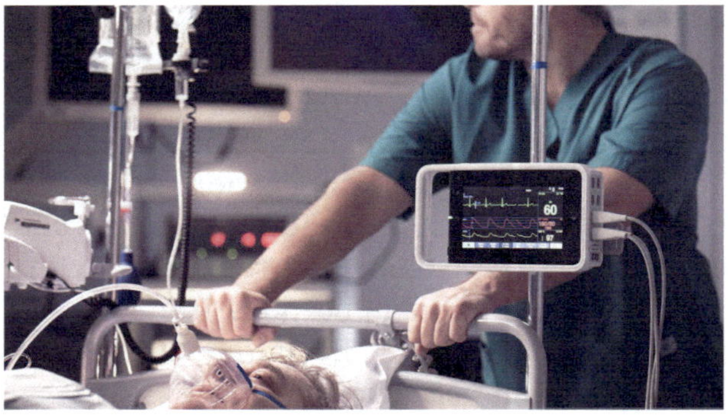

Figure 7.9. Patient monitoring.

Source: https://www.gehealthcare.in/-/jssmedia/carescape-one-landing-callout.jpg?h=1080&iar=0&w=1920&rev=-1&hash=D3F946EF4D29FE6C2256D6C2449B744C.

7.3. Risks and Complications

The ERCP procedure is significant in the diagnosis and treatment of bile duct and pancreatic disease. However, it is not free of risks and complications, which may be mild or severe. Pancreatitis is a frequent complication that occurs in approximately 3%–5% of procedures and is characterized by abdominal pain and elevated pancreatic enzymes. Other possible complications include infections, especially cholangitis, as well as perforations of the gastrointestinal tract that can prove to be life-threatening. Occurrence of these complications requires patient selection, informed consent, and adherence to strict protocols to reduce risk during the procedure (Azab et al., 2019). The above complications must be recognized by both patients and healthcare workers to enhance the advantages of ERCP over the disadvantages thereof (Azab et al., 2019). In addition, certain demographic factors , such as age and comorbidities, may influence ERCP complication risk. Older patients or patients with comorbid illnesses , such as heart disease and diabetes, may have increased complication rates, which makes each patient increasingly individualized in their requirements. For example, studies indicate that patients presenting with acute illness , such as ascending cholangitis or biliary obstruction, can pose a greater risk during the procedure. In assessing these risks, potential predictors of choledocholithiasis, including measurements of total bilirubin levels and liver function test derangement, must be clinically assessed. Subsequent patient stratification into risk groups can then allow for more accurate pre-procedure planning and mitigate adverse outcomes after ERCP, as evidenced by contemporary literature (Magalhães et al., 2015). Finally, despite the associated risks, ERCP remains a particularly effective intervention for various cholangiopancreatic disorders. Continuing technological developments of endoscopic devices and techniques are all aimed at reducing the occurrence of complications. Techniques , such as applications of radiation-free ERCP substitutes also promise to enhance patient safety further, especially in high-risk populations , such as pregnant women, where the use of radiation would lead to fetal complications. Continuing training in endoscopists and following best evidence-based practice can have a significant impact on outcomes. As the medical community comes to appreciate better the risks entailed, the aim remains optimal patient care with the preservation of the effectiveness of this precious diagnostic and therapeutic tool in the management of biliary illness.

7.3.1. Common Complications Associated with Endoscopic Retrograde Cholangiopancreatography (ERCP)

ERCP is a widely utilized investigative and therapeutic intervention in the diagnosis and management of bile duct and pancreatic diseases. However, it is not without complications, and complications may arise during surgery or in the early postoperative phase. Complications like pancreatitis, infections, and perforation are common. Pancreatitis is particularly worrying and is seen in approximately 3%–5% of patients. This is a complication that presents as abdominal pain and may require hospitalization, thus contributing to healthcare costs and patient morbidity. Infections , such as cholangitis also result from manipulation of the bile duct, particularly in patients who have pre-existing biliary obstruction. Understanding of such risks is crucial for practitioners to be able to control and avert potential complications effectively. Aside from the usual complications mentioned, bleeding is also a serious risk in ERCP, especially in patients with coagulopathy or anticoagulant therapy. This complication is precipitated by trauma to the blood vessels with sphincterotomy or cannulation, leading to hematoma or GI bleeding. While the incidence of bleeding is not very significant, the severity of potential hemorrhage warrants vigilance during the procedure. As an added measure, infection after ERCP, especially cholangitis, may be caused due to contamination of the bile duct with bacteria. This emphasizes the requirement for strict aseptic techniques and also antibiotic prophylaxis in high-risk cases. Therefore, efficiency of the operating teams as well as adherence to provided guidelines are critical in the prevention of the rate of complication occurrence. The current literature suggests other diagnostic modalities , such as EUS or MRCP, may potentially decrease the risk of complications of ERCP. By employing these procedures initially, doctors can diagnose diseases like common bile duct (CBD) stones correctly, thereby decreasing the number of unnecessary ERCP procedures. As stated, employing such non-invasive techniques can prevent potential intraoperative complications and decrease patient burden overall. Moreover, assessment of appropriateness of ERCP through thorough imaging studies before the procedure can optimize patient safety and enhance efficient use of healthcare resources (Azab et al., 2019). Lastly, competency in terms of complications of ERCP and evaluating alternative approaches is important to achieve optimal patient outcomes and enhance overall effectiveness of biliary interventions (Morris et al., 2015) (Figure 7.10).

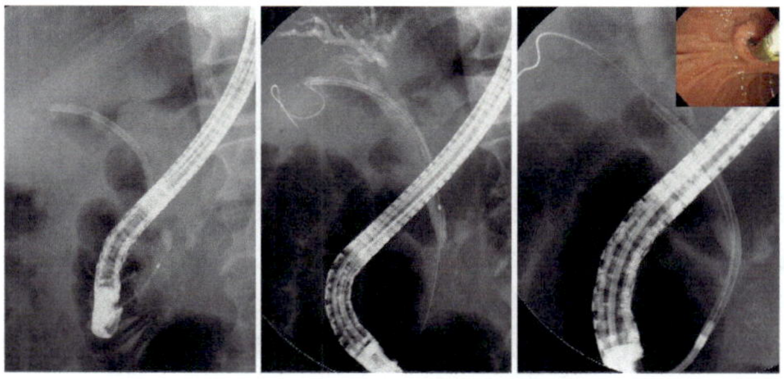

Figure 7.10. Prevention and management of endoscopic retrograde cholangiopancreatography (ERCP)-related complications.

Source: https://oaepublishstorage.blob.core.windows.net/84ea76b5-591a-42b1-b2c8-8193a6c9c7ae/4120.fig.5.jpg.

7.3.2. Risk Factors That Increase Complications

Risk assessment of the risk factors for complications during ERCP is necessary to improve patient outcomes. Patient-specific parameters are particularly important in the risk of adverse events, according to several studies. For instance, demographics like age and comorbid conditions have the potential to predispose patients to post-ERCP complications. As identified by systematic reviews, younger patients are less likely to have complications, whereas older patients or those with comorbidities , such as liver disease, constitute a higher risk category. Furthermore, complicated anatomy is a possibility due to a history of prior surgical procedures. The interplay of the factors requires a detailed pre-procedure workup so that the plan can be tailored and surgeons possess the necessary information for risk management. Apart from patient characteristics, procedural factors also have a significant impact on ERCP safety and effectiveness. Endoscopist experience and skill have a substantial effect on outcomes; proficient operators tend to have higher success rates and fewer complications. In addition, selection of technique—most notably, whether or not to use radiation—is important in terms of both short- and long-term patient safety. Data are provided that procedural non-radiation techniques may decrease the likelihood of certain complications, especially in vulnerable populations , such as pregnant women, as reported from systematic reviews of patient outcomes with ERCP. Appreciation of such procedural nuances is valuable because they may inform guidelines for optimal practice in ERCP and ultimately advance patient safety. Certain clinical presentations could identify increased risks with ERCP. Bile duct stones, associated pancreatitis, or jaundice make the procedure more complex and are contributors to higher complication rates. For example, evidence suggests that several predictive factors occurring together are strongly related to bile duct involvement and would therefore necessitate the detection of these conditions through early preoperative evaluation. According to evidence, patients with three and above risk factors are at high risk and require individualized management strategies to reverse potential complications. Low-risk patients with few predictive factors may be monitored and treated less intensively. This risk stratification is crucial to necessitate complete pre-procedure evaluation to guide ERCP decision-making to adequately adjust the level of care to each patient's unique risk profile (Lakatos et al., 2004; Azab et al., 2019).

7.3.3. Strategies for Minimizing Risks

Good minimization strategies for risks in ERCP are necessary to secure patient safety and optimal outcomes. One of the key techniques is judicious pre-procedure assessments, including a detailed examination of the patients' medical history, medication regimen, and underlying comorbidities. By identifying potential risk factors, healthcare practitioners can adjust their interventions appropriately, for example, pre-procedure imaging studies to accurately define the anatomy of the biliary tree. Pre-emptive detection of risks improves patient safety by preventing complications during the procedure. Further, these assessments may lead to more knowing consent processes, aligning the patient's expectations with procedural realities. A second important strategy includes the incorporation of advanced technology and techniques for optimizing procedural outcomes and their attendant risks. The application of fluoroscopy for ERCP, for instance, allows real-time imaging of the pancreatic and biliary ducts, thus enhancing the likelihood of successful cannulation and diagnosis. While this improves the chances of successful cannulation and diagnosis, it concurrently increases the risk of radiation exposure. Consensus practice based on the safe usage of fluoroscopy, as offered in current studies, focuses on the adoption of educational interventions and guidelines to minimize radiation exposure to patients and health workers (Aberin et al., 2024). In addition to such education interventions, protection devices, such as lead aprons and shielding from radiation, also reflect the dedication to safety while maintaining the procedural advantages of fluoroscopy. With regards to managing complications, having a sound plan for monitoring post-procedure is important. Proper monitoring of patients for signs of adverse effects, including pancreatitis and infection, will significantly influence recovery and long-term patient outcome. It has been found that preoperative biliary drainage may help minimize complications in obstructive jaundice patients before surgery being conducted, but as an across-the-board solution, its efficacy has come into question (van der Gaag et al., 2007). By adopting a very individualized post-procedural care plan depending on patient-specific risk factors and procedural complexity, practitioners can maximize recovery protocols. Hence, an integrated consideration of pre-, intra-, and post-procedural measures is crucial in preventing risks associated with ERCP, ultimately leading to improved patient safety and satisfaction (Figure 7.11).

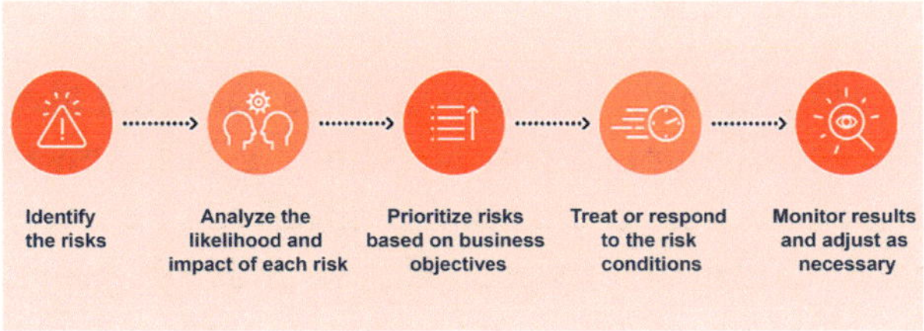

Figure 7.11. Risk management: How to minimize risk and secure success.

Source: https://learn.g2.com/hs-fs/hubfs/G2CM_FI146_Learn_Article_Images-[Risk_management]_Infographic_Image1_V2b.png?width=690.

7.4. Diagnostic Applications

Diagnostic applications of ERCP play a crucial role in the diagnosis and treatment of biliary tract disease. Through imaging of the biliary tree and pancreatic ducts, ERCP is most appropriately able to identify obstructions, strictures, or lesions that will disrupt bile flow. Most often, initial imaging tests , such as ultrasound or MDCT are employed to provide preliminary data regarding the status of the biliary tree. Nevertheless, ERCP offers more accuracy and allows therapeutic maneuvers simultaneously, such as stone removal or stenting. The value of ERCP is also compounded in cases where non-invasive imaging modalities yield equivocal results, necessitating further questioning to confirm diagnoses. The technical success of ERCP, thus, significantly optimizes clinicians' ability to devise appropriate treatment interventions for patients with presenting symptoms related to the biliary system. Ultrasound has always been the initial diagnostic test in the evaluation of biliary tract disease, often determining further application of more invasive techniques like ERCP. As has been noted in recent publications, ultrasound is specifically sensitive for the detection of gallstones, with as much as 100% sensitivity in this particular use case. Its ability to localize lesions or obstructions before ERCP not only assists in laying the groundwork for management of the patient but also facilitates stratification of the patients based on their risk factors and underlying disease complexity. For instance, studies have indicated that the sensitivity of ultrasound compared to ERCP is approximately 92.5%, which demonstrates that precise sonographic examinations have a substantial role to play in the diagnosis process, leading to effective interventions and improved outcomes for patients., 1391). This indicates the plurality of methods involved in modern diagnostic medicine. Also, the improvements in imaging modalities , such as MDCT, have increased the armamentarium of biliary obstruction diagnoses as a main supporting modality to ERCP. Research indicates that MDCT has high specificity and sensitivity in the diagnosis of causes of biliary obstruction with percentages of 94.12% and 87.87%, respectively (Fatehi et al., 2016). The high-resolution imaging provides precise anatomical information about gallstones, strictures, or malignancies of the biliary tree, directing the need for potential early interventions. This places MDCT not only as an option but as an imperative complement to ERCP, particularly in those cases necessitating precise localization and characterization of lesions. The addition of MDCT to the diagnostic process supports the general understanding of biliary pathophysiology, ultimately leading to improved diagnostic accuracy and therapeutic intervention in the clinical setting.

7.4.1. Use of Endoscopic Retrograde Cholangiopancreatography (ERCP) in Diagnosing Cholangitis

ERCP is a key diagnostic and therapeutic intervention in the treatment of cholangitis, an infection of the bile ducts that can be fatal. The technique is particularly valuable in patients with obstructive jaundice, where imaging work-up may suggest the presence of choledocholithiasis or stricture. ERCP allows direct visualization of bile ducts, and physicians are able to visualize the source of cholangitis, such as bile duct stones or neoplastic obstruction. By avoiding these obstacles, ERCP not only makes diagnosis possible but also immediate therapeutic intervention, as it is critical in view of the potential for serious infection and systemic sequelae if untreated. Thus, ERCP has become a first-line technique in clinical practice for the successful diagnosis and treatment of cholangitis. The use of prophylactic antibiotics in ERCP is a topic of special interest, particularly its applicability in the prevention of cholangitis. Gastroenterological centers highly recommend pre-procedure administration of prophylactic antibiotics, particularly in cases of suspected obstructed biliary tree. This is to prevent post-ERCP complications , such as cholangitis and sepsis, thus promoting patient safety during and after the procedure. Current meta-analyses show that prophylactic antibiotic usage would be of great benefit in the prevention of post-procedure cholangitis, with decreases in risk of bacteremia and other biliary obstruction treatment-related infections being reported by studies (Brand, 2011). While it is certain that there are beneficial antibiotics for high-risk patients, more work needs to be done to define their need in uncomplicated cases where successful ERCP is likely to unblock biliary obstruction.

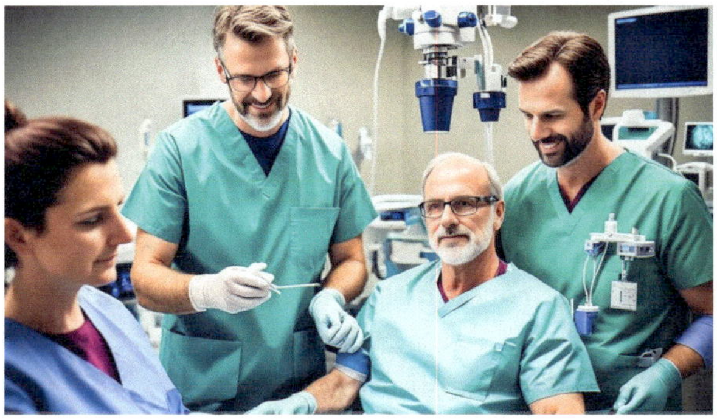

Figure 7.12. Understanding cholangitis.

Source: https://drgooddeed.com/wp-content/uploads/2024/03/Cholangitis-treatment-1024x585.jpg.

Additionally, the effectiveness of ERCP also does not respect the age limit since newer evidence offers the truth that ERCP can be safely conducted in elderly groups even above 90 years. Since biliary disease increases in older groups, the role of ERCP in both diagnosis and cure of cholangitis becomes more important. Studies demonstrate that outcomes in terms of success rate and complications of ERCP for older groups are comparable to outcomes for younger groups, thereby validating that age should not serve as a contraindication for this valuable diagnostic device (Chang & Lei, 2007). With growing confidence in ERCP's safety profile across broad ages, the role must also expand towards individualized pre-procedure assessment and management strategies, especially in cholangitis, where early diagnosis is important in ensuring optimal outcomes among patients (Figure 7.12).

7.4.2. Role of Endoscopic Retrograde Cholangiopancreatography (ERCP) in Identifying Pancreatic Tumors

The role of ERCP in the diagnosis of pancreatic tumors is pivotal, in that it is both diagnostic and therapeutic in function. ERCP is a minimally invasive method of directly visualizing the pancreatic duct and biliary tree, and it offers essential information regarding obstructive pathology. In symptomatic individuals presumed to have pancreatic cancers, such as jaundice or abdominal pain, ERCP is capable of yielding significant results that will chart the course of future management. For instance, cholangiographic images obtained during the procedure may reveal bile duct obstruction by a tumor and enable early treatment and potentially improved patient care. With the increased incidence of pancreatic tumors, the utility of ERCP in ensuring the early diagnosis is still fundamental in enhancing the overall outcome of infected patients. Furthermore, the sensitivity and specificity of ERCP for detecting pancreatic tumors have been highlighted in various studies comparing its effectiveness with other imaging systems. Ultrasound, while commonly employed as a first-line imaging procedure, has been found to be inexact in the determination of the tumor etiology of biliary dilatation, particularly when lesions are intrapancreatic. Research shows that the sensitivity of ultrasound for the detection of such tumors is much lower than with ERCP, and extensive evidence is available to determine that ERCP accurately identifies tumor presence in the majority of cases. Specifically, the incidence of tumors within intrapancreatic ducts was reported at 81.8%, which emphasized ERCP's higher value in diagnosis in such a case. The results show the pivotal function of ERCP in not only being capable of proving the presence of a pancreatic tumor but also in determining the therapeutic option based on the localization and severity of the disease. Even as ERCP has been used to be a very valuable tool in diagnosing pancreatic tumors, the accompanying risks of the procedure must not be downplayed. Side effects, while infrequent, are possible and include perforation or bleeding, which require an understanding of potential results in clinical practice. The frequency of such side effects highlights the importance of operator expertise and experience with immediate treatment. With progressive development in therapeutic modalities and endoscopic technology, an appreciation of the balance between the diagnostic utility of ERCP and complications accrued is vital to clinical practice. In this context, effective application of ERCP for pancreatic tumor detection requires technical proficiency along with an overall strategy for dealing with complications to ensure the optimum provision of care to patients throughout their diagnosis (Figure 7.13).

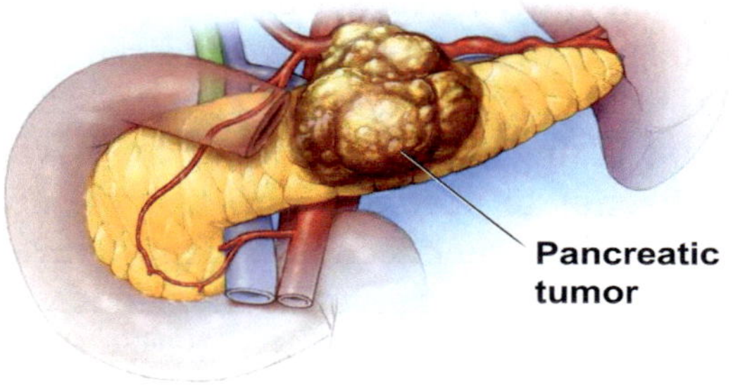

Figure 7.13. Pancreatic cancer.

Source: https://newsnetwork.mayoclinic.org/n7-mcnn/7bcc9724adf7b803/uploads/2016/12/Pancreatic-Cancer-Tumor-Pancreas.jpg.

7.4.3. Evaluation of Biliary Stones Through Endoscopic Retrograde Cholangiopancreatography (ERCP)

The evaluation of biliary stones with ERCP is a cornerstone tool in the diagnosis of suspected CBD stones. Utilizing ERCP not only allows clinicians to visualize but also to effectively treat obstructions caused by these stones. It needs to be understood that even though ERCP has come under wide praise for its therapeutic value, it is also an invasive technique with potential complications. Indeed, the intrinsic risks raise a critical debate on the need for pre-procedure diagnostic workups to minimize unnecessary ERCP procedures. The application of imaging studies , such as EUS or MRCP, can enhance patient safety with the detection of the existence of CBD stones before ERCP, hence reducing complications and conserving healthcare resources, as exemplified in Morris et al. (2015). Furthermore, the success of ERCP can be contrasted with the diagnostic function of ultrasound in detecting biliary disease. Being the initial imaging modality, ultrasound is usually utilized due to its availability and lack of invasiveness. A retrospective study of 53 patients confirmed that ultrasound has high sensitivity with a 100% detection rate for stones and 83.3% for tumors and thereby ensuring its utility in identifying causes of bile duct dilation. Specifically, the correct diagnosis of biliary stones through ultrasound had a 92.5% accuracy level, stressing that initial imaging is viable as a diagnostic device within the diagnostic process before the injection of a more invasive technique like ERCP. This evaluation underscores the necessity for planned diagnostics that are systematic in nature, one that best unites various imaging technologies in a manner that provides better patient outcomes. With the imminent function of ERCP in evaluating biliary stones, there is a harmonious equilibrium regarding how it influences clinical practice. ERCP provides a complete picture and allows intervention, but its emphasis on initial evaluation is needed to minimize procedure burden for patients. Inclusion of ultrasound and MRCP into the armamentarium of diagnostic equipment not only minimizes the dangers of ERCP but also guarantees immediate and perfect treatment of biliary illness. Hence, simplification of the evaluation strategy for biliary stones could have a bearing on improved compliance with best practice in gastroenterology. The simultaneous application of non-invasive imaging modalities with ERCP ultimately leads to better overall management of the patient, as exemplified by the established efficacy in diagnosing biliary tract illnesses (Morris et al., 2015) and (یئاربت et al., 1391).

7.5. Therapeutic Applications

Therapeutic applications of ERCP are important in the management of various illnesses of the biliary and pancreas. ERCP is both therapeutic and diagnostic, hence its supreme role in gastroenterology. Its key advantage is in the diagnosis of obstructions caused by gallstones, tumors, or strictures. After biliary dilatation has been confirmed by imaging studies, ERCP enables physicians to perform interventions that open up these obstructions. With stone removal or stent insertion, ERCP can alleviate symptoms of jaundice and abdominal pain and normalize bile flow. Thus, this endoscopic intervention not only provides information on the underlying pathology but also permits immediate therapeutic maneuvers that can profoundly affect patient outcomes.

Apart from its role in treating obstructive pathology, ERCP has applications in the therapy of pancreatic disease, particularly in the management of complications of pancreatitis. For instance, it has a significant role in the management of pancreatic duct disruptions and strictures that result from complications of chronic pancreatitis. Visualization and destruction of pancreatic duct obstructions may eradicate recurrent episodes of acute pancreatitis and chronic pain. Standards have also come to include ERCP in the standard care of acute biliary pancreatitis, where early decompression will reduce the likelihood of further complications. Laws on the use of ERCP for such medical conditions highlight its therapeutic importance, especially in pediatric patients, as seen in disputes over management strategies outlined in Tringali et al. (2017). In addition, the dynamic growth of therapeutic ERCP has driven it toward broadening applications to other interventional techniques, including the treatment of tumors of the bile duct. According to the results presented by ذکاوت et al. (1391), ERCP can also be utilized to insert biliary stents that decompress obstructions caused by malignant tumors and enhance the quality of life for individuals with advanced diagnoses. The process enables clinicians to manage symptoms , such as cholangitis and pruritus. Technological and endoscopic progress over the last few decades has fostered a broader understanding of ERCP's role, making it a standard part of multidisciplinary therapy for gastrointestinal disorders. ERCP's therapeutic role therefore, highlights its cardinal function in modern medical practice through the provision of timely intervention based on best practice in patient care.

7.5.1. Endoscopic Removal of Bile Duct Stones

Endoscopic bile duct stone extraction is a mainstay of the therapeutic armamentarium following ERCP. The minimally invasive procedure is such that stones are extracted from the CBD, with direct vision and intervention made possible through an endoscope. In choledocholithiasis, or stones that migrate into the CBD, immediate intervention is typically necessary to prevent complications , such as cholangitis or pancreatitis. The duodenum is entered with the endoscope, and cannulation of the CBD and even retrograde contrast injection to screen for stones can be done during the procedure. Efficient retrieval also greatly alleviates obstructive symptoms, from jaundice to severe abdominal pain, so ERCP becomes a prime method of treatment in treating such cases. Together, the extraction of bile duct stones by ERCP not only addresses present clinical concerns but also reduces the risk of long-term complications. A study comparing the long-term outcomes of patients with laparoscopic techniques, along with ERCP, indicated low recurrence of ductal stones, demonstrating the success of endoscopic intervention. The results demonstrate the significance of proper technique and follow-up, as evidenced by the low 2.1% recurrence in a group followed for over 17 years. Moreover, the combination of endoscopic sphincterotomy and stone extraction has been said to produce satisfactory results, with no serious instances of CBD stricture, thus enhancing the overall picture of the procedure in the management of biliary stones (Quaresima et al., 2016).

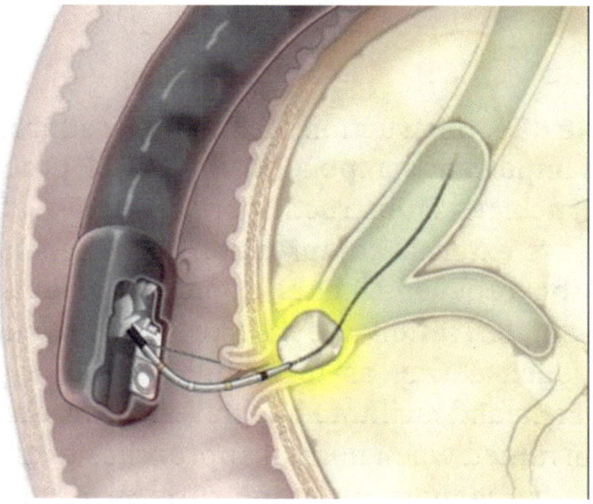

Figure 7.14. Bile duct stone removal.

Source: https://external-content.duckduckgo.com/iu/?u=https%3A %2F%2Ftse1.mm.bing.net%2Fth%2Fid%2FOIP.w YJHWJmTSWPCpVrNThUym AHaFj%3F pid%3 DApi&f=1&ipt=66 9 1a1c6685b d66d8f163af3281b01a79267 09318aa152ba56765e7c2c561c20.

Emergency ERCP is particularly warranted in patients presenting with severe acute cholangitis, where rapid intervention is crucial to prevent deterioration of the clinical condition. Presentation of choledocholithiasis in such cases mandates urgent endoscopic drainage in the form of biliary stenting or stone removal. In a population of patients with severe presentation of cholangitis, forceful ERCP not only alleviated obstructive biliary disease but also proved its efficacy to improve overall rates of survival without the complications of acute pancreatitis. Successful treatment of the patients, with up to 73.7% undergoing biliary drainage procedures, highlights the critical role of ERCP in acute care where timely intervention can have a fundamental impact on patient outcomes (Abdurachman et al., 2010). Generally, endoscopic stone extraction of bile duct stones is a crucial intervention that highlights ERCP's value in treating acute and chronic biliary disease (Figure 7.14).

7.5.2. Stenting Procedures for Bile Duct Obstructions

Bile duct obstruction stenting procedures form an important component of the ERCP procedure, particularly if obstruction of obstructive jaundice due to external compression or malignancies is to be relieved. Stents, typically of plastic or metal derivation, are inserted into the bile duct in such a way as to maintain it as a patent system and facilitate bile flow. This treatment is warranted when normal approaches to drainage are inadequate or other surgical options are limited by the conditions of the patients or tumor invasion. Stenting is highly effective in significantly enhancing the quality of life in patients with biliary obstructions because it relieves symptoms due to jaundice and cholestasis and allows for the administration of concurrent therapies, i.e., chemotherapy in cancer. The success of the stenting procedure is exemplified by its ability to provide a therapeutic result for cholestasis and related symptoms, thereby leading to better patient outcomes. Research indicates that successful cannulation and stenting can record high symptomatic relief rates, but without overlooking the risk of complications. In this regard, post-ERCP complications , such as pancreatitis and cholangitis, are to be monitored closely because they may impair the overall efficacy of the stenting procedure. In a retrospective study of a patient cohort undergoing stenting for malignancy, there was a notable subgroup of patients who experienced post-procedure complications, highlighting the requirement for expertise and patient selection in conducting the procedures (Baruah et al., 2020).

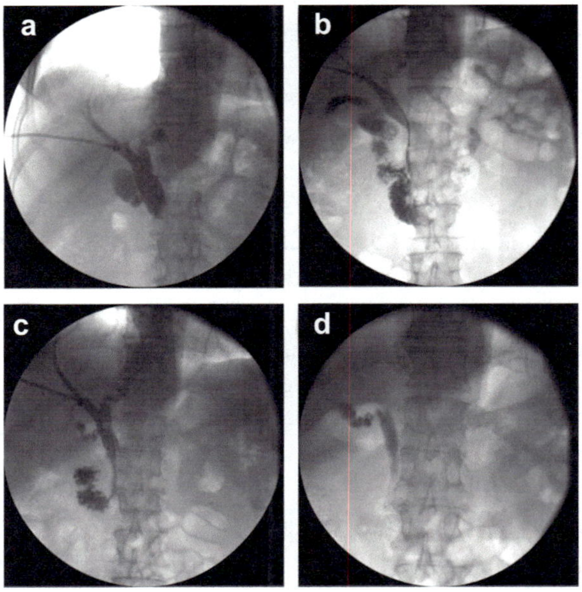

Figure 7.15. Stent placement in a patient with common bile duct obstruction.

Source: https://www.researchgate.net/publication/244948219/figure/fig1/AS:364163357528065@1463834718792/Stent-placement-in-a-patient-with-common-bile-duct-obstruction-with-pancreatic-cancer.png.

The understanding of the risk-benefit balance is therefore important to those operators undertaking ERCP and bile duct stenting. In addition to enhanced patient outcomes, adjunctive use with stenting interventions can also reduce post-procedure complications, such as cholangitis. A study comparing the application of gentamicin blended with contrast media as an adjuvant versus ERCP to determine its influence on cholangitis rates reported that successful drainage with stenting was important, though antibiotic adjuvants were not highly effective in reducing cholangitis cases in their population (Norouzi et al., 2013). This appreciation is valuable since it suggests that the main focus should remain primarily on successful stent deployment and drainage rather than solely on fine-tuning the procedural aids. Through an increasing body of literature, the combination of optimal stenting approaches with complete post-procedure care will likely remain at the center of optimizing ERCP results in patients with bile duct obstruction (Figure 7.15).

7.5.3. Management of Strictures in the Biliary System

The therapeutic approach to strictures of the biliary system is a significant part of therapeutic management made possible through ERCP. Strictures can result due to diverse reasons like chronic inflammation, scarring from prior surgery, or malignancies causing obstruction of the bile ducts. Early identification and therapy of such strictures are important because untreated lesions can lead to cholangitis, biliary cirrhosis, and hepatic failure. The success of ERCP in the therapy of biliary strictures lies in the fact that it is a less invasive procedure and can be combined with sphincterotomy, balloon dilation, and stenting as a single procedure. These procedures enable unblocking and restoration of bile flow, leading to relief from symptoms as well as improved quality of life in patients with the condition. In addition, effective ERCP treatment of biliary strictures has been described in a number of clinical trials, which declare that the result can be greatly determined by the etiology of the stricture. For instance, in strictures resulting from chronic pancreatitis or post-surgical fibrosis, ERCP techniques , such as endoscopic balloon dilation and stenting are beneficial. Advanced imaging techniques coupled with ERCP, such as endoscopic ultrasonography, also play a vital part in proper assessment of the stricture and planning for therapy. However, there are cases when ERCP won't resolve the blockage and other approaches like percutaneous intervention or surgery become inevitable, thereby demonstrating the need for interdisciplinary participation in treating biliary complications (Chen et al., 2009). The application of ERCP has also been maximized with advancements in modern techniques and adjunctive treatments aimed at maximizing the outcomes for patients with biliary strictures. For instance, stent placement with biodegradable stents has emerged as a viable technique to prevent the complications associated with traditional stenting techniques , such as long-term stent maintenance and stent-related infections. The process of patient selection also cannot be overemphasized as a way of maximizing the ERCP outcome, particularly in recurrent or complex strictures. Individualized intervention plans according to specific patient parameters, such as age and overall state of health, can maximize the efficacy of intervention procedures. Specifically, studies indicate that ERCP can lead to successful outcomes in about 60%–90% of patients and, therefore, be a first-line approach to biliary strictures management (Tringali et al., 2017). Thus, continued investigation into new therapies and methods is required for maximizing the treatment of biliary strictures and improving patient prognosis.

7.6. Advances in Endoscopic Retrograde Cholangiopancreatography (ERCP) Technology

Technological development in ERCP has significantly enhanced its application in the diagnosis and management of biliary and pancreatic disease. Old-fashioned ERCP techniques were based on fluoroscopic imaging, good as it is, but risky in the form of radiation exposure and difficulty in visualizing intricate anatomy. More recent advances have introduced high-definition endoscopes and improved imaging technology , such as narrow-band imaging and digital enhancement, for superior, more precise visualization of the bile and pancreatic ductal systems. These developments enable better detection of strictures, stones, and lesions, which ultimately lead to better diagnoses. Additionally, artificial intelligence integrated into image analysis potentially enhances diagnostic correctness and can further render ERCP an even more reliable procedure in the practice of gastroenterology (Raza et al., 2025). Yet another significant development in ERCP is the development of sophisticated accessory devices aimed at securing the safety and effectiveness of the procedure. New balloon dilation techniques and the use of fully covered metal stents have improved therapy of advanced biliary strictures and obstructions. Apart from further widening the scope of relief of obstructions, these devices reduce the rate of complications associated with standard procedures. Moreover, the integration of EUS with ERCP has emerged as an efficacious diagnostic tool that provides real-time imaging and assessment of pancreatic and biliary pathology. EUS gives higher tissue sampling, which is crucial in the differentiation of benign from malignant strictures and better management of patients (N/A, 2022). The above is a case of how integration of different endoscopic skills can optimize treatment outcome. In addition, patient safety is always the utmost concern in ERCP technology development. Advances , such as the development of spasmolytic drugs to minimize pain and the implementation of sedation protocols with decreased adverse events are welcome advances in this field. These advancements lead to a general improvement in patient experience as well as outcomes in ERCP. Continuing education and procedural skill on ever-more advanced technology for gastroenterologists also contribute significantly to higher procedural success rates. As these technologies further develop, the study of long-term impact on patient outcomes and healthcare costs will be essential, providing an avenue for next-generation innovations for ensuring the highest quality of care in endoscopic retrograde cholangiopancreatography (Raza et al., 2025) (Figure 7.16).

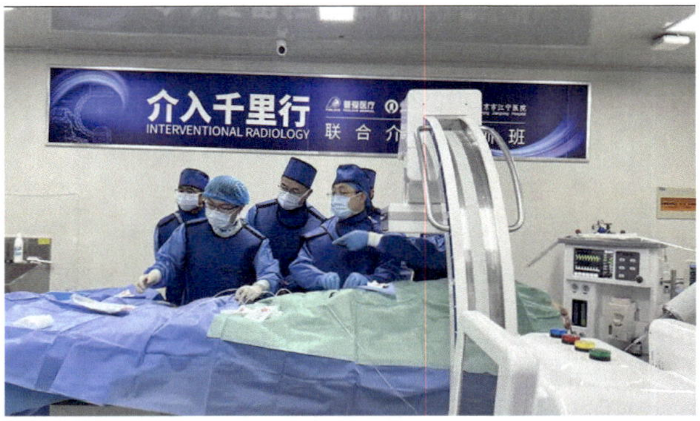

Figure 7.16. Mastering endoscopic retrograde cholangiopancreatography (ERCP) techniques.

Source: https://www.perlove.net/wp-content/uploads/Mastering-ERCP-Techniques-Navigating-Through-the-Realm-of-Interventional-Endoscopy24.webp.

7.6.1. Innovations in Endoscopic Equipment

Endoscopic technology has undergone huge advances that increase the effectiveness of procedures like ERCP significantly. Some of the recent advances include the use of high-definition endoscopes and narrow-band imaging equipment. These two types of technology improve the visualization of biliary structures so that subtle abnormalities that may cause strictures or stones can be detected more efficiently by doctors. Also, technological progress of combined imaging systems that combine EUS with ERCP provides a global approach for biliary disease, enabling diagnostics and therapeutic maneuvers to be achieved at the same time. These systems play an important role, particularly in complicated cases, since they ease the diagnostic process, reducing patients' sedation time and interventions needed. The intersection of endoscopy and technology illustrates the ongoing emphasis on maximizing patient benefit through more precise diagnoses and more efficient treatment. In addition to improved imaging, technological advancements in endoscopic accessories and equipment have transformed ERCP procedures. Access to therapeutic balloons and dilation devices has enabled improved success with the treatment of biliary strictures. These devices facilitate precise access and dilatation of bile duct stenosis at a lower risk of ductal trauma and greater success for procedures. In addition, the use of robotic assistance in endoscopy is gaining more and more popularity and allows greater accuracy for navigating instruments through deep anatomical locations. This new technology not only raises the skill level required for complex procedures but also reduces the risk of injury associated with traditional methods. Therefore, continuous innovation in advanced endoscopic accessories fuels overall ERCP development, empowering gastroenterologists with more potent tools to treat challenging biliary disease. The incorporation of artificial intelligence (AI) into endoscopic technology is a groundbreaking development in gastroenterology. AI technologies are being employed to assist in image interpretation during ERCP procedures, thereby reducing the element of human error and increasing diagnostic accuracy. With the examination of huge datasets and identification of patterns that even experienced clinicians may overlook, AI enhances discrimination between malignant and benign biliary strictures. This comes very close to existing processes in treating such disorders, as noted in recent reviews that emphasize the importance of advanced diagnostic tools in characterizing the etiology of strictures (Raza et al., 2025). The potential to link AI with endoscopic equipment not only accelerates diagnosis but also can individualize treatment planning so that patients receive timely and appropriate care that suits their unique condition. The marriage of AI with endoscopy is a paradigm shift in improving procedural outcomes of ERCP and other interventions.

7.6.2. Development of Imaging Techniques

The development of imaging modalities in medical diagnosis has transformed the treatment of bile duct and pancreatic conditions. Of the innovations in technology, ERCP was a breakthrough. Plain films and ultrasound were the first primary imaging modalities used to image biliary structures. But with the introduction of ERCP, a real-time and dynamic imaging of the pancreatic duct and biliary tree was acquired by using endoscopic techniques supplemented with fluoroscopy. Not only did this method enhance detection of pathological lesions , such as stones and strictures, but also therapeutic procedures on the same visit, thus reducing the number of follow-up surgical visits and improving patient results. Other technological innovations in imaging have also contributed significantly to the safety and efficacy of ERCP interventions. The introduction of non-radiation technologies also represents another great milestone, particularly in susceptible populations , such as pregnant women, where ionizing radiation may pose significant harm. Research has indicated that irradiation-free techniques are still effective in serving diagnostic needs, hence minimizing complications arising from conventional ERCP implementations. In systematic reviews, the necessity for advanced imaging techniques continues to be top of mind, especially in the case of establishing outcomes related to various patient groups, i.e., those undergoing procedures during pregnancy (Azab et al., 2019). This empirical framework demonstrates that improving biocompatible imaging techniques in clinical settings is necessary. As we penetrate further into the area of medical imaging, we realize the future of ERCP is closely tied to imaging technique advancements. The predictive determinants for successful preoperative ERCP have been highlighted through newer studies, with reliance on elaborate imaging evaluations to produce the best outcomes. For instance, identification of certain conditions and symptoms—, such as acute pancreatitis or the formation of bile duct stones—will dictate both the necessity and urgency of the ERCP (Lakatos et al., 2004). The evolution of imaging modalities not only goes beyond improving the precision of diagnoses but also plays an important role in deciding upon regimens of treatment and tailored care of patients. With advancing imaging technology, the disease control of biliary and pancreatic disease will continue to be more and more precisely tailored, opening an era of enhanced patient protection and procedure effectiveness in ERCP.

7.6.3. Future Trends in Endoscopic Retrograde Cholangiopancreatography (ERCP) Procedures

And so the future arrives, and the appearance of ERCP will be radically transformed. Technological advancement will be central to enhancing both the diagnostic and therapeutic capabilities of ERCP procedures. Refinement in imaging technology, such as use of high-definition endoscopes and augmented reality, will enable the clinician to visualize biliary and pancreatic anatomy with heightened precision than ever. These technologies, coupled with the integration of artificial intelligence-based analysis tools for images, will enhance early complication detection rates and overall clinical outcomes. Besides, with advancing methods, attention will increasingly be focused on minimally invasive methods, which will subsequently reduce patient recovery times and result in improved quality of life post-procedure. Furthermore, integrating various multidisciplinary techniques will guide ERCP practices towards an era of personalized medicine. For instance, the combination of ERCP with the development of radiological techniques can facilitate improved detection of biliary pathologies before interventions. Application of robotic assistance in ERCP procedures would also improve techniques with more precise interventions, particularly in difficult anatomy with standard methods of endoscopy. The hybrid model would also increase training for new specialists to maintain expertise with standard and sophisticated techniques, which would result in better procedural success rates. Effective interprofessional working will be central to the translation of these innovations into widespread practice. Patient-centered issues will be paramount in ERCP's future as health systems continue to prioritize holistic models of care. As seen from emerging trends in similar surgical interventions , such as robotic cholecystectomy, factors , such as post-operative complications, recovery time, and patient experience in general will dominate decision-making in ERCP interventions. ERCP doctors will be required to incorporate shared decision-making templates, guiding patients through their options and personal values and health priorities. Furthermore, as research sheds light on different population responses to ERCP, person-centered approaches—considering demographic and clinical characteristics—can optimize procedural success. Adapting ERCP practice in response to evolving patient requirements and outcomes is not only in line with contemporary medical ethos but is ultimately concerned with improving patient care levels in the specialty.

SUMMARY

The conclusion of any scholarly debate on ERCP calls for reconciliation of the findings regarding procedures effectiveness, safety, and new methods. ERCP is currently a core instrument in the diagnosis and therapy of biliary and pancreatic duct disease. The ability of the procedure to facilitate therapeutic maneuvers , such as stone extraction and stenting, puts it at the center of clinical intervention. However, it is essential to consider the innovations in ERCP technology, including nonradiation techniques, which have been introduced to address the concerns of patient safety, particularly in the high-risk population, such as pregnant patients. It is stated in a systematic review that ERCP remains a safe procedure and suggests an adequate risk-to-benefit ratio for managed care among this group of patients (Azab et al., 2019). Safety results reinforce procedural skill and the necessity for patient-by-patient evaluation. Complications are relatively rare if ERCP is performed by experienced doctors, according to a study. Long-term results for procedures that include ERCP, such as laparoscopic transverse choledochotomy, demonstrate a high success rate in treating common bile duct stones. For example, according to a study, the rate of recurrence of ductal stones is extremely low and without evidence of significant complications noted in follow-up examinations (Quaresima et al., 2016). This justifies the role of skilled operators in performing ERCP but emphasizes the importance of sustaining proper training and adherence to guidelines to reduce risks. In summary, the judgment on the use of ERCP at a glance encompasses its status as a vital diagnostic and therapeutic technique, with an unshakable commitment to patient safeguard and process excellence. As further studies increasingly enhance our understanding of its application, particularly in specialized populations, the future of ERCP is promising. The evidence supporting its efficacy, combined with new techniques in avoiding complications, warrants further use in gastrointestinal practice. Lastly, ongoing observation of ERCP outcomes will be a critical factor in its protocol improvement and offering safe, effective, and wholesome care to biliary and pancreatic disease patients.

In determining the most critical issues about ERCP, identification of its participatory role in the diagnosis and treatment of pancreatic and biliary disease is extremely necessary. ERCP combines therapeutic intervention and diagnostic imaging in a single procedure, allowing physicians to see the bile and pancreatic ducts while performing procedures that are necessary, such as stent placement or removal of stones. As gallstones and cancers become more prevalent with an aging population, ERCP is still a valuable tool in the clinical setting. Studies have indicated that the technique offers a minimally invasive alternative to surgery and, therefore, reduces the resulting risks and recovery times for patients. This is particularly well-suited to point out ERCP's growing application in modern medicine, particularly with older individuals, who are likely to present these complex conditions that need successful and trustworthy interventions (Chang & Lei, 2007). Safety profile, especially of ERCP in older patients, is another essential factor in the controversy surrounding ERCP. There has been greater research interest in the therapeutic efficacy and safety of ERCP in patients aged 65 years and older with positive outcomes. It has been keenly observed that the rate of success and complications is not different in elderly individuals from those of their younger counterparts, thereby rejecting the hypothesis that age is a contraindication for the procedure. Against a background of an emergent incidence of biliary disease among the older population, this evidence supports the argument that patient need should be used to underpin clinical decision-making rather than age. The literature implies that critical evaluation and tailored practice should guide the use of ERCP so as not to deprive elderly patients of potentially valuable diagnostic or therapeutic benefit (Chan et al., 2001). Lastly, the ERCP procedure has several significant factors, which include pre-procedure preparation, sedation process, and in-procedure monitoring to ensure patient safety. The medical team must be closely observant of these factors to attain maximum results while minimizing complications, which could be pancreatitis, perforation, or infection. Pre-procedure assessments are commonly a comprehensive review of the patient's general health status, history of medications, and pertinent imaging examinations to determine if ERCP is needed. Moreover, the choice of sedation agents and methods directly influences both procedural success and patient comfort. The greater focus on efficacy and safety, particularly among high-risk patients, highlights the utility of ERCP in treating complex biliary and pancreatic pathologies with certainty of optimal care across diverse populations (Chang & Lei, 2007).

CLOSER LOOK

POST-ANESTHESIA CARE:

Post-anesthesia care (PAC) is a critical phase in perioperative medicine that focuses on monitoring and managing patients immediately after surgery or procedural sedation. This period, often referred to as recovery, occurs in a specialized area known as the post-anesthesia care unit (PACU). The primary goal of PAC is to ensure patient safety while supporting the gradual return of consciousness, vital functions, and physiological stability following anesthesia. Patients in the PACU are at risk for a range of complications stemming from residual anesthetic effects, surgical stress, or pre-existing conditions. Common challenges include airway obstruction, hypoxemia, hypotension, nausea and vomiting, pain, and altered mental status. To address these risks, PAC involves continuous monitoring of vital signs, oxygen saturation, level of consciousness, pain scores, and fluid balance. Nursing staff and anesthesiologists work collaboratively to detect early signs of complications and intervene promptly.

Pain management is a cornerstone of PAC, aiming to provide comfort while minimizing the use of opioids, which can depress respiration and prolong recovery. Multimodal analgesia, incorporating non-opioid medications, regional anesthesia techniques, and adjunct therapies, is increasingly used to optimize pain control and improve patient outcomes. Similarly, prevention and treatment of post-operative nausea and vomiting (PONV) are prioritized, as these symptoms can cause discomfort, delayed discharge, and potential complications such as aspiration.

The duration of PAC varies depending on the type of anesthesia, surgery, and patient factors. Standard discharge criteria are guided by scoring systems such as the Aldrete or Post-Anesthesia Discharge Scoring System (PADSS), which assess consciousness, vital signs, mobility, pain, and surgical site bleeding. Only once patients meet these criteria and demonstrate stability are they transferred to a hospital ward or discharged home if the procedure was outpatient. In addition to immediate physiological care, PAC also emphasizes patient education and communication. Staff provide instructions regarding activity restrictions, pain management, wound care, and signs of complications, ensuring a safe transition from hospital to home.

Modern post-anesthesia care reflects a multidisciplinary approach, integrating anesthesiologists, nurses, and allied health professionals to optimize recovery, enhance patient safety, and improve satisfaction. By combining vigilant monitoring, targeted interventions, and patient-centered education, PAC serves as a crucial bridge between surgery and full postoperative recovery, ultimately supporting better clinical outcomes and reducing perioperative morbidity.

REFERENCES

1. Tringali, A., Thomson, M., Dumonceau, J. M., Tavares, M., Tabbers, M. M., Furlano, R., Spaander, M., Hassan, C., Tzvinikos, C., Ijsselstijn, H., Viala, J., Dall'Oglio, L., Benninga, M., Orel, R., Vandenplas, Y., Keil, R., Romano, C., Brownstone, E., Hlava, Š., Gerner, P., ... Zambelli, A. (2017). Pediatric gastrointestinal endoscopy: European Society of Gastrointestinal Endoscopy (ESGE) and European Society for Paediatric Gastroenterology Hepatology and Nutrition (ESPGHAN) Guideline Executive summary. *Endoscopy, 49*(1), 83–91. https://doi.org/10.1055/s-0042-111002(accessed on 15th July 2025).
2. Abbas, M., Adler, D. G., Affi, A., Alexander, T., Caetano, A. C., Andriulli, A., Apel, D., et al. (2013). *Emergencies after endoscopic procedures.* https://core.ac.uk/download/55625568.pdf (accessed on 15th July 2025).
3. Abdurachman, S. A. (Siti), Agustanti, N. (Nenny), Bestari, M. B. (Muhammad), Djumhana, A., et al. (2010). *The effectiveness of emergency endoscopic retrograde cholangiopancreatography in patients with severe acute cholangitis.* https://media.neliti.com/media/publications/135423-EN-the-effectiveness-of-emergency-endoscopi.pdf (accessed on 15th July 2025).
4. Aberin, T., Adler, D. G., Alkandari, A., Banavage, B., et al. (2024). *Defining standards for fluoroscopy in gastrointestinal endoscopy using a Delphi methodology.* https://core.ac.uk/download/624146839.pdf (accessed on 15th July 2025).
5. Norouzi, A., Khatibian, M., Afroogh, R., Chaharmahali, M., & Sotoudehmanesh, R. (2013). The effect of adding gentamicin to contrast media for prevention of cholangitis after biliary stenting for non-calculous biliary obstruction, a randomized controlled trial. *Indian journal of gastroenterology : official journal of the Indian Society of Gastroenterology, 32*(1), 18–21. https://doi.org/10.1007/s12664-012-0208-yAhuja, V. (2022). *Significance of robotic cholecystectomy over laparoscopic cholecystectomy in the management of cholecystitis: A case study of factors influencing patients' decision at a hospital in Texas, USA.* https://core.ac.uk/download/552518601.pdf (accessed on 15th July 2025).
6. AlAmri, T. A. (2022). *The efficacy of Ringer lactate and sublingual nitrates vs indomethacin to reduce post-ERCP pancreatitis: A review article.* https://core.ac.uk/download/524771648.pdf (accessed on 15th July 2025).
7. Azab, M., Bharadwaj, S., Hong, A. S., Jayaraj, M., et al. (2019). *Safety of endoscopic retrograde cholangiopancreatography (ERCP) in pregnancy: A systematic review and meta-analysis.* https://core.ac.uk/download/286611719.pdf (accessed on 15th July 2025).
8. Azizi, N., Brancatelli, G., Cannella, R., & Khorasanizadeh, F. (2024). *An exploration of radiological signs in post-intervention liver complications.* https://core.ac.uk/download/638998444.pdf (accessed on 15th July 2025).
9. Baak, L. C. (Lubbertus), Besselink, M. G. (Marc), Bhalla, A. (Abha), Bruno, M. J., et al. (2018). *Fluid hydration to prevent post-ERCP pancreatitis in average- to high-risk patients receiving prophylactic rectal NSAIDs (FLUYT trial): Study protocol for a randomized controlled trial.* https://core.ac.uk/download/154410311.pdf (accessed on 15th July 2025).
10. Quaresima, S., Balla, A., Guerrieri, M., Lezoche, G., Campagnacci, R., D'Ambrosio, G., Lezoche, E., & Paganini, A. M. (2016). Results of Medium Seventeen Years' Follow-Up after Laparoscopic

Choledochotomy for Ductal Stones. *Gastroenterology research and practice, 2016*, 9506406. https://doi.org/10.1155/2016/9506406(accessed on 15th July 2025).

11. Baruah, B. J., Bhattachayya, M., Choudhury, B. N., Debroy, A., et al. (2020). *Indications, outcomes and complications of therapeutic endoscopic retrograde cholangiopancreatography procedures in a tertiary care centre in North East India.* https://core.ac.uk/download/539911023.pdf (accessed on 15th July 2025).
12. Beesley, C., Coté, G. A., Hilton, C., Imler, T. D., et al. (2017). *Provider-specific quality measurement for ERCP using natural language processing.* https://core.ac.uk/download/84831430.pdf (accessed on 15th July 2025).
13. Blazeby, J., Blencowe, N., Chalmers, K., et al. (2017). *Methodological overview of systematic reviews to establish the evidence base for emergency general surgery.* https://core.ac.uk/download/79655849.pdf (accessed on 15th July 2025).
14. Raza D, Singh S, Crinò SF, Boskoski I, Spada C, Fuccio L, Samanta J, Dhar J, Spadaccini M, Gkolfakis P, et al. Diagnostic Approach to Biliary Strictures. *Diagnostics*. 2025; 15(3):325. https://doi.org/10.3390/diagnostics15030325(accessed on 15th July 2025).
15. Brand, M. (2011). *Are prophylactic antibiotics indicated for endoscopic retrograde cholangiopancreatography?* https://core.ac.uk/download/39669445.pdf (accessed on 15th July 2025).
16. Chan, F. L., Cheung, S. C. W., & Ng, M. (2001). *Abdominal Pain After Endoscopic Intervention.* https://core.ac.uk/download/45605737.pdf (accessed on 15th July 2025).
17. Chang, W. H., & Lei, W. Y. (2007). *Endoscopic retrograde cholangiopancreatography in elderly patients.* https://core.ac.uk/download/pdf/82371991.pdf (accessed on 15th July 2025).
18. Chen, T. S., Hsia, C. Y., Hung, H. H., Lin, C. C., et al. (2009). *Percutaneous transhepatic cholangiography and drainage is an effective rescue therapy for biliary complications in liver transplant recipients who fail endoscopic retrograde cholangiopancreatography.* https://core.ac.uk/download/pdf/82432377.pdf (accessed on 15th July 2025).
19. Magalhães, J., Rosa, B., & Cotter, J. (2015). Endoscopic retrograde cholangiopancreatography for suspected choledocholithiasis: From guidelines to clinical practice. *World journal of gastrointestinal endoscopy*, *7*(2), 128–134. https://doi.org/10.4253/wjge.v7.i2.128(accessed on 15th July 2025).
20. Morris, S., Gurusamy, K. S., Sheringham, J., & Davidson, B. R. (2015). Cost-effectiveness analysis of endoscopic ultrasound versus magnetic resonance cholangiopancreatography in patients with suspected common bile duct stones. *PloS one*, *10*(3), e0121699. https://doi.org/10.1371/journal.pone.0121699(accessed on 15th July 2025).
21. El-Bahrawy, H., El-Riwini, M., Ghazal, A. H., Sorour, O., et al. (2009). *Single-step treatment of gall bladder and bile duct stones: A combined endoscopic–laparoscopic technique.* https://core.ac.uk/download/pdf/82718403.pdf (accessed on 15th July 2025).
22. Fatehi, D., Gharib, A., Rostamzadeh, A., & Taheri, M. (2016). *Efficacy of multidetector-row computed tomography as a practical tool in comparison to invasive procedures for visualization of the biliary obstruction.* https://core.ac.uk/download/143840623.pdf (accessed on 15th July 2025).

23. Tomoda, T., Kato, H., Miyamoto, K., Matsumi, A., Ueta, E., Fujii, Y., Saragai, Y., Yamazaki, T., Uchida, D., Matsumoto, K., Horiguchi, S., Tsutsumi, K., & Okada, H. (2021). Efficacy of low dose rectal diclofenac for preventing post-endoscopic retrograde cholangiopancreatography pancreatitis: Propensity score-matched analysis. *Digestive endoscopy : official journal of the Japan Gastroenterological Endoscopy Society*, *33*(4), 656–662. https://doi.org/10.1111/den.13828(accessed on 15th July 2025).

24. Hasan, I. (Irsan), Lesmana, L. A., Syam, A. F., Tambunan, M., et al. (2001). *Non-surgical biliary drainage on biliary obstruction due to malignancy.* https://media.neliti.com/media/publications/65934-EN-non-surgical-biliary-drainage-on-biliary.pdf (accessed on 15th July 2025).

25. van der Gaag, N. A., de Castro, S. M., Rauws, E. A., Bruno, M. J., van Eijck, C. H., Kuipers, E. J., Gerritsen, J. J., Rutten, J. P., Greve, J. W., Hesselink, E. J., Klinkenbijl, J. H., Rinkes, I. H., Boerma, D., Bonsing, B. A., van Laarhoven, C. J., Kubben, F. J., van der Harst, E., Sosef, M. N., Bosscha, K., de Hingh, I. H., ... Gouma, D. J. (2007). Preoperative biliary drainage for periampullary tumors causing obstructive jaundice; DRainage vs. (direct) OPeration (DROP-trial). *BMC surgery*, *7*, 3. https://doi.org/10.1186/1471-2482-7-3(accessed on 15th July 2025).

26. Lakatos, L., Lakatos, P. L., Mester, G., Nagy, F., et al. (2004). *Selection criteria for preoperative endoscopic retrograde cholangiopancreatography before laparoscopic cholecystectomy and endoscopic treatment of bile duct stones: Results of a retrospective, single center study between 1996–2002.* https://core.ac.uk/download/11855837.pdf (accessed on 15th July 2025).

27. Lam, S. K., Lau, G. K. K., Ng, M., & Wu, J. C. (1997). *The Use of Endoscopy in Liver Diseases.* https://core.ac.uk/download/37883881.pdf (accessed on 15th July 2025).

28. Ponugoti, S. (2015). *Is a follow-up endoscopic retrograde cholangiography procedure necessary for removal of biliary stent?* https://core.ac.uk/download/230456762.pdf (accessed on 15th July 2025).

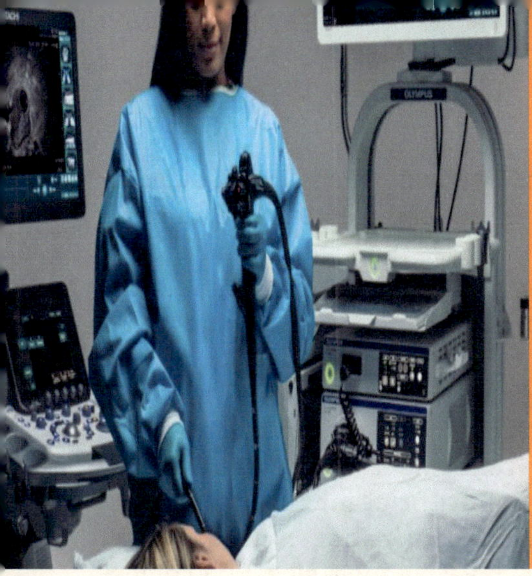

Chapter 8

ENDOSCOPIC ULTRASOUND (EUS)

Contents

Introduction....................217
8.1. Mechanism of Action....................221
8.2. Indications for Endoscopic Ultrasound (EUS)....................224
8.3. Advantages of Endoscopic Ultrasound (EUS)....................227
8.4. Limitations of Endoscopic Ultrasound (EUS)....................231
8.5. Endoscopic Ultrasound (EUS) in Clinical Practice....................234
8.6. Future Directions in Endoscopic Ultrasound (EUS)....................237
Summary....................242
References....................245

Introduction

Endoscopic Ultrasound (EUS) is a significant breakthrough in diagnostic imaging, and particularly in gastrointestinal (GI) imaging. This technique integrates endoscopy and ultrasound such that the layers of the GI tracts and surrounding structures can be imaged with excellent detail. Thus, EUS has become a critical instrument for the diagnosis of numerous GI diseases, with the ability to obtain qualitative and quantitative details, previously not so readily available. With the ability to create high-resolution images of the esophagus, stomach, pancreas, and lymph nodes, EUS is beneficial in identifying abnormalities not visible on traditional imaging techniques. Its application transcends mere visualization since EUS-guided fine needle aspiration (EUS-FNA) enables cytological and histological sampling, thereby increasing diagnostic yield and facilitating therapeutic planning. The clinical utility of EUS is exemplified by its utilization in malignancy staging and treatment planning for gastrointestinal cancers. For instance, studies have shown that EUS can significantly alter management plans in gastric cancer patients, frequently precluding unneeded operations by giving such critical staging information. Laparoscopic ultrasound and diagnostic laparoscopy further complement EUS, adding additional levels of information about tumor behavior and metastasis. With additional study, processes like ultrasound capsule endoscopy (USCE) are poised to revolutionize the discipline by filling in the loopholes of current procedures, allowing for comprehensive bowel wall and even more evaluation. All this forecasts a bright future direction for EUS as being central to future oncology and gastroenterology diagnostic procedures. Also, the development of EUS mirrors a broader trend in medical imaging, with the convergence of technology and clinical practice allowing for more effective, patient-centered care. The ongoing refinement of EUS techniques and instruments, including gains in image resolution and the use of artificial intelligence-driven analysis, heralds a future of precision medicine tailored to the individual patient's needs. With healthcare systems focusing more on early diagnosis and minimally invasive therapies, EUS comes to the fore, facilitating timely interventions that would result in improved patient outcomes. With the development of EUS ushering in to the forefront new medical practices as well as highlighting the need for continuous research and development in this fast-growing field. As the technology of EUS continues to develop and is integrated into clinical practice, it will be a standard of excellence in gastroenterology and beyond (Figure 8.1).

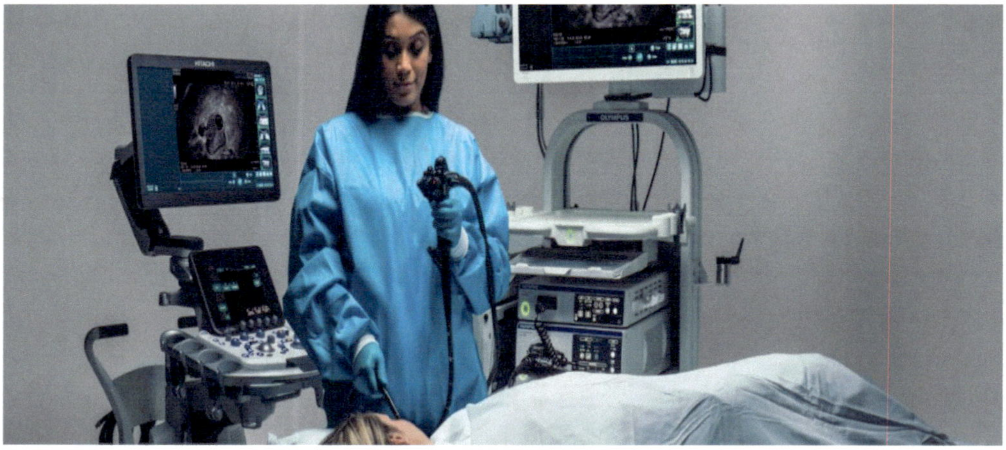

Figure 8.1. Endoscopic ultrasound (EUS).

Source: https://www.pancreaticcancerscreening.com/sites/default/files/styles/hero_image/public/hero-images/EUS_Hero.jpg?h=d1aea52f&itok=2ZIM8MCg.

Definition of Endoscopic Ultrasound (EUS)

EUS is an extremely advanced diagnostic and therapeutic tool that unites endoscopy with ultrasonography. This coupling in an innovative manner allows visualization of inner structures and organs in a minimally invasive procedure, greatly enhancing the capability of clinicians to diagnose many conditions, especially in the gastrointestinal system. During this process, an endoscope with an ultrasound transducer is put into the body, thereby allowing high-resolution images of adjacent anatomical structures , such as the stomach, esophagus, pancreas, and lymph nodes. The ability to obtain real-time images allows clinicians to make knowledgeable decisions regarding future interventions or treatments. As a key instrument for gastroenterology, EUS has become a standard instrument for the evaluation of tumors, cysts, and other pathologies, improving patient outcomes through early detection and intervention. The technological expertise of EUS is not limited to basic visualization, as it can be utilized to assist in fine-needle aspiration (FNA) to allow cytological evaluation of lesions that cannot be accessed by regular methods. This proves useful for patients who have pancreaticobiliary issues, as the procedure can help in biopsying potential malignancies with greater precision. The precision offered by EUS has revolutionized the treatment of gastrointestinal illness, offering a minimally invasive alternative to surgical sampling and lowering patient morbidity. Interestingly, evidence has pointed to the effectiveness of EUS-guided interventions, stating that they offer high diagnostic accuracy rates with lowered complications. Besides, advancements in the technology and practice of EUS implementation have ensured that EUS has become a cornerstone in disease treatment, making it an integral part of modern medicine (Jednačak et al., 2011). EUS is also notable for its evolving technology and techniques, which continue to expand its area of application. Introduction of robotic assistance and enhanced imaging modalities into EUS procedures has unlocked new frontiers in diagnostics and treatment. With the evolution of medical robots, endoscopic ultrasound systems are currently being equipped with more advanced capabilities to provide more precise control and imaging to address some of the limitations experienced with standard EUS procedures. Precisely, the development of advanced robotic systems is a synthesis of endoscopy and new technologies to improve care for patients (Troccaz, 2009). As such systems develop, not only will they further improve the functionality of EUS, but also its effectiveness as an integral part of medical practice, ultimately translating to better diagnostic and treatment outcomes (Figure 8.2).

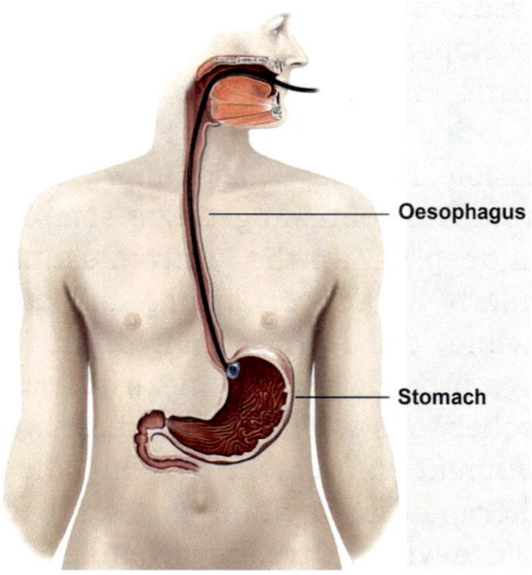

Figure 8.2. Endoscopic ultrasound (EUS).

Source: https://media.healthdirect.org.au/images/inline/original/endoscopic-ultrasound-illustration-b0c37c.png.

Historical Development of Endoscopic Ultrasound (EUS)

The evolution of EUS over the years is a dramatic account that signifies the convergence of advances in endoscopic technology and ultrasound. The development began years ago in the early 1980s when scientists realized that there was a necessity to improve the imaging of gastrointestinal organs. This prompted them to merge the traditional endoscopy with the ultrasound technology. The initial EUS systems utilized high-frequency ultrasound transducers, which provided improved imaging of the submucosal layers and adjacent organs. The intersection of these technologies was a significant step forward in gastroenterology that provided clinicians with technology better than that available with conventional imaging modalities like X-rays and CT scans. As such, EUS soon became an essential diagnostic and therapeutic modality in the assessment of pancreatic and biliary disease, marking a new era of minimally invasive approaches and patient care. As the technology of EUS developed, its applications multiplied, and clinical usefulness increased enormously. As of the mid-1990s, EUS had developed to the point where not only was diagnostic imaging possible, but therapeutic manipulation in the form of FNA biopsies was also feasible. This was a major improvement over the process of obtaining tissue samples from lesions deep within the gastrointestinal tract, particularly for cancer staging and diagnosis. Meanwhile, the introduction of EUS-guided drainage procedures as a means of managing fluid collections was another milestone in the development of EUS. Integrating diagnostic and therapeutic capabilities, EUS became a versatile device in treating complex cases of biliary obstruction and pancreatic disease, as evidenced by retrospective studies comparing EUS procedures with traditional methods in efficacy and safety (Bill et al., 2016). EUS continues to be active today, evolving in accordance with the clinical needs of an active medical environment. Four-dimensional imaging and digital enhancement techniques are more recent modalities that promise further fine-tuning of EUS examinations in terms of accuracy. Enhanced training and promotion of guidelines, as outlined in recent publications, are of important relevance in facilitating continued proficiency among practitioners in conducting these technically challenging examinations (Tringali et al., 2017). With EUS assuming its place in multidisciplinary disease management plans in inflammatory bowel disease and a number of cancers, its position at the forefront of contemporary gastroenterology is increasingly acknowledged. The trajectory of EUS development over time is one not only of technological advancement but also of enhanced diagnostic performance and patient benefit in the gastrointestinal tract.

Importance of Endoscopic Ultrasound (EUS) in Modern Medicine

The function of EUS in contemporary medicine cannot be overemphasized, particularly in gastrointestinal and oncological diagnostics. The benefit of EUS is that it integrates endoscopy with ultrasound to allow high-resolution imaging of the digestive tract and the coverings above. Its ability to see layers of tissue and assess the depth of lesions cannot be equaled by conventional imaging methods. Thus, EUS plays a critical role in diagnosing conditions like pancreatitis, tumors, and cysts, which allows clinicians to make more rational treatment decisions. In acute emergencies like acute non-variceal upper gastrointestinal bleeding ANVUGIB, where timely intervention is essential, EUS becomes extremely useful for prompt assessment and therapeutic intervention. As highlighted in ANVUGIB discussions, devices like EUS can have dynamic scoring systems to risk-stratify and guide management, resulting in better patient outcomes and reduced mortality rates for such life-threatening diseases (Alali & Barkun, 2023). Secondarily, EUS plays a significant role in early diagnosis and therapy of pancreatic cancer, a very aggressive disease with a grim prognosis. As emphasized by contemporary literature, most patients with pancreatic cancer have limited, if any, curative surgical possibilities, so early diagnosis is a critical requirement in an effort to improve survival. EUS excels in this situation by enabling visualization of fine lesions that may not be visible using other imaging methods. Importantly, EUS permits tissue sampling through fine-needle aspiration, which is beneficial in the histopathological diagnosis of pancreatic tumors. This precision not just directs therapeutic strategies but also opens the doors to research on circulating tumor cells (CTCs), which hold promise in the characterization of tumor behavior and treatment decision-making (Pimienta et al., 2017). All of these advances demonstrate the vital role played by EUS in addressing one of medicine's most challenging malignancies. Apart from its use in diagnosis, EUS has emerged as a treatment modality that complements traditional intervention. With advancements in procedures , such as EUS-guided intervention, clinicians can now perform advanced procedures

, such as celiac plexus block and drainage of pancreatic fluid collections with enhanced safety and efficacy. Such minimally invasive procedures reduce the need for more invasive surgical modalities and enhance patients' recovery periods. Additionally, as the practice of medicine becomes more patient-focused and efficient, EUS serves these objectives by facilitating timely and precise interventions. The incorporation of EUS into practice is a paradigm change in the management of gastrointestinal and pancreatic diseases, validating its integral value in contemporary medicine. This evolution not only reflects technological progress but also reflects a broader dedication to maximizing patient care using new, minimally invasive techniques (Figure 8.3).

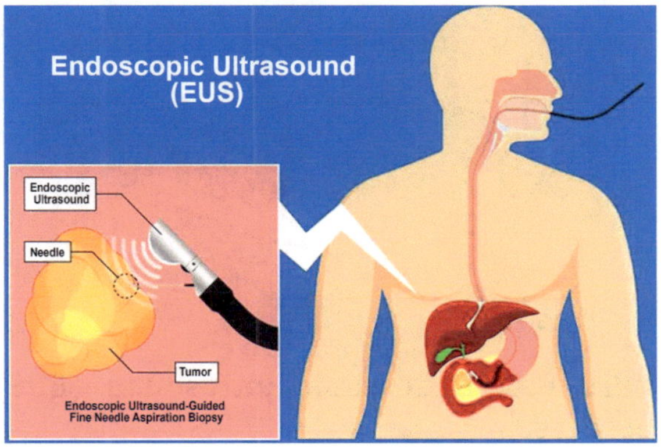

Figure 8.3. Endoscopic ultrasound (EUS).

Source: https://centrefordigestivecare.com/images/departments/endoscopic-ultrasound.jpg.

8.1. Mechanism of Action

The mode of action of Endoscopic Ultrasound (EUS) is based on the ability to utilize high-frequency ultrasound waves to create detailed images of the gastrointestinal tract and surrounding structures. EUS is a combination of endoscopy and ultrasound technology, allowing for minimally invasive imaging of internal organs. The process begins with the insertion of an endoscope with an ultrasound transducer into the digestive tract. When sound waves are generated by the transducer, they travel through tissues and reflect when they reach interfaces of different densities. The reflections are detected and translated to form real-time images, thus providing physicians with critical information regarding anatomical structures and pathological changes, if any. This new imaging capability is particularly important in imaging lesions that are inaccessible to other traditional imaging modalities, thereby enhancing diagnostic success and enabling timely interventions. In pancreatic pathology, EUS has been particularly helpful in the assessment of potential malignancies, i.e., pancreatic carcinoma. The condition is frequently challenging to diagnose since it presents minimal early features and is fatal in a significant percentage of cases; and therefore, correct imaging is crucial in improving patient outcomes. EUS enables early diagnosis of pancreatic cancer through the ability to visualize the size, shape, and nature of pancreatic masses that are undetectable with standard imaging devices , such as CT scans or MRI. Further, the inclusion of fine-needle aspiration using guidance from EUS in procedures enables histologic study of suspicious masses, resulting in more definitive diagnoses. The resolution imaging together with cytological examination puts the position of EUS to occupy a crucial place in multidisciplinary approaches to pancreatic cancer therapy, and thus it becomes the cornerstone in the diagnostic algorithm of high-risk patients (Flores et al., 2009). Moreover, the mechanism of EUS action extends even beyond visualization since it encompasses the role of possible therapeutic interventions. The technique is applied for various therapeutic applications , such as drainage of pancreatic fluid collections, celiac plexus block for pain management, and targeted chemotherapeutic drug delivery. The dual application of diagnostic and therapeutic roles is a reflection of the evolving nature of EUS in gastroenterology. Evolution of techniques , such as probe-based confocal laser endomicroscopy (pCLE) as an adjunct to the EUS platform mirrors the constant effort to enhance diagnostic specificity as well as therapeutic efficacy. By promoting early diagnosis by means of amplified visualization and allowing timely interventions, EUS has a significant impact on patient prognostics and management plans as a whole in gastrointestinal illnesses (Chen et al., 2014). Therefore, it is crucial to comprehend the multidimensional mode of action of EUS to value its revolutionary role in patient care.

8.1.1. Description of the Endoscopic Ultrasound (EUS) Procedure

EUS is a minimally invasive diagnostic method in which endoscopy and ultrasound technology are employed to attain high-resolution images of the internal organs. The procedure involves the insertion of a long, flexible tube with an embedded ultrasound transducer into the gastrointestinal tract via the esophagus, stomach, or duodenum as the common conduit. Insertion of the tube in this way gives proximity to target organs , such as the pancreas, liver, and lymph nodes to attain close-up visualization. EUS is particularly useful when assessing diseases like pancreatic cancer, where the ability to delineate anatomy by EUS is beneficial for staging and treatment. Visualization of structures with the use of the gastric wall decreases the need for more invasive imaging techniques and puts EUS in its correct place as a helpful diagnostic tool in the management of gastrointestinal disease and assisting with successful patient management strategies. The process of the EUS procedure begins with sedation to induce comfort for the patient throughout the process. Following sedation, the endoscope for EUS is inserted gently into the target region, and images are developed in real-time. Radiologists and gastroenterologists utilize these images both for diagnosis and for therapeutic interventions, such as cyst drainage or biopsy. Another important use of EUS is in the celiac plexus neurolysis (EUS-CPN), which is well-suited for reducing abdominal pain related to pancreatic cancers. In this setting, EUS offers an accurate anatomical landmark so that the celiac plexus can be targeted in a chemical ablation that greatly enhances the quality of life of the patient. Therefore, EUS is a procedure not only helpful in diagnosis but also in therapeutic interventions, and it contributes to better patient outcomes. Its heterogeneity extends beyond its direct applications in diagnosing malignancies; it also plays a crucial role in the understanding of complex hepatic conditions.

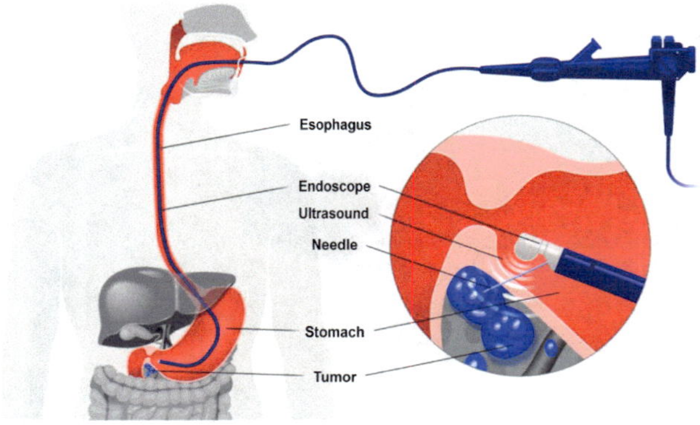

Figure 8.4. Endoscopic ultrasound (EUS): procedure.

Source: https://dims.healthgrades.com/dims3/MMH/8e4f97c/2147483647/strip/true/crop/1024x598+0+0/resize/1600x934!/quality/75/?url=https:%2F%2Fucmscdn.healthgrades.com%2F0b%2F90%2Fa0ae4afb42c9ad04e81ad4bbdf08%2F350778-a-guide-to-endoscopic-ultrasound-body-1296x757-1-1024x598.png.

For example, EUS is increasingly utilized nowadays to assess liver diseases, to obtain accurate imaging of liver segments, and to assist in the diagnosis of focal liver lesions. Furthermore, the procedure assists in assessing collateral circulation in portal hypertension patients, gaining information on potential management strategies. There are advanced technologies that have brought procedures , such as EUS-guided portal vein catheterization, through which direct portal pressure can be measured. As the scientific community keeps extending what is possible with EUS, its clinical use will increasingly simplify the approach to gastrointestinal and hepatic disease and thereby solidify its role as a major diagnostic and therapeutic modality in modern medicine (Al-Haddad et al., 2014; Magalhães et al., 2017) (Figure 8.4).

8.1.2. Types of Ultrasound Waves Used

In EUS, a number of different ultrasound waves play significant roles in enhancing diagnostic yields and treatment modalities. These are divided into two broad categories: continuous wave (CW) and pulsed wave (PW) ultrasound. Continuous wave ultrasound refers to the production of sound waves continuously, which enables the detection of high-speed blood flow. It is particularly beneficial in the assessment of vascular structures, where useful information regarding hemodynamics can be collected by clinicians. Conversely, pulsed wave ultrasound emits the sound waves in a series of discrete pulses, with increased depth resolution. This is a crucial distinction when one is evaluating structures at specific depths, as is often the situation with EUS uses. Choice of the kind of ultrasound wave directly impacts image clarity and accuracy and, ultimately, clinical decision and patient outcome. Of EUS technologies, high-frequency ultrasound waves are generally employed since they offer higher resolution. The frequency range used for EUS is normally 5–20 megahertz (MHz), and the greater frequency is used when imaging superficial lesions, while the lesser frequency is used when imaging deeper structures. The trade-off is depth penetration against spatial resolution; the higher frequency yields better images but has a shallow penetration depth. Above all, developments in ultrasound technology have made it possible to manufacture dedicated transducers that can be set up to operate at various frequencies as per clinical need. Not only does this flexibility enhance diagnostic sensitivity, but it also expands the therapeutic scope of EUS, offering options for intervention beyond plain imaging. Besides CW and PW ultrasound, novel technologies , such as microbubble-enhanced ultrasound are advancing the discipline substantially, particularly towards targeted therapy applications. It has been discovered in research that microbubbles can be engineered to specifically bind to certain tissues, allowing localized therapeutic intervention with the guidance of ultrasound waves. For instance, the integration of microbubbles with ultrasound energies might bring about cavitation effects, and thus lead to fragmentation of unwanted tissue , such as kidney stones, as discovered in recent studies (Bailey et al., 2015). In addition, this method serves as the best example of the future potential convergence of multi-functional ultrasound modalities, which could complement conventional EUS use. With further developments of these innovations, they hold the promise of not only refining imaging accuracy but also optimizing the overall efficiency of interventional applications in EUS to support a wider variety of clinical uses (Kim et al., 2025).

8.1.3. Role of Endoscopes in Endoscopic Ultrasound (EUS)

EUS is an important player in the modern diagnostic environment, particularly in the diagnosis and management of gastrointestinal disorders. EUS is the fusion of endoscopy and ultrasound techniques to achieve excellent visualization of the gastrointestinal tract and surrounding tissues. The technique is not only better at imaging shallow lesions, but also better at imaging deeper structures , such as lymph nodes and the pancreas. As pointed out in recent literature, EUS is particularly good at staging gastrointestinal cancer, better than imaging modalities like CT and MRI in some contexts.

These skills have made EUS a priceless weapon in oncological planning and intervention, allowing for focused treatment protocols adaptable to the needs of individual patients (Azzopardi, 2013). The advantages of EUS go beyond mere visualization; the technology even allows for therapeutic interventions. For instance, EUS-guided FNA achieves histologic diagnosis via the avenue of tissue sampling from otherwise unapproachable lesions. The precise process minimizes the need for more invasive surgical procedures, demonstrating the multifunctional nature of EUS in patient management. EUS also serves as a guide for numerous interventions, such as drainage in pancreatic pseudocysts, again demonstrating the versatility of EUS in therapeutic applications. With advancing procedural techniques, the integration of endoscopic ultrasound with other imaging modalities, such as optical coherence tomography (OCT), promises better diagnostic efficacy and a broader application for EUS in clinical practice (Adams et al., 2006).

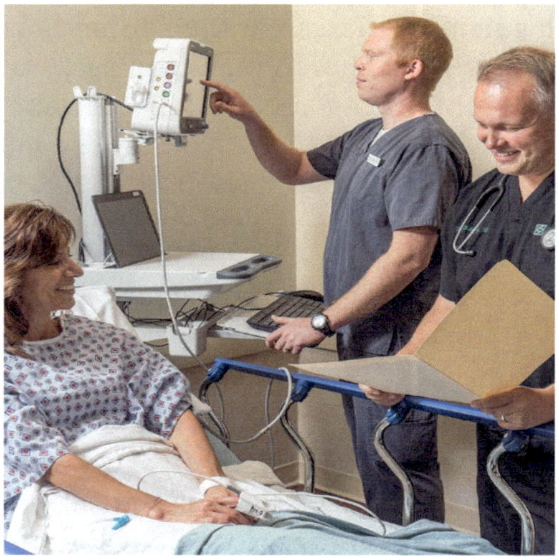

Figure 8.5. Role of endoscopes in endoscopic ultrasound (EUS).

Source: https://www.ssgastro.com/_nuxt/image/d95cc0.jpg.

The evolving nature of EUS technology underscores its pivotal position in gastroenterology. Evolution in endoscope design and imaging capability has allowed for performing complex evaluations and interventions with higher precision. With time, as this technology grows, researchers aim to explore the areas of EUS, such as the efficacy of EUS compared to routine imaging techniques in different clinical presentations. Further studies are also conducted to establish standardized protocols for the use of EUS in different gastrointestinal diseases. The combination of endoscopic techniques with imaging technologies not only enhances diagnostic accuracy but also broadens the scope of application of EUS in other medical specialties, such that improved biopsy techniques and treatment strategies are developed. This combination positions EUS at the hub of a new model in patient management and intervention (Azzopardi, 2013) (Figure 8.5).

8.2. Indications for Endoscopic Ultrasound (EUS)

EUS has emerged as a valuable diagnostic modality in the assessment of a variety of gastrointestinal disorders, predominantly due to its capability to obtain high-resolution images of the gastrointestinal tract and surrounding structures. Of the numerous indications for EUS, one of the most significant is the evaluation of pancreatic lesions, both benign and malignant. Through the integration of the application of EUS with fine needle aspiration (FNA), doctors are in a position to obtain cytological samples for definitive diagnosis, particularly for the purposes of distinguishing pancreatic cancer from chronic pancreatitis. The precision of EUS also allows for the meticulous inspection of the engaged vascular structures, hence enhancing the diagnostic yield in complex situations. With the increasing utilization of EUS in diagnosing pancreatic disease, its relevance to ensuring appropriate care of affected patients becomes increasingly paramount. A further essential utilization of EUS is biliary tract disease assessment, particularly when non-invasive imaging studies cannot provide conclusive diagnostic information. EUS is inherently effective at imaging bile ducts with precise assessment of impending obstruction by stones, strictures, or tumors. EUS possesses the special capability to evaluate the interaction of anatomy between structures and adjacent organs, which is crucial in the planning of surgery or therapy. Forward-viewing echoendoscopes further enhanced the role of EUS in biliary disease management, enabling more precise therapeutic intervention , such as drainage of bile ducts.

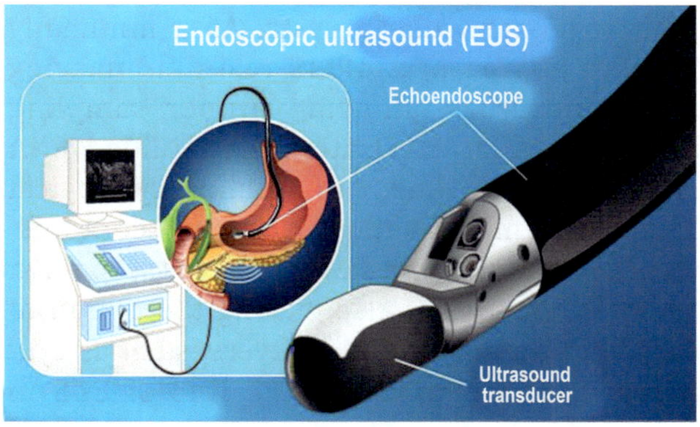

Figure 8.6. Indications for endoscopic ultrasound (EUS).

Source: https://www.animatedpancreaspatient.com/en-pancreas/content.ashx?file=app04/slides/ch11_slide_05.jpg.

The diagnostic yield of EUS-FNA in biliary illness, along with its therapeutic potential, situates it at the core of contemporary management of biliary disease and underscores its position within clinical practice. In addition to its use as a diagnostic tool, EUS has a useful place in the assessment of liver disease, thereby broadening its significance within gastrointestinal medicine. The technique provides accurate imaging of liver parenchyma and aids in the diagnosis and characterization of focal liver lesions, a matter of pivotal significance in understanding cirrhosis and hepatocellular carcinoma. EUS is also crucial in portal hypertension assessment, a critical one in guiding treatment planning and interventions. Secondly, technologies , such as EUS-guided portal vein catheterization facilitate direct portal pressure measurement, a key innovation in hemodynamic comprehension in liver disease patients. All-embracing, this enables clinicians to use EUS not only for the purpose of diagnosis but also to measure the course of liver disease, and therefore, an all-around tool in the management of patients (Araki et al., 2013; Magalhães et al., 2017) (Figure 8.6).

8.2.1. Diagnosis of Gastrointestinal Disorders

The gastrointestinal disorders' multifactorial cause demands advanced diagnostic techniques to make accurate diagnoses and treatment. EUS is a leading diagnostic instrument that allows high-resolution visualization of the gastrointestinal tract and neighboring organs. In contrast to traditional imaging devices, EUS combines endoscopy and ultrasonography to produce close-up views of the esophagus, stomach, pancreas, and intestines. This role is particularly beneficial in the diagnosis of conditions , such as tumors, cysts, and inflammatory conditions. EUS not only enhances visualization but also enables the tissue samples to be retrieved with fine-needle aspiration if necessary. Through the ability to attain precise pictures and biopsies, there is a rise in the overall diagnostic accuracy, hence enhancing the subsequent treatment protocols for individuals with gastrointestinal disorders. In pancreatic disease, the function of EUS comes even more into play. The technique has proven superior to other imaging modalities, such as computed tomography and percutaneous ultrasound, due to its ability to give high-frequency ultrasonic images of both pancreatic tissue and its ductal anatomy in a contemporaneous manner. This volume-full imaging is crucial in differentiating between malignant tumors and benign cystic lesions and its implications are significant for surgical management. EUS-guided fine-needle aspiration is particularly useful as it enables clinicians to aspirate cystic fluid for cytologic assessment and tumor marker testing with further management implications. The reflective capacity of EUS in the management of pancreatic disease reflects its inherent place in the gastrointestinal disorder diagnosis schema, illustrating its vital contribution to the enhancement of patient prognosis through the use of tailored therapeutic measures (Chan et al., 2003). Moreover, evolving guidelines for gastrointestinal endoscopy also reflect the place occupied by EUS in facilitating management plans for disorders from upper gastrointestinal hemorrhage to stricture evaluation. As delineated in current clinical practice guidelines, EUS is indicated for a range of diagnostic and therapeutic applications, including the management of inflammatory bowel disease. The symbiotic relation between diagnosis and therapy is facilitated by the endoscopic capability of EUS to assist in interventions , such as stent placement and therapeutic drainage procedures. Furthermore, as medical technology evolves, practice maintenance and training among EUS practitioners are central to ensuring optimum outcomes. The building evidence base for the efficacy of EUS as a first-line diagnostic modality speaks volumes about its versatility and capabilities in navigating the complex terrain of gastrointestinal disease, ultimately contributing to enhanced quality of patient care (Tringali et al., 2017).

8.2.2. Evaluation of Pancreatic Conditions

Pancreatic assessment has gained significant interest since pancreatic cysts have emerged as a pressing public health concern due to the increasing prevalence of pancreatic cysts. Better cross-sectional imaging techniques have optimized the detection of cystic lesions and thereby better knowledge of their potential malignancy. Of greatest concern, mucinous cysts carry a high risk of the development of pancreatic cancer, a disease of dismal prognosis when it is not diagnosed and treated promptly. Proper evaluation is dependent on the ability to distinguish neoplastic from benign cysts, posing a daunting conundrum for clinicians. Accordingly, research has focused on maximizing diagnostic criteria and techniques in an effort to enhance the quality of the assessments, hoping to provide timely interventions that are commensurate with each condition (Moyer et al., 2019). EUS is now the gold standard method for diagnosing and treating pancreatic pathology, particularly cysts. As a minimally invasive approach, it offers real-time imaging of the pancreas, allowing proper sampling and lesion characterization. EUS-guided FNA is extremely prevalent in yielding cytological and biochemical analysis of cyst contents, thereby making it easier to diagnose benign vs. malignant cysts. Also, having the option to carry out therapeutic maneuvers, such as cyst ablation, also emphasizes the role of EUS in this field. Advances in technology in EUS over the recent years have enhanced its diagnostic yield, reflecting better outcomes for patients. By enabling improved evaluation of pancreatic illnesses, EUS significantly influences clinical decision-making regarding management schemes and potential operations (Scott et al., 2017). As understanding of pancreatic illnesses expands, treatment paradigms are increasingly adopting minimally invasive interventions, indicating shifts in paradigms in management. The ultrasonically guided endoscopic chemoablation of pancreatic neoplastic cysts is one such practice, demonstrating a very promising alternative to historic and long-troubled surgical resection. Recent research shows that the use of non-alcohol-based cocktails of chemoablation is effective in mitigating safety risks inherent in traditional methods, thereby improving the overall risk-benefit ratio for patients. EUS not only provides a vital role in diagnosis but also constitutes a platform of delivery for cutting-edge therapies that can be performed in conjunction with assessment. This convergent approach accelerates patient treatment by combining diagnosis and therapy, resulting in improved outcomes among patients afflicted with many pancreatic disorders, particularly those susceptible to cancer (Moyer et al., 2019).

8.2.3. Staging of Cancers

Staging of the cancers is important in identifying the appropriate therapeutic approach and the prognosis of the disease. For the gastrointestinal cancers, accurate staging is helpful in the assessment of the extent of dissemination of the disease and helps make decisions on future treatment. The standard imaging techniques , such as CT and MRI, are inadequate in providing sufficient information on tumor invasion and lymph node involvement. This is where EUS helps. EUS offers high-resolution imaging, allowing for precise tumor staging through evaluation of the surrounding tissues and establishing whether the cancer has infiltrated surrounding structures. Its staging role is invaluable, particularly in gastroesophageal cancers, as local staging accurately dictates between surgical resection and palliative treatment (Azzopardi, 2013). Besides its imaging advantage, EUS is also used for tissue sampling through FNA which can be utilized for cytological diagnosis and for increasing the accuracy of staging. Direct access to biopsy specimens from lesions enhances the diagnostic advantage of EUS and positions it as a method of first choice in practice. Controversies, however, do exist and primarily regarding the most available techniques and approaches for EUS procedures in cancer staging. For instance, there is considerable controversy over the optimal needle caliber for FNA; there must be a compromise between maximizing tissue yield and patient discomfort. Additionally, contrast agents for EUS are a burgeoning field of research, with potential for improved visualization of lesions and more accurate staging (Trindade & Berzin, 2013). These advances translate the dynamic ability of EUS in cancer treatment and its utility in the treatment of cancer as part of the multidisciplinary approach.

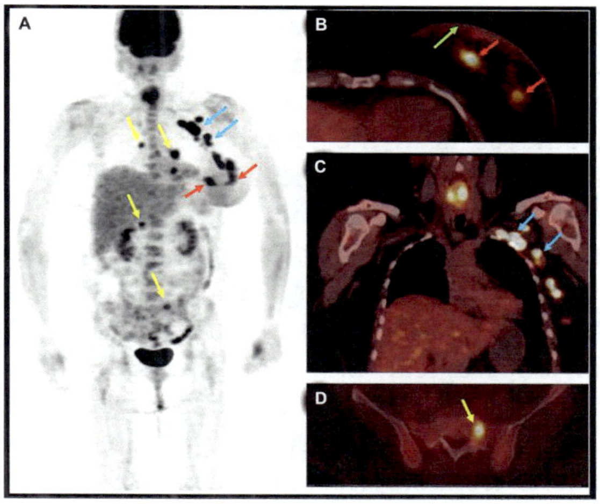

Figure 8.7. Staging of cancers.

Source: https://www.pet.theclinics.com/cms/asset/44717066-889c-4ab0-9cb8-730033693415/gr2.jpg.

8.3. Advantages of Endoscopic Ultrasound (EUS)

EUS offers excellent advantages that enhance its clinical relevance in various gastrointestinal diseases. The most important advantage of EUS is the high resolution of imaging, particularly for organs located close to the gastrointestinal tract. It allows for more detailed visualization of submucosal lesions and lymph nodes, making diagnosis more accurate. Accurate imaging is especially crucial in the differentiation between benign and malignant illness, where a mistake can have profound implications for patient management. Moreover, EUS is a less invasive method that reduces patient discomfort compared to more traditional types of surgery, and is thus a desirable alternative for patients and practitioners alike. By minimizing the demand for bigger incisions and enabling quick recovery, EUS facilitates more patient-friendly diagnosis and treatment of gastrointestinal ailments with increased patient compliance and satisfaction on follow-up. The therapeutic applications of EUS also establish it as a valuable asset in today's medicine. One of the most important advantages is in the FNA biopsy application, which enables the retrieval of tissue samples from inaccessible lesions with a significant augmentation of diagnostic yield. This feature is best evident in biliary strictures, where an accurate tissue diagnosis can guide surgical and oncological management. EUS-guided procedures, such as drainage of pancreatic fluid collections, reflect the versatility of the modality. Modern technological advancements, such as improved imaging software and compatibility with artificial intelligence, further enhance the precision of EUS-guided procedures and interpretations, as seen in studies that explored its application in various pathologies (Raza et al., 2025). Hence, not only does EUS have a role in diagnosis, but it also facilitates therapeutic interventions necessary for effective patient management. Moreover, the role of EUS in encouraging a multidisciplinary diagnostic strategy is a relevant advantage. The integration of EUS with other imaging techniques like MRI and CT scans optimizes the entire diagnostic process, particularly in complex cases of biliary strictures. Biliary strictures, which at times are challenging because of possible benign or malignant pathology, indicate the importance of extensive evaluation methods. Through the combination of EUS use with serum biochemical markers and advanced imaging modalities, clinicians can provide a better, more informed perspective on a patient's condition (Raza et al., 2025). This synergistic process increases diagnostic accuracy and informs clinical decision-making, ultimately leading to better patient outcomes. The capability to integrate diverse specialties ensures timely and proper interventions, further emphasizing the critical role of EUS within the overall scope of gastrointestinal diagnostics and management (Figure 8.8).

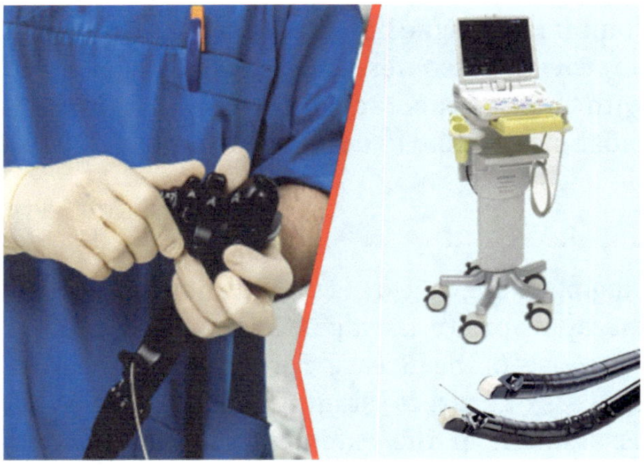

Figure 8.8. Advantages of endoscopic ultrasound (EUS).

Source: https://www.shifa.com.pk/wp-content/uploads/2022/01/EUS-Picture-compressed.jpg.

8.3.1. Minimally Invasive Nature

The minimally invasive nature of EUS has radically changed clinical practice in gastrointestinal medicine. As opposed to traditional surgical approaches, with their usual feature of bulky incisions and prolonged convalescence, EUS uses a thin flexible tube with an ultrasound device. The method offers immediate visualization of internal organs, enabling medical professionals to make precise interventions with little disturbance to neighboring tissues. Through minimizing trauma, patients experience less postoperative pain and reduced hospital stays. Furthermore, EUS's ability to guide interventions , such as biopsies, also goes to reinforce its safety and efficiency, positioning it as a cornerstone of contemporary diagnostic and treatment modalities. Not only does this new technique minimize the physical trauma to patients, but it also optimizes the overall success of the procedure, positioning EUS at the vanguard of minimally invasive procedures. The consequences of EUS extend far beyond the treatment of pancreatic cystic lesions in terms of therapeutic effect and patient safety. With the rising incidence of pancreatic cysts in elderly adults, compounded by increased imaging, it is becoming difficult to determine which lesions to operate on. Traditional pancreatic surgery is hazardous with significant morbidity and lengthy recovery and underscores the need for more conservative therapy. EUS-guided techniques, particularly in the ablation of cysts, are now a viable choice. Recent studies have demonstrated that endoscopic ultrasound-guided chemoablation is a novel, minimally invasive treatment, one that successfully cures neoplastic cysts with fewer complications than more invasive surgery. This new treatment option represents a significant step forward in patient care and is a testament to the success of EUS in managing challenging clinical circumstances (Moyer et al., 2019). As medical technology continues to improve, the implementation of minimally invasive techniques like EUS is evidence of an overall trend toward enhancing procedural safety and patient outcomes. Such enhanced precision provided through EUS is a prime example of new imaging technology facilitating successful intervention with reduced risks associated with traditional surgery. The advent of automation within surgical robotics also supports this trend through offering greater control and precision throughout procedures, as recent research demonstrates (Das & Yip, 2017). The availability of real-time visualization with EUS allows clinicians to make informed decisions rapidly, which is crucial in situations involving pancreatic cyst management and other complex conditions. As newer technologies and approaches are developed, the role of EUS as a gold standard for minimally invasive procedures further solidifies, ultimately seeking to improve the patient experience while reducing the burden of surgical procedures.

8.3.2. High-Resolution Imaging Capabilities

High-resolution imaging capability is a fundamental component of EUS, enhancing diagnosis accuracy and treatment success in all clinical settings. EUS is the combination of endoscopy with ultrasound technology, allowing submucosal layers and surrounding structures to be well-visualized in exquisite detail. The inclusion of high-frequency ultrasound transducers significantly improves the resolution of the images obtained from the gastrointestinal tract and surrounding tissue. Not only does the modality allow for the detection of pathologies , such as tumors and cysts, but it also defines anatomical structures with excellent definition. Therefore, clinicians can make more precise judgments regarding diagnosis and treatment, and the importance of high-resolution imaging in modern endoscopic practice is thus underscored. Outside of the area of visualization, the capabilities of high-resolution imaging in EUS are imperative also in therapeutic procedures. For instance, real-time imaging allows clinicians to carry out minimally invasive treatments more accurately, thus reducing the risks of standard surgery. The ability to see anatomy during procedures helps to enable targeted biopsies and needle aspirations such that tissue sampling is undertaken from the most relevant sites. Further, high-resolution imaging paves the way for innovations , such as self-guided surgical robots, which use precise images to conduct interventions more accurately. By facilitating high accuracy and reduction in human error, these state-of-the-art imaging modalities enhance the safety and effectiveness of EUS procedures in a clinical setup (Das & Yip, 2017). Another significant application of high-resolution imaging facilities in endoscopic ultrasound is neuroendoscopy. New technologies have combined EUS with techniques , such as endoneurosonography (ENS), allowing real-time virtualization of brain structures in 3D. This new combination enables surgeons to produce high-resolution models of brain tumors, enhancing surgical planning and execution. High-resolution imaging also enables the production of neural network algorithms with the ability to interpret and analyze ultrasound data, and thus finally improve tumor morphology modeling. Clinicians are therefore benefited by greater visualization and better understanding of complex anatomy during procedures, hence decreasing invasiveness and improving patient outcomes. These developments illustrate the pivotal significance that high-resolution imaging holds, not only for diagnosis but also for mapping out the future of surgical intervention (Serna & Prieto, 2017) (Figure 8.9).

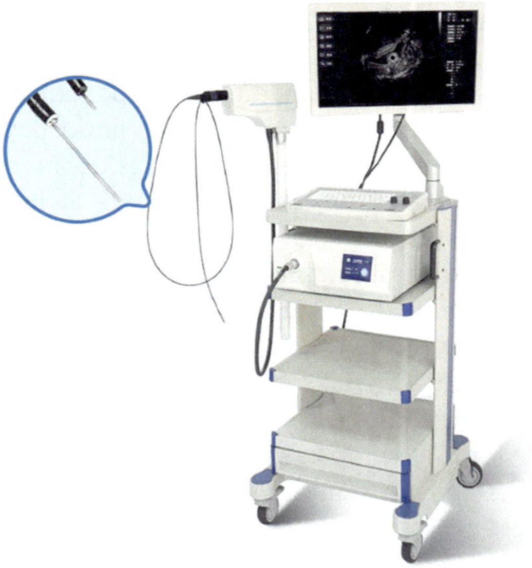

Figure 8.9. High-resolution imaging capabilities of endoscopic ultrasound (EUS).

Source: https://en.lepumedical.com/uploads/image/20220209/11/vsonic-600_1644378197.jpg.

8.3.3. Ability to Perform Fine-Needle Aspiration (FNA)

Having the facility to carry out FNA with EUS enhances the diagnostic facility of this modality. EUS facilitates real-time visualization of the gastrointestinal tract and surrounding structures, hence making it particularly useful for the targeting of lesions that are otherwise not readily accessible. EUS, when combined with FNA, not only facilitates accurate localization of tumors but also permits the acquisition of cytological material for histopathological analysis. This dual function is valuable in initial diagnosis and therapy of gastrointestinal cancers, as it has a tendency to yield more tissue specimens compared to standard methods. Furthermore, technical proficiency required for effective FNA can bear important clinical meaning, thereby increasing the value of training and proficiency in this elegant technique as endoscopic technology proceeds to advance. Current studies have confirmed the proper integration of EUS with FNA techniques as capable of improving the staging of gastrointestinal cancer. The factor of being able to provide cytological samples through FNA makes staging more accurate, which constitutes a central field for determining the best treatment for patients. Evidence shows that the diagnostic efficacy of EUS-FNA is comparable to that of other imaging techniques like CT and MRI and, therefore, a procedure of choice for most practitioners. Through its accurate determination of tumor size and dissemination, EUS-FNA significantly guides oncology patient management algorithms. This capability is particularly significant, as proper staging and classification bear a direct influence on the selection of the therapeutic approach, thus dictating patient prognosis and survival rate (Azzopardi, 2013). In this way, incorporating FNA into EUS not only enhances diagnostic precision but also facilitates decision-making in enigmatic instances of cancer. Moreover, the evolving nature of endoscopy equipment has accelerated innovations in techniques of FNA, thereby guaranteeing better all-around efficacy and safety of treatment. Technical improvements in needles, aspiration techniques, and sampling procedures have improved diagnostic yield, along with reduced complications. Proficiency in these techniques becomes better accepted by clinicians as expertise in FNA is pivotal to ensure optimal benefits to the patients. Enhanced training programs with a focus on technical proficiency of EUS and FNA are proving to be useful in standardizing the quality of care provided across institutions. With the evolving technology, it is necessary that the healthcare professionals keep themselves up to date with the latest techniques and guidelines so that the combination of FNA and EUS remains a cornerstone of the treatment of gastrointestinal illness (Bang et al., 2014) (Figure 8.10).

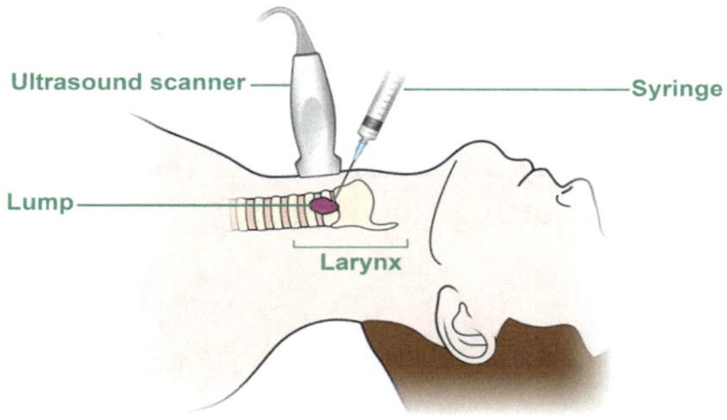

Figure 8.10. Ability to perform fine-needle aspiration.

Source: https://www.macmillan.org.uk/dfsmedia/1a6f23537f7f4519bb0cf14c45b2a629/448-50033/macd273-fine-needle-aspirate-labelled-20181102-1.

8.4. Limitations of Endoscopic Ultrasound (EUS)

Despite its pioneering contribution to the diagnosis and intervention in the gastrointestinal tract, EUS has certain limitations. One of the most significant limiting factors is that the procedure depends on the operator, which significantly contributes to its safety and efficacy. The skill level and experience of the endoscopist are significant deciding factors for obtaining good-quality images and reaching correct diagnoses. Variability in technique can lead to variability in lesion detection or characterization, and ultimately influence patient management. Also, certain anatomical variations, for instance, obesity or previous surgeries, can compromise optimal visualization, further complicating EUS interpretation. Such inherent variability requires rigorous training and continued practice by practitioners to decrease procedural failure and improve clinical results. The other important limitation of EUS is its poor ability to assess the whole gastrointestinal tract in its entirety. While EUS is great at visualizing structures close to the digestive lumen, such as lymph nodes and pancreatic tumors, it is poor at visualizing distal lesions or small bowel disease. Consequently, lesions outside the range of the EUS probe can be entirely missed. This is compounded by the reality that certain conditions, such as pancreatic cysts, require precise distinction of malignant from benign lesions to properly manage them. Several recent papers have shown that while EUS-guided procedures, such as chemoablation of pancreatic cysts, seem promising, their effectiveness could be negated by factors , such as the cysts very precise location or the need for particular skills, which are not ubiquitously available (Moyer et al., 2019). In addition to operator dependence and difficulty with evaluation, its worst feature is also the potential for adverse events due to its procedures. While relatively safe, there is still a potential for complications , such as pancreatitis, infection, or perforation. Particularly with interventional procedures added to EUS, its acute adverse event risk is greater. For instance, EUS-guided FNA is famously known to facilitate tissue sampling but has been reported to be associated with complications in certain situations, particularly with very vascular lesions or lesions that are adjacent to major structures. Therefore, awareness and prevention of these complications are paramount in optimizing the overall safety profile of EUS. Continuing with advances in technology, machinery, and patient selection criteria are needed to maximize the benefits of EUS and minimize potential harms to patients (Scott et al., 2017).

8.4.1. Technical Challenges and Limitations

The benefits of EUS technology, as groundbreaking as it was in its approach to internal imaging, are subject to a multitude of technical challenges and limitations. One of the significant challenges is the quality of the imaging itself, which is prone to influences from operator skill, patient anatomy, and inherent characteristics of ultrasound waves. The contributors can lead to suboptimal visualization of structures, whose impact is expressly evident in compromising diagnostic accuracy. Since EUS employs high-frequency sound waves, interference in transmission may create artifacts or obscure images, complicating clinical assessment. In addition, image interpretation for EUS is highly demanding in terms of expertise, and thus, even with sufficient equipment, there can be diagnostic variations depending on the skill and experience of the practitioners, which have a major impact on patient outcomes. Another severe limitation involves the technical limitations in instrument flexibility and movement. While there have been breakthroughs in robotic devices, navigation in complex anatomies still proves to be tricky. Adding robotic capsule endoscopes has been suggested to improve capabilities but precision in localization within the three-dimensional (3D) gastrointestinal terrain is challenging. Real-time mapping and precise visualization are important for effective intervention during procedures, as presented in the literature (Turan et al., 2017). The need for full 3D mapping emphasizes the issues that arise through the application of static visual information, under which dynamic adaptation is essential to correct medical practice in endoscopy procedures. The absence of standardized datasets and performance metrics for EUS technology makes it even more difficult to evaluate and refine these systems. In fields , such as computer vision, benchmark datasets have significantly powered research and innovation by serving comprehensive points of reference for establishing the efficacy of algorithms (Allan et al., 2019). The EUS field lacks such resources, a limitation that lags developments in robotic surgery and reinforces disparities in technical applications. The initiation of certain initiatives, like the EndoVis workshop for robot image segmentation, has provided an avenue for synergy but has not fully solved the technical obstacles in dataset variability and annotation accuracy. Overcoming these technical obstacles is important in further developing the field of EUS and ensuring the reproducibility and reliability of the results in the clinical setting (Figure 8.11).

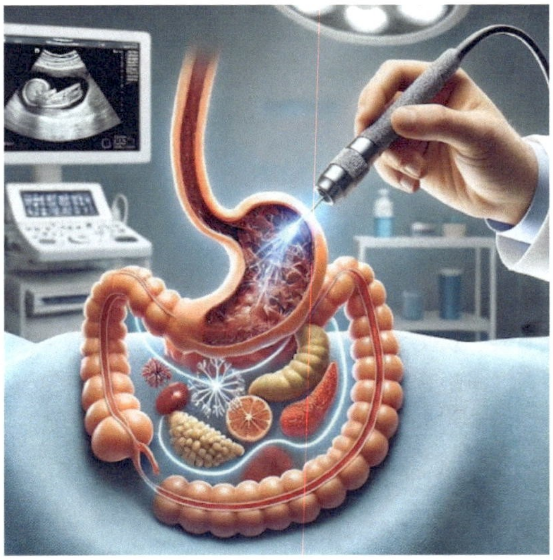

Figure 8.11. Technical challenges and limitations endoscopic ultrasound (EUS).

Source: https://lh4.googleusercontent.com/proxy/hQ3j59cq337elkKGoQ2VV2OXDV5x2LrdTkWKEpJzoIDmAajyLV6-qtEoCDIGQpikZLKpMCyXxa7jKZNjUE6A8ze33QD6Z607u_BUmHj-ntI_LCMLxPdINUPMYmlX4hGd8d2DNzNuLyCnOrAjf2CVJQeJJk780QjsVSH8JxPOtdZt249cU1Iw0Ds.

8.4.2. Patient-Related Factors Affecting Outcomes

When it comes to EUS, patient-related factors are important in the determination of procedure outcomes. These include a myriad of variables ranging from the patient's age, comorbidities, and health status, among other factors that may potentially influence the technical success of EUS as well as the risk for complications. For instance, elderly patients or those with severe comorbidities often present with a higher risk of complications arising from sedation and can exhibit deranged physiological responses to the procedure. Understanding such patient-related variables helps clinicians tailor their practice, enabling pre-procedure evaluation and adjustment of sedation regimens, thereby optimizing patient safety and the potential for successful therapeutic and diagnostic interventions. Furthermore, the psychological status of the patient, including their level of anxiety, can play a significant role in affecting outcomes in EUS. More anxious patients will not be compliant with the procedure as easily, which can lead to less than satisfactory imaging or technical failure. This psychological aspect is not commonly considered in the clinical scenario but plays an important role in patient compliance, acceptance of the procedure, and overall satisfaction with the care received. Utilization of preoperative counseling and stress control measures may mitigate levels of anxiety, ultimately resulting in improved procedural outcomes. Addressing the emotional and psychological needs of patients makes it possible for health practitioners to create a more conducive environment for the optimal utilization of EUS, which provides improved diagnostic accuracy and patient satisfaction. The effects of anatomical and physiological factors cannot be overlooked in evaluating patient outcomes in EUS. Anatomical variation , such as body habitus and anatomical defects, can directly impact visualization and the operators' ability to perform the procedure successfully. For instance, patients with severe obesity or those with a history of abdominal surgery may present with abnormal anatomy that makes access to target organs challenging. Pre-procedure imaging and assessment can therefore help clinicians plan how to proceed while conducting EUS. In addition, patient-related factors , such as underlying gastrointestinal disease may also complicate EUS results, necessitating expertise in each patient's specific condition. Management of such factors is critical in ensuring ideal patient outcomes and underscores the role of tailor-made approaches in the practice of EUS.

8.4.3. Comparison with Other Imaging Modalities

EUS is a useful imaging method, particularly in staging gastrointestinal cancer. When weighed against other conventional imaging techniques , such as computed tomography (CT) and magnetic resonance imaging (MRI), EUS holds advantages. Its resolution is superior in diagnosing small lesions, and it provides real-time imaging that is useful for biopsies and therapy. EUS has been demonstrated to be more precise in tumor staging, and at times it is even superior to CT and MRI in evaluating local invasion of the tumor and nodal involvement. In addition, EUS provides for more extensive evaluation of the surrounding anatomical structures, which is invaluable in therapeutic planning and surgery, and, therefore, enhances the success of patient management. This aspect emphasizes EUS's central role in the diagnostic work-up of patients with suspected gastrointestinal cancer in the context of other imaging modalities (Azzopardi, 2013). Another aspect that differentiates EUS from other imaging modalities is that it is not invasive and can provide for minimizing the exposure of patients to harmful radiation. Unlike techniques , such as CT, where the patient is subjected to a series of radiation exposures, EUS utilizes harmless ultrasound waves with the procedure performed at relatively low risk to the patient. This point can be especially noted in treatment for patients suspected of having common bile duct stones, whereby EUS can be used as an initial diagnostic method. Recent findings have shown that utilization of EUS or Magnetic Resonance CholangioPancreatography (MRCP) before proceeding with invasive interventions like endoscopic retrograde cholangiopancreatography (ERCP) has the potential to significantly reduce the rate of complications of redundant interventions. These findings reveal EUS's role as not only a diagnostic imaging modality but also as one that has the potential to enhance patient safety and reduce the expense of healthcare (Morris et al., 2015).

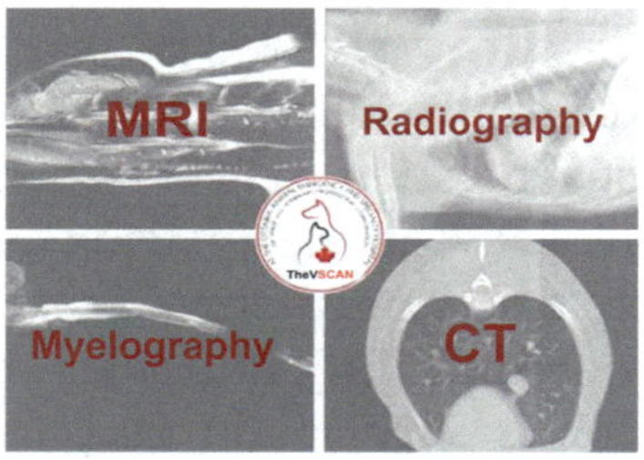

Figure 8.12. Comparison with other imaging modalities endoscopic ultrasound (EUS) serves.

Source: https://static.wixstatic.com/media/425777_3d6010ca435844b78a8495a7cb814fe4~mv2.png/v1/fill/w_528,h_408,al_c,q_85,enc_auto/425777_3d6010ca435844b78a8495a7cb814fe4~mv2.png.

While it is a great modality with many advantages, EUS does have some drawbacks relative to other imaging modalities. As one example, it is operator-dependent and may not necessarily be equally accessible in any clinical setting, leading to unequal access for the patient. While EUS is better at imaging gastrointestinal structures, its decreased ability to diagnose extra-luminal disease may be a drawback when diagnosing some malignancies that have spread outside the gastrointestinal tract. Further, while CT and MRI provide complete evaluation of distant metastases and whole body staging, EUS typically is limited to regional staging. Therefore, it becomes important for the clinician to choose the most appropriate imaging modality according to the individual clinical context of the patient, balancing the particular strengths and limitations of each modality so as to optimize diagnostic yield and treatment planning (Azzopardi, 2013) (Figure 8.12).

8.5. Endoscopic Ultrasound (EUS) in Clinical Practice

The integration of EUS into clinical practice has revolutionized the diagnosis of gastrointestinal and hepatobiliary disease. One of the significant applications of EUS is that it provides high-resolution images of the liver, aiding in the diagnosis and typing of most focal liver lesions and parenchymal liver disease. Unlike traditional imaging techniques, EUS enables direct visualization, and hence clinicians are able to assess liver segments with high accuracy. It also plays a role in demarcating collateral circulation in portal hypertensive patients and has not only diagnostic significance but also prognostic significance. Due to such advancements, EUS has turned into a precious tool for gastroenterologists evaluating patients with complex hepatic pathology, largely bridging the imaging-therapeutics gap in modern medicine (Magalhães et al., 2017). Besides, EUS has gained prominence in clarifying controversies about using it in the staging of malignancies, most notably esophageal and gastric cancers. The nuances of these discussions mirror the multifaceted potential of EUS in actual practice. It is a good example that distinguishing the extent of invasion and nodal involvement profoundly influences treatment plans and outcomes. However, the selection of appropriate techniques, such as FNA gauge and the use of contrast agents, has been contentious among practitioners. These disputes mirror the continuous evolution of EUS methods and foretell a growing appreciation for maximizing diagnostic return with little procedural risk. Attention to these dynamics is essential to providers seeking to exploit EUS in oncologic situations (Trindade & Berzin, 2013). In addition to its diagnostic potential, EUS also has a therapeutic role that enhances its clinical utility. Techniques , such as EUS-guided FNA not only aid in obtaining tissue samples for histological examination but are also of pivotal therapeutic intervention in treating most conditions. For instance, EUS can be employed to drain pancreatic pseudocysts or abscesses that, in other situations, may need more invasive interventions. The ability of EUS to provide real-time imaging makes the procedure more precise and safe during the intervention and, overall, improves patient outcomes. As EUS continues to expand, both in use and technology, its dual role as both therapy and diagnostic tool reminds clinicians of the need for a clear understanding of its applications so that patients can receive appropriate and timely interventions based on their own needs (Magalhães et al., 2017).

8.5.1. Role in Gastroenterology

EUS is a valuable instrument in gastroenterology, and it is largely due to the fact that it can produce high-resolution images of the pancreas, gastrointestinal tract, and surrounding structures. It is a combination of the benefits of endoscopy and ultrasound imaging, allowing doctors to visualize and study numerous forms of gastrointestinal pathology. EUS is also the added advantage of being particularly valuable in evaluating lesions that may be challenging to evaluate with traditional imaging techniques , such as CT scans or MRI. With high-definition images obtained through EUS, diagnostic accuracy is enhanced, which is imperative for treatment planning. For instance, EUS-guided biopsies offer precise tissue sampling, which allows clinicians to diagnose conditions , such as gastrointestinal tumors and pancreatitis. Since it is a non-invasive technique, EUS has gained prominence as a must-have instrument for gastroenterologists, enhancing patient care through early and accurate diagnosis. The use of EUS is not limited to tumor diagnostics; it has also proven to be beneficial in assessing liver disease. The precise imaging features provided by EUS enable physicians to evaluate liver parenchyma and detect a range of focal liver lesions, enlightening their categorization and etiology. The application of EUS in portal hypertension cannot be overstressed since it provides data on collateral circulation and hemodynamics, pertinent factors to liver-impaired patients. Recent advances include the technique of EUS-guided portal vein catheterization which has greatly altered portal pressure measurement practice.

Advances contribute to intensifying the profound understanding of liver disease complexity and enhancing patient management who are affected. This convergence of EUS with liver disease is a classic example of the technique's versatility and usefulness in gastroenterology, demonstrating its increasing relevance in clinical application and study (Magalhães et al., 2017). Additionally, the application of EUS in pancreatic mass diagnosis has been given added strength by recent comparative research that highlights its efficacy compared to alternative imaging tests. For example, SHI research demonstrated that EUS was capable of detecting intratumoral flow with greater contrast-to-tissue ratios than conventional contrast-enhanced EUS. While diagnostic accuracy overall remains a problem, these advancements demonstrate improvement in optimizing the performance of EUS to detect malignant vs. benign masses. Application of such sophisticated techniques points to EUS's growing role in gastroenterology, bringing into focus its potential to enhance diagnostic accuracy and allow better patient management strategies. Continuation of imaging technology advancement under the EUS platform holds much promise for gastroenterologists in the future, as they increasingly rely on these devices to best control gastrointestinal ailments (Eisenbrey et al., 2017) (Figure 8.13).

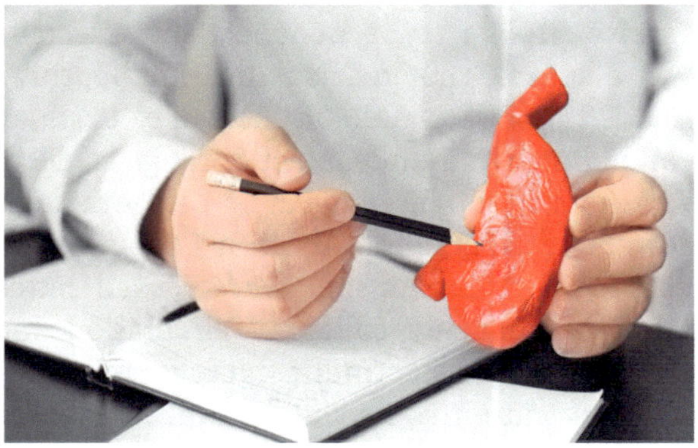

Figure 8.13. Role in gastroenterology.

Source: https://jindalgastroliverhospital.com/wp-content/uploads/2023/03/Understanding-the-Role-of-a-Gastroenterologist-1536x864-1.jpg.

8.5.2. Use in Oncology

EUS is a valuable innovation in the practice of oncology, particularly in the diagnosis and management of pancreatic cancer. The multi-functionality of EUS not only enhances diagnostic sensitivity but also provides crucial staging information that alters treatment planning. The ability of EUS to provide high-resolution images of pathology allows precise measurement of tumor size, location, and proximity to adjacent structures. As such, surgeons can better predict resectability intraoperatively, thus directing treatment instituted accordingly. Such a fundamental EUS role in the preoperative environment underscores its utility not only as a diagnostic modality but also as an integral component in refining cancer management strategies (Scott et al., 2017). Other than its use in the diagnosis, EUS has paved the way for new therapeutic uses, highlighting the role of EUS in oncology. Recent studies have indicated that the utilization of EUS can be optimized as a minimally invasive option for heat treatment , such as focused ultrasound-induced hyperthermia and ablation techniques. Specifically, research has suggested that cancer of various sizes in the pancreas could be treated optimally with transgastric or intraductal ultrasound therapy. These techniques enable physicians to deliver directed thermal energy, which can reduce tumor volume and optimize patient survival while limiting damage to adjacent tissue. This development in EUS technology represents a significant step, giving patients additional less invasive treatment methods that can be used within overall oncological treatment regimens (Scott et al., 2017). Apart from the treatment of established tumors, however, the role of EUS in canceratology also extends to the management of cancer and anticancer therapy complications. For instance, EUS-guided interventions have been employed for pain relief as well as for palliation of other symptoms of malignancies. It has also emerged as a helpful modality in guiding biopsies to reach inaccessible lesions, serving as a minimally invasive technique for obtaining tissue for histological examination. This feature not only confirms the verification of diagnoses but also aids in the assessment of therapeutic responses over the long term. EUS therefore secures its place in the oncology world, making both the diagnostic and therapy methods used in the fight against cancer stronger (Croagh et al., 2018).

8.5.3. Integration with Other Diagnostic Tools

Coupling of EUS with other devices for diagnosis makes pancreatic cancer diagnosis, as well as the treatment of cystic lesions, more accurate. EUS, characterized by its high-resolution imaging capabilities, may be complemented by imaging modalities , such as MRI and CT. If a cystic pancreatic lesion is detected, EUS allows for FNA for cytological sampling, which to be subsequently analyzed to determine the risk of malignancy. By correlating the imaging findings observed on EUS with the anatomical data from MRI and CT scans, clinicians are able to create an integrated image of the appearance of lesions. This multimodal imaging not only aids diagnosis but also makes treatment planning easier, through improved patient outcomes through more effective clinical decision-making. Further, the role of Rapid On-Site Evaluation (ROSE) in EUS-guided procedures is a significant development in bringing diagnostic devices together. Specifically, ROSE provides immediate assessment of aspirated material, providing real-time feedback on cytological features, most useful in the diagnosis of pancreatic cancer. By gaining information in a timely fashion, clinicians can directly determine the necessity of additional sampling or alternative treatment. The combination of EUS and ROSE thus enhances the diagnostic yield of pancreatic lesions significantly. The combination reduces the complexity of the diagnosis, shortening the period between assessment and treatment initiation, hence advancing the patient's diagnostic process and therapeutic outcomes (Carico et al., 2015). In managing pancreatic cystic lesions, combining clinical guidelines with imaging results is necessary. Various cystic neoplasms have varying potentials for malignancy, as highlighted inliterature (Azzopardi, 2013). EUS helps to define key characteristics of these lesions, such as size and septation, which are in accordance with surgical indications. Used in conjunction with serial imaging techniques, such as follow-up by MRI, application of EUS simultaneously enables clinicians to monitor changes and determine whether intervention is required, i.e., in lesions identified as being at high-risk stigmata. This dual application of both techniques makes for an active management approach that seeks to reconcile judicious surveillance with timely surgery, maximizing patient safety and therapeutic effectiveness under the shifting paradigms of pancreatic lesion management.

8.6. Future Directions in Endoscopic Ultrasound (EUS)

With EUS on the rise, perhaps the most optimistic for future research is the design of actively steerable endoscopic capsule robots. These developments represent a radical shift away from the passive capsule endoscopy that has been standard to date because it cannot provide concentrated diagnostic and therapeutic intervention in the gastrointestinal (GI) tract. Recent studies point to the creation of unsupervised real-time odometry and depth learning techniques that enhance motion estimation and depth recovery in such robotic platforms. Advanced algorithms are used in these technologies, which can facilitate real-time navigation and allow for greater localization of lesions and thus enhance diagnostic precision and treatment efficacy in complicated GI disorders (Turan et al., 2018). Integration of such technologies into EUS can lead to enhanced visualization and potential for minimally invasive intervention, ultimately leading to revolutionizing clinical practice. Aside from robotic system technological advancements, the future of EUS will likely be through enhanced imaging modalities that integrate conventional ultrasound with newer imaging modalities, such as elastography and contrast-enhanced EUS. Such methods have the promise of characterizing lesions and tissue parameters better and thus allowing for a more nuanced understanding of many pathologies, especially those involving pancreatic and biliary disease. Contrast-enhanced EUS specifically offers an added dimension of imaging through the capacity to quantify microvascularity in tumors, which should allow for differentiation between benign and malignant lesions. Since these imaging modalities get more advanced and are added to routine practice to utilize, their ability to provide information-rich data will greatly enhance the diagnostic yield of EUS, hence impacting patient management decisions (Portilla et al., 2024). This interdisciplinary approach holds the key to better individualized treatment regimens and better patient outcomes in the future. Further, the ongoing research into the therapeutic applications of EUS will pave the way for its broader acceptance as an integral diagnostic and therapeutic modality for gastroenterology. Advances , such as the development of techniques , such as EUS-guided FNA and EUS-guided tissue acquisition, are already showing to be very valuable for histological sampling of deep locations. Possible future developments may include more accurate and less invasive tissue sampling methods, including integration with real-time molecular diagnostics. Enhanced biomarker detection through EUS technology may also enable earlier diagnosis of cancers and tailor-made treatments, greatly enhancing the therapy of GI cancers. As the utility of EUS grows with innovation, it will increasingly play a key role in multidisciplinary treatment modalities, solidifying its place in contemporary gastroenterological practice (Figure 8.14).

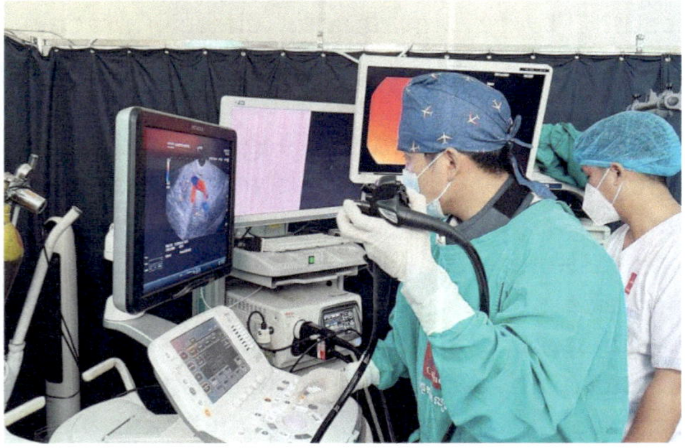

Figure 8.14. Future directions in the field of endoscopic ultrasound (EUS).

Source: http://nkdnews.com/wp-content/uploads/2023/04/ED0CCB06-E6EA-4A5C-BBB8-7ED874749D2E.jpeg.

8.6.1. Technological Advancements

Medical diagnosis has significantly improved with technological advancements, especially with the application of EUS. EUS combines endoscopy and ultrasound to provide a whole picture of the gastrointestinal tract and surrounding tissues, thereby facilitating the diagnosis of diseases. The application of imaging technologies provides real-time visualization of structures and therefore plays an important role in the diagnosis of diseases , such as tumors and pancreatitis. Further developments included optimizing the sensitivity and specificity of EUS, further facilitating its use in gastrointestinal diagnosis. In addition, improved imaging software and image analysis techniques have made enhanced image interpretation possible, leading to more accurate appraisal and better-informed therapy selection. This fusion of technology and medicine not only improves clinical outcomes but is also a revolutionary milestone towards minimally invasive practices with a greater focus on patient comfort and safety. The development of endoscopic approaches has not only revolutionized diagnostic applications but also paved the way for extended therapeutic intervention through the utilization of instruments , such as ultrasonic surgical instruments. These new devices offer an enormous improvement in precision and efficiency in performing surgery on delicate areas, such as the oral and maxillofacial regions. Developments in ultrasonic cutting devices, which operate at certain resonant frequencies, have led to stunning improvements in the outcomes of surgery, particularly in the maintenance of surrounding blood vessel and nerve tissues from injury. Such technology allows for greater control in procedure, enabling surgeons to perform intricate tasks with unprecedented accuracy. Despite this, there exist challenges, most notably the nonlinear dynamic behaviors exhibited by such devices, which affect performance. However, ongoing research and development activity continues to address these challenges to produce a future generation of useful ultrasonic endoscopic surgical devices that will continue to enhance patient care and clinical practice (Cardoni et al., 2015). In addition, the development of steerable endoscopic capsule robots is a cutting-edge innovation in minimally invasive diagnosis. These emerging devices are active, with the potential to move within the gastrointestinal tract, enhancing the capacity to detect diseases and deliver targeted interventions right onto the area of interest. With real-time odometry and depth sensing, such technologies yield more natural and precise diagnoses compared to the traditional passive capsule endoscopy methods. Research demonstrating these improvements has indicated increased motion estimation and depth recovery, demonstrating their application in navigating complex anatomical structures (Turan et al., 2018). With every improvement in the functionalities and capabilities of these endoscopic capsule robots, there arises a greater potential for paradigm-shifting use in gastrointestinal diagnostics. This intersection of robotics with endoscopic practice represents a potentially fertile new field in medical technology, driving advancement toward more effective, patient-centered alternatives.

8.6.2. Potential for New Applications

The potential for novel applications of EUS is one of the greatest advances in diagnostic and therapeutic gastroenterology. EUS has been applied historically to assess a broad spectrum of gastrointestinal disorders, but research is advancing rapidly, which can bring out its potential into more unusual applications. One area of considerable promise is the application of EUS with ultrasonic surgical equipment. These tools, powered by ultrasonic technology, have been impressive in cutting mineralized tissue without causing extensive collateral damage to surrounding anatomical structures. Using new multi-half-wavelength designs, researchers are beginning to find out how to lengthen these tools for use through the endoscope, which could completely revolutionize surgical technique for more advanced procedures, increasing patient safety and procedure efficiency (Cardoni et al., 2015). Moreover, EUS can be an important step towards improving the diagnosis of cancer, particularly pancreatic cancer, which is one of the most malignant cancers. The existing diagnostic approaches are not good, as only a minority of patients can be potential candidates for curative resection, and available treatments offer only modest effects regarding survival. Progress in liquid biopsy technology over the past few years has provided new potential for tumor early detection, primarily by the characterization of circulating tumor cells.

The abilities of EUS to assist in their detection may provide additional information regarding tumor genomics and also contribute to earlier intervention. With evolving research, EUS can be optimally positioned to transform the diagnostic workup of pancreatic cancer by offering non-invasive methods of monitoring disease and response to therapy, thereby bettering patient outcomes (Pimienta et al., 2017). Furthermore, the integration of EUS with emerging technologies has limitless potential. For instance, the use of EUS coupled with artificial intelligence (AI) and machine learning will enhance imaging analysis and diagnostic sensitivity.

Algorithms developed using AI can analyze ultrasound images with increased precision, identifying patterns that are not seen by humans and thus improving the precision of diagnoses. In addition, merging EUS with therapeutic modalities, such as targeted drug delivery systems, can optimize treatment regimens by allowing oncologists to deliver drugs to tumor sites while minimizing systemic exposure and side effects. The recent investigations on these novel applications of EUS stress the need for interdisciplinary partnerships to explore its full therapeutic and diagnostic potential and hold promise for revolutionary enhancements in patient management and improved clinical outcomes in various branches of medicine (Figure 8.15).

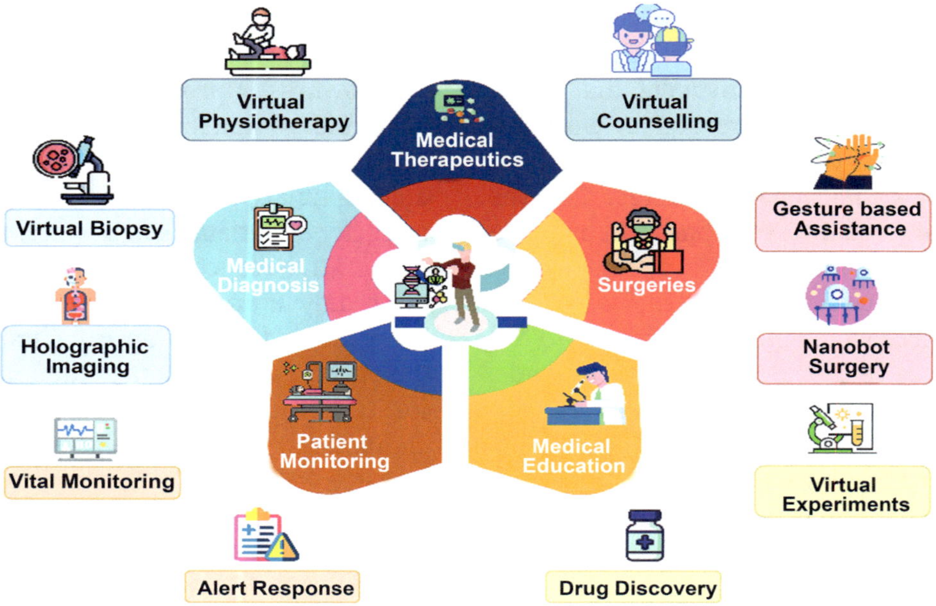

Figure 8.15. Potential for new applications.

Source: https://www.researchgate.net/publication/367971686/figure/fig4/AS:11431281117119233@1675384937760/Potential-Applications-of-the-Metaverse-in-Healthcare.png.

8.6.3. Research and Clinical Trials

Research and clinical trials are key to the innovation and development of EUS, particularly in the management and diagnosis of gastrointestinal disease. EUS has emerged as a fundamental imaging tool, with the ability to visualize inside structures within the body with accuracy. With evolving clinical practice, systematic research must be carried out to not only identify the strengths and limitations of EUS but also to determine the efficacy of EUS in varying clinical scenarios. The trials in recent times have explored the use of EUS for the evaluation of pancreatic lesions, leading to improved diagnostic accuracy and therapeutic intervention. By conducting meticulous clinical trials, researchers are able to obtain solid evidence and create evidence-based treatment protocols that maximize patient outcomes, quantifying the strong impact of research on clinical use of this revolutionary method. The research into the effectiveness of different treatments through EUS has paved the way for revolutionary changes in treatment techniques, particularly in the treatment of pancreatic cystic lesions. With the growing rates of such lesions, research has been drawn towards the line of endoscopic ultrasound-guided therapy, with chemoablation techniques. Endoscopic ultrasound-guided chemoablation has shown promising results as per recent studies for the management of neoplastic pancreatic cysts, offering the advantage of minimal invasive resection over surgical resection.

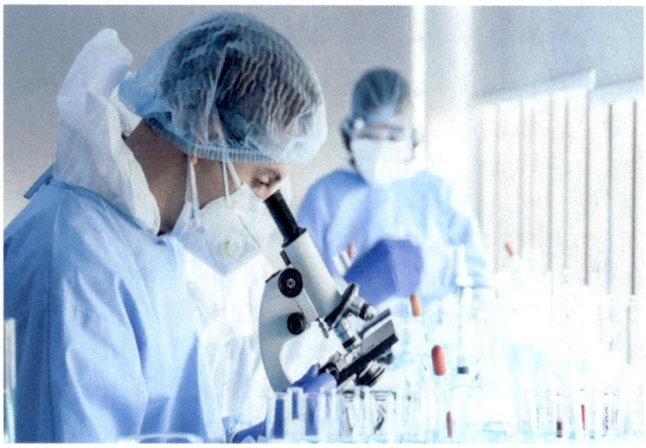

Figure 8.16. Research and clinical trials.

Source: https://altusresearch.com/wp-content/uploads/2021/07/shutterstock_1726134715-scaled.jpg.

This transition towards minimally invasive interventions not only reduces surgery-related morbidity but also highlights the significance of continuous research and clinical trials in refining such methods. For instance, surpassing safety concerns previously linked to alcohol-based ablation methods, innovative drug formulations have emerged that enhance patient safety profiles, justifying the necessity of continuous research in establishing clinical practice (Moyer et al., 2019). In addition to progress in treatment therapies, research in EUS has shown the urgent necessity for devising sound methods for systematic reviews and meta-analyses. Outcomes of these systematic reviews highlight the necessity for high-quality evidence in examining the applications of EUS for therapeutic treatments and the detection of cancer in various clinical conditions. Furthermore, as can be clearly seen through studies on the reliability of electronic databases , such as MEDLINE for retrieving relevant research, clinicians and researchers must make available quality data to inform their practice maximally (Berry et al., 2000). Through the integration of systematic research and clinical trials in the evaluation of EUS, physicians can remain at the forefront of diagnostic technologies and thereby improve patient care and treatment outcomes across medical specialties (Figure 8.16).

SUMMARY

With the development of EUS reaching its conclusion, it is significant to acknowledge its priceless contribution to modern medicine, particularly in optimizing diagnostic and therapeutic interventions. The findings of these studies demonstrate that EUS provides unparalleled insight into gastrointestinal illness anatomy and pathology, thereby enabling precise evaluation and planning for treatment. The ability to image inaccessible structures with standard imaging has established EUS as a mandatory resource for practitioners. With such technology continuing to advance, its use in clinical practice will expand even further, cementing its role as an integral component of endoscopic procedures. Also, variations in learning curves of advanced endoscopy trainees, reported in recent assessments, underscore the need for systematic training and continuous feedback in learning EUS skills. The establishment of a centralized database, according to the study, allows tracking of individual progress and comparison between training congregations. Interestingly, it was shown in the findings that there was high competence attained by most of the trainees at the end of their programs, indicating the capability of EUS training in developing competent practitioners. These realities are crucial not only for the quality improvement of training programs but also to make sure that future practitioners shall be in a position to provide high-quality care in their personal practices (Wani et al., 2017). Passage through the universe of EUS thus helps to demonstrate not only its clinical utility but also that meticulous planning of training and assessment frameworks is vital. As shown, proper utilization of competency assessment tools is pivotal in guaranteeing excellence during surgery. Due to advances in technology, it is possible that EUS may grow more advanced, enhancing its diagnostic capability even more. Consequently, there will be a need to integrate study results into learning systems to equip future generations of endoscopists with the skills needed to tackle the intricacies of gastrointestinal disease (Han et al., 2013). Lastly, EUS's future rests on its adaptive integration into clinical practice, driven by extensive training and ongoing academic investigation.

EUS is now an essential diagnostic and therapeutic tool in gastroenterology, providing high-resolution imaging and access for focal interventions. The evolving paradigms in education and training spell a requirement for a well-delineated competency framework for endoscopy. There have been studies in the recent past showing that there is considerable emphasis on the learning curve development among advanced endoscopy trainees (AETs) with particular importance given to procedures like EUS and ERCP. The evidence indicates that training programs are now increasingly validating EUS competency with formal testing, enhancing the skill set of potential specialists. Data obtained from more than one program is representative of the varied experiences of AETs in progressing toward mastery of EUS and thus providing actionable suggestions for the enhancement of training policies (Wani et al., 2017). In managing the issues of training in EUS, the Joint Advisory Group on GI Endoscopy (JAG) has promoted an evidence-based process for certification. This initiative stems from the knowledge that credentialing practices worldwide range significantly, resulting in variation in EUS competency. By using a Delphi variation process, key stakeholders as a group arrived at essential competencies necessary for independent practice. Recommendations made through this process are to undergo a minimum of 250 hands-on procedures before competency evaluation is conducted, putting formal training protocols first, and implementing mentorship within the first year following certification. These steps are designed to create an evidence-based route that optimizes EUS training quality and safety and, ultimately, patient outcomes in the UK and Ireland (El Menabawey et al., 2023). Specifically, the role of continuous evaluation systems in

EUS training programs cannot be overemphasized. Evidence from various studies indicates that systematic feedback mechanisms facilitate the detection of learning gaps among AETs in real-time, thus allowing for targeted interventions. For instance, applying a competency assessment tool in EUS programs serves as an example of routine monitoring of performance with the facilitation of comparisons between peers. This innovative practice ensures timely counsel to trainees and enables them to particularly address specific issues encountered during training. Lastly, this focus on evidence-based assessment and mentoring secures the foundation for delivering quality EUS services in a manner such that practitioners attain the standard of care needed in clinical practice (Wani et al., 2017).

CLOSER LOOK:

CERTAIN ANATOMICAL VARIATIONS:

Anatomical variations are naturally occurring differences in the structure of body parts that deviate from what is traditionally considered "normal" anatomy. These variations are common and usually benign, but they can have significant implications for clinical practice, surgery, imaging interpretation, and personalized medicine. Understanding these variations is essential for healthcare providers to prevent diagnostic errors, surgical complications, and misinterpretation of radiological studies. Variations can affect virtually any system of the body. In the cardiovascular system, for example, the branching patterns of arteries and veins frequently differ among individuals. The renal arteries may have accessory branches in some people, and the circle of Willis in the brain can exhibit incomplete or asymmetrical formations. Such variations are critical to recognize during procedures like angiography, neurosurgery, or renal transplantation, as unawareness can lead to hemorrhage or inadequate perfusion.

Musculoskeletal variations are also common. Muscles may be absent, duplicated, or exhibit unusual insertions or origins. For instance, the palmaris longus, a forearm muscle, is absent in roughly 14% of the population, which is typically clinically insignificant but may influence tendon grafting decisions. Similarly, variations in the branching of peripheral nerves, such as the median or ulnar nerves, can alter patterns of sensory and motor innervation, impacting outcomes in surgeries or nerve repair procedures.

Visceral anatomy exhibits notable variation as well. The position and morphology of organs like the liver, spleen, or kidneys can differ, sometimes resulting in clinical presentations that mimic disease. For example, a retroaortic left renal vein or a horseshoe kidney may be discovered incidentally during imaging but can influence surgical planning or predispose individuals to complications like obstruction or vascular compression. Awareness of anatomical variations is also vital in radiology. Variants such as accessory fissures in the lungs, cervical rib, or atypical vertebral shapes can be mistaken for pathological lesions if not recognized. Advances in imaging modalities, including CT, MRI, and 3D reconstruction, have improved detection and understanding of these variants, enabling safer interventions.

In conclusion, anatomical variations are a natural and frequent aspect of human biology. While most are asymptomatic, their recognition is crucial in clinical, surgical, and diagnostic settings. A thorough understanding of these differences enhances patient safety, informs surgical planning, and prevents misdiagnosis, highlighting the importance of individualized approaches to anatomy rather than a one-size-fits-all perspective.

REFERENCES

1. Tringali, A., Thomson, M., Dumonceau, J. M., Tavares, M., Tabbers, M. M., Furlano, R., Spaander, M., Hassan, C., Tzvinikos, C., Ijsselstijn, H., Viala, J., Dall'Oglio, L., Benninga, M., Orel, R., Vandenplas, Y., Keil, R., Romano, C., Brownstone, E., Hlava, Š., Gerner, P., ... Zambelli, A. (2017). Pediatric gastrointestinal endoscopy: European Society of Gastrointestinal Endoscopy (ESGE) and European Society for Paediatric Gastroenterology Hepatology and Nutrition (ESPGHAN) Guideline Executive summary. *Endoscopy*, *49*(1), 83–91. https://doi.org/10.1055/s-0042-111002(accessed on 15th July 2025).

2. Adams, A., Alter, M., Berliner, L., Bird, N., Bizheva, K., et al. (2006). *Methods and application areas of endoscopic optical coherence tomography.* https://core.ac.uk/download/77927094.pdf (accessed on 15th July 2025).

3. Serena J. Scott, Matthew S. Adams, Vasant Salgaonkar, F. Graham Sommer, Chris J. Diederich(accessed on 15th July 2025).

4. Al-Haddad, M. A., DeWitt, J. M., & Luz, L. P. (2014). *EUS-guided celiac plexus interventions in pancreatic cancer pain: An update and controversies for the endosonographer.* https://core.ac.uk/download/46963820.pdf (accessed on 15th July 2025).

5. Wani, S., Keswani, R., Hall, M., Han, S., Ali, M. A., Brauer, B., Carlin, L., Chak, A., Collins, D., Cote, G. A., Diehl, D. L., DiMaio, C. J., Dries, A., El-Hajj, I., Ellert, S., Fairley, K., Faulx, A., Fujii-Lau, L., Gaddam, S., Gan, S. I., ... Early, D. S. (2017). A Prospective Multicenter Study Evaluating Learning Curves and Competence in Endoscopic Ultrasound and Endoscopic Retrograde Cholangiopancreatography Among Advanced Endoscopy Trainees: The Rapid Assessment of Trainee Endoscopy Skills Study. *Clinical gastroenterology and hepatology : the official clinical practice journal of the American Gastroenterological Association*, *15*(11), 1758–1767.e11. https://doi.org/10.1016/j.cgh.2017.06.012(accessed on 15th July 2025).

6. Allan, M., Azizian, M., Bodenstedt, S., Duggal, R., et al. (2019). *2017 Robotic Instrument Segmentation Challenge.* https://core.ac.uk/download/196652980.pdf (accessed on 15th July 2025).

7. Turan, M., Almalioglu, Y., Araujo, H. *et al.* A non-rigid map fusion-based direct SLAM method for endoscopic capsule robots. *Int J Intell Robot Appl* **1**, 399–409 (2017). https://doi.org/10.1007/s41315-017-0036-4(accessed on 15th July 2025).

8. Araki, M., Imaizumi, H., Iwai, T., Kida, M., et al. (2013). *Role of a forward-viewing echoendoscope in fine-needle aspiration.* https://core.ac.uk/download/pdf/81162800.pdf (accessed on 15th July 2025).

9. Azab, M., Bharadwaj, S., Hong, A. S., Jayaraj, M., et al. (2019). *Safety of endoscopic retrograde cholangiopancreatography (ERCP) in pregnancy: A systematic review and meta-analysis.* https://core.ac.uk/download/286611719.pdf (accessed on 15th July 2025).

10. Azzopardi, N. (2013). *Endoscopic ultrasound in the staging of gastrointestinal luminal malignancies.* https://core.ac.uk/download/46602401.pdf (accessed on 15th July 2025).

11. Bailey, M., Chi, T., Grubbs, R. H., Kenny, T., et al. (2015). *Targeted microbubbles: A novel application for the treatment of kidney stones.* https://core.ac.uk/download/33121584.pdf (accessed on 15th July 2025).

12. Bang, J., Bellis, M., Collins, D., DeWitt, J., Draganov, P., Farrell, J., et al. (2014). *Techniques for cytologic sampling of pancreatic and bile duct lesions.* https://deepblue.lib.umich.edu/bitstream/2027.42/106695/1/dc23096.pdf (accessed on 15th July 2025).
13. El Menabawey, T., McCrudden, R., Shetty, D., Hopper, A. D., Huggett, M. T., Bekkali, N., Carroll, N. R., Henry, E., Johnson, G. J., Keane, M. G., Love, M., McKay, C. J., Norton, S., Oppong, K., Penman, I., Ramesh, J., Ryan, B., Siau, K., & Nayar, M. (2023). UK and Ireland Joint Advisory Group (JAG) consensus statements for training and certification in diagnostic endoscopic ultrasound (EUS). *Gut, 73*(1), 118–130. https://doi.org/10.1136/gutjnl-2023-329800(accessed on 15th July 2025).
14. Berry, E., Harris, K. M., Hutton, J., Kelly, S., et al. (2000). *Identifying studies for systematic reviews – An example from medical imaging.* https://core.ac.uk/download/58595.pdf (accessed on 15th July 2025).
15. Trindade, A. J. ., & Berzin, T. M (2013). *Clinical Controversies in Endoscopic Ultrasound.* https://core.ac.uk/download/28948200.pdf (accessed on 15th July 2025).
16. Bill, J. G., Darcy, M., Early, D. S., Edmundowicz, S., et al. (2016). *A comparison between endoscopic ultrasound-guided rendezvous and percutaneous biliary drainage after failed ERCP for malignant distal biliary obstruction.* https://core.ac.uk/download/70385846.pdf (accessed on 15th July 2025).
17. Raza D, Singh S, Crinò SF, Boskoski I, Spada C, Fuccio L, Samanta J, Dhar J, Spadaccini M, Gkolfakis P, et al. Diagnostic Approach to Biliary Strictures. *Diagnostics*. 2025; 15(3):325. https://doi.org/10.3390/diagnostics15030325(accessed on 15th July 2025).
18. Cardoni, A., Cerisola, N., Lucas, M., Mathieson, I., et al. (2015). *Understanding nonlinear vibration behaviors in high-power ultrasonic surgical devices.* https://core.ac.uk/download/42360528.pdf (accessed on 15th July 2025).
19. Cardoso, R., Coburn, N. G., Helyer, L., Law, C., et al. (2011). *A systematic review of the accuracy and indications for diagnostic laparoscopy before curative-intent resection of gastric cancer.* https://core.ac.uk/download/37738520.pdf (accessed on 15th July 2025).
20. Carico, E., Carnuccio, A., DI GIULIO, E., Galasso, M., et al. (2015). *Rapid on-site evaluation (ROSE) in pancreatic cancer diagnosis: Doing more with less.* https://core.ac.uk/download/54521845.pdf (accessed on 15th July 2025).
21. Portilla, A. S. P., Portilla, C. S. P., Palacios, G. S. G., Rodríguez, B. S. P., Castillo, S. G. A., Espin, N. E. P., & Pita, G. P. M. (2024). The integration of surgical and dermatological techniques in the treatment of cutaneous aging: multidisciplinary approaches and clinical outcomes - a comprehensive systematic review of current literature. *International Journal of Research in Medical Sciences, 12*(5), 1659–1667. https://doi.org/10.18203/2320-6012.ijrms20240943 (accessed on 15th July 2025).
22. Magalhães, J., Monteiro, S., Xavier, S., Leite, S., de Castro, F. D., & Cotter, J. (2017). Endoscopic ultrasonography - emerging applications in hepatology. *World journal of gastrointestinal endoscopy, 9*(8), 378–388. https://doi.org/10.4253/wjge.v9.i8.378 (accessed on 15th July 2025).
23. Chan, A. C. Y., & Liu, C. L. (2003). *The role of endoscopic ultrasonography in the management of cystic lesions of the pancreas.* https://core.ac.uk/download/37884241.pdf (accessed on 15th July 2025).

24. Chen, Y., Dekker, E., Fockens, P., Lauwers, G., et al. (2014). *Miami classification for probe-based confocal laser endomicroscopy.* https://core.ac.uk/download/28949274.pdf (accessed on 15th July 2025).

25. Cochran, S., Cox, B. F., Cummins, G., Desmulliez, M. P. Y., et al. (2017). *Ultrasound Capsule Endoscopy: Sounding out the Future.* https://core.ac.uk/download/83925812.pdf (accessed on 15th July 2025).

26. Croagh, D., Day, D., McLaren, C. J., Segelov, E., et al. (2018). *Endoscopic Ultrasound in Pancreatic Cancer.* https://core.ac.uk/download/322436464.pdf (accessed on 15th July 2025).

27. Das, N., & Yip, M. (2017). *Robot Autonomy for Surgery.* http://arxiv.org/abs/1707.03080 (accessed on 15th July 2025).

28. Morris, S., Gurusamy, K. S., Sheringham, J., & Davidson, B. R. (2015). Cost-effectiveness analysis of endoscopic ultrasound versus magnetic resonance cholangiopancreatography in patients with suspected common bile duct stones. *PloS one, 10*(3), e0121699. https://doi.org/10.1371/journal.pone.0121699(accessed on 15th July 2025).

29. Moyer, M. T., Maranki, J. L., & DeWitt, J. M. (2019). EUS-Guided Pancreatic Cyst Ablation: a Clinical and Technical Review. *Current gastroenterology reports, 21*(5), 19. https://doi.org/10.1007/s11894-019-0686-5(accessed on 15th July 2025).

30. Eisenbrey, J. R., Forsberg, F., Fox, T., Kowalski, J., et al. (2017). *Subharmonic and endoscopic contrast imaging of pancreatic masses: A pilot study.* https://core.ac.uk/download/213449737.pdf (accessed on 15th July 2025).

31. García Flores, J. R., Mendieta Zerón, H., & Romero Prieto, M. L. (2009). *Limitations in improving detection of pancreatic adenocarcinoma.* https://core.ac.uk/download/635718762.pdf (accessed on 15th July 2025).

32. Han, L., Ho, J. C. M., Ip, M. S. M., Lam, D. C. L., et al. (2013). *Endobronchial ultrasound-guided transbronchial needle aspiration in lung cancer: The first experience in Hong Kong.* https://core.ac.uk/download/38026152.pdf (accessed on 15th July 2025).

33. Jednačak, H., Klarica, M., Miklić, P., Mrak, G., et al. (2011). *The application of ultrasound in neuroendoscopic procedures: First results with the new tool "NECUP-2."* https://core.ac.uk/download/11699986.pdf (accessed on 15th July 2025).

34. Kim, C., Kim, J. Y., Lee, C., Lim, H., et al. (2025). *A PDMS-based 2-axis Waterproof Scanner for Photoacoustic Microscopy.* https://core.ac.uk/download/148822049.pdf (accessed on 15th July 2025).

35. Alali, A. A., & Barkun, A. N. (2023). An update on the management of non-variceal upper gastrointestinal bleeding. *Gastroenterology report, 11*, goad011. https://doi.org/10.1093/gastro/goad011(accessed on 15th July 2025).

36. Pimienta, M., Edderkaoui, M., Wang, R., & Pandol, S. (2017). *The potential for circulating tumor cells in pancreatic cancer management.* https://core.ac.uk/download/323077820.pdf (accessed on 15th July 2025).

37. Serna, A. ., & Prieto, F (2017). *Hacia el modelado 3D de tumores cerebrales mediante endoneurosonografía y redes neuronales.* Towards a 3D modeling of brain tumors by using endoneurosonography and neural networks*

38. Revista Ingenierías Universidad de Medellín, vol. 16, no. 30, pp. 129-148, 2017 https://core.ac.uk/download/84398959.pdf (accessed on 15th July 2025).
39. Troccaz, J. (2009). *Computer- and robot-assisted medical intervention.* http://arxiv.org/abs/0903.4545 (accessed on 15th July 2025).

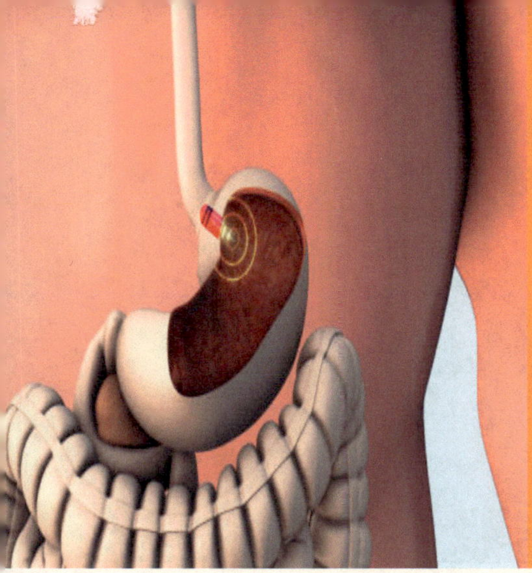

Chapter 9

CAPSULE ENDOSCOPY

Contents

Introduction to Capsule Endoscopy 249
9.1. The Technology Behind Capsule Endoscopy 253
9.2. Indications for Capsule Endoscopy (CE) 257
9.3. Procedure and Patient Experience 260
9.4. Advantages of Capsule Endoscopy 263
9.5. Limitations and Challenges 267
9.6. Future Directions in Capsule Endoscopy 270
Summary 274
References 277

Introduction to Capsule Endoscopy

Capsule endoscopy is a significant advance in gastrointestinal (GI) diagnostics that has revolutionized the visualization and assessment of gastrointestinal disease. Compared to other endoscopic procedures, which are often invasive, capsule endoscopy uses a small, pill-sized camera that can be ingested by patients. This technology has broken down many of the challenges that accompany conventional endoscopic methods, such as discomfort and complications that arise from the need for devices to be delivered through the mouth or anus. The contemporary design of capsule endoscopes has improved patient compliance and the variety of diseases that can effectively be diagnosed by medical practitioners. Hence, the technology became forefront after its discovery, with more and more publications in support of its capacity to identify small intestine pathologies, which are generally hard to reach through ordinary endoscopy. While having numerous advantages, capsule endoscopy has certain disadvantages too. The biggest drawbacks are its reliance on white light imaging, which permits visualization of the mucosal surface alone and does not allow deeper pathologies. This constraint is most critical, especially since many gastrointestinal illnesses reach layers deeper than the mucosa and thus need more thorough imaging methods. For instance, certain illnesses , such as Crohn's disease, present deeper within the GI tract, and transmural imaging is the only means of correctly diagnosing it.

Advances indicate the incorporation of ultrasound technology into capsule endoscopy, which has the potential to create these voids. The potential development of ultrasound capsule endoscopy (USCE) can improve diagnostic capability tremendously by performing high-resolution scanning that allows qualitative and quantitative measurements of the bowel wall, bridging the limitations of current imaging modalities (Cochran et al., 2017). Further research into improved radiation characteristics for capsule endoscopic equipment must be conducted to render them more efficient. Studying has confirmed that traditional methods of diagnosing GI diseases are constrained by the limitations in existing sensor technology, particularly that used in the small intestines, which can be better addressed with wireless sensing advancements (Chirwa et al., 2003). Improved telemetry systems will allow better receipt of data from the capsule during its passage through the GI tract, thereby facilitating real-time observation and analysis. As the technology evolves, future studies will likely equip next-generation capsule endoscopes with enhanced imaging modalities, ultimately making the final decision regarding increased diagnostic accuracy. With such innovations, capsule endoscopy is set to face a revolutionary transformation in the future, promising better outcomes for patients who come with complex GI diseases (Figure 9.1).

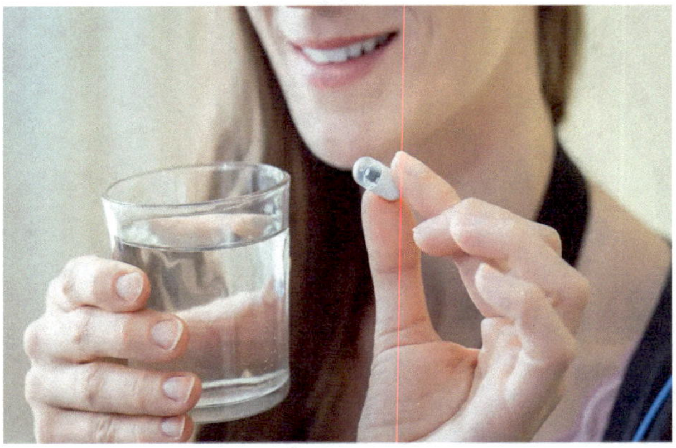

Figure 9.1. Capsule endoscopy.

Source: https://sa1s3optim.patientpop.com/filters:format(webp)/ assets/production/practices/b712dea6a15fd49dab32b645087733271271e3eb/ images/2514766.jpg.

Definition and Purpose of Capsule Endoscopy

The discovery of capsule endoscopy constituted an important leap forward in gastrointestinal diagnosis, bringing an endoscopy facility to visualizing the small intestine in a non-invasive way. In contrast to conventional endoscopic methods involving sedation and invasive procedures, capsule endoscopy entails the patient swallowing a miniature, pill-sized camera that takes high-resolution photos of the digestive system as it passes through the gastrointestinal tract. This new technology is particularly valuable for the diagnosis of cryptic gastrointestinal bleeding and illnesses , such as Crohn's disease. The capsule moves through the digestive tract by itself, transmitting images to an outside recording device. How easy and safe this procedure is makes it an invaluable tool for clinicians who wish to diagnose and monitor gastrointestinal disease quickly, creating new possibilities for early detection and treatment. The function of capsule endoscopy goes beyond plain visualization; it is an extensive diagnostic technique enabling the evaluation of mucosal surfaces. Standard optical methods tend to be limited in their capability to view deeper layers of gastrointestinal tissue, therefore possibly missing vital subtle alterations involved with disease development. In doing so, capsule endoscopy provides a complete assessment of the small intestine, identifying lesions, mucosal lesions, and inflammatory changes that may reflect more sinister underlying processes. The distinct capacity of techniques to obtain wide images of the gastrointestinal tract permits healthcare professionals to make informed decisions regarding further investigation or therapy. As a result, capsule endoscopy not only enhances diagnostic accuracy but also possibly enhances patient outcomes in patients with complex gastrointestinal disease. Advances in technology in recent times have further enhanced the efficiency of capsule endoscopy. The application of computerized processing and sophisticated learning models in analyzing endoscopy images has facilitated the successful extraction and interpretation of texture features from the data obtained.

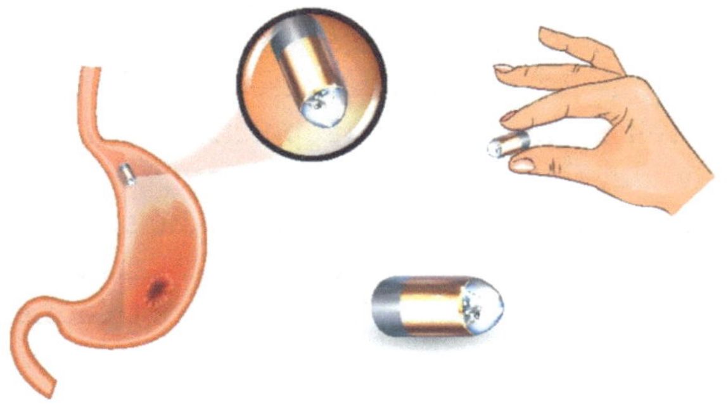

Figure 9.2. Purpose of capsule endoscopy.

Source: https://ghealth121.com/wp-content/uploads/2020/11/Capsule-Endoscopy-Image.jpg.

These technologies have the potential to supplement traditional methods by recognizing patterns typical of disease at an earlier stage, as suggested by new imaging analysis methods (Wadge et al., 2005). Moreover, the study of microultrasound modalities has potential in the identification of cellular changes associated with inflammatory bowel diseases, illustrating the need for complementary modalities for the boost in diagnostic capability within gastroenterology (Lay et al., 2017). With the development in the field, the future could bring about marked change with capsule endoscopy and emerging technologies, revolutionizing the diagnosis and management of gastrointestinal disease and highlighting its pivotal position in modern healthcare (Figure 9.2).

Historical Development of the Technology

The evolution over time of capsule endoscopy is a big step forward in gastrointestinal diagnosis, offering an alternative to traditional endoscopy that is not invasive. This was achieved primarily during the late 20th century, when scientists tried to better visualize the small intestine, which before had been tricky due to the limitations of classical endoscopy. Early development of imaging technologies laid the foundation for capsule design, culminating in the invention of the first ingestible capsule camera by Given Imaging in 2000. This novel device enabled clinicians to take high-quality images of the mucosal lining along the gastrointestinal tract, significantly enhancing diagnostic capabilities for such conditions as Crohn's disease and obscure gastrointestinal bleeding. With increasing clinical applications, the era of capsule endoscopy underwent a transformation, prompting further research in image quality improvement, capsule design, and patient-centered areas that would ultimately enhance the overall healthcare experience. Further advances in capsule endoscopy have included bowel preparation methods and diagnostic algorithms. Research, including studies conducted in multicenter trials, has shed light on the pivotal role played by bowel cleansing regimens to optimize the imaging capacity of capsule endoscopy. For instance, studies have contrasted varied preparation methods in direct comparison, demonstrating that the addition of oral sulfate solutions and diatrizoate agents can significantly increase rates of completion and the overall efficiency of the procedure. As a specific example, application of alternative regimens has provided favorable outcomes in the determination of adequate bowel cleansing, thus sustaining the usefulness of preparation in diagnostic accuracy (Burch et al., 2017). This continued optimization of pre-procedure preparations is proof of the changing nature of capsule endoscopy technology, ensuring not just improved diagnostic returns but also enhanced patient safety and comfort throughout procedures. More importantly, the economic implications of capsule endoscopy have become more highlighted as healthcare systems turn to efficient diagnostic procedures. Use of wireless capsule endoscopy (WCE) has been established as a cost-effective alternative to traditional diagnostic methods for diseases like Crohn's disease. Research indicates that WCE not only provides higher diagnostic yields but also overall decreases the expenditure in healthcare through less repetitive testing and prolonged patient care. By taking up WCE as a first-line diagnostic tool, clinicians are in a position to diagnose gastrointestinal disorders at a lower cost to both patients and healthcare workers (Goldfarb et al., 2004). With continued advances in technology, ongoing tests of its utility and cost-effectiveness will be key to deciding the direction of gastrointestinal diagnostics in the future and improving outcomes for patients.

Role in Modern Gastrointestinal Diagnostics

The advent of capsule endoscopy has revolutionized modern gastrointestinal diagnosis, even more so for the evaluation of the small intestine. Traditional methods often imposed limitations, which posed challenges in the detection of varied conditions , such as small bowel hemorrhage or Crohn's disease. However, capsule endoscopy introduces a less invasive method that provides unobstructed access to the gastrointestinal tract, resulting in enhanced diagnostic potential. This technology has proven to be especially valuable for those patients for whom they cannot apply the usual endoscopic investigation due to anatomical constraints or comorbidities. Through enabling a more complete view into small bowel disease, capsule endoscopy serves not just as a diagnostic tool but also as an integral part of the overall management and treatment plan for gastrointestinal illness, a tremendous advance in clinical practice. In recent years, with the addition of capsule endoscopy to advanced imaging modalities, its use in gastrointestinal diagnostics has further expanded. For instance, the incorporation of capsule endoscopy and balloon-assisted enteroscopy has not only enabled effective visualization but also obtained biopsies from suspicious lesions detected during capsules' passage. This integrated modality enables increased diagnosis of small intestinal conditions, such as Crohn's disease. In accordance with recent research, imaging modalities have not only become essential for the diagnosis of these disorders but also essential for monitoring disease progression as well as therapeutic responses. With every new development in gastroenterology, the utility of these combined diagnostic strategies becomes increasingly apparent, enhancing patient outcomes and shaping future treatment paradigms in the gastrointestinal tract (Hausmann & Albert, 2011). Additionally, the contribution of contemporary diagnostic tools, most notably those acquired through endoscopic practice, is urging a more preventive stance in medicine. The latest developments in endoscopy, best noted with developments , such as chromoendoscopy and magnification endoscopy, highlight early diagnosis as essential for enhancing prognoses in conditions like colorectal cancer. As evidenced in current practice questionnaires, such strategies are essential in rigorous screening modalities for the identification of very small neoplastic lesions that would go unnoticed with standard endoscopic methods (Arebi & Saunders, 2005). This push toward more sophisticated diagnostic technology in endoscopy not only augments detection rates but also reduces the necessity for invasive surgery, giving sound reasons for the requirement of continuous development in gastrointestinal diagnostics. As we continue to embrace these advancements, the landscape of gastrointestinal healthcare is poised for significant improvements, promising a future where patient care is both precise and tailored to individual needs (Figure 9.3).

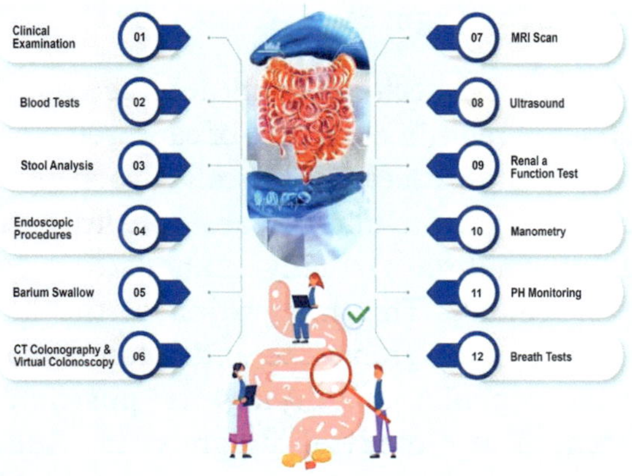

Figure 9.3. Importance in modern gastrointestinal diagnostics.

Source: https://www.reddit.com/media?url=https%3A%2F%2Fpreview.redd.it%2Fa-cool-guide-diagnostic-tests-for-gastrointestinal-v0-jt43ibgi167b1.jpg%3Fwidth%3D1080%26crop%3Dsmart%26auto%3Dwebp%26s%3D10ed70db806e32734289e5d351ad38d8fe3b659f.

9.1. The Technology Behind Capsule Endoscopy

Capsule endoscopy is a revolutionary step in gastrointestinal diagnosis, characterized by non-invasiveness and patient-friendliness. It began with the invention of wireless capsule endoscopy (WCE) in 2000, which enabled visualization of the digestive tract in its entirety without the usual discomfort caused by the standard endoscopic test. Through avoidance of sedation, WCE not only enhanced patient cooperation but has also facilitated easier mass screening programs for intestinal polyps and bleeding. With healthcare systems grappling with increasing digestive system diseases, WCE's innovative design places it at the center as a potential substitute to traditional methods, set to revolutionize diagnosis and treatment of gastrointestinal disease (Turan et al., 2018). Increased technological advancement in capsule endoscopy is shifting towards the integration of active locomotion capabilities, which will greatly enhance the diagnostic capability of capsule endoscopes. Progress in the past few years has resulted in studies on steerable endoscopic capsule robots, which are in development to travel precisely along the gastrointestinal tract. These technologies are driven by the necessity of improving disease diagnosis and enabling targeted treatment, for example, biopsy-like interventions or localized drug therapy. With the application of unsupervised, real-time odometry and depth learning techniques, these advanced capsules are capable of performing sophisticated procedures autonomously, significantly improving diagnostic sensitivity and clinical performance (Turan et al., 2018). With continued progress, these technologies will fundamentally transform the methodological strategy of gastrointestinal imaging. The strength of capsule endoscopy lies not just in its diagnostic feature but also in its therapeutic value within the gastrointestinal tract. The development of robotic capsule endoscopes with micro-robotic functions allows prospective infusion of therapeutic interventions at the site of detection. This paradigm also suggests that future generations of capsule endoscopy may become critical in diagnosis and even treatment, with the potential to possibly reduce the need for individual surgical interventions.

As the technology continues to evolve, the focus on integrating these advanced technologies underscores the challenge of responding to the burgeoning issue created by an aging demographic and rising incidence of digestive disorders. Lastly, ongoing evolution of capsule endoscopy remains crucial, rendering it a pillar of modern gastrointestinal medicine (Ciuti et al., 2016) (Figure 9.4).

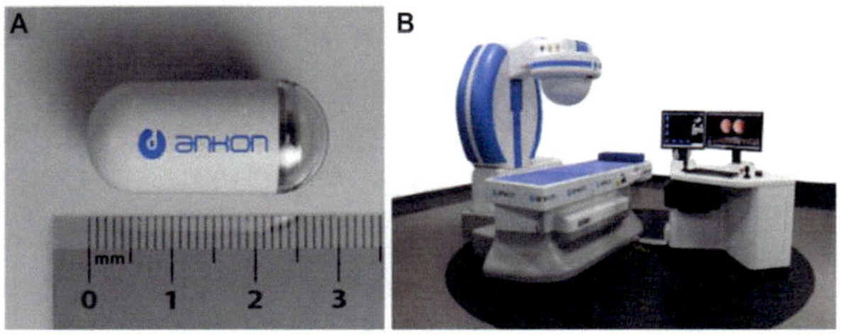

Figure 9.4. Technology behind capsule endoscopy.

Source: https://www.researchgate.net/publication/354865592/figure/fig1/AS:11431281386327872@1745064471594/The-magnetic-controlled-capsule-endoscopy-system-A-The-NaviCam-capsule-endo-scope.tif.

9.1.1. Description of the Capsule Design and Components

The very innovation in capsule endoscopy owes quite a lot to the innovative design of the capsule itself, which has been highly cleverly engineered to carry out a host of diagnostic functions. The focal point of such a design is a tiny, swallowable pill, most often containing a light source, a tiny camera, and a transmitter. The tiny camera snaps high-resolution images of the gastrointestinal tract as it travels naturally through the body, providing physicians with an unprecedented view of inner tissues and pathology. This technological innovation has been able to convert a previously intrusive test into a non-invasive test, minimizing pain for the patient while enhancing diagnostic accuracy. Furthermore, the incorporation of an image compressor allows for effective data storage, allowing maximum data during the transit through the body (Intzes et al., 2015). The capsule design also incorporates advanced wireless communication technologies, which are necessary for real-time data transmission. Operating in the main at the 2.45 GHz Industrial, Scientific and Medical band provides improved data rates with high-definition video streaming that supports gastrointestinal visuals' real-time monitoring. Frequency choice not only supports higher bandwidth on which data can be carried but also optimizes antenna performance, important to prevent signal loss through the human body (Agneessens et al., 2013).

These high-tech communication components enable the real-time passage of captured images to an outside receiver, typically worn by the patient, so that clinicians are able to review the information virtually immediately after the procedure. This integration of the latest technology also grants the entire functionality of the capsule, solidifying its position in contemporary medical diagnostics. Adding to the utility of the capsule is its power management system, designed to deliver long-term operation with consistent performance. Power sources, typically in the form of batteries incorporated into the capsule, are designed for extended use without discomfort or additional intervention to the patient. Efficient energy usage, along with the capsule being lightweight and aerodynamically shaped, enables it to pass smoothly through the gastrointestinal tract. This careful design of components leads to a versatile and user-friendly device, which not only meets its primary diagnostic purpose but also opens the door for further development of gastrointestinal imaging. By merging innovative design features with state-of-the-art technology, capsule endoscopy provides doctors with an effective and informative tool for assessing gastrointestinal wellness, emphasizing the wider importance of its innovative design (Intzes et al., 2015) (Figure 9.5).

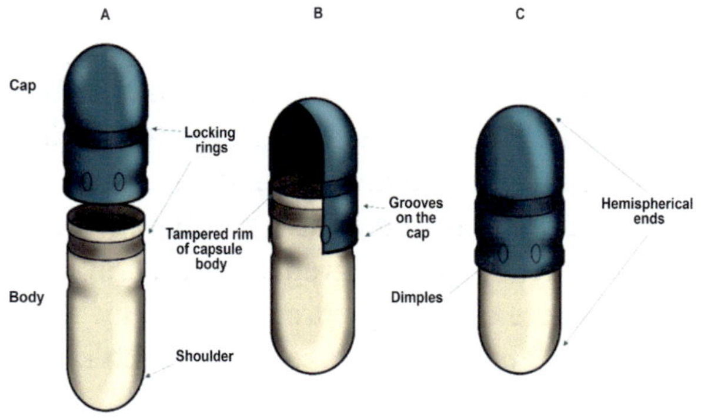

Figure 9.5. Description of the capsule design and components.

Source: https://pub.mdpi-res.com/pharmaceuticals/pharmaceuticals-15-01398/article_deploy/html/images/pharmaceuticals-15-01398-g001.png?1668761426.

9.1.2. Mechanism of Action During the Procedure

The general mechanism of action during the performance of capsule endoscopy is the utilization of sophisticated imaging technology for capturing high-quality images of the gastrointestinal tract. A capsule with a tiny camera is propelled through the GI system by a battery that allows it to traverse on its own for a period of time. As the capsule passes through the intestine, it photographs at a fixed interval and transmits this information to an external receiver that is held by the patient. In comparison to standard endoscopic evaluation, this method circumvents the discomfort associated with such procedures and therefore improves patient compliance and diagnostic yield. Furthermore, the strategic design of the capsule improves its navigational capabilities such that the capsule will be able to travel through the complicated anatomy of the GI tract without direct operator control, making capsule endoscopy a revolutionary breakthrough in diagnostic medicine. The second important aspect of capsule endoscopy is how the capsule is transported through the GI tract. The most recent developments have explored hybrid locomotion, where internal actuation systems are combined with external magnetic dragging. This new method allows the capsule to alter its profile through an internal legged system that assists in traversing collapsed regions of the gastrointestinal tract. When the capsule encounters regions where passage is restricted, the legs are capable of actively reshaping themselves to provide necessary clearance.

To complement this mechanism, small permanent magnets contained in the capsule react to an external magnetic field such that a dragging movement provides sufficient mobility even in challenging anatomical positions (Quaglia et al., 2010). This innovation not only enhances the capsule's ability to access complex barriers but also the overall efficiency of the imaging process. The combination of these technologies not only improves the efficiency of capsule endoscopy but also suggests the need for continuous research in automatic navigation techniques. Computer vision-based navigation algorithms that seek to enable more natural flexible endoscope steering are one of the promising research areas. Such algorithms utilize techniques , such as lumen centralization and visual odometry, thus providing enhanced control over the devices path (Van der Stap et al., 2013). Although the current potential of capsule endoscopy is impressive, finding commercialization for automated systems remains a long-term challenge. Therefore, research planning in economical mechatronics and in formulating robust algorithms will be essential to realize the maximum potential of this technology in clinical use to transform the science of gastrointestinal diagnostics (Figure 9.6).

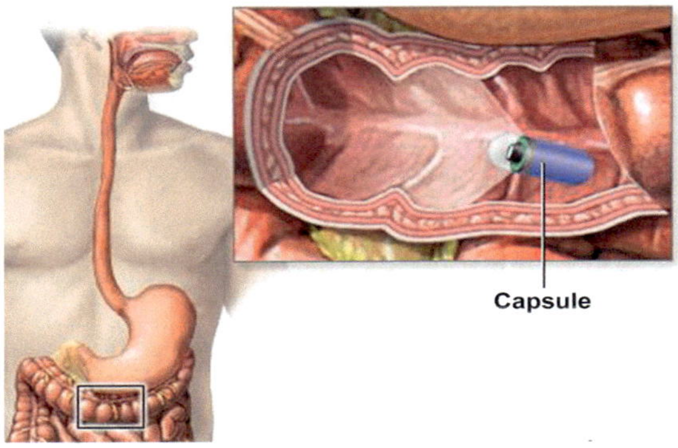

Figure 9.6. The mechanism of action during the procedure of capsule endoscopy.

Source: https://medlineplus.gov/ency/images/ency/fullsize/24352.jpg.

9.1.3. Comparison with Traditional Endoscopic Methods

The advent of capsule endoscopy has been a stunning evolution in the context of gastrointestinal diagnosis and is a fundamental departure from traditional endoscopic methods. The traditional endoscopy, typically with the utilization of a flexible scope, is patient-discomforting and sedation-dependent. In comparison, capsule endoscopy involves no invasive process as patients swallow a tiny capsule with a camera chip implanted in it that photographs the digestive system. Not only has this technology enhanced patient comfort, but it has expanded access to gastrointestinal testing for patients who might have otherwise resisted traditional techniques because they were afraid or uncomfortable.

By eliminating the need for sedation and invasive techniques, capsule endoscopy allows for a more patient-friendly alternative that can lead to increased compliance and a better overall diagnostic experience. Despite the clear advantages of capsule endoscopy, standard methods continue to be valuable in the diagnostic process. Methods , such as routine endoscopy provide for instantaneous visualization and the ability for intervention, including biopsies and polypectomies, which is not available with capsule endoscopy. Furthermore, the risk of lesion miss owing to the capsules' relatively fast passage time within the intestines continues to be an issue. As highlighted in recent articles, while capsule endoscopy provides a high volume of information in many respects better than the traditional methods, the inability to control image acquisition and the lack of capability to carry out immediate interventions during the procedure can undermine its effectiveness in certain clinical situations.

Consequently, capsule endoscopy practice translation must be balanced carefully with proven effectiveness by traditional practice to yield the highest patient benefits. Progress in image processing technology can consolidate the gap between capsule endoscopy and traditional methodology even further. Time-consuming wireless endoscopic image analysis has long been a doctor's issue, as seen, and solutions were needed to enhance image registration and interpretation. Recent advances in image stitching methods, such as those based on the PCA-SIFT algorithm, enable more accurate gastrointestinal image reconstruction, which would offer more insight and diagnostic capability with capsule endoscopy (Attar et al., 2018). These technological revolutions, thus, can elevate the grade of capsule endoscopy in clinical practice from merely an add-on to potentially a primary method of gastrointestinal tract visualization, particularly for obscure bleeding and small bowel assessment (Intzes et al., 2015). Lastly, innovations in such techniques could yield a total system that integrates the merits of conventional and capsule endoscopic modalities to achieve maximum diagnostic methods in gastroenterology (Figure 9.7).

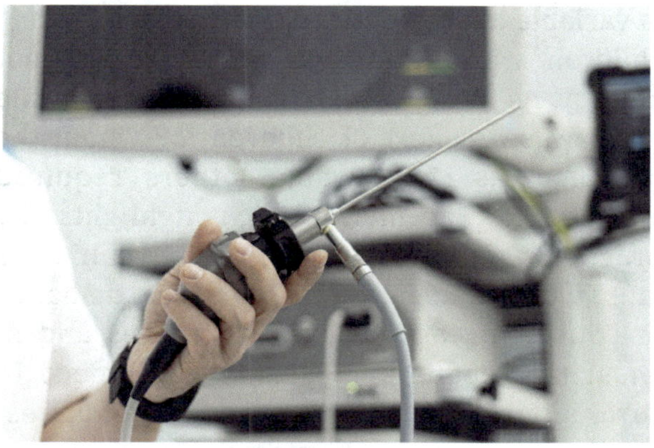

Figure 9.7. Comparison with traditional endoscopic methods.

Source: https://www.curasia.com/wp-content/uploads/2025/04/man-holds-a-medical-endoscope-on-the-background-o-2024-10-18-09-25-55-utc-scaled.jpg.

9.2. Indications for Capsule Endoscopy (CE)

Application of CE has revolutionized diagnosis and treatment of numerous gastrointestinal diseases. Notably, indications for this minimally invasive technique include obscure gastrointestinal bleeding, suspected Crohn's disease, and small bowel tumors, among others. Obscure gastrointestinal bleeding, typically resistant to diagnosis through conventional means, is one of the most frequent indications for CE. With the technique now widely used as the gold standard for the examination of the small intestine, it enables physicians to diagnose conditions , such as ulcers, polyps, and vascular malformations quite effectively. Additionally, as CE can offer real-time imaging of the mucosal surface, it offers timely interventions and a more individualized approach to treatment for such patients with unexplained gastrointestinal bleeding (Bufler et al., 2009). The effectiveness of the procedures in revealing pathologies confirms its position in contemporary gastrointestinal diagnostics. Additionally, the functionality of CE is also present in pediatric patients, and its feasibility and safety have been increasingly discussed among younger populations. A study done on children ranging from 1.5–7.9 years demonstrated that CE was feasible to perform, revealing widespread pathologies—like Crohn's disease—previously undetected using traditional diagnostic methods. Gastrointestinal bleeding was indicated in 83 patients as the primary indication, with various positive findings confirmed through capsule studies. The variation in indications between old and young patients considers the developmental parameters that affect gastrointestinal disorders (Bufler et al., 2009). For instance, while obscure bleeding is always significant in all age groups, presentations of diseases , such as Crohn's may vary, necessitating the application of age-specific approaches in pediatric gastroenterology. Lastly, growing uptake of capsule endoscopy not only addresses its therapeutic capability but is an indicator of the advancements in technology that improve patient care. Better capsule and imaging device designs have evolved as a result of innovation, minimizing discomfort and increasing overall procedure success rates. The introduction of CE has also created new possibilities for its use outside the small intestine, to esophageal and colonic disease, therefore broadening its indication and enhancing its clinical usefulness (Muñoz-Navas et al., 2008). The implications are far-reaching, as they indicate a trend towards more comprehensive, or whole-gastrointestinal, assessment, allowing diagnosis at an earlier stage and intervention in other diseases. Finally, the expanding indications of capsule endoscopy are a turning point in the history of the development of gastrointestinal diagnostics.

9.2.1. Diagnosis of Small Bowel Disorders

Small bowel disease diagnosis is achieved through a range of methods, but capsule endoscopy has been a significant tool for decades. This non-invasive diagnostic technique allows for wide evaluation of the small intestine, particularly in patients with unexplained gastrointestinal hemorrhage or suspected Crohn's disease. It is best suited for pediatric patients, as evidenced in a systematic study of children between 1.5 and 7.9 years old, in which the safety and effectiveness of WCE in this patient population were demonstrated. Surprisingly, the research was able to reveal most of the pathologies like polyps, ulcerative jejunitis, and Meckel's diverticula, testifying to the diagnostic potential of this technique compared to other negative studies in the past (Bufler et al., 2009). Through technological advancements, capsule endoscopy has maximally increased the potential for diagnosing small bowel disease, enabling practitioners to investigate previously challenging areas of the gastrointestinal tract. While capsule endoscopy has a central role, its performance is often augmented if complemented by other imaging techniques and interventional treatments. For instance, balloon-assisted enteroscopy not only improves biopsy retrieval but also maximizes visualization of the small bowel, particularly in Crohn's disease. This two-way strategy allows one to investigate small bowel disease in depth as well as any possible extra-intestinal disease, which is crucial for total patient care. Additionally, integration with magnetic resonance imaging (MRI) contributes to the diagnosis and provides a broader background for the effectiveness of disease treatment and management (Hausmann & Albert, 2011). Thus, the combination of capsule endoscopy with other recent imaging technologies forms a robust diagnostic process, ensuring better resolution of clinical data and facilitating the development of specialized therapy measures for patients suffering from small bowel diseases. Despite its advancement, there are hindrances in the application of capsule endoscopy for diagnosing small bowel disease. For example, reliability in capsule introduction techniques is variable among patients, particularly among children, where swallowing capsules may not be easy. As in the research stated above, while there was a cohort of children for whom the capsule was swallowable, others required endoscopic placement, which highlights the practical limitation within which clinicians must work (Bufler et al., 2009). Also, demands in countering age-specific difficulties and in ensuring adequate recording equipment to cover all pediatric age ranges remain of utmost significance. Ongoing development of diagnostic techniques and blending with newer technology is the way to overcome these challenges, keeping capsule endoscopy moving in the diagnosis and management of small bowel disease (Figure 9.8).

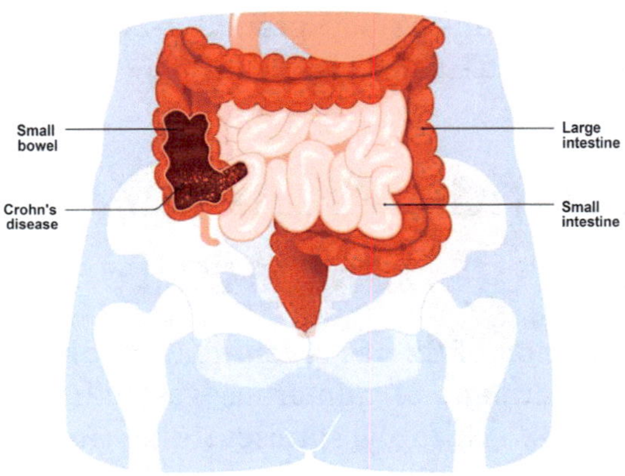

Figure 9.8. Diagnosis of small bowel disorders.

Source: https://post.medicalnewstoday.com/wp-content/uploads/sites/3/2022/12/2352107-Crohn's-disease-in-the-small-bowel_1296x1147body-1024x906.png.

9.2.2. Evaluation of Gastrointestinal Bleeding

Evaluation of gastrointestinal bleeding is a complex process for which comprehensive knowledge of different diagnostic modalities is essential. Of these, capsule endoscopy has been a 21st-century breakthrough technique, particularly in the assessment of occult gastrointestinal bleeding, a condition much in the business of self-description as vague. Intraoperative enteroscopy was traditionally considered to be the gold standard for the examination of the small intestine, but with its invasiveness and the morbidities that ensue, the trend has turned to less invasive techniques like capsule endoscopy and balloon-assisted enteroscopy. These new techniques not only enhance the diagnostic yield but also create a less traumatic experience for patients. This changing scenario brings into focus the need for medical professionals to adopt advanced diagnostic devices with the ability to achieve well-visualized and focused identification of lesions that cause gastrointestinal bleeding. Further, inclusion of trained personnel in the procedure of capsule endoscopy has also proven effective, particularly in maximizing the efficiency of the test. Studies reveal pre-reading video capsule recordings by experienced nurses to be effective, allowing identification and classification of suspected abnormalities that would otherwise go undetected. Guarini et al (2018) indicates that before analyzing time by the gastroenterologist, nurses selecting relevant lesions for evaluation reduces the time taken to interpret considerably, thus maximizing the diagnosis process. This teamwork not only enhances the work process but also allows gastroenterologists to concentrate on essential analysis and the management of patients. Through the promotion of interdisciplinary collaboration in healthcare facilities, the diagnostic process of gastrointestinal bleeding can be streamlined and become increasingly patient-centered, leading to improved outcomes. Although capsule endoscopy has enhanced detection of gastrointestinal bleeding, its results have to be put into context against other modes of investigation , such as intraoperative enteroscopy. Although studies demonstrate a 70% association between capsule endoscopy and intraoperative enteroscopy for lesion identification, the latter's high diagnostic yield cannot be overlooked—particularly in cases where obscure bleeding presents, where brevity and accuracy are paramount. (Monsanto et al., 2012) observes that intraoperative enteroscopy can achieve a high level of lesion detection in the small intestine, enabling timely intervention strategies for patients. However, intraoperative enteroscopy also has the potential for harm in the form of elevated procedure-related mortality. Clinical decision-making, therefore, should involve cautious evaluation of each patient's case, weighing the benefits of various diagnostic methods and also considering the inherent risks of invasive methods. A balance of these factors is required for the best management of gastrointestinal bleeding (Figure 9.9).

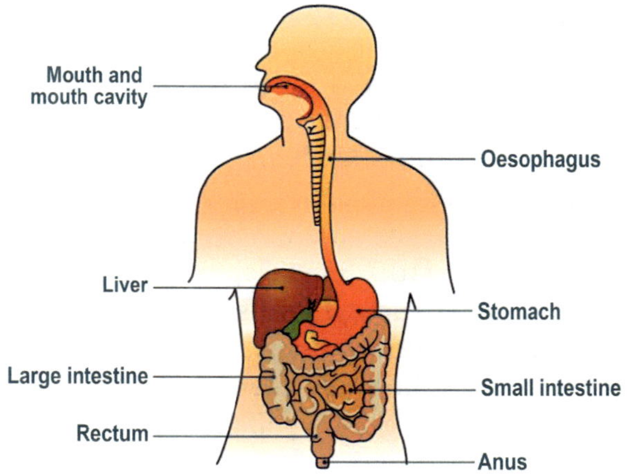

Figure 9.9. Evaluation of gastrointestinal bleeding.

Source: https://media.healthdirect.org.au/images/inline/original/hrxt4a_gastrointestinal-bleeding-62e7f4.png.

9.2.3. Assessment of Inflammatory Bowel Diseases (IBD)

Diagnosis of IBD has changed through the years, particularly in reference to diagnostic evolution. Historically, IBD has been prevalent in Western countries, with a tremendous increase in incidence since the 1950s. However, a significant change in the world epidemiology of IBD has been noticed wherein regions previously shown to have low prevalence , such as Eastern Europe and Asia, are now facing rising rates of incidence. This new trend indicates the power of augmented diagnostic knowledge and with it. Additionally, variation in the quality of epidemiologic studies supports a greater understanding of IBD in this regard to establish strong measurement frameworks. Hence, increased awareness and advanced diagnostic methods must be employed to effectively quantify the burden of IBD and explore environmental determinants of disease onset (Lakatos, 2006). Capsule endoscopy is a new technology in the assessment of IBD, particularly for small intestine visualization. Traditional endoscopic tests, while helpful, are often plagued by problems of access and patient discomfort. Advances in capsule endoscopy offer a non-invasive way to comprehensively investigate the gastrointestinal tract and enhance surveillance and diagnosis. High-resolution imaging throughout the small bowel is crucial in the detection of inflammation, lesions, and abnormalities of IBD. Endoscopic visualization of anatomically challenging-to-see regions makes it easier for doctors to make more informed decisions regarding treatment options. Hence, capsule endoscopy is a significant development in the diagnostic technology for IBD, acting as a bridge between clinical interventions and symptoms (Arebi & Saunders, 2005). Moreover, the integration of these emerging endoscopic technologies has transformed the treatment strategies for patients with IBD. Through developments , such as chromoendoscopy and magnifying endoscopy, clinicians can effectively diagnose small neoplastic lesions, which is crucial for the identification of early cancer and preventive therapies. In addition, the therapeutic procedures by means of devices like double balloon enteroscopy allow for targeted interventions that can minimize the need for invasive surgical procedures. The diagnostic evaluation made possible by such high-tech endoscopic modalities supports a personalized approach to IBD management in which interventions are performed in line with individual patient profiles. As more is discovered about the complexities of IBD through research, health practitioners must learn new technologies to enhance patient outcomes and general assessment methods in this field (Arebi & Saunders, 2005) (Figure 9.10).

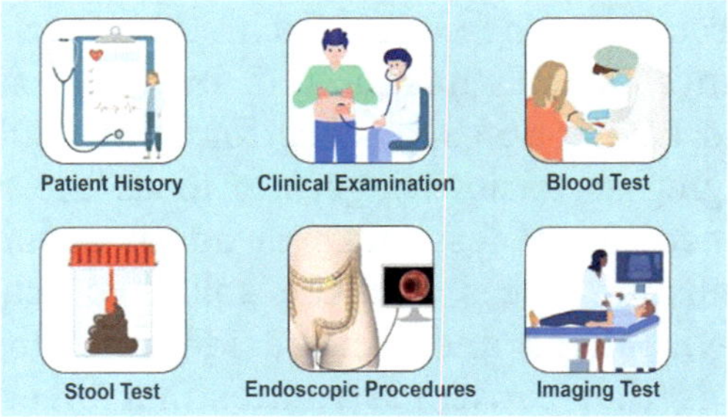

Figure 9.10. Assessment of inflammatory bowel diseases (IBD).

Source: https://www.hexahealth.com/condition/inflammatory-bowel-disease.

9.3. Procedure and Patient Experience

The integration of capsule endoscopy into routine gastrointestinal practice has significantly affected the patient experience through the availability of a non-invasive method to supplant routine endoscopic evaluation. The most significant advantage is the ability to view the small intestine completely without the associated discomfort of conventional methods. Patients typically report a less stressful encounter because they can swallow a capsule and go about their normal activities while the device captures pictures. This autonomy not only improves patient satisfaction but also underscores the importance of comfort to patients in the clinical setting. Furthermore, the visual representation of gastrointestinal wellness offered by capsule endoscopy diminishes patient anxiety because the patient can engage more actively in the planning of their treatment options and health-care discussions, making better-informed decisions about their treatment. Apart from its ability to increase patient comfort, procedural effectiveness at capsule endoscopy improves significantly with trained specialists participating in viewing the recordings. The cooperation between gastroenterologists and nurses, as demonstrated from certain recent research studies, highlights that nurses can effectively perform initial reading of capsule images for the identification of lesions before medical examination. Pre-reading not only preserves the quality of care by preventing lesions from being overlooked but also leads to a significant reduction in the time for evaluation, which is critical in high-use settings.

By shortening the time taken for medical evaluations from approximately 49 minutes to just 10 minutes, health professionals are able to spend additional time with patients and conduct follow-up treatments, thereby enhancing the overall patient experience in capsule endoscopy (Guarini et al., 2018). As the realization of the benefits of capsule endoscopy sets in, so does the need to address the bowel preparation process preceding the procedure. Recent studies have shown that the safety and efficiency of bowel cleansing regimens directly affect patient outcomes in capsule endoscopy. For instance, the addition of diatrizoate solution to bowel preparation has been reported to have promising results as regards completion rates as well as transit times, which are significant to successful studies. There is a compromise, however, in that some preparation regimens can lead to a higher incidence of gastrointestinal side effects, which diminish patient satisfaction (Burch et al., 2017). Therefore, there must be a balance between maximizing preparation and maintaining patient comfort, with the acknowledgment of well-informed decision-making in planning and performing capsule endoscopy procedures.

9.3.1. Preparation Required Before the Procedure

Patients need to adhere to specific guidelines that are preparatory before capsule endoscopy to ensure the efficacy of the procedures. The most significant of these is dietary adjustment, which usually commences at least 24 hours before the test. Patients are usually instructed to have a clear fluid diet, excluding solid foods and possibly irritating substances , such as alcohol and caffeine. This pre-procedure food restriction permits visualization of the small intestine to be accurately seen throughout the procedure, permitting monitoring with better images to be captured by the capsule. A well-cleaned gastrointestinal tract is critical in ensuring accurate interpretation of findings, making it a primary justification for following pre-procedure strictures and guidelines. In addition to dietary restrictions, bowel preparation is also crucial in this regard. Doctors can also prescribe an enema or a laxative to thoroughly clean the intestines, and this reduces the likelihood of having retained stool that can hide significant findings. This is particularly important, given that capsule endoscopy can identify lesions and abnormalities of the small bowel. A well-prepared bowel not only enhances the image quality obtained but also limits the necessity of follow-up procedures that can increase costs and discomfort to patients. Adequate bowel preparation is in conformity with best practice in gastroenterology, and it serves to enhance the diagnostic capability of this emerging technology, as encapsulated in recent information indicating the efficacy and success of capsule endoscopy (Muñoz-Navas et al., 2008). The medical professional's role, involving trained nurses, is also significant during pre-procedure preparations. The professional expertise of assessing a patient's readiness and providing corresponding instructions can significantly enhance the overall efficacy of the procedure. Studies have indicated that nurses can efficiently identify lesions and classify them when involved in pre-viewing the video capsule, facilitating the gastroenterologist's evaluation (Guarini et al., 2018). This common approach not only conserves review time but also improves the quality of diagnosis, so it is crucial to be thoroughly prepared before the procedure. The application of such techniques is characteristic of the commitment to advancing patient results and the research in gastrointestinal diagnosis with capsule endoscopy.

9.3.2. Step-by-Step Overview of the Capsule Ingestion Process

The procedure of swallowing the capsule begins with the preparation of the patient, which is fundamental to achieve accurate results during a capsule endoscopy. Patients are normally instructed by medical practitioners to starve for some hours before intake to clear the gastrointestinal tract. Fasting is important because it minimizes any interference that will distort the images taken by the capsule. Furthermore, patients can also be subjected to an initial screening to rule out contraindications to the procedure, such as gastrointestinal obstructions. Preparation not only enhances the quality of captured images but also enlightens the patient's expectations and reduces anxiety levels toward the procedure. After these initial steps have been established, the responsibility then rests upon the patient, who must strictly follow the guidelines presented to optimize their experience after capsule ingestion. Once prepared appropriately, the patient swallows the capsule, which is roughly the size of a large vitamin. It is simple to do this by swallowing the capsule down with a small amount of water, so that it can pass unimpeded through the esophagus. The capsule will pass through the entire gastrointestinal tract, taking images as it goes. The pictures are transmitted wirelessly to a recorder carried on the patient's belt, which is connected to electrodes carried on the body to monitor the capsule's passage. As it passes through the digestive tract, it captures two images every second, creating a close-up visual record. It should be ensured that the capsule begins properly; improper ingestion could result in poor imaging, which would interfere with the effective detection of gastrointestinal pathologies. After being ingested, patients are typically advised to continue their regular daily activity, unrestricted movement, while allowing capsules to be excreted by the gastrointestinal tract. The process takes approximately 8–12 hours, depending on digestive rates. During this time, the patients are required to observe some post-ingestion guidelines, such as avoiding some fluids or food that may hinder the working of the capsule. Once the capsule completes its transit, typically by being naturally expelled, the data needs to be synchronized, enabling healthcare providers to examine the taken images in detail. Prompt and accurate analysis is of paramount importance in diagnosing diseases , such as gastrointestinal bleeding or inflammatory bowel disease, again highlighting the importance of a proper ingestion process as highlighted by Tringali et al. (2017) and Reingruber et al. (2009) (Figure 9.11).

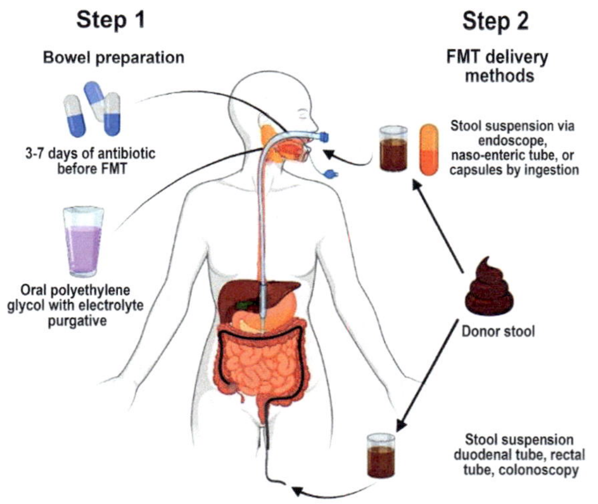

Figure 9.11. Step-by-step overview of the capsule ingestion process.

Source: https://pub.mdpi-res.com/cancers/cancers-14-00691/article_deploy/html/images/cancers-14-00691-g001.png?1644310918.

9.3.3. Post-Procedure Monitoring and Data Retrieval

The post-procedure monitoring time is quite crucial in capsule endoscopy since it encompasses collection and evaluation of data acquired during the process. Continuous monitoring for confirmation that the device is passing through the gastrointestinal tract without retention or blockage follows ingestion of the capsule. This phase includes monitoring of the patient's symptoms, but also real-time assessment of the capsule position to facilitate interventions if necessary. Doctors must critique the information obtained in a bid to identify any abnormality or complications, hence enhancing patient safety and procedure success. A keen understanding of the monitoring process notably contributes to the overall assessment of gastrointestinal status in patients and informs subsequent medical decisions regarding treatment, follow-up, etc. Retrieval of data is a significant aspect of the capsule endoscopy process that has a direct bearing on the outcome of the monitoring process. Used to test conditions , such as small bowel bleeding and Crohn's disease, the capsule transmits a significant amount of visual data that must be systematically recorded and interpreted. The development of highly advanced telemetry microsystems, as seen in recent literature, is one evidence of technological innovation that improves data fidelity and transmission reliability. The integration of several sensors and wireless interfaces can make the collection of high-quality images in real-time possible, which are critical to precise diagnosis (Cooper et al., 2005). Furthermore, precise training of medical staff in the interpretation of the sets of data is necessary to get the maximum benefit of capsule endoscopy, ultimately resulting in improved patient management and targeted intervention. Under post-procedure monitoring and data recovery conditions, ensuring adequate communication between the capsule and the receiving base station is of critical importance. Communication success or failure directly affects the quality of data acquisition and analysis that follows. Design strategies effective at reducing power consumption while increasing data transmission capabilities have been designed to optimize the performance of the capsule. For instance, the application of a feedback clock control loop and mixed-signal sensor circuits has been instrumental in minimizing errors when transmitting data, and in maintaining the telemetry system reliable, as observed in experiments (Cooper et al., 2005). This technology efficiency emphasis not only raises the quality of monitoring but also influences the patient experience, with on-time data retrieval supporting the speedup of diagnosis and treatment planning to ultimately improve clinical outcomes (Figure 9.12).

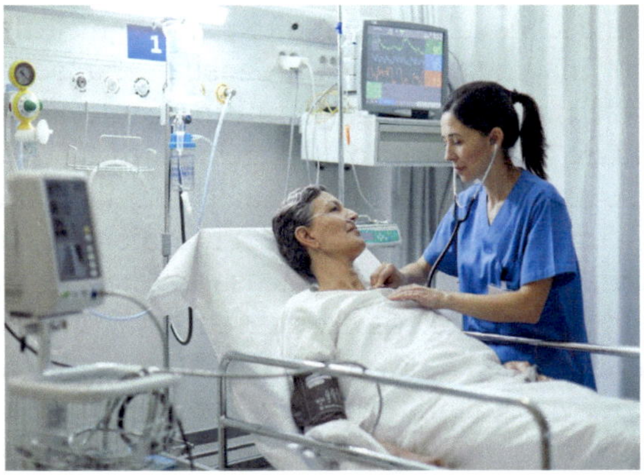

Figure 9.12. Post-procedure monitoring and data retrieval.

Source: https://radiusky.com/wp-content/uploads/2020/12/postanesthesiamonitoring.jpg.

9.4. Advantages of Capsule Endoscopy

Capsule endoscopy has revolutionized gastrointestinal diagnosis with a number of advantages over endoscopy. In the first place, capsule endoscopy is less invasive, which significantly reduces the danger associated with routine endoscopy, such as bleeding or infection. This advantage is sought by patients, as there is no invasive procedure, therefore less discomfort and fear associated with the diagnostic process. Moreover, because the capsule is swallowed, it allows for an end-to-end examination of the entire gastrointestinal tract, specifically the small intestine, which is often not possible to visualize with conventional endoscopic methods. Such wide accessibility is valuable in the diagnosis of such diseases as obscure gastrointestinal bleeding, Crohn's disease, and small bowel tumors. Therefore, the aspect that capsule endoscopy is a non-invasive process not only enhances patient comfort but also elevates diagnostic accuracy, making it a giant step ahead for gastrointestinal treatment. The second obvious advantage of capsule endoscopy is the advanced visualization it offers through cutting-edge imaging technology. Capsule endoscopes have a number of high-definition cameras that capture thousands of images as they travel through the gastrointestinal tract. This real-time imaging provides gastroenterologists with detailed knowledge of mucosal pathology that could be overlooked with conventional methods. The use of such advanced technologies is part of today's demand for precision medicine and contributes to improved diagnostic outcomes. In addition, as the use of endoscopic vision technology evolves, it enhances the ability for individualized patient assessment. With the implementation of advances in computing and imaging modalities, doctors can successfully track lesions and administer targeted therapy, illustrating the clinical utility of capsule endoscopy in modern practice (Fu et al., 2021). Last but not least, the accessibility and ease of capsule endoscopy should not be overemphasized. The procedure can be conducted on an outpatient basis, which reduces hospital stays and lowers healthcare costs for providers and patients alike. Because no sedation is required for the capsule, patients resume their normal life in hours after the procedure, a striking contrast with other endoscopic techniques that typically involve anesthetics and days of convalescence. The ease of use also makes it possible for more comprehensive screening opportunities, possibly leading to earlier diagnosis of gastrointestinal disease in asymptomatic individuals. Besides, the burgeoning interest in research in magnetically actuated bio/soft robots suggests future development will continue to advance capsule technology, improving navigation and imaging capability, thereby advancing overall utilization of this technology (Ebrahimi et al., 2020). To this extent, capsule endoscopy is a diagnostic technology giant step, uniting safety, efficiency, and precision (Figure 9.13).

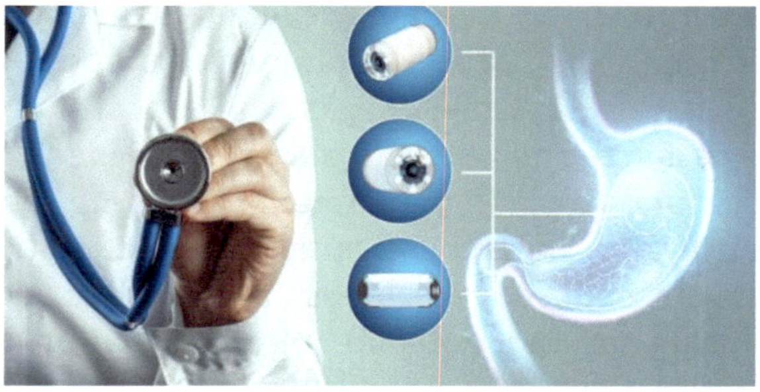

Figure 9.13. Advantages of capsule endoscopy.

Source: https://www.ibihealthcare.com/wp-content/uploads/2022/10/image-2.jpg.

9.4.1. Non-Invasive Nature of the Procedure

The capsule endoscopy is a new, non-invasive technology that has transformed gastrointestinal diagnosis, particularly for the diseases of the small intestine. It differs from traditional endoscopy, which often involves sedation and invasive equipment, because it uses a pill-sized capsule carrying an onboard camera that photographs as it travels through the gastrointestinal tract. This method alleviates patient discomfort with the provision of visual access to previously difficult-to-reach regions through conventional techniques. The comparative lack of invasiveness not only makes the procedure more acceptable to patients but also reduces the risks of sedation and body trauma. As such, patients are easily able to resume normal activities immediately after consuming it, which indicates the unique benefit of such a method in clinical settings, most notably in illnesses like small bowel Crohn's disease, where traditional methods would be wanting in diagnostic potential (Arebi & Saunders, 2005). In addition to the non-invasiveness of its nature, capsule endoscopy is also supported by the simplicity of preparation, another factor that expands its practicality in clinical practice. The procedure is minimally prepared compared to other endoscopic invasive methods, significantly lowering the barrier to patient entry. Patients need only fast for several hours before consumption of the capsule, and this allows for natural and unobstructed transit through the gastrointestinal system. This functional advantage is particularly important in the outpatient setting, where patients are anxious about convenience and minimal disruption of their normal routines. Furthermore, as the technology supports increasingly advanced imaging capacity, it can produce high-resolution images capable of supporting accurate diagnosis and prompt intervention, enhancing the quality of patient care overall (Arebi & Saunders, 2005). Therefore, the non-invasive nature of capsule endoscopy is central to encouraging patient compliance and minimizing anxiety for those receiving gastrointestinal assessment. Further, the capabilities of capsule endoscopy are being taken into the therapeutic field, thereby enhancing patient care. While primarily for diagnosis, the technological innovations have led to additional methods, such as balloon-assisted enteroscopy, whereby therapeutic interventions can be performed where indicated. This is a paradigm shift in the treatment of gastrointestinal disorders. For instance, in the case of small bowel Crohn's disease patients, the non-invasive character of capsule endoscopy enables routine monitoring and disease activity assessment without the complications associated with surgical exploration or repeated invasive testing (Hausmann & Albert, 2011). This combined ability highlights the potential of capsule endoscopy to not just enhance diagnostic accuracy but also drive and optimize treatment streams in an individualized approach, showing how the non-invasive nature of the technology may define future gastroenterology clinical practice (Figure 9.14).

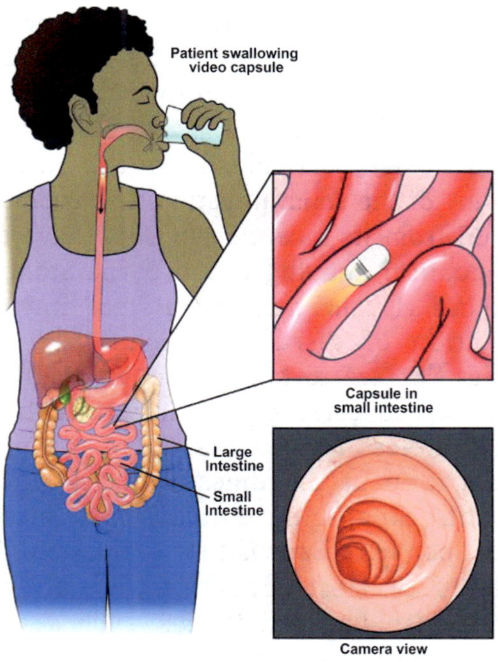

Figure 9.14. Non-invasive nature of capsule endoscopy in gastrointestinal diagnostics.

Source: https://patient.gastro.org/wp-content/uploads/2021/09/CGH-Patient-Ed-2019-Capsule-792x1024.jpg.

9.4.2. Enhanced Visualization of the Small Intestine

The revolutionary capsule endoscopy procedure has introduced a vast change in the area of gastrointestinal diagnostics, particularly in the case of the small intestine. The traditional endoscopic studies are unpleasant and require the use of sedatives, which can prove to be a deterrent to patients from undergoing necessary investigations. Capsule endoscopy, on the contrary, employs a miniature camera ingestible that captures excellent images of the gastrointestinal tract and is non-surgical with little ease of administration. This disruption-free approach encourages more participation in screening programs, thereby improving the likelihood of detection of diseases , such as small bowel adenocarcinoma, although rare, remains a relevant problem in the context of undiagnosed gastrointestinal hemorrhage (Berger et al., 2010). Increased visualization features here not only improve the patient's comfort level but also improve the accuracy of diagnosis, particularly in the intricate anatomy of the small intestine. The evolutions in WCE from its inception in 2000 have been astronomical, making it the cornerstone for enhanced visualization of the small intestine. Utilization of disruptive technology, WCE enables doctors to break through traditional limitations concerning gastrointestinal studies. Being wireless implies that there is ongoing visualization of the digestive tract without sedation, thus being enticing to a broader patient population to visit for evaluation (Ciuti et al., 2016). Most importantly, the ability of WCE to visualize pathologies, such as small bowel tumors, can result in early treatment, thereby improving clinical outcomes. The ability to acquire full visual information without compromising the comfort of the patient reflects the multi-dimensional utility of capsule endoscopy and highlights its very significant role in modern digestive health care. Future capsule technologies promise further advances in the visualization of the small intestine. The integration of microrobotics with advanced imaging functionality is on the horizon, and it can further transform the field of gastrointestinal diagnosis and treatment. The potential for active locomotion, in which the capsule navigates complex intestinal topographies actively, exists to significantly enhance image acquisition and analysis (Ciuti et al., 2016). Additionally, the development of embedded therapeutic modules can transform the capsule into a therapy platform from a diagnostic tool, allowing real-time therapeutics in the course of the examination. These envisioned advances indicate the vibrant future of capsule endoscopy in gastrointestinal medicine as it can potentially have an active role in screening, diagnosis, and therapeutic interventions, providing unparalleled visualization and control over small intestinal disease.

9.4.3. Increased Patient Comfort and Compliance

Within the context of capsule endoscopy, the concept of increased patient comfort and compliance is the core to the achievement of effective diagnostic outcomes. Patients have traditionally been worried about the level of discomfort that generally accompanies standard endoscopic procedures, which are invasive in nature and involve sedation. Capsule endoscopy, however, addresses these concerns by offering a less invasive solution that alleviates such anxieties. The new design involves patients swallowing a small capsule containing a camera, which can traverse the gastrointestinal tract whilst patients carry out their routine activities. The radical departure from the conventional method is not only causing increased comfort but also increased willingness to have the procedure done, hence enhanced overall rates of compliance. The process of preparation for capsule endoscopy plays an important role in guaranteeing patient satisfaction and comfort. Research has indicated that a clear liquid diet before the procedure leads to adequate intestinal cleanliness without being as well tolerated as more severe bowel preparation protocols. Arguello-Viudez et al. (2011) describe that patients were most compliant when they were subjected to this less severe preparation protocol compared to others, like polyethylene glycol solutions, which were less well tolerated. The findings show that eliminating the preparation requirements significantly enhances patient acceptability for the procedure and consequently increases the overall utility of capsule endoscopy for diagnosis. Furthermore, technological advancements in capsule endoscopy enhance patient comfort as a result of increased communication between the capsule and the outside monitoring equipment. Research has investigated radio frequency (RF) communication to transmit data to an external receiver, with promising consequences for patient comfort.

According to Joseph et al. (2014), the realization of efficient and easy-to-use wireless body area networks enables smooth interaction throughout the procedure. By minimizing potential disturbances and discomfort related to equipment, patients are better positioned to attend to the examination process itself as opposed to the technicalities involved. The meeting of comfort-focused technologies with patient protocols actually creates an environment that invites compliance, thus supporting the overall success of capsule endoscopy (Figure 9.15).

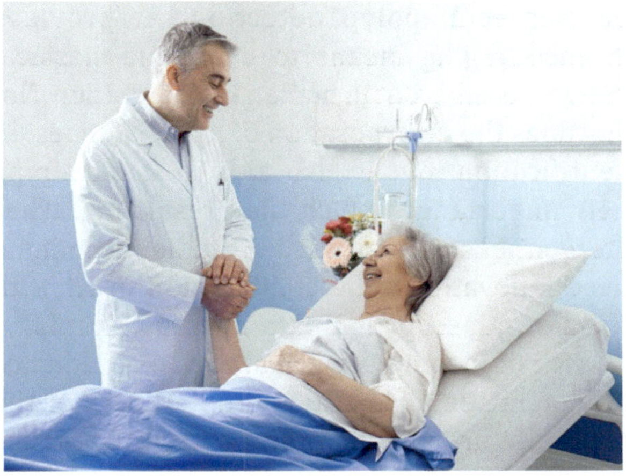

Figure 9.15. Increased patient comfort Increased patient comfort and compliance and compliance.

Source: https://www.rightpatient.com/wp-content/uploads/2023/11/The-Importance-of-Patient-Comfort-and-How-Biometrics-Can-Help-1030x772.jpg.

9.5. Limitations and Challenges

CE has significantly advanced gastrointestinal (GI) disease diagnosis, but it also poses many limitations and challenges that must be examined carefully. One of the limitations is that the imaging capability of existing capsule technologies has limitations. Specifically, the devices primarily rely on white light imaging, which has the limitation of only inspecting the mucosal surface. As Woods & Constandinou (2011) have said, this limitation severely restricts the evaluation of root pathologies, since it is greatly dependent on evident signs of illness. Therefore, the inability to obtain transmural imaging hinders the effective evaluation of diseases like inflammatory bowel disease. Such ignorance of deeper information about the GI tract can lead to misdiagnosis or delayed diagnosis, hence decreasing the utility of CE to physicians. Another major challenge of capsule endoscopy includes the power efficiency and space constraints within the capsule. Recent developments, including the development of a micropositioning mechanism for directed drug delivery, speak volumes about attempts to enhance CE functionality (Woods & Constandinou, 2011). These developments typically come with sophisticated engineering constraints that undermine the overall performance of the device. While the micropositioning mechanism both offers targeted drug delivery and miniaturization, it occupies valuable space inside the capsule, making further integration of sophisticated imaging technology more complicated. This joining of therapeutic and diagnostic activities, promising as it is, has to be achieved with very fine-tunings so that both activities can be made effective without either detracting from the other. Finally, image interpretation of capsule endoscopy is a significant challenge because the volume of information generated can overwhelm physicians. The current reliance on manual review protocols translates into extended interpretation times, which could lead to delays in diagnosis and treatment plans. Cochran et al. (2017) argue that there is potential for the incorporation of quantitative ultrasound (QUS) technology to enhance diagnostic speed and accuracy. By partially automating image interpretation, clinical professionals can not only improve efficiency but also reduce the possibilities of human errors in interpreting the intricate information captured during the test. However, integrating such advanced technologies into existing CE systems involves stringent validation and training to ensure that their benefits are achieved to the fullest extent in real practice.

9.5.1. Potential for Incomplete Visualization

Incomplete visualization with capsule endoscopy remains a significant problem in its clinical application. Unlike traditional optical colonoscopy, capsule endoscopy is fortunate to be noninvasive and to have the potential for visualization of the entire gastrointestinal tract. However, its effectiveness can be hindered by a number of factors, including bowel preparation, transit time, and limitations of the capsule itself. Inadequate bowel preparation may lead to residual fecal load, which obscures significant lesions and biases diagnostic evaluation. Transit times between patients may also vary widely, affecting the extent to which the capsule is able to examine the intestinal lumen and hence introducing the risk of missed diagnosis. Together, these restrictions highlight the need to comprehend the circumstances in which capsule endoscopy fails to visualize large lesions, especially in colorectal cancer screening. Even if the potential of capsule endoscopy is high, its ability to achieve total visualization is still questionable. Conventional methods, including optical colonoscopy, have been discovered to possess increased sensitivity for the detection of pre-malignant lesions due to their ability to permit direct visualization and therapeutic interventions. While capsule endoscopy might find a niche in screening regimens, particularly in patients who are at risk or who are unable to tolerate routine colonoscopy, the absence of an interventionist's capability for immediate visualization and intervention upon detected anomalies presents a barrier. The great difference in capsule endoscopy performance and optical colonoscopy (OC) underscores the need for additional research focused on detecting and minimizing incomplete visualization risk. With developments in capsule technology, an understanding of its limitations and an attempt to enhance visualization capability are essential when considering its use in screening programs for colorectal disease. AI development may address some of the deficiencies in the visualization of capsule endoscopy. AI algorithms have been shown over recent years to significantly enhance image processing, detection, localization, and characterization of lesions along the course of capsules through the gastrointestinal tract. With reported sensitivity rates rising to 99.9% for colorectal polyp detection, AI provides an encouraging means to overcome classical limitations inherent in human interpretation. Not only does the incorporation of AI assist in lesion identification, but it also aids in determining their importance, which may result in earlier interventions. As explained in studies examining these innovations, the combination of AI with capsule endoscopy is a path toward minimizing the risk of incomplete visualization, and hence the diagnostic yield and overall efficacy of the minimally invasive method in clinical practice (Baatrup et al., 2024).

9.5.2. Risk of Capsule Retention in the Gastrointestinal Tract

The development of capsule endoscopy has transformed the practice of gastrointestinal diagnostics, offering a non-invasive means of observing the mucosal surface of the gastrointestinal tract. But one key concern associated with this technology is the capsule retention. Capsule retention occurs when the device cannot pass along the gastrointestinal tract, which can lead to various complications , such as obstruction or the need for surgery. Risk factors for retention include previous treatment with strictures, malignancies, or inflammatory bowel disease like Crohn's disease, which can derange the usual transit of the capsule. Of utmost importance to clinicians is that they carefully assess the appropriateness of capsule endoscopy in specific patients and implement preventive measures to prevent this risk. Recent studies have also attempted to quantify capsule retention risk among different patient groups and conditions. For instance, in a multicenter trial of obscure gastrointestinal bleeding (OGIB) and Crohn's disease patients, the overall rate of retention was found to be very low, approximately 0.6% in a total of 172 patients. This low rate is comforting, and it suggests that with due application of criteria and taking pre-existing gastrointestinal disease into account, capsule endoscopy can be effective as well as safe. However, the risk of retention is an important consideration, particularly in those with known strictures or other anatomical abnormalities known to place them at risk for complications. Thus, strict patient evaluation before capsule ingestion is essential to minimize risks of retention. In addition to patient-specific factors, advances in capsule technology have also assisted in improving retention-related safety profiles. More contemporary designs of capsules, such as those with panoramic images, might make diagnosis more accurate while simultaneously reducing the risk of retention through faster passage through the gastrointestinal tract. Moreover, the evolving trend of further development in more sophisticated imaging technology assists in easier visualization of potential obstructions before capsule ingestion, allowing for better-informed decision-making for clinicians. In spite of the low retention rate found in many studies, vigilant vigilance and absolute compliance with best practices are necessary to pre-emptively manage and prevent capsule retention at clinics. The synergy of patient histories in detail and high technology will ultimately enhance the safety and effectiveness of capsule endoscopy as a gastroenterologic diagnostic tool (Figure 9.16).

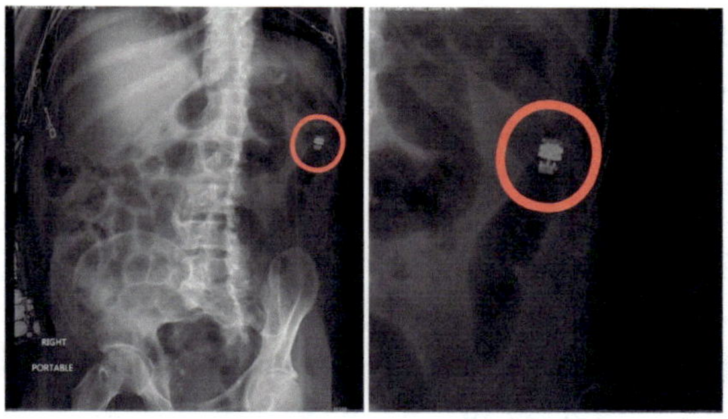

Figure 9.16. Risk of capsule retention in the gastrointestinal tract.

Source: https://static.wixstatic.com/media/e35976_d606489c7f1546e28cd1912751e4ad16~mv2.jpg/v1/fill/w_980,h_551,al_c,q_85,usm_0.66_1.00_0.01,enc_auto/e35976_d606489c7f1546e28cd1912751e4ad16~mv2.jpg.

9.5.3. Limitations in Diagnostic Capabilities Compared to Traditional Methods

The future of capsule endoscopy is a tremendous leap forward in gastrointestinal diagnostics, but diagnostic limitation compared to traditional methods still exists. One key concern is in the passive aspect of the capsules, which restricts the physicians control over the examination process. As opposed to standard flexible endoscopy, where manipulation of the endoscope can be controlled by the clinician for focused observation, capsule endoscopy relies exclusively on the capsule's natural transit through the gastrointestinal tract. This loss of control could lead to missed lesions or an incomplete examination, with the potential omission of significant pathologies that would have been otherwise identified using conventional methods.

Thus, while capsule endoscopy provides a painless alternative, it cannot fully replace conventional means of precise diagnostics through interactive interaction (Cosmas et al., 2014). The second major shortcoming of capsule endoscopy is localizing and mapping within the gastrointestinal tract. Current technology is not able to provide real-time three-dimensional (3D) imaging, which is essential to achieve accurate diagnosis and navigation. Compared to traditional methods, where precise lesion targeting and biopsy acquisition are made possible by doctors, the passive capsule only has a linear series of images with no means to add spatial context. Modern advances in robotic capsule endoscopy work towards enhancing the current shortcomings, but combining precision localization technologies , such as visual SLAM, is still in development. With raw instruments to undertake accurate 3D mapping, physicians are stopped from working with the visualized lesions and accurate anatomical positions, which obstructs the diagnostic process (Turan et al., 2017).

Finally, capsule endoscopy image interpretation poses its challenges compared to traditional methods of diagnosis. The capsule captures a high volume of images, which may overwhelm the examining physician and lead to potential oversights or misinterpretations. As compared to conventional endoscopy, where a doctor can see and evaluate findings in real time, capsule endoscopy requires serious analysis of recorded data, frequently due to human error on the basis of distraction or fatigue. Additionally, the absence of immediate feedback during the procedure may limit the doctor's ability to investigate further based on visual inspection. These observations point towards the imperative for improved data analysis tools and procedures in capsule endoscopy to complement rather than substitute the accuracy of traditional diagnostic processes (Cosmas et al., 2014).

9.6. Future Directions in Capsule Endoscopy

The future of capsule endoscopy is very promising as advancements in technology continue to enhance its functionality and flexibility in gut diagnostics and therapies. Developments in imaging technology in recent years, particularly the incorporation of high-definition and narrow-band imaging, have greatly improved the visual acuity as well as the detection rates of mucosal lesions. This kind of improvement is pivotal in early detection and treatment of conditions , such as vascular lower GI bleeding, which has proved difficult in the past with its diverse etiology and complexity. As per current literature, the integration of these new imaging techniques into capsule endoscopy is likely to increase diagnostic effectiveness and therapeutic outcomes, leading to increased opportunities for a personalized approach in patient management (Alomair, 2024).

With medical practitioners embracing these advancements, the potential for capsule endoscopy to provide complete information regarding GI health will definitely maximize patient management strategies. Other than advancements in imaging technology, the development of remotely controlled capsule endoscopes represents a major breakthrough. Overcoming the limitations of passive motion, researchers are designing novel control methods and dynamic system modeling for propelling guided motion through the gastrointestinal tract. The ability of active navigation of the gastrointestinal tract will further enhance the diagnostic capability of capsule endoscopy, enabling physicians to more conveniently observe and assess distant sites. As explored in recent studies, the addition of artificial intelligence to such systems further enhances their function, making autonomous direction and live feedback available to experts

(Abdollahi et al., 2024). Consequently, further development of capsule endoscopes that move on their own could dramatically change how medical professionals approach diagnosing and treating gastrointestinal disease, with solutions previously impossible. More importantly, the future of capsule endoscopy is not only about advances in technology but also about what it implies for patient-centered care. The scope for hybrid methods combining capsule endoscopy with other modalities, including endoscopy and angiography, highlights a revolutionary pathway in the treatment of GI disorders. Such combinations could provide treatment plans with a complete spectrum of all three modalities, each bringing its own set of strengths to the table to obtain maximal benefit for patients. The combination of new embolic materials with improved endoscopic technique can mark a paradigm shift, aimed at an even more collaborative and multi-faceted approach to the control of gastrointestinal bleeding (Alomair, 2024). Ultimately, as technology and research further progress, capsule endoscopy will become part of a more tailored, streamlined, and coordinated model of gastrointestinal care (Figure 9.17).

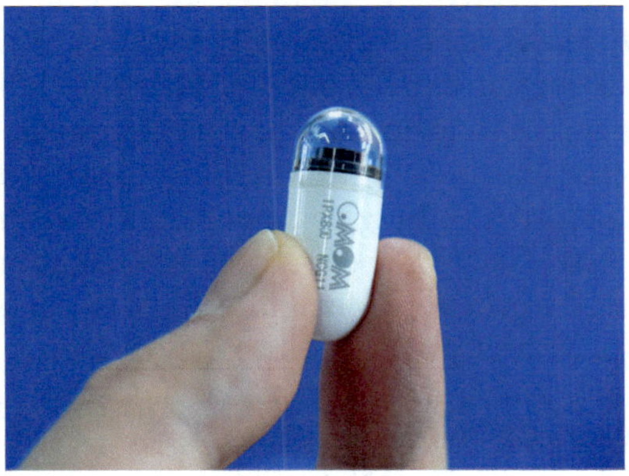

Figure 9.17. Future directions in capsule endoscopy.

Source: https://source.ichongqing.info/2021/11/Future-Capsule-Endoscopy-Technologies-Applied.jpg.

9.6.1. Technological Advancements on the Horizon

The introduction of capsule endoscopy has revolutionized the diagnosis of the GI tract, primarily because it is non-invasive and very tolerable in patients. Advances of the future will introduce Artificial Intelligence (AI) with the potential to dramatically enhance diagnostic capability. AI systems, with the aid of advanced machine learning algorithms , such as convolutional neural networks (CNNs), are being designed to support the identification and classification of lesions found under capsule endoscopy. This technology not only seeks to improve the sensitivity of lesion detection but also seeks to minimize the errors clinicians typically overlook with traditional examinations. With automated endoscopic image analysis, AI would streamline clinical workflows and eventually help healthcare professionals make more precise and timely diagnoses (Burczyk et al., 2025). The future of capsule endoscopy is thus set to benefit immensely from these AI-driven advancements, with the outcome being improved patient outcomes. In parallel with AI development, technology advancements in imaging modalities are also set to enhance capsule endoscopy efficacy. The merging of 3D modeling methods from image sequences obtained using wireless capsule endoscopes is a thrilling idea. Recent research indicates that 3D form reconstruction from images obtained using capsule endoscopy can help gastroenterologists gain a better understanding of the GI tract, particularly in complex cases. By embracing methods , such as shape from shading (SFS) and shape from focus (SFF), the study can overcome the challenges of non-uniform lighting in traditional capsule images. Such methods have shown the capability of reconstructing thin 3D models successfully, thus making better diagnosis and visualization possible for areas of interest (Ahmad et al., 2023). The emergence of such techniques is symptomatic of the future in which capsule endoscopy becomes an increasingly impactful diagnostic tool, combining visual data with sophisticated modeling.

Furthermore, as there are more technological environment shifts, the ethical considerations of AI embedding in medical diagnostics become increasingly important. The application of algorithms to decision-making in capsule endoscopy makes it difficult to assign responsibility and legitimacy to AI-based assessments. Even as these technologies add precision and effectiveness, the requirement of big, diverse data sets for model training remains a challenge to be addressed to achieve complete and equitable healthcare outcomes. Additionally, integration of AI tools demands regulation mechanisms to guarantee their trustworthiness and safety of use in clinical practice (Burczyk et al., 2025). With capsule endoscopy technologies advancing, a balanced strategy has to be employed so that AI aids, rather than detracts from, the clinician's hand in patient care. Such merging of innovation and ethical management will define the future of capsule endoscopy and its impact on gastrointestinal diagnostics (Figure 9.18).

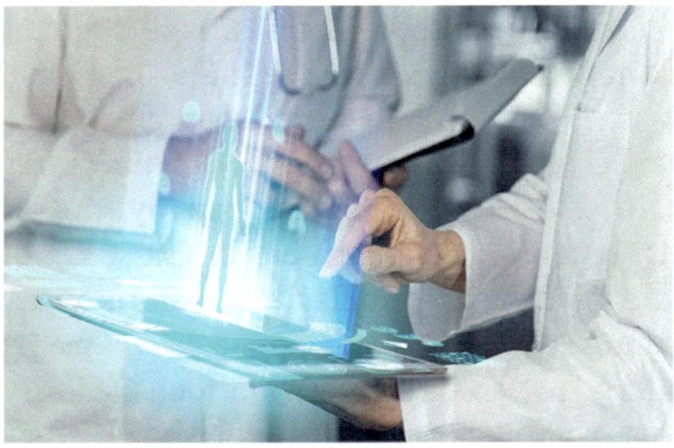

Figure 9.18. Technological advancements on the horizon.

Source: https://www.talktomedic.com/blog/wp-content/uploads/2022/11/Impact-Of-Technological-Advancements-In-The-Healthcare-Industry.jpg.

9.6.2. Potential Integration with Artificial Intelligence (AI)

Future potential to integrate AI into capsule endoscopy offers transformative potential to significantly enhance diagnostic function for gastroenterology. Capsule endoscopy, in the past, has struggled with image review being manual in nature, and major findings may be overlooked due to the sheer volume of images captured. However, these challenges can be addressed through the application of advanced machine learning algorithms, i.e., CNNs, for computerized detection and classification of gastrointestinal tract lesions. These technologies can have implications leading to improved sensitivity and specificity in pathological abnormality detection, hence streamlining clinical processes and facilitating early interventions. By employing AI in this novel field, physicians can not only lower the rate of undiagnosed cases but also improve the overall results of the patients, aiding the ongoing pursuit of precision medicine in clinical practice. Besides, research proves the possibility of fully incorporating AI into the capsule endoscopy procedure. A study observed the development of an AI recognition network with outstanding diagnostic performance of 99.9% sensitivity and 99.4% specificity in the detection of colorectal polyps. It offers the possibility of the automatic processing of large groups of images, wherein only interesting images are further analyzed for characterization, i.e., measurement of size and distinction between neoplastic and non-neoplastic polyps. These advancements point to the real-world implementation of AI to enhance the diagnosis process, ultimately bridging the existing gap between capsule endoscopy and conventional optical colonoscopy. The effects of integrating AI into routine clinical practice are vast, as they hold the promise of refining conventional practices and pushing the door open to more detailed examination techniques in gastroenterology. However, the journey towards the successful integration of AI in capsule endoscopy comes with its own set of obstacles. The reliance on big, heterogeneous data sets to train AI algorithms is a turning point inhibitor since the success of such algorithms greatly relies on the quality and diversity of input data. Secondly, there are ethical concerns surrounding AI-facilitated clinical decision-making that must be carefully weighed by stakeholders in the medical fraternity. Setting up open regulatory frameworks and moral guidelines that regulate the use of AI technologies will be essential in maintaining trust and ensuring patient safety. Additionally, studies on algorithmic optimization and the development of universal protocols will be essential in achieving the full potential of AI applications in capsule endoscopy. In overcoming these challenges, the medical profession can work to optimize the synergy of AI, thereby optimizing diagnostic accuracy and patient care in gastroenterology.

9.6.3. Expanding Applications in Gastrointestinal Health

Capsule endoscopy has significantly widened the use of diagnosing various GI illnesses, particularly among those previously under- or unserved populations, such as children. As indicated in recent studies, the possibility of applying WCE in children aged 1.5 years allows using a non-invasive technique for the diagnosis of diseases like Crohn's disease, gastrointestinal bleeding, and malabsorption syndromes. The result of the multicentric European study presented differed pathologies in a series of 83 children, with visible differences as a function of age. Fortuitously, complications were minimal, and the majority of cases showed effective diagnosis without adverse consequences. This not only reflects the safety of the technique but also implies the need for pediatric adaptation in endoscopic technology, further promoting the use of capsule endoscopy in the protection of pediatric patients from invasive techniques (Bufler et al., 2009). In addition to the development of diagnostic technologies in pediatric gastroenterology, applications of capsule endoscopy are also being enhanced with new technology , such as microultrasound (μUS). *Ex vivo* studies of porcine gastrointestinal tissue reveal that μUS is more effective in identifying early cellular changes in diseases , such as Crohn's disease than traditional optical imaging technologies. These advancements not only promise better accuracy in the earlier diagnosis of disease but also address the existing need for less invasive diagnostic technology. Through the synergy of quantitative and qualitative tissue characteristic analysis via μUS, doctors may soon be able to leverage sophisticated tools that view incipient disease development that traditional capsule endoscopy cannot measure. Such a symbiotic association between capsule endoscopy and emerging imaging technologies is bringing in a new era of comprehensive gastrointestinal health testing (Lay et al., 2017). Ongoing evolution of capsule endoscopy in the backdrop of increasingly broad applications in gastrointestinal health is essential to bettering patient outcomes. The integration of mucosal imaging with techniques like μUS and the consideration of unique patient populations enable both early treatment and diagnosis for the individual patient. Clinical practices in the future must be such that flexibility and innovation are prioritized, so that technology remains competitive with the complexity of GI disease. As the specialty matures, it may be anticipated that ongoing R&D will lead to increasingly sophisticated capsule designs and imaging modalities able to address more fully the many facets of gastrointestinal disease. The implementation of these technologies has the potential to transform gastroenterological management, ultimately leading to the advantage of a large number of patients and revalidating the merits of minimally invasive treatments (Bufler et al., 2009; Lay et al., 2017).

SUMMARY

In encapsulating the study of capsule endoscopy, its pioneering role in diagnosing and treating gastrointestinal illness, particularly those that are hard to access, like the small intestine, must be appreciated. The technique is a painless alternative to traditional endoscopic testing, which otherwise is fraught with much discomfort and danger for the patient. As mentioned, pairing capsule endoscopy with cutting-edge imaging technologies—e.g., balloon-assisted enteroscopy—enhances its diagnostic potential. These complementary modalities allow for direct harvest of biopsy and provide an entire view of the gastrointestinal tract, which substantially improves disease control of chronic diseases like Crohn's disease. The growing body of evidence suggests the necessity of integrating these new-age imaging modalities into practice to maximize patient outcomes and develop more efficient treatment algorithms (Hausmann & Albert, 2011). Moreover, the progress in wireless sensor technology is a major turning point in gastrointestinal diagnosis. Conventional approaches are based on cannulae that are painful for patients and have restrictions to access. Wireless capsule endoscopy, by comparison, provides a simplified method with much improved patient experiences. Nonetheless, as stated, issues surrounding radiation properties in the complicated human physiology require constant innovation. Finite-difference time-domain is an essential aspect in the design optimization of the telemetry system, which allows enhanced transmission and image quality. As research continues to address issues of antenna efficiency and radiation pattern, there is still hope for capsule endoscopy to be a significant player in gastrointestinal healthcare (Chirwa et al., 2003). Lastly, this chapter illustrates the tremendous developments and ongoing challenges in the field of capsule endoscopy. The applicability of the technology continues to expand, particularly with the growing demand for minimally invasive diagnostic technologies. As scientists and health professionals further develop these methods, careful attention must be paid to improve diagnostic quality and patient comfort. Directed research into how these imaging technologies affect clinical outcomes could establish new standards for patient care and treatment. Emphasizing the integration of capsule endoscopy with both traditional and emerging technologies will be paramount since the discipline is nurturing developments aimed at enhancing the overall effectiveness of gastrointestinal diagnosis and management (Chirwa et al., 2003; Hausmann & Albert, 2011).

In touching on the developments described in the current chapter, several significant considerations are apparent in identifying the diagnostic tool in the medical field. Above all, capsule endoscopy is an option for visually examining the GI tract in cases where other avenues, like colonoscopies, are risky or problematic for patients. The process requires the use of a tiny, swallowable capsule that contains cameras that record video footage of the intestines as it moves through. This innovation not only contributes to the patient's comfort but also extends the scope of gastrointestinal diagnostics, allowing for an in-depth examination of hard-to-reach areas where ordinary endoscopies may fail. The implications of the early diagnosis of conditions , such as colorectal polyps and cancer highlight the need for more development of this technology in the fight against serious medical issues, as the source material describes how effective the algorithms are in diagnosing polyps with high accuracy (Figueiredo et al., 2014). Another distinct feature of the chapter is the mention of sophisticated algorithms that facilitate the analysis of large amounts of data generated by capsule endoscopy. These algorithms play a central role in the detection of polyps and other abnormalities with geometrical analysis and assessment of texture content to categorize video frames. In particular, the proposed algorithm demonstrates very high sensitivity and specificity, at a sensitivity rate of over 81% per polyp at 90% specificity (Figueiredo et al., 2014). Such a measure of performance shows an impressive reduction in the volume of workload for human operators, along with ease of facilitation of the frame analysis process. This computerized approach not only minimizes error associated with fatigue during long analyses but also optimizes global diagnostic accuracy, making capsule endoscopy a more sensitive and reliable diagnostic tool in the assessment of the gastrointestinal tract. Finally, the chapter describes some of the latest advances in capsule endoscopy technology, such as 3D reconstruction and localization capabilities that are built into actively controlled capsule endoscopic robots. Such advancements could revolutionize the discipline of navigating the GI tract, increasing the effectiveness of the procedure through real-time feedback and adjustment during scans. The methods discussed here show promising results in prototype tests, leading the way to feasibility for precise, real-time mapping and adjustment for non-rigid deformations in the gastrointestinal tract. As research continues to evolve and these technologies improve, it is clear that capsule endoscopy will play an increasingly key role in modern gastrointestinal diagnosis and treatment, aiding clinical outcomes as well as patient experience.

CLOSER LOOK

BOWEL PREPARATION:

Bowel preparation is a critical component of gastrointestinal procedures, particularly colonoscopy and certain colorectal surgeries. Its primary goal is to cleanse the intestines of fecal matter, ensuring optimal visualization, reducing procedural complications, and improving diagnostic accuracy. Adequate bowel preparation is associated with higher polyp detection rates, shorter procedure times, and a decreased risk of infections or perioperative complications. The process of bowel preparation typically involves a combination of dietary modifications, oral laxatives, and sometimes adjunctive measures. Patients are often advised to follow a low-residue or clear-liquid diet for 24–48 hours prior to the procedure. Clear liquids such as water, tea, and broth are encouraged, while high-fiber foods, dairy, and solid meals are restricted to minimize residue in the bowel.

Oral laxatives form the cornerstone of bowel cleansing. Polyethylene glycol (PEG) solutions are commonly used due to their efficacy and safety, particularly in patients with electrolyte imbalances or renal insufficiency. Other options include sodium phosphate preparations, magnesium citrate, and stimulant laxatives like bisacodyl. The regimen may be administered as a single dose or split-dose, with the latter shown to improve bowel cleanliness and patient tolerance. Adjunctive measures may include enemas or prokinetic agents in selected cases.

Patient adherence and comfort are crucial for effective bowel preparation. Large volumes of PEG solutions and the unpleasant taste of some laxatives can reduce compliance. Strategies to improve adherence include flavoring agents, chilled solutions, smaller split doses, and clear, written instructions. Additionally, adequate hydration throughout the preparation period is important to prevent dehydration and electrolyte disturbances. Proper bowel preparation is assessed using standardized scoring systems, such as the Boston Bowel Preparation Scale, which evaluates cleanliness across different segments of the colon. Inadequate preparation can necessitate repeat procedures, increase procedural risk, and reduce diagnostic yield.

While generally safe, bowel preparation is not without potential complications. These include nausea, vomiting, bloating, abdominal pain, and rare electrolyte imbalances, particularly in elderly or medically complex patients. Careful patient selection, education, and monitoring are therefore essential to minimize risks and optimize outcomes.

In conclusion, bowel preparation is a foundational step in the success of colonoscopy and certain colorectal surgeries. Effective preparation relies on patient adherence, appropriate selection of cleansing agents, and clear communication regarding dietary and hydration guidelines. By ensuring optimal bowel cleanliness, clinicians enhance procedural safety, accuracy, and overall patient outcomes.

REFERENCES

1. Tringali, A., Thomson, M., Dumonceau, J. M., Tavares, M., Tabbers, M. M., Furlano, R., Spaander, M., Hassan, C., Tzvinikos, C., Ijsselstijn, H., Viala, J., Dall'Oglio, L., Benninga, M., Orel, R., Vandenplas, Y., Keil, R., Romano, C., Brownstone, E., Hlava, Š., Gerner, P., ... Zambelli, A. (2017). Pediatric gastrointestinal endoscopy: European Society of Gastrointestinal Endoscopy (ESGE) and European Society for Paediatric Gastroenterology Hepatology and Nutrition (ESPGHAN) Guideline Executive summary. *Endoscopy*, *49*(1), 83–91. https://doi.org/10.1055/s-0042-111002(accessed on 15th July 2025).
2. Abdollahi, F., Shaheed, M. H., Thaha, M. A., Vepa, R., et al. (2024). *A review of modeling and control of remote-controlled capsule endoscopes.* https://core.ac.uk/download/603254382.pdf (accessed on 15th July 2025).
3. Agneessens, S., Castel, T., Joseph, W., Rogier, H., et al. (2013). *Improved reception of in-body signals by means of a wearable multi-antenna system.* https://core.ac.uk/download/55806400.pdf (accessed on 15th July 2025).
4. Ahmad, B., Farup, I., Floor, P. A., Hovde, A., et al. (2023). *3D reconstruction of gastrointestinal regions using single-view methods.* https://core.ac.uk/download/646150506.pdf (accessed on 15th July 2025).
5. Hausmann J, Albert JG (2011) Detecting and Managing Small Bowel Crohn's Disease – Capsule Endoscopy Becoming a First Line Diagnostic Method? J Gastroint Dig Syst S1:002. doi:10.4172/2161-069X.S1-002(accessed on 15th July 2025).
6. Turan, M., Almalioglu, Y., Araujo, H. *et al.* A non-rigid map fusion-based direct SLAM method for endoscopic capsule robots. *Int J Intell Robot Appl* **1**, 399–409 (2017). https://doi.org/10.1007/s41315-017-0036-4(accessed on 15th July 2025).
7. M. Turan et al., "Unsupervised Odometry and Depth Learning for Endoscopic Capsule Robots," 2018 IEEE/RSJ International Conference on Intelligent Robots and Systems (IROS), Madrid, Spain, 2018, pp. 1801-1807, doi: 10.1109/IROS.2018.8593623.(accessed on 15th July 2025).
8. Monsanto, P., Almeida, N., Lérias, C., Figueiredo, P., Gouveia, H., & Sofia, C. (2012). Is there still a role for intraoperative enteroscopy in patients with obscure gastrointestinal bleeding?. *Revista espanola de enfermedades digestivas*, *104*(4), 190–196. https://doi.org/10.4321/s1130-01082012000400004(accessed on 15th July 2025).
9. Alomair, O. A. (2024). *New trends in management of vascular lower GI bleeding between endoscopy and angiography: Literature review.* https://core.ac.uk/download/640070005.pdf (accessed on 15th July 2025).
10. H S Lay et al 2017 J. Phys.: Conf. Ser. **797** 012003(accessed on 15th July 2025).
11. Guarini, A., De Marinis, F., Hassan, C., Manta, R., De Francesco, V., Annibale, B., & Zullo, A. (2018). High concordance between trained nurses and gastroenterologists in evaluating recordings of small bowel video capsule endoscopy (VCE). *Journal of gastrointestinal and liver diseases : JGLD*, *27*(2), 271. https://doi.org/10.15403/jgld.2014.1121.272.bch(accessed on 15th July 2025).
12. Arebi, N., & Saunders, B. P. (2005). *Endoscopy: An evolving specialty.* https://core.ac.uk/download/46602009.pdf (accessed on 15th July 2025).

13. Ciuti, G., Caliò, R., Camboni, D., Neri, L., Bianchi, F., Arezzo, A., Koulaouzidis, A., Schostek, S., Stoyanov, D., Oddo, C. M., Magnani, B., Menciassi, A., Morino, M., Schurr, M. O., & Dario, P. (2016). Frontiers of robotic endoscopic capsules: a review. *Journal of micro-bio robotics*, *11*(1), 1–18. https://doi.org/10.1007/s12213-016-0087-x(accessed on 15th July 2025).

14. Arguello-Viudez, L. (Lidia), Balanzo-Tintore, J. (Joaquin), Carballo-Alvarez, F. (Fernando), Espinos-Perez, T., et al. (2011). *Evaluation of different bowel preparations for small bowel capsule endoscopy: A prospective, randomized, controlled study.* https://core.ac.uk/download/83574169.pdf (accessed on 15th July 2025).

15. Attar, R., Wang, Z., Xie, X., Yue, Y., et al. (2018). *2D reconstruction of small intestine's interior wall.* http://arxiv.org/abs/1803.05817 (accessed on 15th July 2025).

16. Baatrup, G., Blanes-Vidal, V., Braun, J. M., Nadimi, E. S., et al. (2024). *Towards full integration of artificial intelligence in colon capsule endoscopy's pathway.* http://arxiv.org/abs/2406.09761 (accessed on 15th July 2025).

17. Berger, A., May, A., Moglia, A., Postgate, A., Ross, A., Tocchi, A., Neugut, A. I., et al. (2010). *Duodenal carcinoma at the ligament of Treitz: A molecular and clinical perspective.* https://core.ac.uk/download/78918848.pdf (accessed on 15th July 2025).

18. E. Wadge, M. Boulougoura and V. Kodogiannis, "Computer-assisted diagnosis of wireless-capsule endoscopic images using neural network based techniques," CIMSA. 2005 IEEE International Conference on Computational Intelligence for Measurement Systems and Applications, 2005., Messian, Italy, 2005, pp. 328-333, doi: 10.1109/CIMSA.2005.1522889.https://core.ac.uk/download/161114235.pdf (accessed on 15th July 2025).

19. van der Stap, N., van der Heijden, F., & Broeders, I. A. (2013). Towards automated visual flexible endoscope navigation. *Surgical endoscopy*, *27*(10), 3539–3547. https://doi.org/10.1007/s00464-013-3003-7(accessed on 15th July 2025).

20. Bufler, P., Fritscher-Ravens, A., Milla, P., Nuutinen, M., et al. (2009). *The feasibility of wireless capsule endoscopy in detecting small intestinal pathology in children under the age of 8 years: A multicenter European study.* https://core.ac.uk/download/12175824.pdf (accessed on 15th July 2025).

21. Burch, W. C., Jr., Kashyap, P. K., Kastenberg, D., et al. (2017). *Multicenter, randomized study to optimize bowel for colon capsule endoscopy.* https://core.ac.uk/download/155271589.pdf (accessed on 15th July 2025).

22. Burczyk, R., Duszyński, K., Iglewski, P., Jarych, A., et al. (2025). *Automated recognition of abnormalities in gastrointestinal endoscopic images – Evaluation of an AI tool for identifying polyps and other irregularities.* https://core.ac.uk/download/656518186.pdf (accessed on 15th July 2025).

23. Chirwa, L. C., Cumming, D. R. S., Hammond, P. A., Roy, S., et al. (2003). *Electromagnetic radiation from ingested sources in the human intestine between 150 MHz and 1.2 GHz.* https://core.ac.uk/download/1393541.pdf (accessed on 15th July 2025).

24. Cochran, S., Cox, B. F., Cummins, G., Desmulliez, M. P. Y., et al. (2017). *Ultrasound capsule endoscopy: Sounding out the future.* https://core.ac.uk/download/83925812.pdf (accessed on 15th July 2025).

25. Woods, S. P., & Constandinou, T. G. (2011). Towards a micropositioning system for targeted drug delivery in wireless capsule endoscopy. *Annual International Conference of the IEEE Engineering in Medicine and Biology Society. IEEE Engineering in Medicine and Biology Society. Annual International Conference, 2011*, 7372–7375. https://doi.org/10.1109/IEMBS.2011.6091717Cooper, J. M., Cui, L., Cumming, D. R. S., Hammond, P. A., et al. (2005). *A programmable microsystem using system-on-chip for real-time biotelemetry.* https://core.ac.uk/download/1394255.pdf (accessed on 15th July 2025).

26. Cosmas, J., Intzes, I., & Meng, H. (2014). *Technology of swallowable capsule for medical applications.* https://core.ac.uk/download/29139345.pdf (accessed on 15th July 2025).

27. Ebrahimi, N., Bi, C., Cappelleri, D. J., Ciuti, G., Conn, A. T., Faivre, D., Habibi, N., et al. (2020). Magnetic actuation methods in bio/soft robotics. *Advanced Functional Materials, 31.* https://doi.org/10.1002/adfm.202005137 (accessed on 15th July 2025).

28. Figueiredo, I. N., Figueiredo, P. N., Mamonov, A. V., Tsai, Y. H., et al. (2014). *Automated polyp detection in colon capsule endoscopy.* http://arxiv.org/abs/1305.1912 (accessed on 15th July 2025).

29. Fu, Z., Jin, Z., Zhang, C., He, Z., Zha, Z., Hu, C., Gan, T., et al. (2021). The future of endoscopic navigation: A review of advanced endoscopic vision technology. *IEEE Access, 9*, 41144–41167. https://doi.org/10.1109/access.2021.3065104 (accessed on 15th July 2025).

30. Goldfarb, N. I., Pizzi, L. T., Fuhr, J. P., Jr, Salvador, C., Sikirica, V., Kornbluth, A., & Lewis, B. (2004). Diagnosing Crohn's disease: an economic analysis comparing wireless capsule endoscopy with traditional diagnostic procedures. *Disease management : DM, 7*(4), 292–304. https://doi.org/10.1089/dis.2004.7.292(accessed on 15th July 2025).

31. Intzes, I., Meng, H., & Vassios, V. (2015). *Design of wireless swallowable capsule with minimum power consumption and high-resolution images.* https://core.ac.uk/download/30340135.pdf (accessed on 15th July 2025).

32. Joseph, W., Martens, L., Lopez-Linares, K., Thielens, A., et al. (2014). *Characterization of path loss and absorption for a wireless radio frequency link between an in-body endoscopy capsule and a receiver outside the body.* https://core.ac.uk/download/55888533.pdf (accessed on 15th July 2025).

33. Koulaouzidis, A., Annese, V., Ben-Soussan, E., Clarke, J., Cotton, J., Rondonotti, E., Esaki, M., et al. (2016). *Small-bowel capsule endoscopy with panoramic view: Results of the first multicenter, observational study (with videos).* https://core.ac.uk/download/46565102.pdf (accessed on 15th July 2025).

34. Lakatos, P. L. (2006). *Recent trends in the epidemiology of inflammatory bowel diseases: Up or down?* https://core.ac.uk/download/11855817.pdf (accessed on 15th July 2025).

35. Muñoz-Navas, M. (Miguel). (2008). *Capsule Endoscopy.* https://core.ac.uk/download/83573528.pdf (accessed on 15th July 2025).

36. Quaglia, C., Dario, P., Menciassi, A., Simi, M., et al. (2010). *Design, fabrication, and testing of a capsule with hybrid locomotion for gastrointestinal tract exploration.* https://core.ac.uk/download/54929724.pdf (accessed on 15th July 2025).

37. Reingruber, H., Universitat Autònoma de Barcelona. Escola d'Enginyeria, Vilariño Freire, F. (2009). *Intestinal content detection in capsule endoscopy using robust features.* https://core.ac.uk/download/13302198.pdf (accessed on 15th July 2025).

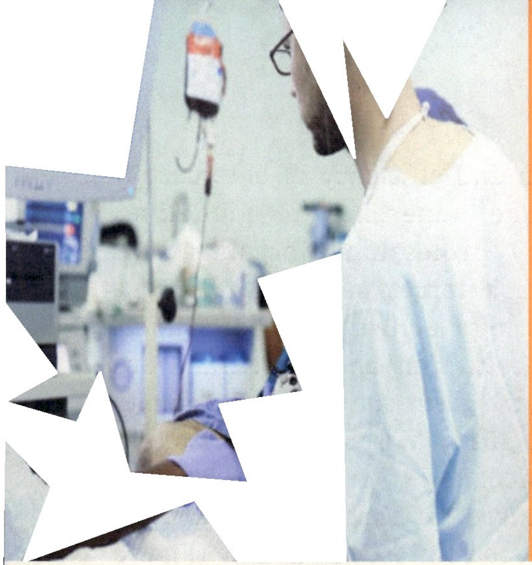

Chapter 10

ENTEROSCOPY TECHNIQUES

Contents

Introduction 281
10.1. Historical Background 284
10.2. Types of Enteroscopy 287
10.3. Indications for Enteroscopy 291
10.4. Preparation for Enteroscopy 294
10.5. Enteroscopy Procedure 297
10.6. Complications and Risks 300
Summary 304
References 307

Introduction

Enteroscopy has grown more prominent as an area of gastrointestinal medicine, and its utility is largely based on the fact that it provides direct visual and intervention in the small intestine. Because patients present with a myriad of gastrointestinal symptoms, the demand for improved diagnostics has driven the evolution of enteroscopy modalities. This process involves highly specialized endoscopic techniques to overcome the complexity of the small bowel, a region normally not easily approached by conventional endoscopy. The role of enteroscopy techniques becomes more important in light of increasing numbers of small bowel pathology cases, prompting advancements both in terms of technology as well as clinical practice to optimize patient outcomes. Thus, this essay tries to explore the different aspects of enteroscopy with special reference to evolution, technique, and clinical usefulness of enteroscopy in the present era. The convergence of methods of enteroscopy gives clinicians excellent tools for a number of therapeutic procedures, including biopsy acquisition, polypectomy, and even foreign body retrieval. Advances in technology in instrument and imaging design have taken endoscopists' reach to regions that were not initially accessible for intervention. The success of these approaches is further supplemented by the inclusion of ultrasound imaging, which has been explained by the European Federation of Societies for Ultrasound in Medicine and Biology. The establishment of the Gastrointestinal Ultrasound (GIUS) task force indicates an operational change toward the application of these advanced imaging modalities in practice, which paves the way for better-informed healthcare professionals' decisions (Nylund et al., 2017).

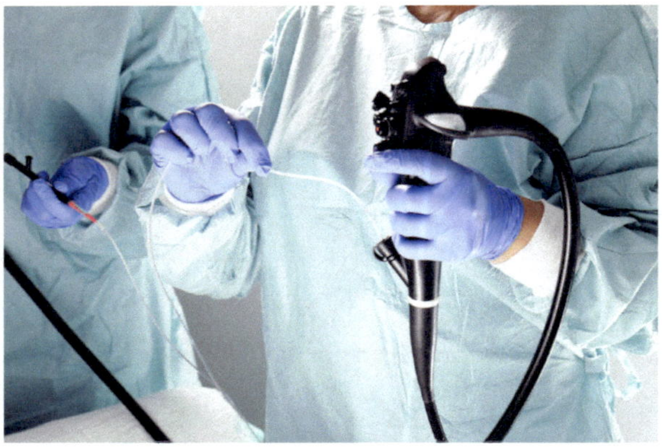

Figure 10.1. Enteroscopy techniques.

Source: https://www.rockymountaingastro.com/wp-content/uploads/2018/08/Double-Balloon-Enteroscopy.jpg.

These developments underscore the necessity to maximize enteroscopy procedures to deliver the optimal diagnosis and treatment of small bowel disease. In addition, the impact of evolving enteroscopy techniques goes beyond plain intervention; it bears high stakes in research and clinical education training. As healthcare turns towards evidence-based practice, the incorporation of empirical evidence into clinical practice guidelines ensures practitioners are adequately informed with current methodologies. The following essay will discuss the impacts that evolving research and technology have on the standardization and efficiency of enteroscopy techniques. The adherence to guidelines established by professional organizations and clinical task forces serves to improve practice uniformity across different clinical environments, cultivating a spirit of teamwork and learning in the gastroenterology community (Balzarini et al., 2011). Most significant, lastly, is the development of new enteroscopy technology, one that promises to transform therapeutic paradigms in gastrointestinal health (Figure 10.1).

Definition of Enteroscopy

Enteroscopy is a type of endoscopic procedure that enables the visualization and assessment of the small intestine, a field that was previously not considered accessible to direct intervention. Enteroscopy is an essential diagnostic tool for evaluating many gastrointestinal conditions, especially obscure gastrointestinal bleeding and inflammatory bowel diseases , such as Crohn's disease. With the use of advanced technologies, enteroscopy allows practitioners to obtain high-quality images and, if desired, therapeutic interventions , such as biopsies or cauterization. With the introduction of newer equipment in the form of balloon-assisted enteroscopes and capsule endoscopes, the scope and applications of enteroscopy have been enhanced manyfold, allowing greater in-depth assessment of pathology in the small bowel. Therefore, not only does this process enhance diagnostic yield, but it also plays an important part in the overall management of gastrointestinal symptomatology by informing the planning of subsequent treatment. The utility of enteroscopy is seen by its use in the investigation of obscure gastrointestinal bleeding (OGIB). In this case, small bowel capsule endoscopy (SBCE) has proven to be a useful asset since it allows practitioners to see the small intestine without invasion. This new technique has transformed the diagnostic process by providing sharp images that can reveal a potential source of bleeding. While SBCE's negative results may complicate the clinical picture—raising the specter of the risk of rebleeding—enteroscopy remains crucial in patients whose initial examinations are unable to identify bleeding lesions. The requirement for follow-up by enteroscopy in patients with adverse SBCE results is emphasized by studies demonstrating a high rate of patients likely to suffer from rebleeding events. As such, the coupling of SBCE and enteroscopy provides an example of how modern imaging can enhance diagnostic quality and management interventions in gastroenterology (Castro et al., 2014). On another note, enteroscopy has evolved significantly, with technological advances enhancing its efficiency and ease. Double-balloon enteroscopy and other endoscopic modalities have now transformed the practice of clinicians in diagnosing the small bowel. These modalities allow for deeper intubation of the small intestine, and diagnosis in previously elusive conditions is now possible. Enteroscopy techniques are especially important in the treatment of chronic disease , such as Crohn's disease, as highlighted in literature on the application of imaging for the assessment of treatment. These advances allow clinicians to take biopsies and perform therapeutic maneuvers directly in the small bowel, thus transforming potential surgical procedures into non-interventional or minimally interventional ones. As practitioners further develop the procedures, enteroscopy continues to be a cornerstone of current gastroenterological practice, providing essential information on the treatment of complex small bowel disease (Hausmann & Albert, 2011).

Role of Enteroscopy in Gastrointestinal Diagnostics

The role of enteroscopy in the diagnosis of the gastrointestinal tract has come more into favor, particularly for its sole capability for scoping and assessing the small bowel. Traditional endoscopic techniques have frequently been disappointing in addressing pathology of this segment of the gastrointestinal tract due to its length and intricacies. Enteroscopy, employing methods , such as double balloon enteroscopy (DBE) and device-assisted enteroscopy (DAE), has revolutionized the concept of approaching small bowel diagnosis. DBE can travel through the whole small bowel through both the anterograde and retrograde routes, making complete visualization and treatment of mid-gastrointestinal bleeding, polyps, and tumors possible. As research would show, its diagnostic value is significant, with DBE offering a broader view of the small bowel than hitherto possible, thus facilitating more effective clinical decisions. Use of small-bowel capsule endoscopy highlights the importance of enteroscopy in the diagnosis of gastrointestinal disease even more. Being a non-invasive technique, this is particularly useful for patients with suspected small-bowel bleeding since it photographs the entire mucosa of the intestine safely and effectively. New guidelines incorporate capsule endoscopy as a first-line test owing to its excellent safety profile and tolerance by patients (Pennazio et al., 2022). In addition, its use on time within 48 hours of bleeding raises the chances of detection of potential sources of hemorrhage. Capsule endoscopy's flexibility is also demonstrated in its use in the evaluation of diseases like Crohn's disease and iron-deficiency anemia, and hence becomes a critical tool in the diagnostic arsenal. Therefore, the evolution of enteroscopic modalities represents a paradigm shift in the assessment of small intestinal diseases. Also, enteroscopy has been useful, especially in therapeutic as well as diagnostic applications, especially in the treatment of lesions discovered through preliminary tests. Device-assisted enteroscopy allows experts not only to observe but also to cure various conditions, including vascular lesions, tumors, and other abnormalities inside the small intestine itself (Fılı, 2015). This twofold capability makes enteroscopic techniques even more valuable, thus making them preferred for use over surgery. The expanding evidence base in favor of enteroscopy further highlights its clinical applicability, especially with decreased complication rates as practitioners gain more experience. In totality, the incorporation of enteroscopic techniques into gastrointestinal diagnosis represents a remarkable progress, with enhanced diagnostic precision and therapeutic benefit, ultimately for the patient in a wide range of gastrointestinal illnesses (Figure 10.2).

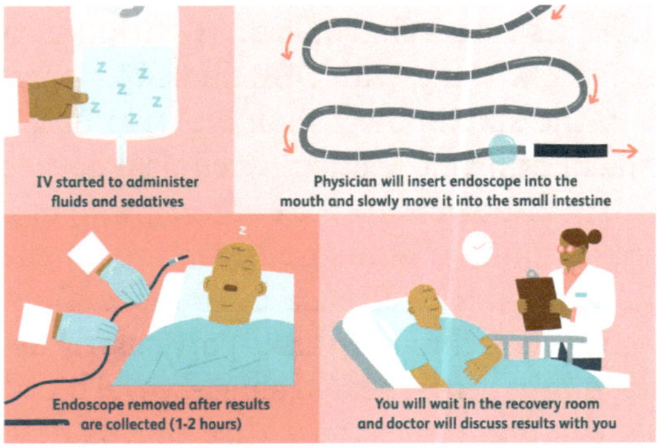

Figure 10.2. Importance of enteroscopy in gastrointestinal diagnostics.

Source: https://www.verywellhealth.com/thmb/MM26UTp9W2EZMm0uV2O1KnzbDhs=/1500x1000/filters:no_upscale():max_bytes(150000):strip_icc()/enteroscopy-procedure-4588157-01-c2c9f2535552483db13412f43e6aaec4.png.

10.1. Historical Background

The development of enteroscopy techniques through the years is one of the milestone events in gastroenterology history, reflecting improvements in technology, medical science, and treatment practice. Enteroscopy, or endoscopic investigation of the small intestine, has become an indispensable diagnostic and therapeutic tool for gastrointestinal disease. The early days of this specialty were very rudimentary, settling with simple endoscopic instruments and cursory visual investigations. But the advancement of endoscopic technology since the mid-20th century has brought more advanced tools, enabling gastroenterologists to see and engage with the digestive system in ways previously unimaginable. The adaptation of techniques like endoscopic hemostasis and polipectomy in the 1970s turned the tide, moving from observation to active intervention, making the seeds of contemporary enteroscopy methods (Pennazio et al., 2022). With the evolution of enteroscopy, the complexity of the procedures necessitated the requirement for higher expertise and training among gastroenterologists. Initially, the procedures were largely focused on diagnosis; subsequent advances in endoscopic procedures added therapeutic applications as well. The advent of endoscopic sphincterotomy highlighted this shift and exemplified the dual potential of endoscopy in diagnosing and actually treating conditions. In addition, advances like plastic and metal stents for biliary palliation are also key milestones in interventional endoscopy. They highlight the necessity of ongoing education and change in the industry, as interventionalists now need to have a versatile skill set extending far beyond standard diagnostic procedures (Pennazio et al., 2022). Therefore, the history of enteroscopy procedures is a story of medical development, an image of how gastroenterology practice evolved over time. From the crude gastrointestinal examinations to the sophisticated interventions is a testament to the relentless search for improved patient care and outcomes. With the advancement of methods, so did the gastroenterologists' work advance, since they had to learn a complete set of procedures that require high expertise. This indicates the need for ongoing learning and training so that practitioners can keep up with the old setting and new advancements in enteroscopy. The convergence of these elements brings more insight into the function of enteroscopy in modern gastrointestinal medicine to the fore (Pennazio et al., 2022).

10.1.1. Development of Enteroscopy Techniques

The evolution of enteroscopy methods significantly enhanced the capacity to diagnose gastroenterology, enabling doctors to see and assess the small intestine effectively. Routine endoscopic examinations were largely limited to the upper and lower regions of the gastrointestinal tract, and in-depth studies of the small bowel were not possible. Fiberoptic technology enhanced the evolution of enteroscopy methods, allowing for more extensive enteroscopy methods, including deep enteroscopy, which provides longer viewing and intervention in the small bowel. Innovations have made it possible for physicians to diagnose conditions that were hard to diagnose in the past, such as small bowel tumors or occult gastrointestinal bleeding, thereby improving patient prognosis. Thus, understanding of these advances is crucial for healthcare practitioners and educators as a way of enhancing diagnostics and therapy strategies in small bowel disease. Wireless capsule endoscopy (WCE) represents a significant advance in enteroscopy techniques, achieving minimally invasive visualization of the small intestine. The technique involves swallowing a capsule containing a camera, which transmits images to a recording device as it travels through the digestive tract. The introduction of WCE was welcomed enthusiastically because it removes most of the disadvantages of conventional endoscope examination, particularly in terms of patient tolerance and diagnostic yield. Evidence shows a gradual rise in the use of WCE in different medical centers, evidence of the method's increasing popularity among the clinical community (Ghunaim & Bach, 2014). The possible delayed diagnosis, in addition to capsule retention issues, points towards the need for continuous research and development in enteroscopic procedures to maximize their use in clinical practice. Endoscopic treatment has evolved into a significant component of the treatment of diseases like Crohn's disease, particularly in stricture or obstruction. Endoscopy in this setting is a less invasive intervention that makes diagnostic evaluation compatible with therapeutic intervention, thereby providing a less invasive alternative to more conventional surgical treatments. The introduction of novel techniques, such as balloon dilation and strictureplasty, has added efficacy and safety to the procedures, offering personalized treatment strategies in line with the principles of precision medicine (Bartocci et al., 2024). Moreover, ongoing research continues to bridge gaps in evidence to further enhance outcomes in therapeutic enteroscopy. As the specialty progresses, understanding of the interaction between these new techniques and traditional approaches will be central to optimizing treatment methods for complex gastrointestinal disease (Figure 10.3).

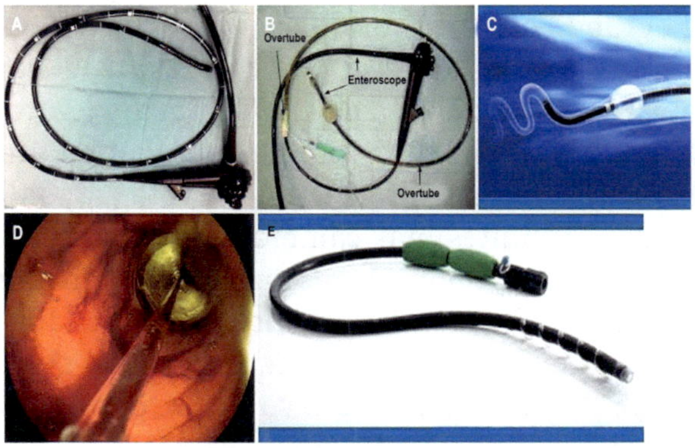

Figure 10.3. Development of enteroscopy techniques.

Source: https://f6publishing.blob.core.windows.net/8e101209-539c-486d-91f5-fc7ec33518b4/WJGE-5-476-g003.jpg.

10.1.2. Key Milestones in Enteroscopy

The historical development of enteroscopy methods has been framed by major milestones that have defined the future of gastrointestinal diagnostics and therapy. One of the greatest advancements was the advent of the double-balloon enteroscopy (DBE) procedure in the early 2000s, allowing for deeper access to the small bowel than traditional procedures. The new method allowed clinicians to visualize and treat small intestinal pathology, formerly highly inaccessible. The introduction of DBE not only carried with it a technological improvement but also paved the way for higher standards and procedures of training for enteroscopic procedures. As reported in recent studies, advances in training designs have had positive effects on the overall quality of endoscopic practice, further enhancing the capacity to perform complex enteroscopic interventions (Alrubaiy et al., 2018). Thus, critical milestones in enteroscopy also influence the safety and efficacy of treatment of the gastrointestinal tract. The next and most important milestone in the development of enteroscopy technology was the introduction into clinical practice of video capsule endoscopy (VCE). That minimally invasive technology, first introduced towards the end of the 1990s, provides for detailed visualization of the small intestine through the use of a swallowable capsule with an infinitesimal camera. VCE has found a particularly beneficial application in the diagnosis of occult gastrointestinal bleeding, Crohn's disease, and other diseases of the small bowel. The minimally invasive nature of this test has greatly improved patient compliance and comfort, but still provides high-quality diagnostic imaging. Furthermore, the development of endoscopic ultrasonography (EUS) has further expanded the horizon for the assessment of gastrointestinal conditions and the delivery of therapeutic interventions. These developments have highlighted the need for rigorous training programs, ensuring that gastroenterology professionals are properly qualified to utilize these advanced devices effectively (Pennazio et al., 2022). Training and certification in advancing enteroscopy procedures are crucial and cannot be overstated. Thorough training programs have come into being, emphasizing the need for proper training to navigate the rising complexities of these interventions. A recent survey brought to light that while training satisfaction has improved, there remains an issue with variable access to training lists and the ineffectiveness of offered training in certain regions of priority (Alrubaiy et al., 2018). As a response to the issues, there are initiatives being proposed to standardize training approaches and boost accessible resources. These updates are required to maintain high standards of care. Because enteroscopy is now constantly evolving with emerging innovations and interventions, ongoing focus on training and procedural precision will ensure that practitioners can make the most of the innovations, ultimately having a positive impact on patient outcomes in gastrointestinal health.

10.1.3. Evolution of Technology in Enteroscopy

Technological progress in enteroscopy has been a significant advancement in gastrointestinal diagnostic and therapeutic interventions. Traditionally, endoscopic procedures were only able to image parts of the gastrointestinal (GI) tract, thereby precluding the assessment of small intestine conditions. The arrival of capsule endoscopy in 2000 revolutionized the practice by offering a painless way to investigate the entire small intestine. This technique, employing a tiny camera in a capsule, facilitates viewing of otherwise inaccessible locations, thereby assisting in the diagnosis of uncommon gastrointestinal bleeding, Crohn's disease, and small bowel tumors. The broad acceptance of capsule endoscopy as a gold standard examination test is testimony to the broad impact of technological advances on patient outcomes as well as the diagnostic quality of enteroscopy techniques (Muñoz-Navas et al., 2008). Moreover, the evolution in wireless capsule technology has further expanded its uses in clinics. The contribution of Gavriel Iddan in 1981, who introduced the wireless camera pill, enabled gastroenterologists to gain clear images of the GI tract without an invasive procedure. Despite the limitations of the technology in the early period, the subsequent development in optical sensors and communication systems has greatly enhanced the performance and diagnostic application of such capsules. New technologies in multi-wavelength optical sensors enable a greater number of chemicals to be detected, significantly increasing diagnostic specificity. Furthermore, the application of advanced optical communication links has overcome the bandwidth limitations inherent in radio frequency systems and increased data transmission rates.

These breakthroughs underscore a development that not only improves visualization but also enhances the overall worth of enteroscopy in the clinic (Katsafadou, 2023). Further development and research in the field of enteroscopy, which is continually growing, seek to integrate new technology , such as artificial intelligence and machine learning, to optimize diagnostics and therapeutic interventions. These technologies have the promise to enhance image analysis and decision-making during enteroscopic procedures and potentially deliver real-time gains in clinical outcomes.

The convergence of computational capabilities with advanced imaging modalities promises unprecedented potential for the detection of diseases earlier in gastrointestinal diseases. There are also new developments to develop intelligent capsules that have enhanced sensor technology to detect certain biomarkers for numerous GI conditions. Hence, enteroscopy's future lies in both the evolution of existing methods as well as the revolutionary use of technology that encourages patient-centered approaches to gastrointestinal treatment.

10.2. Types of Enteroscopy

Enteroscopy techniques have undergone evolution and have come up with many different methods that cater to various diagnostic and therapeutic roles within the gastrointestinal tract. Of these techniques, traditional push enteroscopy remains a cornerstone procedure, offering access to the proximal small bowel. While useful, its shortcoming is that it cannot access the distal segments. To improve upon this, balloon-assisted enteroscopy in the form of the double-balloon technique and single-balloon technique has been developed and introduced, offering deeper examination. Balloon-assisted systems offer better maneuverability with the endoscope and better visualization, and these play a central role in the diagnosis of small bowel disorders. Notably, these new methods have significantly enhanced the diagnostic yield on the examination of unexplained lesions or gastrointestinal hemorrhage, and this captures the evolving nature of enteroscopy practices in enhancing patient results through enhanced accessibility (Fernandez et al., 2020). Wireless capsule endoscopy has completely revolutionized small intestine visualization, offering a non-invasive alternative to traditional enteroscopic interventions. The capsule, which consists of small cameras attached to it, moves through the gastrointestinal tract, snapping photographs that provide highly useful information on small bowel pathologies. This technology is particularly helpful in the diagnosis of small intestine tumors, which is challenging due to the slippery nature of the tumors and the unavailability of the bowels for access. With continued improvement in imaging, the sensitivity and specificity of diagnoses have sharply risen, allowing better surveillance in high-risk groups. While wireless capsule endoscopy is a significant advantage, its lack of ability to provide therapeutic intervention is a limitation, making other methods more essential in the clinic (Hausmann & Albert, 2011). Spiral enteroscopy is another emerging technology in enteroscopy procedures that utilizes a new overtube to allow the endoscope to be advanced in a spiral manner. This method is aimed at effective engagement of the small intestines intricate anatomical features to achieve a longer reach compared to traditional methods. Through enhancement of scopes propulsion capability by the use of flexible overtubes, spiral enteroscopy has a potential benefit for patients requiring extensive small bowel access. This method is particularly suited in the management of small bowel tumors, where accurate positioning is highly significant in diagnosis and management. The continuous investigation and incorporation of various enteroscopy modalities emphasize the importance of individualized approaches in gastroenterology, allowing practitioners to optimize their approaches to secure effective diagnosis and intervention of gastrointestinal diseases (Fernandez et al., 2020) (Figure 10.4).

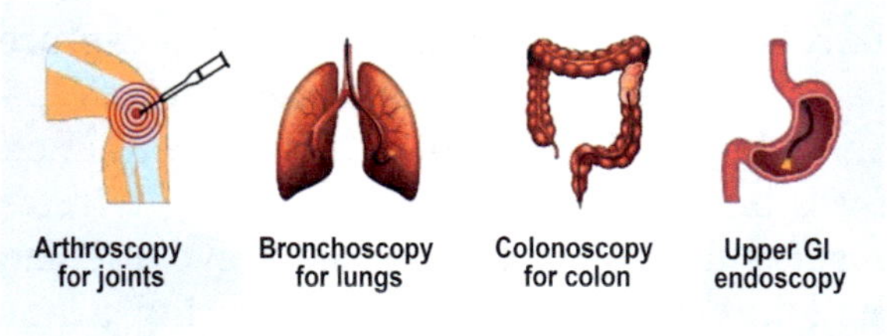

Figure 10.4. Types of enteroscopy.

Source: https://image.slidesharecdn.com/endoscopy-190724124710/95/endoscopy-types-preparation-diagnosis-procedure-and-risks-4-638.jpg?cb=1563972496.

10.2.1. Push Enteroscopy

Push enteroscopy is a key milestone in gastrointestinal diagnostic technology, particularly for the small bowel. The small bowel used to be a no-go zone for regular endoscopic investigation, stifling doctors' capacity to diagnose a treasure trove of ailments that may be found here, including bleeding, Crohn's disease, and tumors. Push enteroscopy was a breakthrough, allowing further investigation of the small bowel. This technique employs a long, flexible endoscope that is "pushed" beyond the scope of standard endoscopy, enabling the visualization and therapeutic intervention of previously inaccessible pathologies. Push enteroscopy, especially, has proven beneficial for evaluating small bowel bleeding, enabling physicians to visualize sources of bleeding that are not visualizable by non-invasive imaging or upper endoscopy modalities. A systematic review refers to the comparative effectiveness of push enteroscopy, particularly with reference to its comparison with single balloon enteroscopy, two important balloon-assisted enteroscopic interventions. While both have established safety and minimal rates of complications, findings reveal that single balloon enteroscopy can provide greater diagnostic and therapeutic success rates than push enteroscopy. The review indicates that push enteroscopy remains relevant, especially for direct intervention or management of small bowel disease. Also important are ongoing reviews of these techniques as they complement a physician's tool set in the management of gastrointestinal diseases. With new evidence being discovered, the medical community continues to evaluate the specific indications and effectiveness of push enteroscopy in the overall framework of enteroscopic interventions (Abdulaziz et al., 2022). Of particular interest is the contemporary management of small bowel diseases, particularly Crohn's disease, which includes the application of push enteroscopy as part of an extended diagnostic modality. While capsule endoscopy is an endoscopic technique that is permissive for initial visualization, push enteroscopy allows for biopsies and therapeutic maneuvers to be directly done, and this can be of paramount significance in managing active disease or assessing complications. Current technical improvements in imaging further enhance push enteroscopy, optimally enhancing the therapeutic potential of observing disease activity and therapeutic reaction, particularly in patients who have undergone surgical intervention. Through integration of these techniques, clinicians can provide an integrated treatment regimen for the treatment of small bowel disorders, ultimately leading to improved patient outcomes and individualized therapeutic protocols (Hausmann & Albert, 2011).

10.2.2. Balloon-Assisted Enteroscopy

The new technique of balloon-assisted enteroscopy has brought gastrointestinal diagnostics into a new era, particularly in the visualization and intervention of small bowel disease. As opposed to traditional endoscopic methods that have the tendency to encounter difficulties in moving through the twisting anatomy of the small intestine, balloon-assisted enteroscopy employs a specialized balloon tip with added flexibility and maneuverability. This technique facilitates deep intubation of the small intestine, which provides a better opportunity to enter segments that are otherwise hard to evaluate. The increased maneuverability facilitated by the balloon system enhances the endoscopist's precision to diagnose such entities as Crohn's disease, small bowel tumors, and obscure gastrointestinal bleeding. Using this new method, physicians are capable of acquiring critical biopsy specimens and performing therapeutic maneuvers, hence improving patients' outcomes and reducing the need for more invasive surgical intervention. Balloon-assisted enteroscopy is of particular significance in the management of complex disorders , such as Crohn's disease. Current studies have highlighted the integration of the technique with other imaging technologies to further increase diagnostic yields and successful treatment. For instance, studies prove that integration of balloon-assisted enteroscopy with capsule endoscopy will significantly improve the diagnostic yield for small intestinal lesions, which is essential for tailoring patient management programs. Contemporary studies indicate that imaging and treatment of small bowel lesions make it possible to create a balanced plan of care for chronic inflammatory illnesses and therefore, facilitate more effective treatment plans. Also, the procedure's capacity to acquire biopsies from otherwise inaccessible sites enables clinicians to establish definitive diagnoses, thereby leading to maximally effective therapeutic intervention and improved long-term health outcomes for patients with such multifactorial disorders (Hausmann & Albert, 2011). While many advantages are associated with balloon-assisted enteroscopy, the procedure mandates careful attention to patient selection and procedure risk. While it is well noted for having a low rate of complications compared to traditional intraoperative enteroscopy, certain patient groups are at increased risk for procedure-related morbidity.

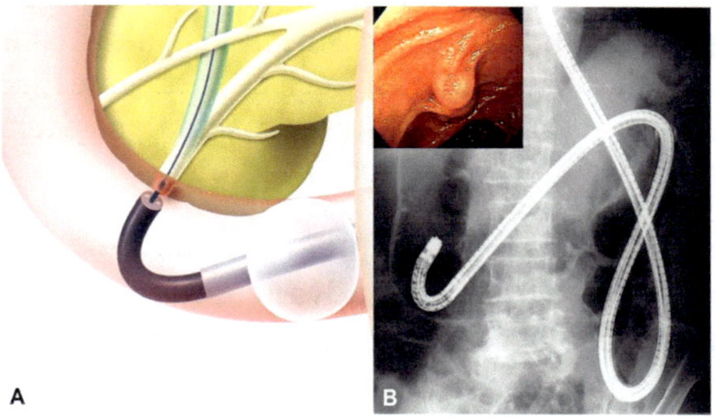

Figure 10.5. Balloon-assisted enteroscopy.

Source: https://els-jbs-prod-cdn.jbs.elsevierhealth.com/cms/attachment/ee3718f0-4ada-4d79-ac1a-ff6800394ebc/gr4_lrg.jpg.

Its safety profile has been evaluated through studies and noted that, though infrequent, complications can include bleeding or perforation. Indications for this modality are also important to understand; it is employed primarily when other diagnostic means have been unsuccessful. Nevertheless, the cumulative success of balloon-assisted enteroscopy in the diagnosis and management of small bowel pathology validates its crucial role in modern gastrointestinal practice. As evidenced in publications, adequate training and clinical experience are essential to optimize the success of this new endoscopic technique (Monsanto et al., 2012) (Figure 10.5).

10.2.3. Double-Balloon Enteroscopy

Double-balloon enteroscopy, a new modality of enteroscopy, has become popular due to its ability to visualize and intervene on the pathology of the small bowel. In this modality, two balloons are positioned on the endoscope, one at the tip and one on the overtube, such that the endoscopist has the convenience to traverse the tube-like yet individually challenging anatomy of the small bowel. The two-way inflation of the balloons allows for segmental push of the endoscope, creating a deep access into the area distal to the duodenum. This capability is particularly useful in diagnosing and treating conditions , such as gastrointestinal bleeding, tumors, or strictures that regularly happen within this part of the body.

The new technique of double-balloon enteroscopy is an advancement beyond enteroscopic techniques, especially overcoming the limitations of traditional endoscopy. Double-balloon enteroscopy has proven to be a helpful tool in clinical practice, especially in the geriatric patient population, as they often present with complicated gastrointestinal diseases. Evidence points toward the fact that almost 35%-40% of the elderly present to medical centers with gastrointestinal symptoms annually, many of whom have gastrointestinal hemorrhage (Cengiz & Oğuz, 2019). Such diseases have an added prevalence in older patients due to antiplatelet and anticoagulant therapy which is common in older patients. Double-balloon enteroscopy facilitates the easy identification of the site of bleeding, via prompt therapeutic measures , such as cauterization or clipping. Accordingly, this procedure not only aids in diagnosis but plays a central role in the prevention of morbidity and mortality due to untreated gastrointestinal illness in the geriatric patient, a testament to its worth as a specialty use within the enteroscopic arsenal. The addition of double-balloon enteroscopy to the collective pool of enteroscopy procedures speaks to a profound achievement in gastrointestinal diagnosis and treatment. Its minimally invasive nature is attractive to both patients and practitioners alike as it offers shorter recovery periods and fewer complications than traditional surgical techniques. It also allows access to distal small bowel lesions, elevating detection rates of otherwise unattainable lesions and therefore enhancing clinical results. With the growing population in older age groups and an aging population, effective and safe diagnostic modalities become increasingly significant. The advent of double-balloon enteroscopy into everyday practice equips healthcare providers with an effective instrument to deal with the complexity of gastrointestinal illness, particularly in older patients who stand a greater chance of being crippled by unchecked hemorrhage (Cengiz & Oğuz, 2019) (Figure 10.6).

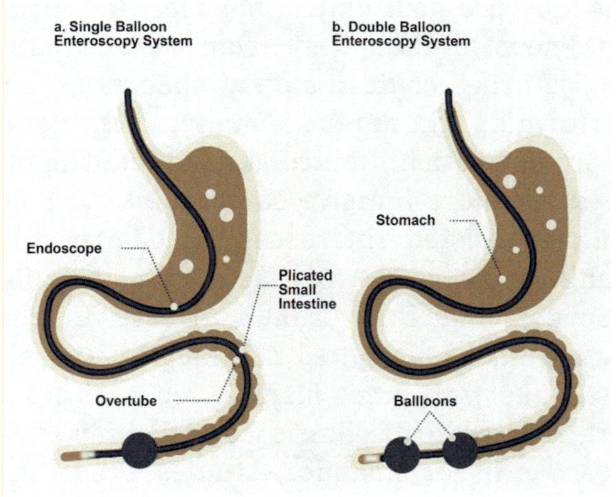

Figure 10.6. Double-balloon enteroscopy.

Source: https://gastrohealth.com.sg/wp-content/uploads/2022/11/Gastro-Health_V3-01-1536x1246.png.

10.3. Indications for Enteroscopy

In the contemporary armamentarium of gastrointestinal diagnosis, enteroscopy has emerged as the prime modality to manage many indications within the small bowel. Small bowel disease typically presents special challenges due to the native anatomy and limitations of usual endoscopy. Enteroscopy indications are primarily centered on the examination of small bowel bleeding, potential Crohn's disease, and small bowel tumors. For example, patients who present with unexplained gastrointestinal bleeding, where initial investigations yield no results, can benefit significantly from enteroscopic procedures. Apart from facilitating proper visualization, these techniques provide therapeutic modalities like biopsy and cauterization, thus maximizing patient outcomes and impacting further management plans. With advances in enteroscopy technology, its use in the diagnosis and management of diseases of the small bowel is on the rise. Crohn's disease is an important indication for enteroscopy due to its multi-factorial pathology in the small intestine. Despite its occult features, a successful endoscopic and imaging examination is warranted. Recent evidence indicates that imaging examinations, i.e., magnetic resonance imaging, are complementary to enteroscopy by giving a global view of enteral and extra-intestinal manifestations of Crohn's disease. Enteroscopy, particularly in combination with techniques , such as balloon-assisted endoscopy, has been successful in the detection of inflammation, strictures, and lesions that are not easily found using regular scopes. As noted by present clinical evidence, this comprehensive approach leads to early diagnosis, which is essential for the initiation of appropriate therapeutic regimens and improved long-term patient management outcomes, thus reiterating the importance of enteroscopy in modern gastroenterology (Hausmann & Albert, 2011). Furthermore, enteroscopy has gone far beyond being a simple diagnostic procedure. Modern advancements like double balloon enteroscopy have revolutionized small bowel access such that not only can diagnosis be established, but also therapeutic procedures can be achieved. This has particular relevance in large adenomatous polyps of the colon and submucosal tumors, where surgical alternatives might otherwise have been deemed. Since endoscopic mucosal resections and hemostatic procedures can now be performed, enteroscopy decreases the reliance on surgical interventions, thus minimizing patient morbidity and recovery periods. With the development of the technique, systematic training programs and advanced technologies must be used by endoscopists interested in becoming proficient and enhancing the effectiveness of enteroscopy in challenging cases, placing it in a central role for gastrointestinal therapeutics of the future (Arebi & Saunders, 2005).

10.3.1. Diagnosis of Small Bowel Diseases

The diagnosis of small bowel disease has also been revolutionized with advances in enteroscopy technology, bringing in new modalities of visualization and evaluation of the small bowel. The earlier methods were also limited by the inability to access the distal ends of the gastrointestinal tract, which posed challenges in diagnosis in conditions , such as Crohn's disease, cancer of the small bowel, and obscure GI bleeding. Enteroscopy now provides the opportunity to not only inspect but also obtain biopsies from otherwise inaccessible sites, thus permitting histological evaluation. This has proven particularly significant in small bowel inflammatory disease, where accurate diagnosis is crucial for making appropriate decisions about treatment. As a result, enteroscopy is now a standard procedure that can help increase our knowledge of complex gastrointestinal disorders, refine diagnosis accuracy, and, in turn, lead to early medical interventions (Akerman et al., 2013). In diagnosing small intestine disease, therapeutic interventions made possible by enteroscopy, such as stricture dilation, have become basic procedures. With techniques like hydrostatic balloon dilation of strictures complicating Crohn's disease, endoscopists can alleviate obstruction and minimize the need for surgical intervention. Not only does this preventive approach address acute clinical manifestations, but it also contributes significantly to improved management of chronic conditions. The potential for immediate visualization and control of small bowel lesions on enteroscopy supports a dual purpose: making a diagnosis, along with simultaneously providing immediate therapeutic options.

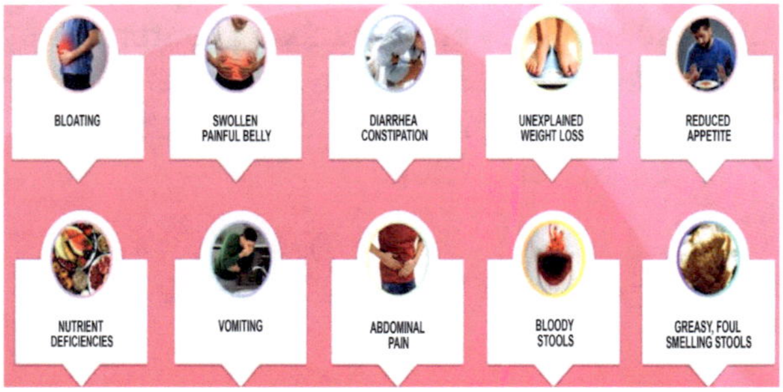

Figure 10.7. Diagnosis of small bowel diseases.

Source: https://thegastrosurgeon.com/wp-content/uploads/2025/04/Common-Symptoms-of-Small-Bowel-Disorders-at-Dr.-Patta-Radhakrishnan-1024x696.jpg.

This is a change of paradigm in practice in the field of gastroenterology, with the differentiation between diagnosis and treatment becoming increasingly less distinct, improving quality of care as well as patient outcomes (Akerman et al., 2013). Furthermore, the enlarged list of enteroscopy techniques points to an evolutionary period for endoscopy that is expanding the possibilities for small bowel diagnosis. Advances in double balloon enteroscopy and capsule endoscopy have not only made the small intestine more accessible but also enhanced diagnostic practice, namely the identification of small neoplastic lesions. The application of advanced imaging equipment assists in identifying delicate abnormalities, allowing early diagnosis that is essential to be able to take good care. As endoscopic procedures evolve, they have the potential to redefine standards of care. The shift to more comprehensive, interventional enteroscopy practice is a significant step in gastroenterology with the promise of increased diagnostic yield and treatment of small bowel disease (Figure 10.7).

10.3.2. Management of Gastrointestinal Bleeding

Gastrointestinal bleeding management has been transformed with advancements in enteroscopic procedures, which combine advanced diagnostic and therapeutic capabilities. Historically, gastrointestinal bleeding has been primarily managed with invasive surgery; however, the advent of technical improvements , such as endoscopic mucosal resection and a range of balloon-assisted enteroscopy technologies, has altered this paradigm. These procedures give clinicians an overview of the entire gastrointestinal tract, allowing them to intervene in a focused manner that not only diagnoses but also cures diseases that may lead to hemorrhage. Improved training programs and the incorporation of simulators in training have improved the competencies of specialists, thus improving patient outcomes and reducing complications during intervention (Arebi & Saunders, 2005). Of the enteroscopy techniques, balloon-assisted enteroscopy and capsule endoscopy have emerged as pillars in diagnosing elusive gastrointestinal bleeding. Balloon-assisted enteroscopy has the potential for both diagnostic evaluation and therapy, in contrast to the confines of earlier measures. For instance, in accordance with studies, intraoperative enteroscopy (IOE) has been found to be of high diagnostic yield in that it detected bleeding lesions in approximately 79% of cases when standard endoscopic measures are indecisive (Monsanto et al., 2012). This indicates a critical point of transition between diagnosis and emergency management, demonstrating how the technologies enable efficient intervention to stem the risks associated with prolonged bleeding events. Beyond this, the ethos of doing multimodal management is at the heart of the whole treatment of gastrointestinal bleeding. Perhaps the best means of maximizing patient outcomes is collaboration between gastroenterologists, surgeons, and radiologists. Recognition of the source of bleeding is often required to result in an interaction between endoscopic and surgical approaches for effective resolution. Current evidence highlights the importance of an individualized approach, wherein minimally invasive techniques are afforded priority but are added to surgical intervention as needed. With the evolving landscape of enteroscopic procedures, continued research and trials will hopefully refine the algorithms for the management of gastrointestinal bleeding to more adequately equip health care workers with the most suitable modalities of treatment (Arebi & Saunders, 2005) (Figure 10.8).

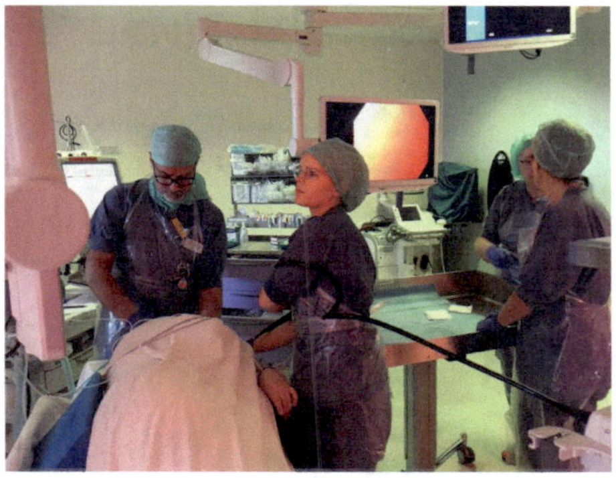

Figure 10.8. Management of gastrointestinal bleeding.

Source: https://www.bmj.com/sites/default/files/sites/defautl/files/attachments/bmj-article/2019/03/gastrointestinal_bleeding_surgery.jpeg.

10.3.3. Evaluation of Suspected Malignancies

The diagnosis of GI tract suspected malignancies is a challenging task for gastroenterologists and is done by using advanced enteroscopic techniques. Enteroscopy, particularly when combined with the most recent technologies like colon capsule endoscopy (CCE), has significantly altered the diagnostic approach to potential malignancies. CCE offers total visualization of the entire GI tract and detection of suspicious lesions. A more recent study emphasized that dual-camera analysis, a feature of advanced CCE, resulted in the detection of far greater findings compared to single-camera methods, which bears testimony to its effectiveness in malignancy detection (García Montes et al., 2013). Such capability assumes a critical role as timely detection can have a profound bearing on prognosis and treatment results for patients. Furthermore, the complexity of small intestinal tumor diagnosis reinforces the need for state-of-the-art enteroscopic techniques. These tumors have typical presentations sometimes lost, and therefore challenging to diagnose using standard methods. Some of these approaches , such as balloon-assisted enteroscopy, have been proven to be viable solutions with enhanced access to direct visualization and biopsy capacity in the small bowel. Recent studies have indicated that integration of new endoscopic and imaging technologies has greatly improved diagnostic sensitivity and accuracy in the detection of small intestinal tumors, thus facilitating timely clinical intervention (Hausmann & Albert, 2011). These advances highlight the central role of enteroscopy techniques in the systematic evaluation of malignancies. By integrating these enteroscopic advances, clinicians can develop personalized surveillance protocols for patients with heightened risk of malignancies, particularly those with familial susceptibility or previous GI illness. An enteroscope-directed approach not only aids in the specific examination of suspected malignancies but also aligns with current optimal preventive care practice. Instituting an organized approach to surveillance can substantially enhance rates of early detection of colorectal and small bowel cancers, raising the standard of overall patient care. With ongoing research revealing the capabilities of new enteroscopic methods, clinicians need to stay updated and flexible to ensure maximal effectiveness in their diagnostic work concerning suspected malignancies.

10.4. Preparation for Enteroscopy

Preparation for enteroscopy is highly significant in the sense that it helps ensure the best possible outcome from the procedure. Before the procedure, patients typically receive a complete assessment performed upon them, including a review of their medical history and recent symptomatology. This helps identify any pre-existing conditions that may complicate the procedure. Dietary preparation is also typically instituted, with instructions for a liquid diet for 24–48 hours before the procedure. Additionally, bowel preparation with enemas or laxatives is required to have an unobstructed view of the gastrointestinal tract on enteroscopy. Well-prepared bowel significantly enhances the visualization of pathology and, hence, diagnostic yield and therapeutic success. Where other imaging techniques, such as capsule endoscopy, have been employed, results of these initial tests can inform enteroscopy preparation so that focus is solely on the most pertinent small intestine segments (Muñoz-Navas et al., 2008). Patient education is also an important component of enteroscopy preparation. Reassurance that the patient understands the procedure, purpose, potential risks, and outcome is likely to minimize anxiety and maximize cooperation. Pre-procedure appointments are where the practitioner typically describes potential complications, the use of sedation, and what to do after the procedure. They are advised to have a companion drive them home after the procedure, particularly when they have received sedation. Patient education regarding post-procedure signs and symptoms to report is also crucial because early complication reporting can significantly influence the safety of patients. It is not only the duty of healthcare workers to educate but also to instill confidence and trust, thus ensuring that the enteroscopy procedure is a success (Attwell et al., 2025). Newer methods of enteroscopy also call for specialized preparations in patients with altered gastrointestinal anatomy. This population comes with unique challenges that must be addressed for the intervention to be successful. For example, for patients who undergo surgeries , such as Roux-en-Y gastric bypass, some modification of the standard preparatory procedure, such as the utilization of specialized endoscopic methods, is required. Literature indicates that the selection of suitable endoscopes and procedures in such patients has a significant effect on the success of interventions, hence the importance of pre-procedure planning (Attwell et al., 2025). Lastly, meticulous preparation, both physical and academic, forms the foundation of a successful enteroscopy so that health practitioners can deliver the best care possible while minimizing patients' discomfort and risk (Figure 10.9).

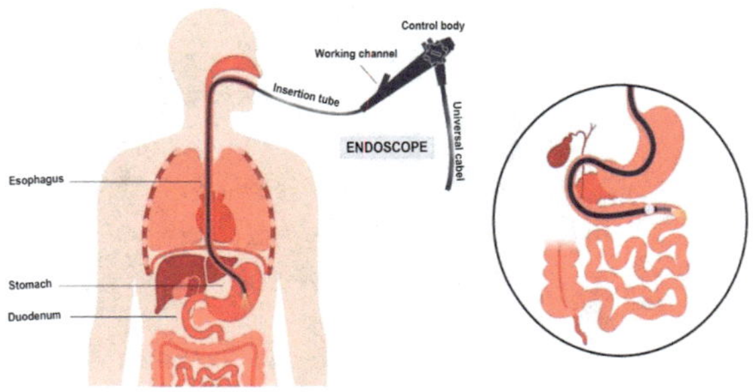

Figure 10.9. Preparation for enteroscopy.

Source: https://www.gigeorgia.com/app/uploads/2024/05/enteroscopy-procedure-960x557-2.jpg.

10.4.1. Patient Assessment and Selection

Effective patient assessment and selection are critical factors in the performance of enteroscopy procedures, particularly in guaranteeing both the precision of diagnoses and procedure safety. Comprehensive assessment starts with a comprehensive medical history, including the patient's onset of symptoms, illness course, and previous gastrointestinal disease. In the treatment of Crohn's disease and other diseases, medical practitioners need to employ adequate imaging techniques to ascertain a firm knowledge of the extent of the disease. Studies have indicated that modalities like magnetic resonance enterography (MRE) are more specific and sensitive in the diagnosis of small bowel pathology compared to routine ultrasound, indicating the need for accurate modality selection at the stage of diagnosis (Taylor et al., 2018). Such initial investigations form the basis on which a patient's candidacy for enteroscopic intervention and treatment planning in general is decided. Secondly, patient selection for enteroscopy is determined clinically in addition to potential contraindications. For instance, the complexity of the procedure to be expected, the overall health status of the patient, and existing medical conditions should all be thoroughly considered. Adherence to sedation protocols, as outlined in the present guidelines, is also a critical aspect of patient selection. Patients may have varying degrees of sedation from minimal to deep sedation depending on the complexity of the procedure (Abdullah et al., 2017). Adequate sedation management is not only crucial to optimize patient comfort but also to ensure procedural success at the lowest risk. Therefore, a proper evaluation that considers these factors ensures an improved outcome for enteroscopy. Besides sedation concerns and clinical evaluation, ongoing communication with the patient is also required for building trust and cooperation throughout the study. Patient education on the enteroscopy procedure, what it is intended for, and potential complications can significantly minimize anxiety and facilitate informed decision-making. In addition, open communication helps determine that patients are fully aware of preparation and post-procedure care, which is essential in minimizing complications. By engaging the patient in discussion on treatment and personal issues, clinicians enhance patient satisfaction and adherence to medical recommendations. This combined approach of assessment and decision-making ultimately leads to improved results in enteroscopy practice by adding clinical sense to patient-centered thinking (Figure 10.10).

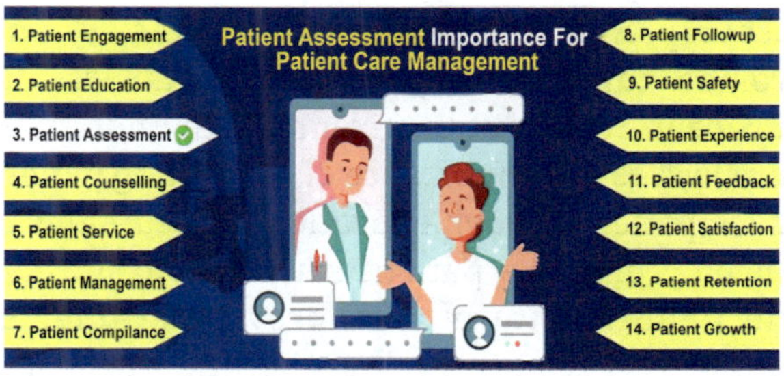

Figure 10.10. Patient assessment and selection.

Source: https://images.drlogy.com/assets/uploads/img/admin/blog/patient-assessment.webp.

10.4.2. Pre-procedural Instructions

Proper pre-procedure instructions are highly essential for the successful performance of enteroscopy procedures and have an impact on patient outcomes as well as procedure efficiency. Instructions are usually provided to include diet restriction, medication adjustment, and preparation protocol to be followed before the procedure. For instance, patients can be asked to hold a clear liquid diet for 24 hours before the procedure to decrease bowel content and enhance visualization during enteroscopy. In addition, some medications , such as anticoagulants or antiplatelet drugs, might have to be adjusted or temporarily discontinued to minimize the risk of complications from the procedure. Thus, meticulous communication of the guidelines not only enhances patient compliance but also aligns with best practice outlined in contemporary literature, such as the rigorous assessment in professional texts for endoscopic procedures that underpin fastidious pre-procedure planning to optimize outcomes. Beyond diet and medicine-related concerns, patient education in relation to the enteroscopy process itself is an essential aspect of pre-procedure instructions. It is critical that patients understand not just the rationale for the procedure, but what to expect during and after their enteroscopy. Simple explanations about the technology involved, potential discomfort, and recovery techniques can alleviate anxiety and promote adherence to pre-procedure advice. The European Society of Gastrointestinal Endoscopy emphasizes the importance of motivating patient participation through educational discussions to not only enhance patient satisfaction but also affect the quality of care provided (Adler et al., 2019). Second, the incorporation of visual aids or educational brochures will assist in enhancing verbal information so that patients will be more adequately prepared for their procedure. Last but not least, patient individual factor assessment and potential risks before enteroscopy are a critical part of the pre-procedure protocol. That entails thorough medical history screening and identification of any contraindications necessitating an alternative method or extra precautionary measures. For example, patients with past experience of gastrointestinal hemorrhage or severe cardiovascular disease would require special guidance to ensure safety during the procedure. As documented in the latest small-bowel endoscopy quality measure guidelines, one must quantify service and practitioner competencies against accepted performance indicators. These stringent measurements induce a safety culture and climate of improvement in endoscopy services that ensures patient preparation is rigorously founded on state-of-the-art practice guidelines (Adler et al., 2019). This offers a balanced approach to enteroscopy, focusing on patient safety while maximizing procedural outcome (Figure 10.11).

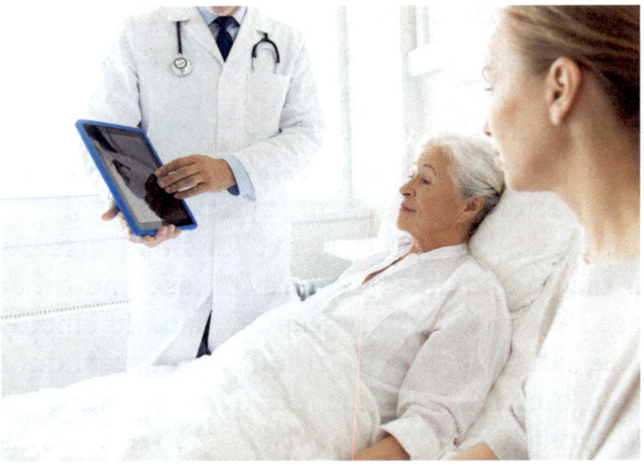

Figure 10.11. Pre-procedural instructions.

Source: https://www.dralinajafi.com/wp-content/uploads/2018/09/post-op.jpg.

10.4.3. Sedation and Anesthesia Considerations

Effective management of sedation and anesthesia is a significant factor in enteroscopy practice, particularly in light of physiological and psychological sequelae of such procedures. Enteroscopy typically involves the confrontation of friable structures of the gastrointestinal tract, and as such, there is a requirement for careful attention to patient safety and comfort. Deep sedation or general anesthesia may be required in some patients to prevent anxiety, pain, or discomfort from the procedure. The choice between sedation and general anesthesia typically hinges on the individual policies of the health facility and the complexity of the procedure. For example, for complex interventions, increased levels of sedation may be required to guarantee immobility and compliance from the patient. Additionally, the prevalence of comorbidities in patients could further determine how the anesthetic should be conducted, necessitating individualized protocols designed by the clinical team to adhere to best practice in enteroscopic procedures, as outlined in recent guidelines on practice in sedation (Tringali et al., 2017). Apart from patient comfort, vigilant observation under sedation is essential to avoid risks due to potential adverse effects. Anesthesiologists and the medical staff must be competent in recognizing symptoms of compromise during enteroscopic procedures, given the dynamic nature of patient response to sedatives. Constant monitoring of vital signs, oxygen saturation, and level of consciousness is important to ensure patient safety.

Equipment for preservation of airway patency and management of respiratory distress must be readily available in any center where sedation is employed. Moreover, best practice requires establishing clear protocols for recovery after the procedure, with careful observation to gauge patients' return to baseline status. By enforcing rigorous sedation practices, medical practitioners not only ensure a less painful procedure experience but also ensure utmost patient safety and care (Tringali et al., 2017). Sedation decision-making in enteroscopy also extends to post-procedure stages, with consequences transferring to recovery procedures. Half-lives of sedatives used in procedures should be known, so recovery times can be approximated and patients appropriately monitored during the postoperative period. These considerations are especially relevant to discharge procedures, as patients may not be cleared for discharge until they have met specific discharge criteria, including stable vital signs and sufficient recovery from sedation. Patient communication about these factors can help to alleviate fear and increase global satisfaction with the process. Patient education on side effects and the necessity of coordinating post-procedural support is also critical, reminding us that sedation not only affects the experience of the procedure itself but also profoundly affects the entire patient experience. Thus, protocols of integrated sedation in enteroscopy are crucial in ensuring optimum patient outcomes and safety throughout the continuum of care (Tringali et al., 2017).

10.5. Enteroscopy Procedure

The enteroscopy procedure has significantly developed in modern medicine, particularly as a significant diagnostic and therapeutic procedure for exploring the small intestine. Historically, intraoperative enteroscopy was the gold standard but has been transformed by innovations , such as capsule endoscopy and balloon-assisted enteroscopy. These have enhanced patient safety and comfort by reducing the need for invasive surgical intervention. The application of enteroscopy, particularly where unexplained gastrointestinal bleeding is at issue, still holds center stage despite the advent of non-invasive technologies. Research has demonstrated intraoperative enteroscopy to have a diagnostic yield of 79% for identifying bleeding lesions, confirming its worth in instances in which non-invasive modalities remain inconclusive (Monsanto et al., 2012). Collectively, enteroscopy techniques have been transformed by the confluence of several modalities within the treatment of small bowel diseases. For instance, capsule endoscopy is generally the first line of investigation as it is non-invasive and can see the entire small bowel. But once lesions have been detected, balloon-assisted enteroscopy can take biopsies and therapeutic interventions, effectively bridging the gap between diagnosis and treatment. Such a dual approach not only enhances diagnostic potential but also allows for personalized management of diseases , such as Crohn's disease and small bowel tumors. Moreover, imaging tests like magnetic resonance imaging are increasingly utilized to assess enteral involvement and track treatment in patients, which illustrates the complexity of today's enteroscopy procedures (Hausmann & Albert, 2011). Regardless of advances in enteroscopy techniques, challenge remains, particularly with regard to accompanying risks and complications. The intraoperative enteroscopy procedure, while effective, is fraught with a high risk of complications, including procedure-related mortality and postoperative complications. It has been reported to be associated with 5% mortality and 21% postoperative complications (Monsanto et al., 2012). These statistics emphasize the requirements of meticulous selection of patients and clear indications for its use. Enteroscopy, and particularly in the context of therapeutic intervention, should thus be reserved for those cases where other methods of diagnostic modalities have been unsuccessful. Careful use of these techniques is critical to an optimal outcome for patients, whereby the benefits of enteroscopy are optimized against the risks of this invasive treatment (Figure 10.12).

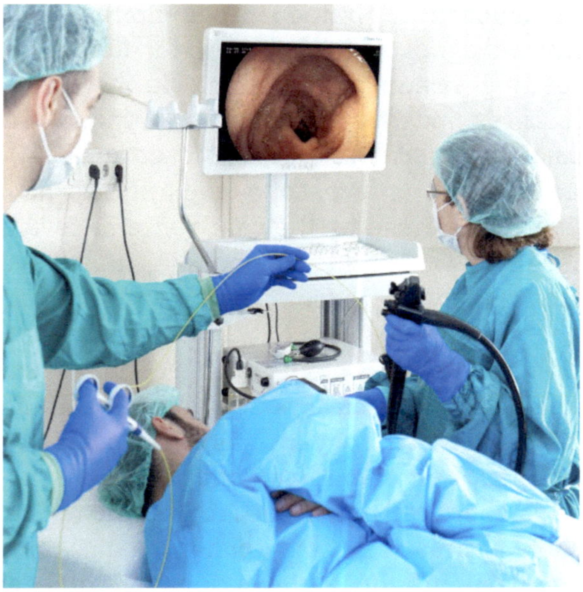

Figure 10.12. Enteroscopy procedure.

Source: https://gastro-md.com/wp-content/uploads/2020/01/UGIE-Graphics3-min-1024x1024.jpg.

10.5.1. Step-by-Step Overview of the Procedure

The enteroscopy intervention begins with thorough patient examination, which plays an important role in achieving optimal safety and success of the procedure. Patient history will be gathered before proceeding with the procedure, including previous gastrointestinal symptoms, and patients are usually advised to starve for several hours. Starvation reduces gastrointestinal contents that can interfere with visualization during the procedure. The patient can then be sedated to minimize discomfort, which minimizes the process. Adequate sedation is so important because it allows the medical team to perform the enteroscopy in such a manner that minimizes pain and anxiety, thus making the whole process successful. The initial step of the actual process is the accurate insertion of the enteroscope, equipped with a camera and therapeutic devices suited for the intervention, marking the transition from preparation to active intervention. Following insertion, the enteroscope is advanced beyond the small intestine to the target region, typically with the assistance of fluoroscopy or other imaging modalities. This procedure requires precise maneuverability to negotiate the curvatures of the small bowel to visualize strictures, masses, or mucosal abnormalities. Advanced techniques like double-balloon and single-balloon enteroscopy, as mentioned in the literature, achieve deep enteral access and greatly improve diagnostic yield (Aktas et al., 2009). During this phase, the physician can use various tools attached to the enteroscope, such as biopsy forceps or polypectomy snares, to deliver two-way diagnosis as well as treatment. This aspect refers to the extent of enteroscopy procedures in not only diagnosing but also delivering instant treatment, especially beneficial in strictures or polyp management. The final step in enteroscopy is the withdrawal of the enteroscope and careful inspection of the biopsies or therapeutic intervention done. Post-procedure monitoring is necessary to ensure that the patient is stable and complication-free, as enteroscopic procedures, although largely innocuous, can be associated with some risk (Aktas et al., 2009). After observation, results , such as histopathology of biopsies are typically presented in a follow-up subsequently completing the procedure cycle. This broad-based approach is a significant milestone in gastrointestinal intervention and diagnostics, reducing the extent of more invasive surgical methods in cases , such as those for Crohn's disease or other serious gastrointestinal diseases. By understanding these systemic processes, doctors can increase procedural results along with the standard of patient care significantly within the framework of enteroscopy procedures.

10.5.2. Role of the Endoscopist

The endoscopist's role within modern gastrointestinal medicine is vital, especially within the framework of enteroscopy procedures. These specialists possess the training necessary to perform intricate procedures, which enables them to visualize and manipulate the gastrointestinal tract accurately. Since they conduct diagnostic and therapeutic procedures with varying endoscopic modalities, the skill of endoscopists is most crucial. They assume complex cases, such as elusive gastrointestinal bleeding or suspected inflammatory bowel disease, which quite frequently demand superior techniques like balloon-assisted enteroscopy or capsule endoscopy. Not only does the procedure get done by the endoscopist, but they also report the findings, which determine subsequent management that can have a significant impact on patient outcomes. Moreover, the endoscopist's role is more than just technical execution; it encompasses a complete comprehension of patient care. The endoscopists are tasked with choosing the appropriate indications for their procedures and should possess a good grasp of the broad spectrum of conditions that can be diagnosed through enteroscopy. For instance, they not only deal with cases regarding such mundane conditions as Crohn's disease but also recognize severe though less frequent conditions like enteropathy-associated T-cell lymphoma or even infections like Whipples disease, reflecting their diagnostic expertise and clinical acumen.

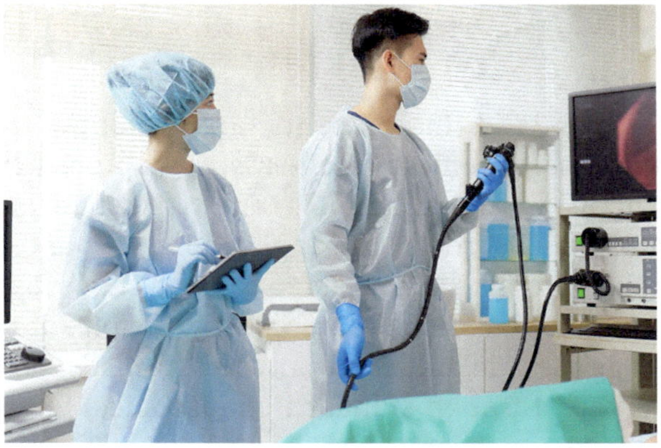

Figure 10.13. Role of the endoscopist.

Source: https://detrox.com.tr/en/wp-content/uploads/2025/01/The-Role-of-Endoscopy-Nurses-in-Infection-Control.webp.

The ability of the endoscopist to navigate such complexities assures timely as well as appropriate interventions, critical in preventing complications arising due to untreated gastrointestinal afflictions, as reflected in the guidelines (Tringali et al., 2017). In addition to technical and clinical responsibilities, maintenance of skills and ongoing education are imperative components of the role of the endoscopist within a dynamic health care environment. Ongoing education is part of it, as developments in enteroscopy technology and devices introduce variations in best practices. Endoscopists need to be proficient in these skills in a bid to deliver multiple procedures with efficacy and safety at optimal levels. Besides, they tend to co-work with multidisciplinary teams, sharing information and outcomes culminating in team-based learning. Such commitment to professional progress not only enhances the endoscopist's personal practice but ultimately improves surgical and patient care quality in general, as a reflection of the significance of their contribution to the management of gastrointestinal health (Fry et al., 2013) (Figure 10.13).

10.5.3. Use of Imaging and Tools During Enteroscopy

Imaging and instruments are essential in enhancing the efficacy of enteroscopy, a procedure central to the diagnosis and treatment of intestinal disorders. The application of advanced imaging tools , such as video capsule endoscopy and balloon-assisted enteroscopy, enables it to image the small intestine, an area normally hard to reach through standard endoscopies. Video capsule endoscopy, first introduced by Gavriel Iddan in 1981, revolutionized gastroenterology with the provision of a modality to visualize the entire GI tract in a non-invasive way. While these technologies augment the enteroscopic armory, the need for expert interpretation on the part of the gastroenterologist is more than ever before. The endoscopist must not only be well-versed in standard endoscopic practice but also proficient in accurately interpreting complex images from newer modalities, reflecting the evolving requirements of this specialty (Monsanto et al., 2021). In addition to imaging technology, enteroscopy is facilitated by novel devices intended to enhance diagnostic yield and therapeutic intervention. The introduction of EUS has gone a long way in enhancing the possibility of diagnosis, allowing imaging and tissue sampling to be performed simultaneously. EUS uses ultrasound waves to inform doctors about the anatomy of surrounding tissues, enhancing the visibility of lesions and the potential for fine-needle aspiration biopsies. Moreover, advances in wireless capsule technology have ushered in new methods of detecting lesions that conventional endoscopy cannot visualize. Such capsules have gone beyond their initial optical sensor limitations as research goes on with multi-wavelength optical sensors and high-bandwidth communications to counter much improving the detection rate of various GI diseases, consequently, streamlining the diagnostic process (Katsafadou, 2023).

Ongoing innovation in imaging tools and techniques in enteroscopy is key to satisfying the complexities of gastrointestinal diseases. With emerging technology, integration of technological advances and physician capability is at the heart of optimizing patient outcomes. Training gastroenterologists to cope with both the conventional and innovative aspects of endoscopic examination is paramount. With profound knowledge of image interpretation coupled with skill in new technologies's application, like high-resolution optical systems, health care professionals are capable of delivering timely and accurate diagnosis. The combination of these advanced imaging modalities and devices and the endoscopist experience and expertise will ultimately enhance the value of enteroscopy as a part of modern gastroenterology (Monsanto et al., 2021).

10.6. Complications and Risks

There are inherent complications and risks involved with the application of enteroscopy techniques, particularly small bowel capsule endoscopy (SBCE), and these must be carefully weighed. One of the serious complications of capsule endoscopy is mucosal trauma. In children, introduction using a Roth net resulted in mucosal trauma in 50% of cases, reflecting a significant problem in terms of the safety of this method, especially in at-risk groups. Additionally, while SBCE is not usually invasive, the risk of capsule retention in the gut is a major risk and may necessitate further surgery. Such complications only emphasize the importance of rigorous patient selection and follow-up so that the benefits of using enteroscopy modalities are more than the risks involved in their application (Bufler et al., 2009). Complications have also been reported due to other enteroscopic methods, such as balloon-assisted enteroscopy, which, despite being extremely beneficial in diagnosing and managing small bowel pathology, can lead to complications. According to recent evidence, complications of these procedures can be perforation, bleeding, and pancreatitis.

Depending on the technique and overall condition of the patient, it is determined. In enteroscopies, identification of the strengths and limitations of other imaging techniques , such as CT enterography (CTE) and MRE, becomes important. Although these modalities are typically non-invasive, they also carry complications , such as contrast material allergy and radiation exposure, making it important to give a critical assessment of risks for different diagnostic procedures (Carvalhoa & Cotter, 2015). Importantly, the decision-making process regarding the utilization of enteroscopy methods requires a critical assessment of potential contraindications and complications. For instance, patients with a past history of bowel obstruction or with certain gastrointestinal anomalies may not be eligible for particular enteroscopic procedures, and risk poor outcomes. In addition, a blend of various enteroscopy procedures may require specially conceived protocols for maximizing efficacy with minimizing complications. Patient-specific variables like age and the nature of the gastrointestinal disorder are to be known for maximizing the choice of technique. By appropriately weighing the potential risks against the desired diagnostic or therapeutic outcomes, doctors can better handle the enteroscopy challenges, making patient encounters safer and enhancing health outcomes (Bufler et al., 2009; Carvalhoa & Cotter, 2015) (Figure 10.14).

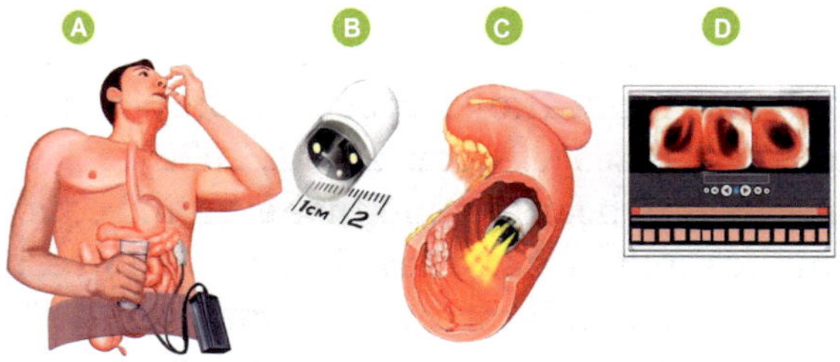

Figure 10.14. Complications and risks use of with capsule enteroscopy techniques.

Source: https://www.gutworks.com.au/wp-content/uploads/JAYA-videocapsule-endoscopy-perth-murdoch.jpg.

10.6.1. Common Complications Associated with Enteroscopy

Where enteroscopy is performed, information concerning general complications is necessary for both practitioners and patients because these can have a direct impact on procedure success and patient safety. Single balloon enteroscopy and push enteroscopy are among the methods that have been proven to successfully view and treat small bowel pathology. Despite their ease of access of the small intestine, such procedures come with risks. Of great importance are the complications in the shape of perforation and significant hemorrhage, even though they do not occur with a high level of frequency. The following elements might influence the development of such complications during enteroscopy: preconditions, technical proficiency of the operator, and intra-procedural issues (Abdulaziz et al., 2022). Preparedness and expertise are what the operators require to handle these risks adequately and react effectively when they do occur. Another great aspect of the complications of enteroscopy. This is the recognition of the great variability in patient outcomes with such procedures. Some studies indicate that, while modalities , such as single balloon enteroscopy can yield greater diagnostic and therapeutic success rates than push enteroscopy, the overall rate of adverse events is relatively low. For example, a systematic review found that the two procedures are, in general, considered safe, though complications arose in only a small number of cases (Abdulaziz et al., 2022). Yet, it is important to bear in mind that even infrequent complications, when they do arise, can result in serious and life-threatening conditions. This reinforces the need for the practitioner to not only be aware of the procedural techniques but also to learn about the type of complications that may occur with each technique. Additionally, the management and prevention of enteroscopy complications are part of good patient care management. Risk-minimization measures entail the application of detailed patient assessment before the procedure, and the application of cautious technique during the endoscopy. For instance, proper knowledge of risks , such as embolization and infection may promote the creation of targeted prophylactic action based on the individual patient's requirement (Abbas et al., 2013). Further, it is essential to have standardized clinical protocols for promptly responding to emergencies that may occur during enteroscopy. By doing this, the medical staff can enhance the overall safety profile of enteroscopy so that it can be an effective diagnostic and therapeutic instrument for small bowel disorders without posing significant complications.

10.6.2. Risk Factors for Adverse Events (AEs)

The frequency of AEs with enteroscopy procedures creates issues that necessitate thorough familiarity with the risk factors involved. Pinned to the top of these is simply the sheer technical sophistication of the procedures themselves, particularly in the wake of such innovations as device-assisted enteroscopies (DAEs). The more sophisticated the techniques involved get, the greater the risk of complications of differing intensities thereby rising. Operator skill, procedural guidance, and patient-specific variables have crucial effects on AE frequency. Awareness of the operator regarding potential complications, along with observation skills in early detection, has been shown to critically affect the outcome, ultimately resulting in improved patient safety during procedures (Abbas et al., 2013). Patient selection is also key in reducing risks due to enteroscopic interventions. Certain medical histories like coagulopathy, previous abdominal surgery, and tumors are known to augment the risk of adverse effects. For example, obscure gastrointestinal bleeding (OGIB) and inflammatory bowel disease patients are destined to undergo more severe treatment and evaluation protocols, thereby increasing the level of intervention that is being carried out. One review assessing DAEs observed that diagnostic success and subsequent therapeutic success are equally dependent on the proper selection of candidates for the procedure. In that regard, one must balance maximizing diagnostic information with possible complications (Monsanto et al., 2016). Last, resources and infrastructure utilized at each procedure can significantly contribute to the likelihood of complications. A well-organized facility that can handle emergent complications, such as perforations or heavy hemorrhaging, will be necessary to improve patient outcomes after the procedure. Good risk management is not only about understanding current conditions, but also the availability of proper equipment and trained personnel for immediate implementation. Recent reviews emphasize the importance of an efficient strategic plan for preventive methods and emergency preparedness that, complemented with soundly informed operator experience, can significantly reduce the incidence of serious complications during enteroscopies (Abbas et al., 2013).

10.6.3. Strategies for Minimizing Risks

In the case of enteroscopy methods, effective risk minimization strategies are instrumental to patient safety and best results. One of the principal methods involves meticulous pre-procedure examinations to find potential risk factors, i.e., comorbidities or previous gastrointestinal problems. By appropriate measurements, clinicians can tailor the procedure based on the patient's immediate health status, thereby avoiding complications. Additionally, patient discussion about the benefits and risks of enteroscopy encourages informed consent, enabling them to make well-informed decisions regarding their care. The synergy of advanced imaging modalities, such as the complementary utility of endoscopic retrograde cholangiopancreatography (ERCP) and EUS, is also pivotal in advancing diagnostic accuracy at the cost of reduced adverse events, as both modalities are employed to effectively illuminate the underlying pathologies of biliopancreatic disease (Macedo et al., 2017). Finally, the implementation of standard protocols and guidelines goes a long way in minimizing risk in enteroscopy procedures. These existing policies oversee patient preparation, procedure conduct, and postoperative care, such that best practices are followed by all staff. For instance, enforcing improved recovery after surgery (ERAS) guidelines for enteroscopy can facilitate reduced stays in the hospital and improved recovery time through minimization of stress reactions and optimal fluid optimization. Training and education form the cornerstones of this plan; endoscopists must go through intensive training with a concentration on technical skills as well as management of potential complications. More training courses, following the concurrent initiative in both ERCP and EUS, can yield endoscopists proficient in crisis management and preventive strategies, enhancing the overall safety paradigm under which such procedures are administered (Carvalhoa & Cotter, 2015). Finally, the necessity of continuous data collection and analysis cannot be overemphasized in the quest for risk reduction with enteroscopy. Continuous procedural outcome audits allow for the identification of trends, complications, and opportunities for improvement, leading to evidence-based optimization of techniques and protocols. Moreover, utilization of technology for quality improvement activities, e.g., tracking adverse events and corrective action in a timely fashion, fosters a culture of safety and accountability. By operating in interdisciplinary teams, health professionals can share knowledge and best practice, hence maximizing the aggregate knowledge of risk factors of enteroscopy enhances their comprehension of the dual role of ERCP and EUS as diagnostic modalities and also therapeutic means to enable a more sophisticated patient pathway comprehension, optimizing care to avoid risks of invasive examinations (Macedo et al., 2017; Katsafadou, 2023) (Figure 10.15).

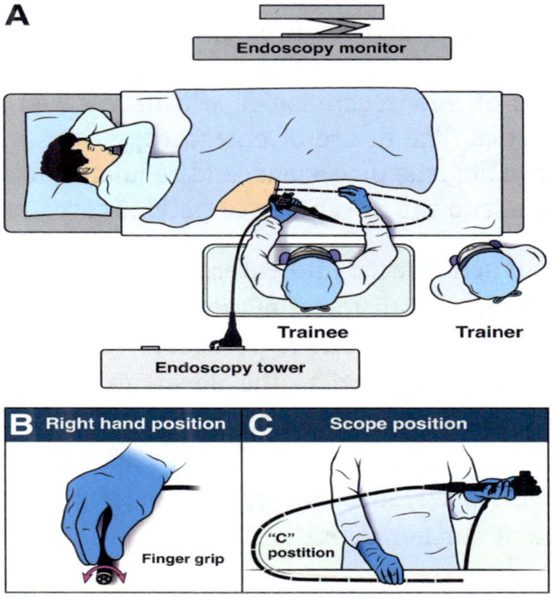

Figure 10.15. Strategies for minimizing risks of enteroscopy techniques.

Source: https://www.cghjournal.org/cms/10.1016/j.cgh.2022.12.036/asset/5b4e27cf-d653-42be-bbb4-7e3c1e4b3cf5/main.assets/gr2_lrg.jpg.

SUMMARY

Overall, the advancements in enteroscopy procedures mark a defining moment in gastrointestinal diagnosis. Traditional endoscopic procedures often failed, particularly in reaching the small intestine where important pathology may be overlooked. Wireless capsule endoscopy, developed by Gavriel Iddan, revolutionized this setting by providing full visual inspection of the entire gastrointestinal system. However, as indicated in existing literature, the new wireless capsules' limitations include low wavelength detection and low data transfer capability through radio frequency communication (Katsafadou, 2023). Addressing these challenges becomes an important aspect in enhancing the diagnostic capability of enteroscopy techniques since achieving high specificity and bandwidth in imaging solutions remains a central issue. Furthermore, the integration of new-generation technologies, such as artificial intelligence, is emerging as a revolutionary component of endoscopy. By leveraging machine learning-based computer programs, i.e., convolutional neural networks, doctors are capable of accelerating lesion detection rates, thereby limiting the chances of missed diagnosis. This objective is indispensable because AI has the potential to support clinician decision-making in real-time settings, supported by recent studies (Burczyk et al., 2025). The synergy of bringing together AI applications and novel imaging modalities is such that one can almost envision future advancements in enteroscopy propelling breakthroughs in diagnosis and outcomes to lead a new standard of care. Finally, while the future promises so much, there is a need to appreciate the challenges that accompany these advances. Regulatory frameworks, ethical concerns with AI-based diagnostics, and requirements for massive training datasets are technical challenges that need to be overcome to use the full capacity of these approaches. In addition, conducting standardized tests of new technologies will have a central role in assessing their effectiveness and safety in practice. The future of enteroscopy thus rests in the pursuit of research and cooperation among technologists, physicians, and regulatory bodies to ensure that innovation translates into tangible benefit to the advantage of patient care and medical practice in general.

The research into enteroscopy techniques reveals a variety of methods aimed at catching and detecting small intestine conditions. Of these techniques, classical endoscopy is the historically significant one, but it possessed glaring limitations, particularly concerning the small bowel. The deficiency led to the development of techniques , such as colonoscopy, which significantly revolutionized gastrointestinal diagnosis by providing a non-invasive means of viewing the small intestine. The transition from standard endoscopic methods to progressively more advanced technologies, such as deep enteroscopy, illustrates ongoing advances in diagnostic modalities, which enable further depth and accuracy of observation. As the future unfolds, integration of diagnostic modalities—in contrast to being as they are different from standard monitoring methods to high-technology imaging systems—will be most important to maximizing patient outcome, illustrating the paradigm shift of gastrointestinal disease diagnosis and management. Observation of disease activity in diseases , such as Crohn's disease illustrates the necessity of using strong enteroscopy procedures. Since clinical decision-making is ever more reliant on quantitative measurement, the effectiveness of enteroscopy becomes part of determining treatment strategies. The Annual Exchange on the Advances in Inflammatory Bowel Disease (IBD Ahead) 2011 training program emphasized this by advocating the application of a combination of symptom assessments, endoscopic evaluations, biomarker assays, and imaging for more effective disease monitoring (Albert et al., 2013). Not only do these multi-disciplinary approaches enable accurate diagnosis, but they also help in prognosis prediction and treatment effectiveness assessment. Furthermore, standardized reporting of these examinations allows for longitudinal assessment, thus optimizing patient management over time. Consequently, the complementary strategy involving several enteroscopic procedures in combination with advanced monitoring equipment optimizes the clinician's capacity to adequately confront patient needs promptly and efficiently. Enteroscopy's future is achieved through subsequent technological advancements, principally wireless capsule endoscopy, which makes up for the shortcomings of conventional techniques. Successful development of multi-wavelength optical sensors and advanced optical communications links is a revolutionary leap in the capability to capture high-quality images of the gastrointestinal tract. Such developments make possible more widespread detection capabilities and faster data transmission, effectively culminating in more accurate diagnosis. Such improvements can augment real-time image delivery, which has the potential to revolutionize the management of acute gastrointestinal bleeding, a common but severe problem (Katsafadou, 2023). Moreover, as these new technologies are incorporated further, there will be an enhanced comprehension of their clinical applications, bringing them closer to the needs of gastrointestinal diagnostics. Thus, the ongoing increases in enteroscopy techniques are not only significant but are necessary to revolutionize the nature of care provided in gastroenterology.

CLOSER LOOK

BOTH PHYSICAL AND ACADEMIC DIMENSIONS:

Human development and performance are shaped by multiple interrelated dimensions, among which physical and academic aspects play central roles. Both areas contribute to an individual's overall well-being, cognitive growth, and long-term success, yet they often influence each other in complex ways. Understanding these dimensions can inform educational strategies, health interventions, and personal development approaches. The physical dimension encompasses factors such as growth, fitness, motor skills, nutrition, and general health. Regular physical activity supports cardiovascular and musculoskeletal health, enhances muscular strength, and improves endurance. Beyond the physiological benefits, physical development also contributes to mental well-being. Exercise has been shown to reduce stress, anxiety, and depressive symptoms, while enhancing mood, alertness, and energy levels. Proper nutrition and sleep are integral to this dimension, as they underpin both physical growth and cognitive function. Early identification of physical limitations or health issues can prevent long-term complications and optimize daily functioning.

The academic dimension involves intellectual growth, learning, and cognitive performance. It includes the development of skills such as reading, writing, numeracy, problem-solving, and critical thinking. Academic success is influenced by both intrinsic factors, such as motivation, attention, and memory, and extrinsic factors, including teaching quality, home environment, and access to resources. Cognitive engagement fosters neural development and strengthens executive functions, which are essential for planning, decision-making, and goal-directed behavior. Additionally, academic achievement often shapes social opportunities and future career prospects, emphasizing its broader societal significance.

Importantly, the physical and academic dimensions are interconnected. Regular physical activity has been linked to improved concentration, memory retention, and classroom performance in children and adolescents. Conversely, academic demands and stress can affect sleep patterns, energy levels, and overall physical health. This interplay highlights the need for holistic approaches that integrate both dimensions. Programs that combine physical education with cognitive challenges or incorporate active learning strategies exemplify how physical and academic development can reinforce each other.

In conclusion, focusing on both physical and academic aspects provides a comprehensive understanding of human development. Optimizing physical health through exercise, nutrition, and rest can enhance cognitive function, while supporting academic growth fosters critical thinking and lifelong learning skills. Recognizing and nurturing the synergy between these dimensions allows individuals to achieve balanced development, improved well-being, and greater long-term success in personal, educational, and professional spheres.

REFERENCES

1. Tringali, A., Thomson, M., Dumonceau, J. M., Tavares, M., Tabbers, M. M., Furlano, R., Spaander, M., Hassan, C., Tzvinikos, C., Ijsselstijn, H., Viala, J., Dall'Oglio, L., Benninga, M., Orel, R., Vandenplas, Y., Keil, R., Romano, C., Brownstone, E., Hlava, Š., Gerner, P., ... Zambelli, A. (2017). Pediatric gastrointestinal endoscopy: European Society of Gastrointestinal Endoscopy (ESGE) and European Society for Paediatric Gastroenterology Hepatology and Nutrition (ESPGHAN) Guideline Executive summary. *Endoscopy*, *49*(1), 83–91. https://doi.org/10.1055/s-0042-111002(accessed on 15th July 2025).

2. Abbas, J., Adler, D. G., Affi, A., Alexander, S., Caetano, A. C., Andriulli, A., Apel, D., et al. (2013). *Emergencies After Endoscopic Procedures.* https://core.ac.uk/download/55625568.pdf (accessed on 15th July 2025).

3. Abdulaziz, A., Alrezuk, M., & AlAmri, T. (2022). *Single balloon enteroscopy versus push enteroscopy for small bowel bleeding assessment: A systematic review and meta-analysis.* https://core.ac.uk/download/524771605.pdf (accessed on 15th July 2025).

4. Abdullah, M. (Murdani), Daldiyono, D., Fauzi, A. (Achmad), Makmun, D., et al. (2017). *National consensus on the use of sedation drugs in the gastrointestinal endoscopic procedures.* https://media.neliti.com/media/publications/238028-national-consensus-on-the-use-of-sedatio-8d053ad4.pdf (accessed on 15th July 2025).

5. Adler, S., Bellisario, C., Bennett, C., Bisschops, R., et al. (2019). *Performance measures for small-bowel endoscopy: A European Society of Gastrointestinal Endoscopy (ESGE) quality improvement initiative.* https://core.ac.uk/download/604668316.pdf (accessed on 15th July 2025).

6. Akerman, P. A., Bizzotto, A., Costamagna, G., Galasso, F., et al. (2013). *Enteroscopic balloon dilation of multiple ileal strictures in suspected Crohn's disease.* https://core.ac.uk/download/pdf/82136116.pdf (accessed on 15th July 2025).

7. Aktas, H., & Mensink, P. B. F. (2009). *Therapeutic Balloon-Assisted Enteroscopy.* https://core.ac.uk/download/19187573.pdf (accessed on 15th July 2025).

8. Albert, A., Ignjatovic, A., Sturm, A., Baert, F., Best, L., Boirivant, F., Borthne, A., et al. (2013). *Optimizing monitoring in the management of Crohn's disease: A physician's perspective.* https://core.ac.uk/download/pdf/81981383.pdf (accessed on 15th July 2025).

9. Hausmann J, Albert JG (2011) Detecting and Managing Small Bowel Crohn's Disease – Capsule Endoscopy Becoming a First Line Diagnostic Method? J Gastroint Dig Syst S1:002. doi:10.4172/2161-069X.S1-002(accessed on 15th July 2025).

10. Albert, J., Arai, H., Bailey, A., Beggs, J., Bernstein, D., Bessette, R., et al. (2011). *Current Advance in Small Bowel Tumors.* https://core.ac.uk/download/pdf/8733535.pdf (accessed on 15th July 2025).

11. Taylor, S. A., Mallett, S., Bhatnagar, G., Baldwin-Cleland, R., Bloom, S., Gupta, A., Hamlin, P. J., Hart, A. L., Higginson, A., Jacobs, I., McCartney, S., Miles, A., Murray, C. D., Plumb, A. A., Pollok, R. C., Punwani, S., Quinn, L., Rodriguez-Justo, M., Shabir, Z., Slater, A., ... METRIC study investigators (2018). Diagnostic accuracy of magnetic resonance enterography and small bowel ultrasound for the extent and activity of newly diagnosed and relapsed Crohn's disease (METRIC): a multicentre trial. *The lancet. Gastroenterology & hepatology*, *3*(8), 548–558. https://doi.org/10.1016/S2468-1253(18)30161-4(accessed on 15th July 2025).

12. Pinho, R., Mascarenhas-Saraiva, M., Mão-de-Ferro, S., Ferreira, S., Almeida, N., Figueiredo, P., Rodrigues, A., Cardoso, H., Marques, M., Rosa, B., Cotter, J., Vilas-Boas, G., Cardoso, C., Salgado, M., & Marcos-Pinto, R. (2016). Multicenter survey on the use of device-assisted enteroscopy in Portugal. *United European gastroenterology journal, 4*(2), 264–274. https://doi.org/10.1177/2050640615604775 (accessed on 15th July 2025).

13. Monsanto, P., Almeida, N., Lérias, C., Figueiredo, P., Gouveia, H., & Sofia, C. (2012). Is there still a role for intraoperative enteroscopy in patients with obscure gastrointestinal bleeding?. *Revista espanola de enfermedades digestivas, 104*(4), 190–196. https://doi.org/10.4321/s1130-01082012000400004 (accessed on 15th July 2025).

14. Alrubaiy, L., Biswas, S., British Society of Gastroenterology Trainees' Section, China, L., et al. (2018). *Trends in UK endoscopy training in the BSG trainees' national survey and strategic planning for the future.* https://core.ac.uk/download/195307861.pdf (accessed on 15th July 2025).

15. Pedro Boal Carvalhoa,* , José Cotter (2016). Contrast-Enhanced Cross Sectional Imaging and Capsule Endoscopy: New Perspectives for a Whole Picture of the Small Bowel https://core.ac.uk/download/132797620.pdf (accessed on 15th July 2025).

16. Arebi, N., & Saunders, B. P. (2005). *Endoscopy: An Evolving Specialty.* Malta Medical Journal. 2005, Vol.17(3), p. 32-36 https://core.ac.uk/download/46602009.pdf (accessed on 15th July 2025).

17. Attwell, A., Augustin, H., Edmundowicz, S., Hammad, H., Han, D., et al. (2025). *The success and safety of endoscopic retrograde cholangiopancreatography in surgically altered gastrointestinal anatomy.* https://core.ac.uk/download/649474413.pdf (accessed on 15th July 2025).

18. H Ghunaim, C Bach - Medicine, 2014 (2014). *Implementing wireless capsule endoscopy (WCE) in digestive system diagnostics.* https://core.ac.uk/download/52955742.pdf (accessed on 15th July 2025).

19. Balzarini, M., Orsello, M., & Del Piano, M. (2011). *Therapeutic uses of Spiral Enteroscopy.* https://core.ac.uk/download/322399930.pdf (accessed on 15th July 2025).

20. Bartocci, B., Cammarota, G., Capobianco, I., Del Gaudio, A., Di Vincenzo, F., Lopetuso, L. R., Papa, A., et al. (2024). *Endoscopic management of strictures in Crohn's disease: An unsolved case.* https://core.ac.uk/download/655042021.pdf (accessed on 15th July 2025).

21. Bufler, P., Fritscher-Ravens, A., Milla, P., Nuutinen, M., et al. (2009). *The feasibility of wireless capsule endoscopy in detecting small intestinal pathology in children under the age of 8 years: A multicenter European study.* https://core.ac.uk/download/12175824.pdf (accessed on 15th July 2025).

22. Burczyk, R., Duszyński, K., Iglewski, P., Jarych, A., et al. (2025). *Automated recognition of abnormalities in gastrointestinal endoscopic images – Evaluation of an AI tool for identifying polyps and other irregularities.* https://core.ac.uk/download/656518186.pdf (accessed on 15th July 2025).

23. Nylund, K., Maconi, G., Hollerweger, A., Ripolles, T., Pallotta, N., Higginson, A., Serra, C., Dietrich, C. F., Sporea, I., Saftoiu, A., Dirks, K., Hausken, T., Calabrese, E., Romanini, L., Maaser, C., Nuernberg, D., & Gilja, O. H. (2017). EFSUMB Recommendations and Guidelines for Gastrointestinal Ultrasound. EFSUMB-Empfehlungen und Leitlinien des Gastrointestinalen Ultraschalls - Teil 1: Untersuchungstechniken und Normalbefund (Langversion). *Ultraschall*

in der Medizin (Stuttgart, Germany : 1980), *38*(3), e1–e15. https://doi.org/10.1055/s-0042-115853(accessed on 15th July 2025).

24. Campillo Fernandez, A. J., Pons-Beltrán, V., Santonja, A., Sánchez-Díaz, M., et al. (2020). *Analysis of the 'Endoworm' prototype's ability to grip the bowel in in vitro and ex vivo models.* https://riunet.upv.es/bitstream/10251/171701/1/TobellaPons-BeltranSantonja%20-%20Analysis%20of%20the%20Endoworm%20prototypes%20ability%20to%20grip%20the%20bowel%20in%20in.pdf (accessed on 15th July 2025).
25. Castro, F. D., Cotter, J. de A. B., Gonçalves, T. C., Moreira, M. J., et al. (2014). *Small bowel capsule endoscopy in obscure gastrointestinal bleeding: Normalcy is not reassuring.* https://core.ac.uk/download/55633380.pdf (accessed on 15th July 2025).
26. Cengiz, C., & Oguz, D. (2019). *Gastrointestinal hemorrhage and its management in geriatric age group.* https://core.ac.uk/download/275898723.pdf (accessed on 15th July 2025).
27. Fry, L. C., Mönkemüller, K., Olano, C., Safatle-Ribeiro, A. V., et al. (2013). *Unusual findings in the small bowel.* https://core.ac.uk/download/pdf/82312026.pdf (accessed on 15th July 2025).
28. García Montes, J. M., Hergueta Delgado, P., Herrerías Gutiérrez, J. M., Jiménez García, R., et al. (2013). *Application of colon capsule endoscopy (CCE) to evaluate the whole gastrointestinal tract: A comparative study of single-camera and dual-camera analysis.* https://core.ac.uk/download/51386982.pdf (accessed on 15th July 2025).
29. Katsafadou, M. (2023). *Towards an endoscopic capsule for the detection of gastrointestinal bleeding: Spectroscopic sensing and optical data communications.* https://core.ac.uk/download/640805988.pdf (accessed on 15th July 2025).
30. Macedo, G., Moutinho-Ribeiro, P., & Peixoto, A. (2017). *CPRE e ecoendoscopia: Um mesmo viajante em estradas convergentes.* https://core.ac.uk/download/223219191.pdf (accessed on 15th July 2025).
31. Muñoz-Navas, M. (Miguel). (2008). *Capsule Endoscopy.* https://core.ac.uk/download/83573528.pdf (accessed on 15th July 2025).
32. Pennazio, M., Rondonotti, E., Despott, E. J., Dray, X., Keuchel, M., Moreels, T. G., Sanders, D. S., et al. (2022). Small-bowel capsule endoscopy and device-assisted enteroscopy for diagnosis and treatment of small-bowel disorders: European Society of Gastrointestinal Endoscopy (ESGE) guideline – Update 2022. *Endoscopy, 55*, 58–95. https://doi.org/10.1055/a-1973-3796 (accessed on 15th July 2025).
33. Saygılı, F. (2015). *Examining the whole bowel, double balloon enteroscopy: Indications, diagnostic yield and complications. World Journal of Gastrointestinal Endoscopy, 7*, 247–247. https://doi.org/10.4253/wjge.v7.i3.247 (accessed on 15th July 2025).

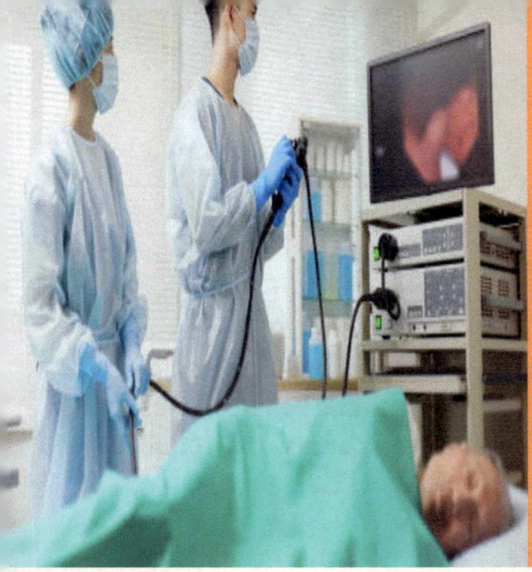

Chapter 11

THERAPEUTIC ENDOSCOPY

Contents

Introduction....311
11.1. Historical Background....314
11.2. Types of Therapeutic Endoscopy....318
11.3. Indications for Therapeutic Endoscopy....321
11.4. Techniques and Procedures....324
11.5. Risks and Complications....327
11.6. Future Directions in Therapeutic Endoscopy....331
Summary....335
References....338

Introduction

The last decades have seen therapeutic endoscopy dramatically change with the integration of advanced technologies to enhance diagnostic and therapeutic capabilities. Previously limited to visualization, flexible endoscopes today find applications in a broad array of advanced intraluminal therapeutic procedures. Endoscopic procedures are explained by the advancement in the incidence of gastrointestinal disease, which calls for new modes of intervention. Although highly effective, the design of the flexible endoscopes has not moved much in 50 years and is a challenge in navigating complex anatomical structures. To address this shortcoming, researchers are now venturing to automate the navigation of endoscopes, a change that is likely to yield better accuracy and user-friendliness in therapeutic procedures (Van der Stap et al., 2013). Understanding the importance of navigation technology in therapeutic endoscopy is important, as it directly influences the success of interventions. Applications of image-based navigation algorithms have shown potential for the enhancement of endoscope steering. Techniques , such as lumen centralization and visual odometry provide the foundation for the automation of endoscope motion, overcoming the limitations introduced by present nonintuitive steering mechanisms. While there have been promising studies done, their application as commercially viable solutions remains high on the horizon. The growing level of sophistication in endoscopic procedures will create the need for automation and improved navigation tools that will reshape therapeutic endoscopy in the future (Van der Stap et al., 2013).

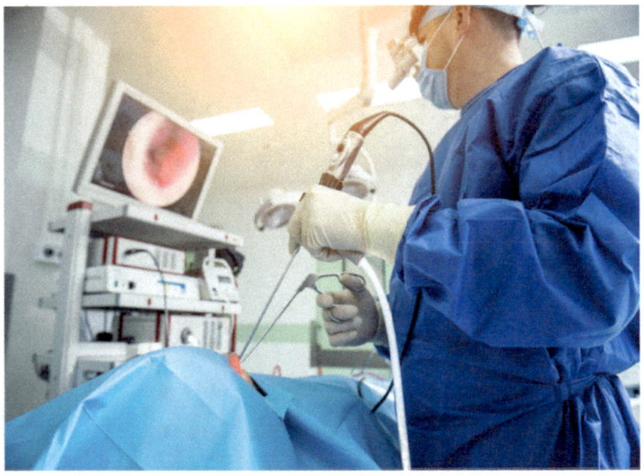

Figure 11.1. Therapeutic endoscopy.

Source: https://external-content.duckduckgo.com/iu/?u=https%3A%2F%2Fchblob.icloudhospital.com%2Fimagecontainer%2F7-509e53cd-f9a1-4b07-aa4e-702327cb0838.jpg&f=1&nofb=1&ipt=578743d36fb1ee3a2609a43803810482f7f48dcc988cde7ce50f722c6eb8e1db.

Further, the development of new technology, such as actively controlled capsule endoscopic robots, introduces a paradigm change in minimally invasive surgery. Such technologies require high-performance real-time 3D reconstruction and localization, which is crucial to ensure successful navigation along the gastrointestinal tract. Current studies demonstrate the feasibility of combining magnetic and vision-based localization to enhance system accuracy. Real-time intraoperative registration of maps, adapting to non-rigid deformations, demonstrates a remarkable leap in the complexity of sophistication of endoscopic techniques and their therapeutic applications. As research continues towards developing new solutions, the integration of such advanced technologies will not only streamline the workflow of endoscopic procedures but also enhance patient care through more accurate outcomes and reduced intervention times (Figure 11.1).

Definition of Therapeutic Endoscopy

Therapeutic endoscopy is an important breakthrough in the practice of minimally invasive medical interventions, whose principal function is to diagnose and treat various gastrointestinal illnesses. Therapeutic endoscopy is a collection of interventions that utilize endoscopic techniques to deliver therapeutic medications or mechanical devices directly into a particular location of the gastrointestinal tract. The primary aim of therapeutic endoscopy is to deliver safer, more effective alternatives to traditional surgery, allowing for quicker recovery and less patient morbidity. This modern discipline combines diagnosis with immediate therapeutic potential, typically increasing patient outcome and satisfaction. It therefore addresses a variety of conditions, including malignancies, strictures, and bleeding ulcers, reflecting its similarly diverse profile throughout gastroenterology and beyond. At the very center of therapeutic endoscopy are the set of instruments and technologies that lead to its efficiency. For instance, the use of self-expanding metal stents (SEMS) has become an integral modality in the management of obstructions and other complications. Comparative analyses have shown to identify that, although both bare SEMS and cSEMS are effective in small bowel obstruction, the latter has been shown to possess a higher rate of stent migration, which would affect therapeutic decision-making. This technological advancement is indicative of an overall trend in medical robotics and computer-assisted interventions for the purposes of improving accuracy and control in therapeutic interventions. As emphasized in recent publications, the success of such interventions in most instances relies on the character of the stent used, emphasizing the reality of good decision-making in therapeutic endoscopy (Albert et al., 2013). Furthermore, the area of therapeutic endoscopy continues to develop, with very promising future prospects in the practice of medicine. The integration of robotics and computerized systems into endoscopic practice is an expanding interest in refining procedural accuracy, a key to success in the clinic. The application of assistive robots in endoscopy, for instance, has been proven to diminish the influence of human error, thereby maximizing patient outcomes. This type of advancement is reflective not only of technological advances but also of ongoing interest in maximizing therapeutic technique within gastroenterology. In the years to come, more investigation of these developments will certainly expand the utility of therapeutic endoscopy, providing doctors with improved tools to increase diagnostic effectiveness and treatment success (Troccaz, 2009).

Relevance in Modern Medicine

Therapeutic endoscopy is a revolutionary advancement in modern medicine that has dramatically altered the management of some gastrointestinal disorders. By reducing invasive procedures, this technique maximizes diagnostic accuracy at the same time as patient recovery is minimized. Its ability to intervene directly in the gastrointestinal tract, such as polypectomy, stricture dilation, and stenting, points to its significance in contemporary medical procedures. Therapeutic endoscopy also plays a significant role in treating diseases that in the past were accessed through open surgery, thereby decreasing patient risk and discomfort. The use of technology, such as advanced imaging, also goes further to advance these procedures by improving visualization and enabling precise interventions. As highlighted by recent literature, effective control of conditions like Crohn's with endoscopy is a model case for the broader impact of this discipline on patient outcomes and health care effectiveness as a whole (Albert et al., 2011). In addition to its therapeutic use, the relevance of endoscopy in current medicine is also accentuated by value-based health care approaches. A patient-centered model of care emphasizes maximum health benefits at sustainable costs. Therapeutic endoscopy follows these principles, as it can truncate the requirement for more risky, more invasive surgery, lowering healthcare costs while enhancing patient satisfaction. The conservativism offered by such approaches enables healthcare providers to provide comprehensive care that is both effective and efficient. Therefore, by incorporating endoscopic interventions into daily treatment procedures, healthcare systems can improve access to necessary interventions, ease the burden on surgical units, and eventually provide an even more responsive health milieu (Böbel & Martis, 2009). On top of this, emerging technologies revealed in therapeutic endoscopy highlight its central position in shaping medicine's future. Techniques , such as capsule endoscopy and balloon-assisted enteroscopy are transforming diagnostic and therapeutic models, particularly for intricate gastrointestinal disorders. These advances facilitate further thorough examinations and therapies that were once found to be too risky or unfeasible. As healthcare continues to evolve, the ongoing development of therapeutic endoscopy to incorporate new technology will continue to be instrumental in optimizing patient benefits. This is not only directed towards effective therapy but also towards long-term surveillance and treatment of chronic diseases, which are needed to improve quality of life. Therapeutic endoscopy thus serves as a vindication of the application of innovation in clinical practice, which proves its persistent value in modern medicine (Hausmann & Albert, 2011) (Figure 11.2).

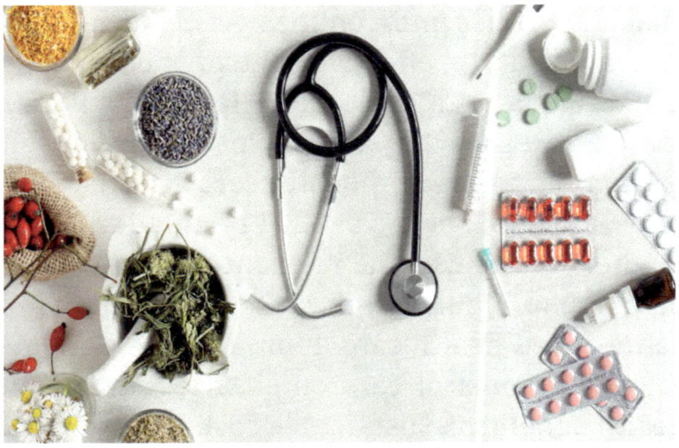

Figure 11.2. Importance in modern medicine.

Source: https://www.autoimmuneinstitute.org/wp-content/smush-webp/2024/02/Holistic-vs-Modern-Western-Medicine.jpg.webp.

11.1. Historical Background

The evolution of therapeutic endoscopy has been significantly shaped by advancements in technology and the growing understanding of gastrointestinal pathology. Early endoscopic techniques, which can be traced back to the 19th century, were rudimentary and primarily diagnostic in nature. However, the potential for therapeutic interventions became evident as endoscopic tools improved. With the introduction of the flexible endoscope in the 1960s, the physician began to explore therapeutic applications as well as visualization of the gastrointestinal tract. These advancements laid the foundation for modern-day techniques, making procedures , such as polypectomy and foreign body removal possible, eventually leading to better patient outcomes and safety. The recognition of therapeutic potential, with increasing incidences of gastrointestinal disease, has propelled research and development in this field, making it a vital component of contemporary medical practice. As the applications of therapeutic endoscopy have increased, so have the methods involved. The evolution of newer technologies , such as endoscopic mucosal resection (EMR), is a case in point. EMR is now an essential technique of resection for lesions to allow en bloc resection of large adenomas and polyps. New evidence has shown that extended EMR is as good as TEM for large rectal adenomas, with cost benefits and fewer complications compared to EMR. These findings mirror the continued quest for quality in therapeutic endoscopy techniques, balancing efficacy, patient safety, and healthcare expense. This bridge of clinical efficacy with cost-effectiveness is particularly pertinent within the present healthcare environment, and hence, there is a need for practitioners to transform and adapt their therapeutic endoscopy styles. The historical trajectory of therapeutic endoscopy demonstrates the reciprocating relationship between diagnostic innovation and therapeutic application. Success with techniques like the CLOtest® in detecting *H. pylori* also shows how developments in diagnostic technology have paved the way to effective treatment programs, vastly influencing patient management protocols. Studies have reported that reused CLOtest® is more accurate for diagnosis compared to other testing methods, with practice implications in resource-constrained settings. The intersection of diagnostic modes and treatment possibilities is crucial; as knowledge about gastrointestinal disease grows, so does the potential to implement directed interventions. The progressive historical background of therapeutic endoscopy is an ongoing endeavor to merge technological innovation with therapeutic efficacy, ultimately enhancing patient treatment and care and treatment outcomes within an increasingly changing medical landscape.

11.1.1. Development of Endoscopic Techniques

The development of endoscopic methods has been revolutionary in the field of therapeutic medicine, significantly augmenting diagnostics and therapeutic interventions. Earlier, endoscopy was in a basic visualization mode only, with invasive methods needing to be employed to receive proper diagnoses. Advances have since introduced high-definition visualizations and light filtering tools, which spurred further sophisticated procedures. These advances make it possible for improved visualization of internal structures and lesions, allowing therapists to make more informed therapeutic decisions. Further, the introduction of autofluorescence imaging (AFI) is an innovation that pushes the boundaries of endoscopic interventions beyond traditional limits. New research explains AFI as a way to distinguish cancerous tissue from healthy tissue, thereby enhancing the efficacy of surgical interventions and indirectly influencing patient outcomes positively (Wizenty et al., 2020). Besides, the therapeutic role of endoscopic interventions has increased significantly, particularly in the management of diseases once addressed by surgery. Endoscopic mucosal resection and endoscopic submucosal dissection represent new modalities for tumor and polyp excision with minimal risk and recovery compared to conventional surgery. Accompanying these interventions are advancements in hemostatic instrumentation that have enhanced the control of effective gastrointestinal bleeding. In diseases like vascular lower gastrointestinal bleeding, the complementarity of angiographic and endoscopic modalities has been shown to optimize patient care by providing integrated treatment regimens. These developments underscore the growing appreciation of the role of endoscopy as a foundation stone for therapy, with ongoing research continually improving techniques and equipment to further push the standards of care in this area (Alomair, 2024). The development of endoscopic technology reflects a general direction towards precision and customization of therapeutic options. Modern endoscopy includes an increasingly AI and machine learning functionality to maximize decision-making and procedural productivity. By being able to process vast amounts of data, AI-based systems can assist physicians in diagnosing abnormalities with greater accuracy and more quickly, thereby maximizing workflows and improving diagnostic precision. As the specialty evolves further, multidisciplinary collaboration will be essential to incorporate new forthcoming technologies and treatment regimens. Analysis by peer-reviewed assessment of new techniques will be crucial for establishing their safety and efficacy profiles. So the future is bright for endoscopic techniques, poised to go further in therapy indications and reestablish the standard in patient care for the subspecialty of therapeutic endoscopy (Figure 11.3).

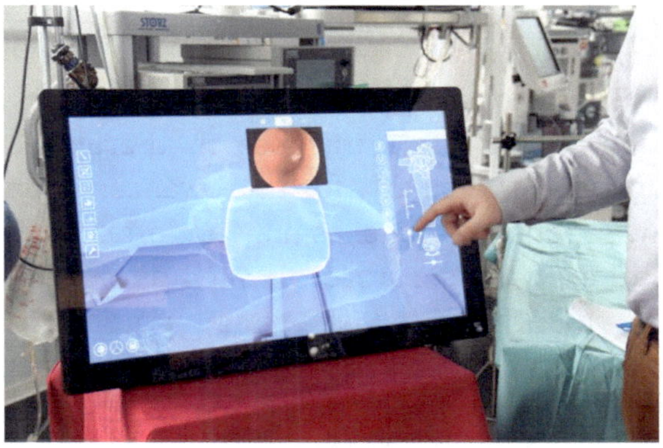

Figure 11.3. Development of endoscopic techniques.

Source: https://www.surgicalroboticstechnology.com/wp-content/uploads/2021/09/Endoscopy-simulation-modules-740x493.jpg.

11.1.2. Milestones in Therapeutic Endoscopy

Therapeutic endoscopy has evolved considerably since its origin, with significant milestones achieved that have revolutionized patient care in the practice of medicine. The development of endoscopic procedures , such as endoscopic retrograde cholangiopancreatography (ERCP) has revolutionized the treatment of biliary and pancreatic illnesses, providing less invasive alternatives for traditional surgery. ERCP facilitates diagnosis and clearance of the obstruction, allowing for timely intervention of diseases like cholangitis and pancreatitis. It not only enhances the recovery of patients but also minimizes the risk of more extensive operations. With the evolution of technology, other advancements like the use of endoscopic ultrasound and newer imaging technologies have led therapeutic endoscopy to an integrated approach towards complex gastrointestinal disease. These milestones reflect the position of endoscopic therapy as pillars in the entire horizon of minimally invasive gastrointestinal treatment. Another hallmark of therapeutic endoscopy is the use of photodynamic therapy (PDT) that utilizes photosensitizers in the selective cancer therapy.

The procedure has become popular as it serves a twofold purpose in therapy and diagnosis, particularly for those cancers where conventional approaches may not offer the full solution. Photosensitizers , such as hypericin have demonstrated excellent potential in photodynamic diagnosis (PDD) as molecular contrast agents to enhance tumor visualization during endoscopy. Progress in optical imaging modalities and the development of artificial intelligence for diagnostic algorithms have further improved the efficacy of PDT. Minimally invasive methods provided by PDT and PDD, in addition to facilitating easy identification of tumors, have also enhanced surgical clearance, thereby playing a crucial role in cancer therapy. This innovative method illustrates how therapeutic endoscopy not only progresses but also embraces new-age technology to better the lives of patients. Finally, the achievement of multidisciplinary team success in therapeutic endoscopy is an affirmation of the fundamental principle of modern healthcare. This co-management often includes multidisciplinary experts like gastroenterologists, radiologists, oncologists, and pathologists working synergistically to address intricate medical issues. An outstanding innovation in this context has been the development of nanotechnology which has opened up immense possibilities of therapeutic endoscopic applications. Use of a drug or imaging agent-delivering biocompatible nanoparticles permits targeted therapy and enhanced therapeutic efficacy. Furthermore, the aforementioned technologies are readily integrated into existing endoscopic approaches, making them even more therapeutically beneficial. With further increase in interdivisional cooperation among the branches of therapeutic endoscopy, the promise of personalized treatment modalities is building steam. With the incorporation of innovations from other medical disciplines, therapeutic endoscopy is set to revolutionize patient management in gastroenterology and beyond, beating the challenges of modern medicine (Figure 11.4).

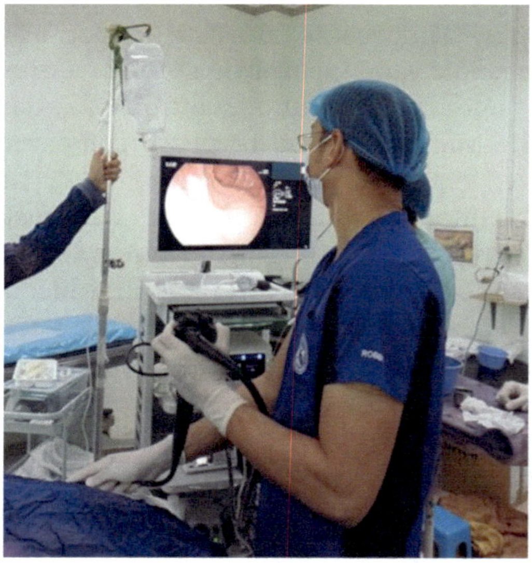

Figure 11.4. Milestones in therapeutic endoscopy.

Source: https://external-content.duckduckgo.com/iu/?u=https%3A%2F%2Ftse2.mm.bing.net%2Fth%3Fid%3DOIP.p6uW2o_5pGbrfErSGLJR3gHaHu%26pid%3DApi&f=1&ipt=6fae231b0916672429156d67f900b9c09acf255b44d293a476a9c9b75e661c09.

11.1.3. Evolution of Technology in Endoscopy

Technological evolution in endoscopy has played a crucial role in improving diagnostic and therapeutic results substantially. Conventional endoscopic techniques commonly had drawbacks like invasive procedures, patient discomfort, and limited visualization potential. Yet, recent developments have ushered in newer, more advanced instruments like high-definition imaging and narrow-band imaging, which have radically reshaped the domain of gastrointestinal (GI) diagnostics. With these developments come new hemostatic devices that maximize therapeutic efficiency in healing disorders like vascular lower gastrointestinal bleeding. Not only does the implementation of these sophisticated instruments increase diagnostic accuracy, but it also minimizes invasiveness, further maximizing patient comfort as well as recovery. With the advancement of technologies, the field of therapeutic endoscopy is evolving at a very rapid pace towards less invasive techniques that are effective in treatment and adequate response to patient needs (Alomair, 2024). Furthermore, the arrival of wireless capsule endoscopy (WCE) is a significant step in the development of endoscopic technology. This ground-breaking procedure enables practitioners to image the GI tract without causing damage, offering a contrast to traditional endoscopic examination, which is sometimes necessary with sedation and can be uncomfortable. Since its advent in 2000, WCE has indicated potential as an agent of mass screening and patient compliance with the avoidance of much of the anxiety associated with traditional endoscopic examination (Ciuti et al., 2016). Not only does the technology make visualization of the small intestine possible in bulky volumes, but it also opens doors to new advancements. The continuous merging of microrobotics into WCE, with features like active motion and therapeutic modules included, hints at a bright future for endoscopic assistance, thereby enhancing both diagnostic accuracy and therapeutic efficiency. In the future, the infusion of AI into endoscopic technology presents an intriguing horizon in the evolution of therapeutic endoscopy. Systems based on AI have begun to aid in real-time image interpretation and decision-making during diagnosis, significantly improving the accuracy and speed of endoscopic interventions. Such integration will enhance the ability to detect abnormalities and provide patient-specific interventions, ultimately establishing a more individualized trend in GI tract management. In conjunction with emerging treatments and hybrid technologies that converge endoscopy with angiography or robotic intervention, the future of therapeutic endoscopy appears both revolutionary and patient-centric. While investigation keeps growing in this domain, the potential for improved results and more acceptable patient experiences is made to wait just over the horizon by the insatiable quest for technological excellence (Ciuti et al., 2016; Alomair, 2024) (Figure 11.5).

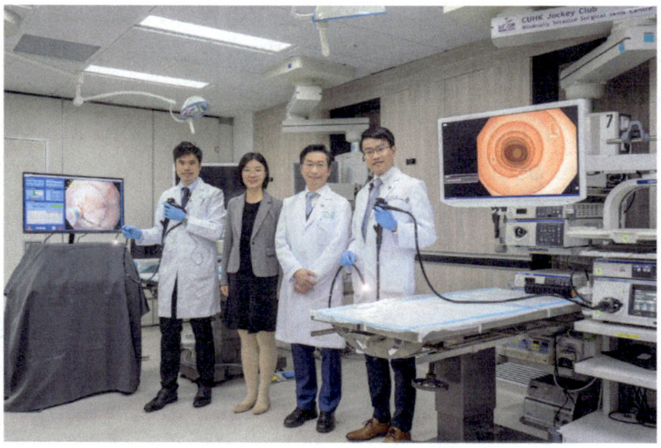

Figure 11.5. Evolution of technology in endoscopy.

Source: https://external-content.duckduckgo.com/iu/?u=https%3A%2F%2Fcdn.opengovasia.com%2Fwp-content%2Fuploads%2F2023%2F12%2FArticle_26-Dec-2023_4-HK-main-1271.jpg&f=1&nofb=1&ipt=1d2a2973b044c5eaa3b3520e31f8036b6ecd466bba937c735bdcb2ba09ed5601.

11.2. Types of Therapeutic Endoscopy

Therapeutic endoscopy consists of a variety of procedures aimed to diagnose and cure GI conditions. ERCP is one of the numerous types used primarily to diagnose and treat conditions of the bile ducts and pancreas. During ERCP, a flexible endoscope is advanced through the mouth into the duodenum so that contrast dye may be injected into the bile ducts for imaging. ERCP may identify blockage, stones, or strictures and facilitate therapeutic intervention in the form of stone removal or stenting. The capacity to perform these advanced maneuvers increases the value of therapeutic endoscopy in the management of complex GI diseases, with the advantage of diagnostic precision and direct therapy. Endoscopic mucosal resection (EMR) is another useful type of therapeutic endoscopy that offers a minimally invasive procedure for removing early cancers or pre-cancerous lesions from the GI tract. EMR involves injecting a substance to elevate the lesion, followed by the removal of the target tissue with specialized devices through the endoscope. The method minimizes morbidity associated with incision in comparison to traditional surgery and allows for more precise excision. With the advancement of the technique, scientists have researched incorporating newer imaging and navigation technology, bringing about innovations , such as real-time 3D reconstruction into the science. All such advancements would render procedures like EMR more efficient, enabling improved localization and excision of lesions with the help of actively controlled, steerable capsule endoscopic robots that can deliver targeted interventions (Turan et al., 2018). Lastly, stenting endoscopically is also a similarly beneficial therapeutic intervention, particularly in obstructed or strictured gastrointestinal patients. This procedure involves the placement of a stent—a tube that is inserted to keep the passageway open—within the obstructing site itself, thereby opening up regular flow or function. Stenting is an effective treatment for symptoms due to tumors, inflammation, or other intestinal obstructions. Endoscopic stenting, as opposed to traditional surgical techniques, is less invasive and sometimes gives faster patient recovery times. Besides, the advent of navigation technologies, including real-time visual guidance, enhances stent deployment accuracy in challenging anatomical conditions. The integration of these sophisticated technologies with therapeutic endoscopy defines its evolution as a robust and adaptable intervention technique in modern medicine.

11.2.1. Gastrointestinal Endoscopy

Endoscopy of the gastrointestinal tract has revolutionized the practice of diagnosing and treating gastrointestinal disorders. This minimally invasive method allows for direct visualization of the gastrointestinal tract, permitting the health professionals not only to diagnose pathological conditions but also to intervene therapeutically. Endoscopy has a purpose beyond mere diagnosis; it has a variety of therapeutic applications , such as polypectomy, foreign body removal, and hemostasis of bleeding lesions. The ability to combine diagnostic and therapeutic procedures shortens the course of patient care, erases signs and symptoms, and prevents complications of untreated gastrointestinal illness. Gastrointestinal endoscopy is thus a central part of modern therapeutic practice, ensuring that patients are subjected to successful and timely interventions consistent with their own personal disease. Sedation during gastrointestinal endoscopy cannot be overstated in its significance because it is heavily influential over the overall patient experience and success of the procedure. Patient safety and comfort during endoscopic procedures require careful assessment of sedation techniques based on patient and procedure factors. Practice of sedation is a continuum from light to deep sedation, and agents , such as midazolam and propofol are most frequently used to facilitate. Specifically, moderate sedation is applied in simple diagnostic endoscopic procedures, whereas more invasive procedures are warranted for deeper sedation. The consensus guidelines point to prudential sedation selection that has a direct influence on recovery and satisfaction for the patient, finally leading to enhanced therapeutic endoscopy efficacy (Abdullah et al., 2017). Pediatric endoscopy of the gastrointestinal tract presents unique challenges and opportunities, particularly in complex healthcare settings , such as Nigeria. A recent retrospective study highlights the common indications for endoscopic procedures among pediatric patients, indicating upper abdominal pain and GI bleeding are the most frequent indications for these procedures, particularly in teenagers (Atimati et al., 2022). This age-specific difference also necessitates age-specific endoscopic methods with consideration of age-specific anatomical and physiological differences. In this regard, therapeutic endoscopy is of utmost significance to tackle cases , such as variceal bleeding, where timely intervention can significantly improve patient outcomes. By taking into account the particular needs of children, gastrointestinal endoscopy can be utilized more effectively to diagnose and treat a variety of gastrointestinal diseases so that children get the best treatment in the therapeutic field (Figure 11.6).

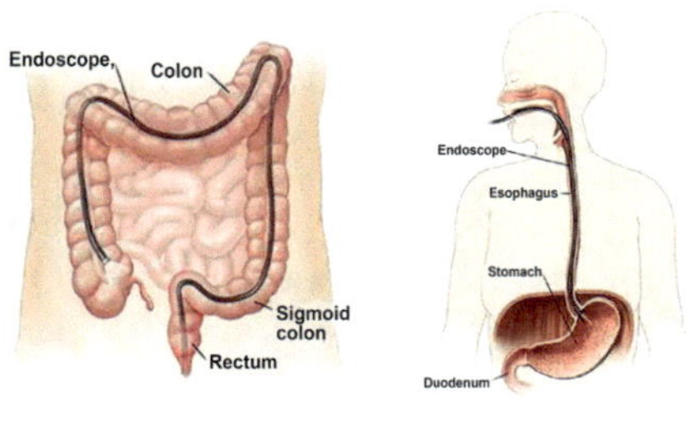

Figure 11.6. Gastrointestinal endoscopy.

Source: https://drruchitpatel.com/images/upper-lower-gi.webp.

11.2.2. Bronchoscopic Procedures

Bronchoscopic procedures are a significant component of therapeutic endoscopy, particularly for the diagnosis and treatment of many pulmonary diseases. This less invasive intervention allows direct visualization of the airways such that clinicians can intervene where otherwise more invasive surgical approaches would be required. For example, flexible bronchoscopy is widely utilized for the therapy of tumors or foreign bodies obstructing the airway and can administer therapeutic agents, i.e., laser therapy or cryotherapy, directly to the site. The technology of bronchoscopy continues to advance, and with each advancement, the accuracy of procedures increases, which is key to improving the outcomes of patients and reducing morbidity rates from traditional surgery. One of the significant advances in bronchoscopic procedures is the research on autonomous systems that would ease navigation and manipulation of flexible endoscopes. The current issues pertain to ergonomics and intuitive control functions, which have the potential to make mastering endoscopic skills difficult. Research on image-based navigation algorithms is an intriguing area; however, as suggested in recent publications, no commercially viable autonomous flexible endoscopy system has been developed. As these technologies continue to develop, there's potential for drastic change in the way bronchoscopic procedures are performed, with wider availability and effectiveness for more patients, ultimately leading to better overall provision of healthcare in thoracic medicine (Van der Stap et al., 2013). In addition, the intricacies of bronchoscopic interventions extend beyond procedure effectiveness into complications for various techniques. One study of the assessment of transtracheal thoracic exploration provided insight into potential risks, including adhesions and the need for proper post-procedure observation. In these situations, the study indicated that with increased bronchoscopic technology and enhanced surgical skill, complications could be reduced and healing and recovery rates optimized for patients. The inherent challenge of performing bronchoscopic procedures underscores the importance of ongoing education and skill development in physicians for optimal patient outcomes. With the advancement of technology in therapeutic endoscopy, efforts are directed at standardizing technical skill with novel practice to expand the role of bronchoscopic use in the treatment of thoracic disease (Chang et al., 2011).

11.2.3. Urological Endoscopy

Urological endoscopy is an innovation in therapeutic endoscopy to facilitate visual examination and treatment of urological conditions directly. It is a non-surgical intervention facilitated through the application of endoscopes, which are advanced instruments with cameras and diagnostic and treatment instruments. Urologic endoscopy is applied to a range of operations, such as removal of kidney stones, management of bladder tumors, and assessment of urinary tract pathology. The primary advantage of this procedure is that it minimizes trauma to adjacent tissues significantly, thus shortening recovery times and complications compared to traditional surgical procedures. By wise utilization, urological endoscopy has transformed into a treatment of urological disease, providing clinicians and patients with functional options in the realm of efficacy and safety. In recent years, urological endoscopic technology has strengthened its position as a therapeutic device further, as shown in the development of the JakoscopeTM and related instruments utilized for this new method. As stated, this new method involves the use of a retractorscope with fiberoptic high-intensity light to allow for improved visualization of the site. By utilizing this minimally invasive procedure, surgeons can perform intricate procedures , such as nephrectomy and ureterolithotomy, via small incisions, which are sometimes just 3–6 cm in size. With the cost-effectiveness of the instrument paired with procedure efficiency, urological endoscopy is a feasible alternative to more invasive surgical procedures. The reality that the operations can be carried out with little postoperative pain and the same rates of morbidity as laparoscopic surgery points to the great clinical benefits of such technological advancements (Frang et al., 2011). Furthermore, urologic endoscopy is not only for surgery but also encompasses diagnostic studies that can guide treatment (Frang et al., 2011). The use of endoscopic procedures allows for biopsies and *in situ* assessment of multiple urological anomalies , such as prostatitis and urinary incontinence. The multi-modal method of diagnosis optimizes the clinician's capability to tailor treatment protocols to suit precise diagnoses, which ultimately results in enhanced patient outcomes. The quick possibility of diagnosis and treatment minimizes patient waiting time to undergo treatment and relieves both physical and emotional symptoms of urological disease. As therapeutic endoscopy continues to advance, the associated implications for urology highlight the need for ongoing development and design evolution to further increase the success of patient care strategies in this field (Kazimierczak & Skea, 2015) (Figure 11.7).

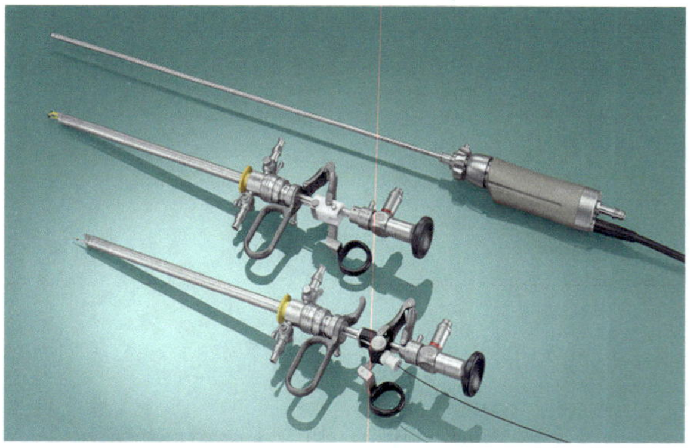

Figure 11.7. Urological endoscopy.

Source: https://sciexaminer.com/wp-content/uploads/2020/03/Urology-Endoscopes.jpg.

11.3. Indications for Therapeutic Endoscopy

Therapeutic endoscopy is one of the most important treatments in the management of many gastrointestinal diseases, and its indications are numerous and highlight its clinical importance. Among all its indications, control of gastrointestinal bleeding is most important because therapeutic endoscopy can be applied to identify the source of bleeding and obtain hemostasis. The ability to visualize and act on lesions , such as ulcers, varices, and angiodysplasias not only aids in the diagnosis but also acts on life-threatening conditions directly. Therapies , such as endoscopic hemostasis using clipping or band ligation have become procedures of first choice and have significantly improved the prognosis of patients with upper and lower gastrointestinal bleeding. The use of endoscopy in this context cannot be overstated since it often avoids the need for invasive surgical procedures, advancing patient safety and reducing hospital stays (Tringali et al., 2017). Besides its use in hemorrhage control, therapeutic endoscopy is utilized in the case of patients with structural irregularities like stricture and stenosis. Conditions , such as inflammatory bowel disease, esophageal stricture, and caustic injury need balloon dilatation or stent insertion procedures for the relief of obstructing symptoms and improved quality of life. Endotherapy allows for the treatment of these lesions directly without the risk associated with more aggressive surgical approaches. For example, the ability to dilate strictures under direct visualization can lead to immediate relief of symptoms , such as dysphagia, significantly enhancing patient comfort and function. Advances in endoscopic technology and technique have made clinicians able to overcome these problems with success, marking a revolution in the treatment of gastrointestinal disease (Deesomsak et al., 2013). Moreover, foreign body removal by therapeutic endoscopy is a critical indication that must not be overlooked. Of particular interest in children is foreign object ingestion, leading to severe health outcomes and gastrointestinal distress. Therapeutic endoscopy allows safe removal of the objects without the risk of inducing complications like perforation or obstruction. The very high level of versatility of endoscopic procedures helps clinicians address the complexity of various pathologies, ranging from impaction of food to sharp objects. The speedy and effective management of such presentations with the assistance of endoscopic intervention determines its significant relevance in emergency conditions. All in all, the range of therapeutic endoscopy indications clearly points to its definitive place in the management of the gastrointestinal tract in the modern era, offering alternatives that are both less and more effective (Tringali et al., 2017) (Figure 11.8).

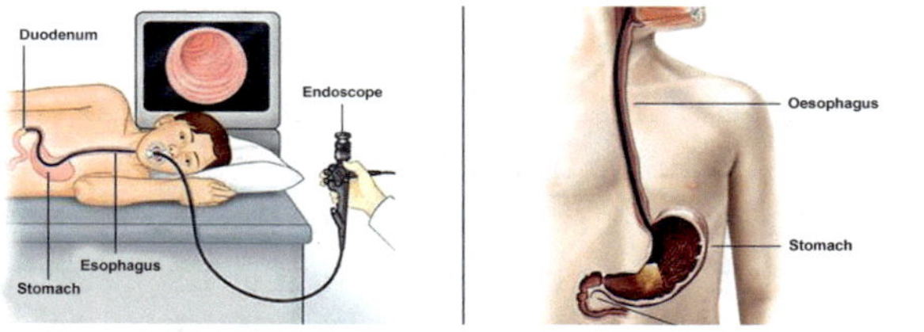

Figure 11.8. Indications for therapeutic endoscopy.

Source: https://drsamitjain.com/images/services/pediatric-endoscopy1.jpg.

11.3.1. Diagnosis of Gastrointestinal Disorders

The diagnosis of gastrointestinal disorders has significantly shifted with the advancement in medical technology, particularly with the use of therapeutic endoscopy. This minimally invasive procedure has transformed the discipline of gastrointestinal diagnosis by providing the ability to visualize the gastrointestinal tract directly. Through the application of fiber-optic technology, physicians can obtain high-resolution images and take biopsies during the same encounter, enhancing diagnostic accuracy as well as therapeutic results. The global increase in the incidence of gastrointestinal diseases has accelerated the need for appropriate diagnostic strategies, which has spurred a remarkable increase in the utilization of endoscopy. According to reports, endoscopy exhibits a higher diagnostic yield than conventional techniques, making it a vital instrument in the diagnosis and treatment of several gastrointestinal disorders, ranging from common conditions to uncommon diseases (Eke, 2021). In children, gastrointestinal endoscopy has emerged as a key diagnostic modality, adapted to the specific requirements of younger patients. A Nigerian tertiary hospital retrospective study found the most common indications for pediatric endoscopy and revealed that the most common reasons for referral were upper gastrointestinal bleeding and upper abdominal pain (Atimati et al., 2022). These findings highlight the importance of early diagnosis of gastrointestinal disease, particularly in children, in which timely intervention can greatly influence the outcome. The study further showed that the majority of the cases were diagnosed with diseases , such as gastritis, hiatus hernia, and duodenitis, demonstrating the broad spectrum of gastrointestinal diseases that could be adequately assessed by endoscopic examination. In addition, the indications of therapeutic endoscopy do not remain limited to diagnosis but also extend to a form of treatment for many gastrointestinal diseases. The blend of therapeutic treatments with diagnostic potential allows real-time treatment of pathologies diagnosed during the endoscopic procedure itself, thus promoting efficiency and patient gain. For instance, therapeutic treatments , such as variceal banding for esophageal varices may be performed alongside diagnosis, illustrating how therapeutic endoscopy justifies the treatment of complex gastrointestinal disease. Growing acceptance and utilization of endoscopic interventions highlight the dynamic nature of pediatric gastroenterology and emphasize the need for continued research and progressive endoscopic practice to meet new healthcare demands (Eke, 2021).

11.3.2. Treatment of Malignancies

Malignancy therapy through therapeutic endoscopy is a significant leap in the management of oncologic care, revolutionizing the treatment of most gastrointestinal malignancies. Conventional procedures like open surgical resection are usually accompanied by a high degree of morbidity and long recovery times. With the entry of minimally invasive endoscopic procedures, though, precise intervention is made possible that can overcome these limitations. A major solution comes in the form of endoscopic submucosal dissection (ESD), where early-stage tumors are removed, leaving behind healthy tissue intact. This technique is particularly worthwhile for gastric and esophageal lesions, where careful removal is followed by excellent long-term outcomes. The ability to be so precise is testimony to the worth of adding endoscopic technologies to treatment protocols for malignancies, providing patients with alternatives to healing and a better quality of life. Besides, the management of intestinal cancers, particularly complicated by perforation, demonstrates the significance of therapeutic endoscopy in today's oncology. For instance, small bowel lymphomas are uncommon and may evolve into nonspecific presentations such that timely treatment becomes extremely difficult. Under these circumstances, endoscopic therapy can be used to provide diagnostic clarity as well as therapeutic relief. As suggested by case reports, an intestinal T-cell lymphoma patient had perforation, and laparotomy followed by segmental enterectomy was the treatment. However, the priority remained systemic disease control by adjuvant therapy, as surgical intervention is not always in accordance with the best long-term prognosis. This illustrates that while endoscopy might permit critical interventions, the overall management strategy first needs to prioritize holistic oncologic care involving systemic therapies to cure the underlying malignancy effectively (Banu et al., 2016). In addition, the therapeutic benefit of endoscopy is not limited to the identification and treatment of malignant lesions but also to pivotal roles in the prevention of adverse consequences due to complications from systemic diseases. For instance, acute esophageal necrosis (AON) can be used to show how emergent endoscopy may be invaluable for recognizing serious underlying conditions , such as concomitant malignancies. The literature indicates that many patients diagnosed with AON, typically under emergency procedures for gastrointestinal bleed, also have serious comorbidities that complicate their overall management of general health. Of interest, there were cases where AON occurred as a manifestation of Zollinger-Ellison syndrome, an expression of the interplay between gastrointestinal cancer and endoscopic therapy. Under these circumstances, endoscopy serves not only as a diagnostic tool but also plays a crucial role in planning an integrated strategy for the treatment of both the acute presentation and the basal cancers, emphasizing its key position in modern oncologic practice (Annibale et al., 2019) (Figure 11.9).

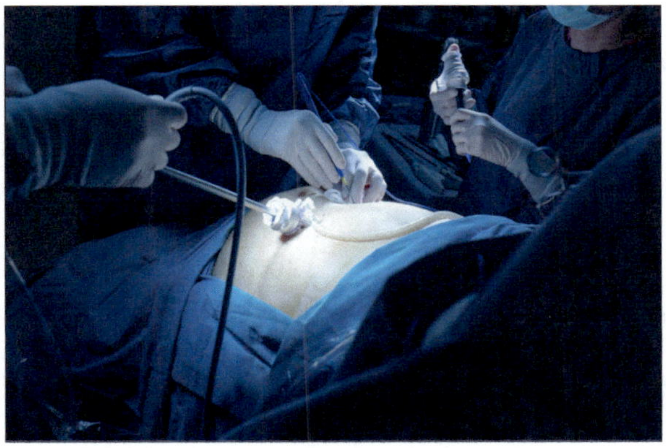

Figure 11.9. Treatment of malignancies.

Source: https://spineina.com/content/uploads/2019/05/iStock-939284920.jpg.

11.3.3. Management of Bleeding and Obstructions

Bleeding and obstruction control in therapeutic endoscopy is a critical undertaking that depends on intimate acquaintance with underlying anatomical and pathological factors. Acute gastro-intestinal bleeding, for instance, can be caused by numerous varied sources , including peptic ulcers, malignancies, and vascular anomalies. Effective management begins with a thorough evaluation, possibly necessitating the use of endoscopic techniques that allow direct visualization and intervention. Bleeding can be controlled by sclerotherapy or clipping. Development of special complications that can occur in the postoperative period must also be considered in creating a treatment plan, especially in patients having deranged anatomy secondary to bariatric surgery. Surgeons should understand the risk of structural complications and should also be able to identify the symptoms clearly so that they can provide timely and effective interventions, as mentioned in Beekley et al. (2018). Obstruction in the gastrointestinal tract is another challenging area in therapeutic endoscopy management, and it may be caused by many etiologies , including neoplasms, strictures, or inflammatory disease. The initial treatment of such obstructions is usually diagnostic imaging or endoscopic evaluation to identify the nature and severity of the obstruction. Therapeutic endoscopy is then performed to excise the obstruction through balloon dilation or stenting. All these procedures are aimed at restoring patency of the lumen using minimal invasive surgery. Furthermore, ongoing assessment and control of the root cause, such as stricturing conditions like Crohn's disease, are required to prevent recurrence. The understanding of the complexities inherent in each case facilitates individualized management methods that can significantly enhance patient outcomes. Beyond the technical maneuvers, the causes responsible for bleeding and obstructions need to be adequately dealt with. For example, *Helicobacter pylori* infection has been implicated in mucosal damage that results in bleeding disorders and potential obstructive lesions. The clinician thus must attack this not just by addressing the acute presentation via therapeutic endoscopy but also by embracing prevention of recurrence. Systematic surveillance of the pattern of antibiotic resistance and rigid adherence to treatment protocols is a hallmark of chronic care for conditions like *Helicobacter pylori*, as emphasized in Ciorbagiu et al. (2016). Such an integrated approach goes to emphasize the necessity of counterbalancing acute therapeutic measures with general systemic therapy such that patient treatment is holistic and effective in countering the threats of gastrointestinal pathologies (Figure 11.10).

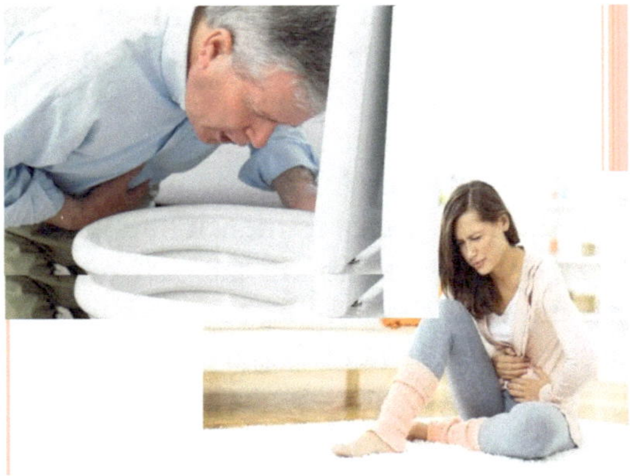

Figure 11.10. Management of bleeding and obstructions.

Source: https://image.slidesharecdn.com/gasrtointestinalbleedingobstruction-141231160142-conversion-gate02/75/Gasrtointestinal-bleeding-obstruction-12-2048.jpg.

11.4. Techniques and Procedures

In therapeutic endoscopy, the techniques and procedures employed are essential to safety and efficacy. Other techniques, such as ERCP, demonstrate the advanced skill set employed in tackling the intricacy of the gastrointestinal tract. ERCP in particular is focused on both diagnosis and treatment of pancreatic and biliary disorders, necessitating an acute awareness of anatomy and potential complications. The availability of non-radiation techniques revolutionized the procedure, with clinicians trying to limit exposure to the barest minimum while providing maximum safety to the patient. Such innovations highlight the importance of continued education and adaptation in therapeutic endoscopy procedures as a measure of training with an emphasis on these new techniques. Moreover, practices in sedation during therapeutic endoscopy are important considerations in patient comfort and the success of the procedure. Historically, there have been alarming accounts of excessive use of sedative medication, particularly in vulnerable populations , such as the elderly. There is evidence that large doses of opioids and benzodiazepines can lead to an undesirable outcome and there are severe ethical considerations regarding the use of sedation. With newer guidelines that guide doses of sedation, it appears that it is improving among healthcare professionals. Adherence to these recommendations can decrease risks of avoidable morbidity and mortality from unguided sedation procedures, thereby enhancing patient outcomes and overall procedural safety (Lord et al., 2006). Therapeutic endoscopy growth is also established by evidence-based assessment of methods utilized, particularly when addressing specific patient populations. There has been a growing body of literature seeking to evaluate procedures among special populations, such as pregnant women undergoing ERCP. The conditions offered by pregnancy necessitate vigilant concern for maternal as well as fetal safety, leading to the use of comparative research between radiation and non-radiation techniques during the procedure. Through the application of meta-analyses and systematic reviews, there has been a lot of information collected on the outcomes of ERCP in pregnant patients, with specific emphasis on the employment of modified techniques to ensure safety and efficacy. Such constant evaluation of endoscopic intervention not only improves procedural techniques but also underlines the ever-present emphasis on patient-oriented care in therapeutic endoscopy (Azab et al., 2019).

11.4.1. Endoscopic Mucosal Resection (EMR)

EMR has now assumed a pivotal role in the field of therapeutic endoscopy, particularly for the removal of superficial neoplasms of the gastrointestinal tract. By enabling dysplastic or malignant lesions to be endoscopically removed in a minimally invasive environment, EMR is a pivotal intervention that preserves adjacent normal tissue and reduces the requirement for more extensive surgical interventions. The technique employs submucosal injection followed by circumferential mucosal incision to enable precise excision of lesions.

This not only aids in accurate diagnosis but also enhances the effectiveness of treatment, thereby leading to favorable patient outcomes. Having undergone proper training and strict adherence to predetermined standards, the application of EMR in clinical practice has completely changed the treatment scenario of gastrointestinal cancers, thereby proving its worth as an effective therapeutic modality in gastroenterology. While having its advantages, EMR cannot be void of risk and complications, and it is this that warrants the practice of trained operators to perform the procedure. Bleeding, perforation, and incomplete resection remain pertinent issues that must be properly addressed. These have been documented by research to be contained, however, through adherence to best practice , such as selective lesion treatment and technical expertise in resection. In addition, development of endoscopic equipment, including better visualization technologies and innovation of endoscopes specialized in certain applications, has contributed to the outcomes and safety profiles. For instance, over-the-scope clips (OTSC) can be applied in the event of a complication like perforation during EMR, as documented in studies , such as reporting on outcomes of iatrogenic gastrointestinal tract perforations treated with OTSC insertion (Antonucci et al., 2016). Therefore, understanding these intricacies is of the utmost importance in the realization of effective EMR procedures. Integration of EMR into therapeutic endoscopy not only promotes the development of treatment methods but also allows ongoing research with a focus on maximizing technique as well as for the criteria of patient selection. Clinical studies continue to aim at long-term results, including rates of recurrence and the value of electromagnetic coagulation of combined treatments, such as radiofrequency ablation, to further enhance therapeutic success. The exploration of these synergistic practices will aid in creating effective protocols that effectively treat lesions and also promote general patient health. Such studies are needed to bridge existing knowledge gaps and create more sophisticated EMR practice. As therapeutic endoscopy continues to develop, continuing professional education and adherence to evidence-based guidelines will be crucial in maintaining the very best level of care, ultimately leading to improvements that have profound impacts on patient populations (Figure 11.11).

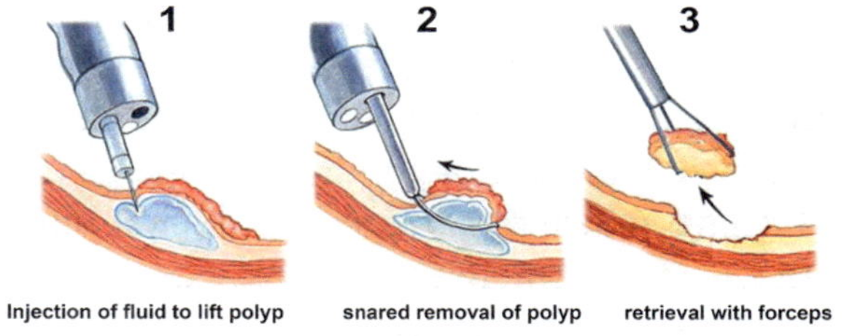

Figure 11.11. Endoscopic mucosal resection (EMR).

Source: https://www.gastromedicine.com.au/images/endoscopic-mucosal-resection-img.jpg.

11.4.2. Endoscopic Retrograde Cholangiopancreatography (ERCP)

ERCP is a valuable asset in the therapeutic endoscopy arsenal, namely for the treatment of pancreatic and biliary conditions. The technique is known for its double function of both diagnostic assessment and therapeutic treatment, such as the removal of bile duct stones and the treatment of strictures. Its effectiveness can be highlighted by the technique's capacity to merge visualization of the pancreatic and biliary ducts with therapeutic measures, thus presenting a minimally invasive option to surgery. However, ERCP is technically demanding and may be associated with complications, and thus stringent procedural expertise and selection criteria for the patient are needed to guarantee the best results. Safety and efficacy assessment in heterogeneous patient groups, specifically the obviously vulnerable pregnant and elderly subjects, is of particular interest since these groups are likely to pose extra challenges and risk factors for the procedural results. Discussion of ERCP in special populations , such as pregnant women, is relevant and poses considerable safety profiles and clinical implications. Current systematic reviews have indicated that while pregnancy makes the course of presentation of biliary disease more complicated, ERCP remains a possibility for intervention. Hormonal changes during pregnancy can predispose to cholelithiasis, and therefore, care must be taken during this period. Studies have shown ERCP with nonirradiative techniques can be accomplished with minimal hazards to mother and fetus. Outcomes of pregnancy patients after ERCP have shown remarkable therapeutic effects with few inconveniences, indicating the need for procedure-specific approaches to preparation and counseling of patients. These observations are important not only for enhancing procedural safety but also for guiding clinical practice in treating pregnant patients with biliary disorders (Azab et al., 2019). In addition, ERCP use among elderly patients deserves further study because the incidence of biliary diseases rises with age. Research has demonstrated that elderly patients, including those aged more than 90 years, could be safely submitted to ERCP without an increased risk of complications compared to younger patients. Since the elderly population is on the rise, it is crucial to understand the specific implications of carrying out ERCP in such individuals. The literature has indicated a high success rate with few complications, lending support to the argument that age should never be a reason for not employing ERCP as a therapeutic agent. Hence, clinical decision-making has to be reduced to specific patient needs and individual indications for ERCP and not presumption by age. Overall, these findings support ERCP as a treatment option in various patient populations, affirming its position in therapeutic endoscopy (Chang & Lei, 2007) (Figure 11.12).

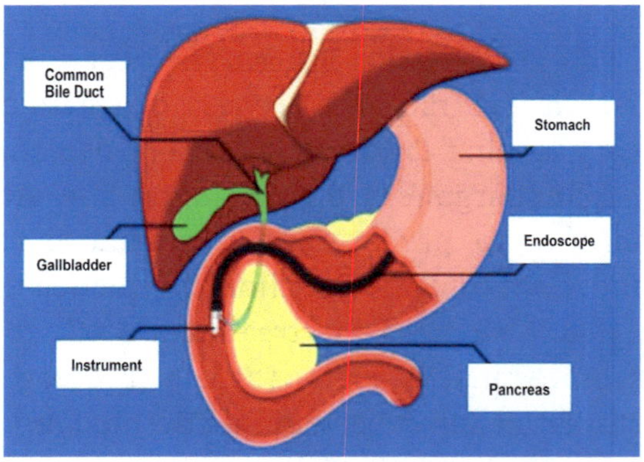

Figure 11.12. Endoscopic retrograde cholangiopancreatography (ERCP).

Source: https://www.regencymedicalcentre.com/wp-content/uploads/2021/03/Why-ERCP-1024x684.jpg.

11.4.3. Endoscopic Ultrasound (EUS)

EUS has played a significant role as a therapeutic endoscopy technology, enhancing diagnostic capability and facilitating minimally invasive intervention. EUS takes advantage of the alliance between endoscopy and ultrasound to visualize gastrointestinal organs and surrounding tissues in real time. Seeing these tissues in detail helps clinicians diagnose several conditions , including tumors and inflammatory conditions. Moreover, EUS is invaluable in fine-needle aspiration biopsy guidance, enabling cell samples to be obtained from lesions that could otherwise be hard to diagnose. The precise test imaging by EUS significantly enhances the accuracy of diagnostic testing, making it an extremely useful tool in modern therapy treatment protocols. Apart from its role in diagnosis, EUS is now also valuable in several therapeutic interventions, particularly in the treatment of pathologies of the biliopancreatic system. EUS-guided drainage of pancreatic fluid collections and fiducial marker placement for stereotactic radiotherapy are but a few examples of the modality's versatility. EUS can also decrease the invasiveness of procedures that used to be done more invasively. For instance, with methods , such as OTSC insertion, EUS can be immediately engaged in the management of complications , such as gastrointestinal perforations, which occur infrequently but with significant consequences. Studies indicate that successful closure by OTSC provides a high clinical success rate, which has implications regarding the role of EUS in enhancing patient outcomes within the therapeutic process (Antonucci et al., 2016). The future of EUS is bright for continued innovations, particularly through the addition of AI technologies. As AI continues to advance in endoscopic research, improved risk stratification, report generation, and quality measures with EUS procedures are feasible. Coupled with these technologies, patient care is likely to become more customized through optimizing the diagnostic process and therapy planning. These developments are essential, given the rising sophistication of gastrointestinal disease and need for precision in intervention method (Ahmad et al., 2021). Biliopancreatic endoscopists, hand in hand with AI researchers, will be at the forefront in translating such advancements into the clinical environment, further solidifying the role of EUSs as a pillar of therapeutic endoscopy (Ahmad et al., 2021) (Figure 11.13).

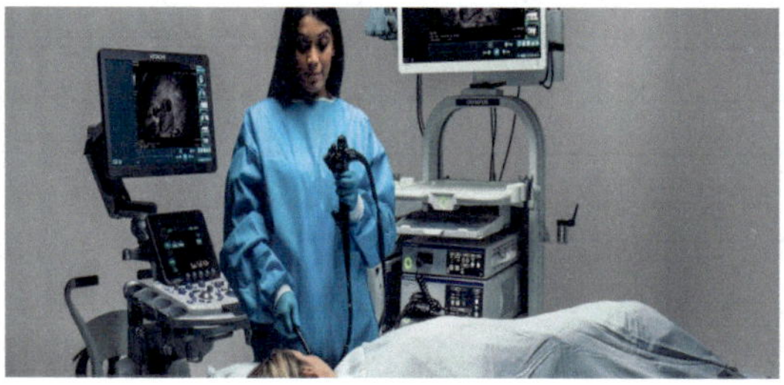

Figure 11.13. Endoscopic ultrasound (EUS).

Source: https://www.pancreaticcancerscreening.com/sites/default/files/styles/hero_image/public/hero-images/EUS_Hero.jpg?h=d1aea52f&itok=2ZIM8MCg.

11.5. Risks and Complications

Therapeutic endoscopy, as useful as it is in managing the majority of gastrointestinal conditions, is not without complications and risks. These unwanted effects can be classified into three general categories: fetal, maternal pregnancy-associated, and maternal non-pregnancy-associated complications. Familiarity with these risks is especially relevant when endoscopic treatment is contemplated in a high-risk patient, such as a pregnant patient. A systematic review of the safety of ERCP in this population has shown that while the procedure is, in most cases, effective, the rate of complications can be extremely variable based on techniques used and underpinning the need for customized strategies in clinical practice. Being vigilant on the incidence and type of such complications is also crucial for practitioners to control effects both on mothers and on fetuses in the course of procedures like ERCP (Azab et al., 2019). Anesthesia-related complications are also a serious challenge for therapeutic endoscopy. The nature of an anesthetic regimen may considerably influence patient outcomes and the overall safety of the procedure. Complications , such as post-operative nausea, vomiting, and longer recovery periods have been noted with certain anesthetic combinations. For instance, in a study comparing propofol and etomidate, it was discovered that the use of these medications among elderly patients resulted in varying recovery periods and levels of patient satisfaction. Specifically, the prevalence of injection pain and the frequency of myoclonus were significantly higher in specific groups, which indicates the significance of careful selection and dosing of anesthetic medications during endoscopic procedures (Meng et al., 2016). The recognition of these intricacies enables practitioners to enhance their competencies, thus enhancing safety and overall procedural efficacy. Moreover, issues related to the endoscopic procedure itself, including potential perforation, bleeding, and infection, represent pertinent concerns. These complications have the potential to alter the patient's management markedly and could lead to longer hospitalization or the need for additional operative procedures. The risk of such complications parallels the increasing complexity of the endoscopic procedure being performed. For example, therapeutic procedures, such as endoscopic mucosal resection, are inherently riskier than diagnostic endoscopies. Therefore, it is of the utmost importance for physicians to weigh the risks against the benefits thereof, particularly in the case of patients with co-morbid illnesses or other complicating factors. Lastly, fostering an overall understanding of the range of risks and complications of therapeutic endoscopy enables clinicians to optimize patient results and make optimal use of these technological developments.

11.5.1. Common Complications Associated with Procedures

Therapeutic endoscopy, as useful as it is in the diagnosis and treatment of numerous gastrointestinal afflictions, does come with its complications. One particular issue relates to the use of sedatives in procedures. Traditionally, the excessive use of benzodiazepines and opioids for sedating older patients has resulted in high morbidity and mortality through respiratory depression and cardiac instability. Such unsafe practices have been noted, leading to a re-examination of sedation protocols. New guidelines have emerged, which advocate more conservative dosing strategies, particularly in high-risk populations like the elderly. This new practice supports the necessity of ongoing assessment of sedation practices to minimize the risks of therapeutic endoscopy without compromising patient safety (Lord et al., 2006). Aside from sedation-related complications, therapeutic endoscopy predisposes to an array of procedural complications, particularly with procedures , such as ERCP. The advanced intervention, primarily utilized in the management of bile duct obstruction, carries a low but significant complication rate. These complications include pancreatitis, perforation, and infections, significantly impairing the outcomes of patients. Patient and protocol choice is crucial, especially in pregnant women who may have unique complications due to hormonal changes influencing the development of gallstones. Recent literature suggests that ERCP in pregnant women needs to be performed with increased awareness of the potential maternal and fetal complications, as well as with consideration of maintaining radiation-free techniques (Azab et al., 2019). These complications necessitate pre-procedure planning as well as aftercare. Complications due to therapeutic endoscopy can also extend beyond immediate procedural complications. Long-term effects like stricture or obstruction of the bowel can follow therapeutic measures like balloon dilation or stent placement. Such complications may arise days or even weeks following the procedure, rendering the clinical situation complicated and necessitating further intervention. It then becomes important for medical professionals to implement careful follow-up procedures to monitor for late complications and educate patients on potential symptoms requiring early medical intervention. Through the development of a patient education and monitoring culture with the potential hazards, the overall safety of therapeutic endoscopy can be enhanced, thereby improving the satisfaction and results of the patients in the long run (Figure 11.14).

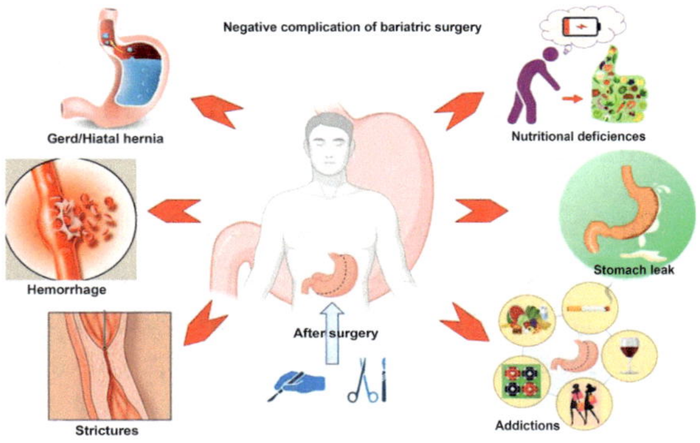

Figure 11.14. Common complications associated with procedures.

Source: https://www.researchgate.net/profile/Milena-Peruhova/publication/372518758/figure/fig2/AS:11431281175792680@1689869130263/Early-and-late-complications-of-bariatric-procedures.ppm.

11.5.2. Risk Factors Influencing Complications

The awareness of the numerous risk factors that influence complications is most critical in ensuring patient safety and improving the rates of procedural success in therapeutic endoscopy. One of the most critical factors is patient age, as older patients have more intricate medical and comorbid histories that complicate endoscopic procedures. For instance, studies affirm that aging patients develop altered pharmacokinetics that may affect the action and safety of anesthesia. Moreover, in case there are pre-existing conditions , such as cardiovascular disorders or diabetes, then this can amplify risks for complications during as well as after the procedure. These age and health-related risk factors necessitate thorough pre-procedure assessments as well as tailored precautions against potential adverse outcomes, hence improving worldwide patient care. The second pertinent risk factor is the technique applied per se for therapeutic endoscopy. ERCP, for example, has comparatively more complications than most endoscopies. This is especially true for pregnant women who may have special complications due to hormonal changes that predispose them to conditions , such as cholelithiasis. A systematic review has revealed that while inherent risks exist, the use of nonradiation ERCP techniques in pregnancy is a safer alternative, validating the need for selecting appropriate methodologies based on individual patients' profiles. The procedural complexity demands that health professionals pay attention to various techniques and the risk implications of each, so that they opt for the most suitable interventions for their own respective patients' specific clinical situations (Azab et al., 2019). Finally, the choice of anesthetic regimen is also a critical determinant of complications in therapeutic endoscopy. Anesthetic agents vary in terms of safety profiles, particularly in vulnerable populations , such as the elderly. An assessment of the safety and efficacy of sedation by etomidate and propofol with gastroscopy showed considerable differences in recovery rates and complication rates of different anesthetic regimens. Surprisingly, propofol, though effective for inducing sedation quickly, has a higher rate of myoclonus and postoperative nausea compared to etomidate, which exhibits a more stable hemodynamic profile (Meng et al., 2016). This awareness of anesthetic risk factors is an indication of the necessity for clinicians to take careful consideration of the benefits and limitations of all forms of sedation to ensure that the selected anesthetic plan is suitable for each patient's individual needs and risk profiles for therapeutic endoscopy (Figure 11.15).

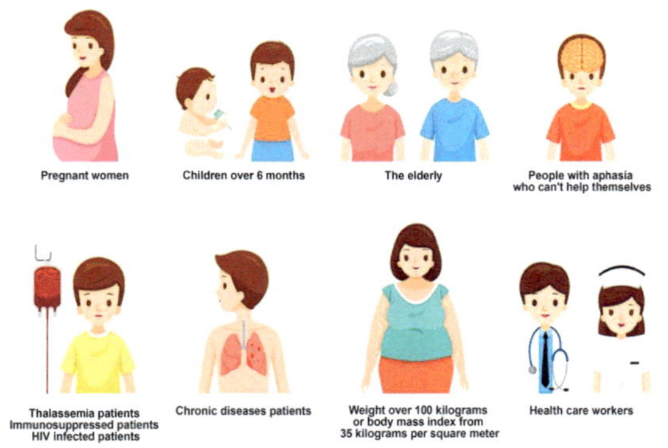

Figure 11.15. Risk factors influencing complications.

Source: https://duckduckgo.com/?q=Risk+factors+influencing+complications&t=h_&iar=images&iaf=size%3ALarge&iai=https%3A%2F%2Fcdn1.vectorstock.com%2Fi%2F1000x1000%2F39%2F05%2Fpeople-at-high-risk-for-flu-complications-vector-27503905.jpg.

11.5.3. Strategies for Minimizing Risks

During therapeutic endoscopy, implementation of effective measures for risk minimization is key to patient safety and optimization of outcomes. Amongst the most significant are the detailed pre-procedure assessments, which assist in identifying patient-related risk factors likely to affect procedural success. A thorough assessment , including medical history, physical examination, and relevant imaging studies, helps clinicians tailor the strategy based on individual needs. Furthermore, informed consent processes should include the clear articulation of potential risks associated with the procedure to empower patients in decision-making about healthcare. Such meticulous preparatory processes, combined with advanced planning, can significantly reduce risks of complications, thereby leading to increased patient satisfaction as well as improved clinical results. Moreover, the selection of appropriate endoscopic procedures also plays a critical role in reducing risks. For example, employment of high-definition imaging and narrow-band imaging technology facilitates clearer visualization during interventions, allowing for more precise interventions and minimizing the risk of injury to surrounding tissues. Application of advanced hemostatic devices in endoscopic procedures can directly manage unforeseen bleeding complications, thereby optimizing therapeutic efficacy while simultaneously minimizing exposure to danger. Secondly, the integration of artificial intelligence devices into endoscopic procedures is a new development that can potentially contribute to real-time decision-making, and even reduce procedural flaws.

Such advancements result in an environment of controlled practice in procedures and ultimately improved quality and outcomes of patient care. Care after procedure is the other vital component of therapeutic endoscopy's risk management chain. Having sharp surveillance for any indication of side effects after the procedure will lead to early diagnosis and treatment of complications, thus enhancing patient safety significantly. Having adequate postoperative procedures, such as such routine follow-up visits and education of the patient on signs of complications, is essential. Particularly, research indicates that tailored follow-up care can minimize the incidence of complications , such as infections or bleeding complications. Addressing patient concerns and educating them regarding expectations of recuperation not only increases satisfaction but also allows them to take on an active role in their own treatment. Therefore, the incorporation of pre-procedure assessment, advanced techniques, and robust post-procedure measures represents a comprehensive strategy toward limiting risks of therapeutic endoscopy, which ultimately aids better patient and healthcare outcomes (Alomair, 2024; Andrade et al., 2025).

11.6. Future Directions in Therapeutic Endoscopy

Directions for future therapeutic endoscopy are also illuminated by advancing technological advances that center on optimizing the efficacy and precision of less-invasive treatments. One promising direction is the development of actively steerable capsule endoscopes, which transform the traditional passive diagnostic instrument into an active one with more control that can travel along the GI tract. This is assisted by sophisticated technologies in real-time odometry and depth estimation, enabling such capsules to perform complex maneuvers like targeted drug delivery and biopsy-like procedures independently. All of these inventions have the potential to revolutionize diagnosis and patient management by facilitating clinicians to effectively visualize inaccessible locations with less physical stress on the patient inherent in conventional endoscopy, eventually leading to patient-centered treatment in therapeutic procedures (Turan et al., 2018). Additionally, incorporating AI into therapeutic endoscopy is a promising horizon. The technologies of artificial intelligence are being deployed to enhance diagnostic accuracy and therapeutic decision-making with innovative imaging modalities , such as high-definition and narrow-band imaging. Machine learning algorithms can sort through vast datasets and identify patterns that may elude the human eye, facilitating earlier diagnosis of GI pathologies and improved outcomes on average. Moreover, AI-based technologies can predict potential complications during procedures, integrate operational efficiencies, and optimize techniques. This prognostic ability is most critical in that it complements the personalization of treatment planning based on patient profiles, thereby allowing for more tailored therapeutic endoscopy in harmony with current trends towards personalized medicine (Alomair, 2024). The future of therapeutic endoscopy also embraces the possibility of hybrid approaches combining various methodologies for optimal care for the patient. For instance, the integration of endoscopic modalities with new angiographic techniques in the management of vascular lower gastrointestinal bleeding is one of such developments. This hybridization exploits the advantage of the two modalities to provide treatment where one would not be adequate. Innovations like computed tomographic angiography (CTA) and superselective embolization complement endoscopic techniques and are employed selectively based on patient characteristics and clinical contexts. As they evolve and converge, the technologies provide an opportunity for the development of personalized treatment protocols sensitive to the diverse etiologies of conditions managed by therapeutic endoscopy, with a focus on interdisciplinary teamwork in achieving better patient outcomes (Alomair, 2024) (Figure 11.16).

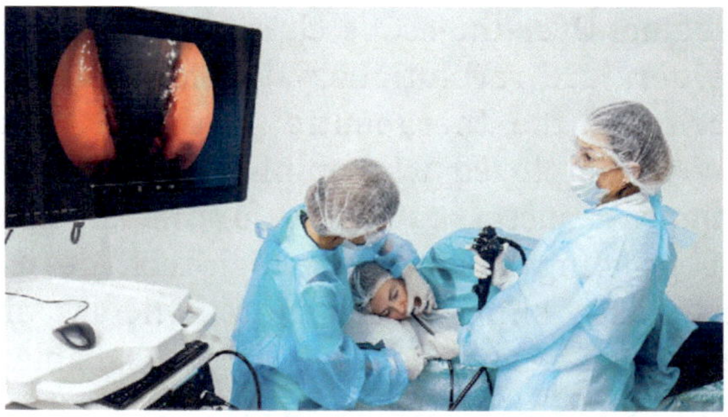

Figure 11.16. Future directions in therapeutic endoscopy.

Source: https://www.medicalbuyer.co.in/wp-content/uploads/2019/12/Untitled-1.jpg.

11.6.1. Innovations in Endoscopic Technology

Endoscopic therapy has undergone great improvements that have revolutionized diagnosis and treatment. A significant such development is the high-definition imaging technology, which provides enhanced quality visualization of gastrointestinal architecture. Clinicians can now detect lesions and vascular anomalies that had otherwise been undetectable. Furthermore, narrow-band imaging (NBI) enhances the visibility of mucosal and vascular patterns and facilitates the identification of dysplastic tissue. These advances not only enable earlier detection but also contribute to more precise therapeutic interventions, ultimately resulting in improved patient outcomes. The enhanced abilities made possible by these technologies identify the potential of personalized approaches to the treatment of such disorders as vascular lower gastrointestinal bleeding, a disorder treated by recent endoscopic advances documented in the literature (Alomair, 2024). Another major endoscopic technology advancement is the advent of new hemostatic devices with specificity for use in emergent situations. Conventional endoscopic techniques are often time-consuming and require highly skilled operators to achieve successful hemostasis, particularly in instances of gastrointestinal bleeding. Over-the-scope clips and hemostatic powders are revolutionary technologies that accelerate the therapeutic procedure. They may be employed with minimal convenience to improve success rates even for difficult cases. The growing use of such high-tech devices portends a shift toward more efficient and responsive management techniques, capable of easily being integrated into a broader spectrum of patient needs and clinical contexts. Thus, with changing technologies in therapeutic endoscopy, integration of these sophisticated tools is bound to make a huge difference in patient treatment in acute non-variceal upper GI bleeding and associated morbidity and mortality (Alali & Barkun, 2023). Aside from enhancements in imaging and hemostatic techniques, the potential for incorporating AI in therapeutic endoscopy is revolutionary. AI algorithms can review vast amounts of endoscopic images and provide real-time assistance in identifying abnormalities and suggesting possible intervention strategies. The technology enhances the efficiency of endoscopy and can cut down examination times, significant in emergency cases where rapid decision-making is crucial. Moreover, AI's predictive capabilities would further aid risk stratification among patients, guiding treatment decisions on the basis of individual clinical parameters. With the amalgamation of AI continuing to develop, it has the potential to not only optimize therapeutic interventions but also establish a new collaboration among clinicians and technology, ultimately fostering improved patient outcomes and a more individualized journey to care in therapeutic endoscopy (Alomair, 2024).

11.6.2. Potential for Robotic-Assisted Endoscopy

The use of robotic assistance in endoscopic interventions is a major advance in therapeutic endoscopy. Using robotics, medical professionals can enhance precision and control during the performance of diagnostic and therapy procedures. Robotic systems are designed to support clinicians so that complex procedures become easier, minimizing patient discomfort as well as recovery time. The advancement of computer-aided medical procedures, as observed in the discussion on medical robotics, demonstrates the potential of robotics in transforming traditional endoscopy procedures into more efficient and effective processes (Troccaz, 2009). With improvements in the robotic system, their therapeutic use in endoscopy seems promising as they seek to improve clinical performance and patient satisfaction. One of the most exciting areas of investigation for robotic-assisted endoscopy is the development of actively propelled capsule endoscopes. Unlike passive capsules that pass through the gastrointestinal tract, such newer technologies are capable of moving with precise control, even facilitating the possibility of aimed therapeutic interventions. Greater mobility via sophisticated means, such as magnetic actuation, is highly promising for enhancing the efficacy of capsule endoscopic procedures (Slawinski et al., 2015). The blending of sensor data with robot control not only aims to surpass conventional invasive methods but also promises less invasive treatment of gastrointestinal pathology.

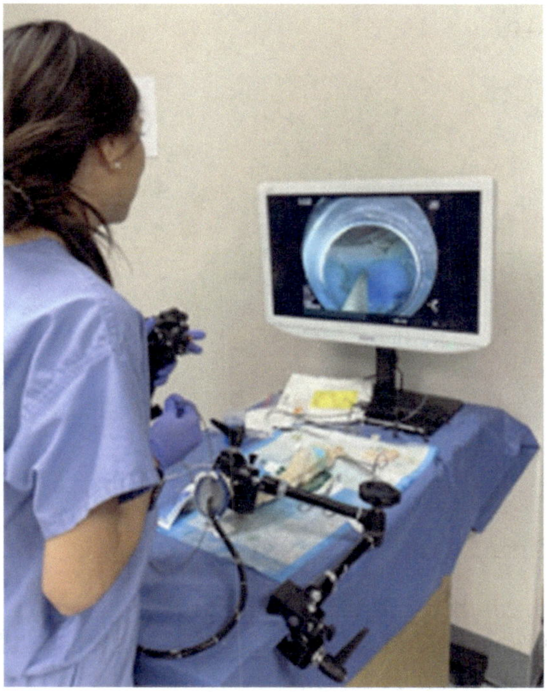

Figure 11.17. Potential for robotic-assisted endoscopy.

Source: https://www.giejournal.org/cms/10.1016/j.gie.2024.04.1464/asset/88fb6562-91b8-4f2a-b4bd-b657f71abebe/main.assets/fx2_lrg.jpg.

This shift from passive surveillance to active intervention puts robotic-assisted endoscopy as a therapeutic revolution instrument in a position to overcome current limitations and pave the way for future advancements. Second, the extent of robotic endoscopy is not confined to simple mobility augmentation but encompasses the introduction of sophisticated functions that hold the potential to transform patient care. Innovative drug delivery systems incorporated within robotic capsules are a step forward in therapeutic capability, facilitating targeted treatment in therapeutically hard-to-reach locations (Slawinski et al., 2015). With continued advancements in robot technologies, the potential to automate endoscopic procedures brings efficiency and accuracy to procedures, in line with the growing demand for minimally invasive interventions. With further development of such technologies towards clinical translation, they have the potential to revolutionize therapeutic endoscopy, providing patients with safer and more effective interventions and, at the same time, easing pressure on health systems (Figure 11.17).

11.6.3. Research Trends and Clinical Trials

The evolving pattern of therapeutic endoscopy is a reflection of escalating trends in research and clinical trials towards better patient outcomes. The most recent research has focused on the use of modern endoscopy equipment, such as the Endocuff Vision, that assists in improving mucosal vision during colonoscopy. Randomized trial demonstrated that Endocuff Vision use significantly reduced examination time without compromising lesion detection rates compared with standard colonoscopy. The wide-ranging implications of the technology are profound because, in addition to making procedures easier, it has the potential to enhance the early detection of gastrointestinal lesions, a cornerstone of improving patient prognoses. Thus, the information gathered through such clinical trials plays a crucial role in guiding clinical practice as practitioners use new instruments to further improve their diagnostic and therapeutic skills (Garcia et al., 2019). Clinical trials into various therapeutic modalities also highlight the importance of individually tailored treatment approaches in endoscopy. For instance, a critical appraisal of rates of recurrence of intestinal metaplasia and dysplasia in Barrett's esophagus patients after complete eradication focused on the extent of variation in treatment techniques, such as radiofrequency ablation (RFA) and stepwise complete endoscopic mucosal resection (SRER). The findings indicated higher rates of recurrence when RFA was used compared to SRER, and this points to the need for strict patient selection and post-treatment follow-up. These observations point towards the evolving perception of treatment results and patient care protocols in therapeutic endoscopy, hence calling for a more advanced policy of care that centers on individually tailored treatment regimens (Cinnor et al., 2017). Moreover, the emphasis on strict clinical trials is necessary to confirm the efficacy and safety of emerging endoscopic treatments. With the emergence of new technologies and therapeutic approaches, i.e., novel imaging techniques and minimally invasive surgery, their verification by large-scale clinical investigations becomes necessary. The data generated through such investigations not only guide clinical suggestions but also supply practitioners with the best practices in patient care within an ever-changing medical environment. Additionally, with the trend towards evidence-based practice, ongoing research will be pivotal in shaping the future of therapeutic endoscopy and aligning it with the highest standards of patient safety and treatment efficacy. Therefore, integration of clinical trials into routine practice is key to encouraging innovation and optimizing therapeutic outcomes in endoscopic procedures (Cinnor et al., 2017; Garcia et al., 2019) (Figure 11.18).

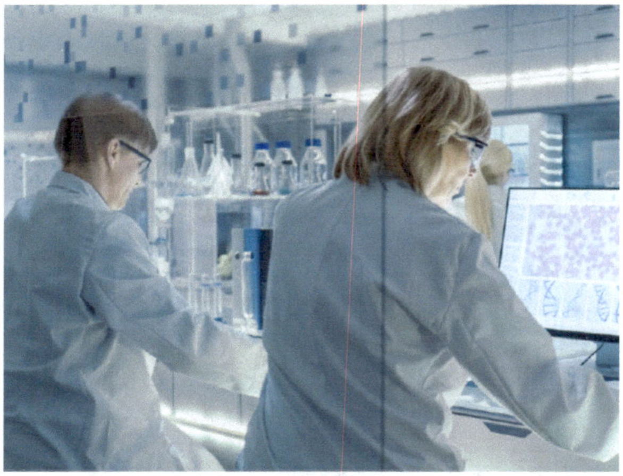

Figure 11.18. Research trends and clinical trials.

Source: https://clarkstonconsulting.com/wp-content/uploads/2023/12/2024-Clinical-Trials-Trends_FEATURED.png.

SUMMARY

In summarizing this analysis of therapeutic endoscopy, it is essential to acknowledge the strong implications that this treatment has for the treatment of gastrointestinal disease. As discussed in the essay, therapeutic endoscopy does not simply exist as a diagnostic tool but rather as a driving mechanism of effectiveness in treatment. The significance of endoscopic practice in treating conditions like ulcerative colitis and Crohn's Disease is increasingly becoming more prominent, highlighting the need for uniform assessment methods. For instance, various endoscopic scores have been developed to measure disease activity, but the absence of uniform validation reflects the existing challenges in clinical practice. A renewed focus on mucosal healing as a therapeutic strategy places additional importance on precise endoscopic evaluation. As research in the area continues to evolve, it is imperative that physicians adopt standardized scoring systems to ensure the best patient care and personalized treatment strategies (Corleto et al., 2016). Additionally, findings from nurse-implemented endoscopy provide a state-of-the-art model for the operational dynamics of gastrointestinal endoscopy. The evidence presented in the form of trained nurses being able to perform diagnostic endoscopy safely disrupts traditional hierarchies within clinical settings. Scores for patient satisfaction and quality of test both suggest that nurse-applied procedures are equal to, if not superior to, physician-performed procedures, making services more accessible and efficient in patient care. This endoscopic democratization not only creates an open model of healthcare but also inspires the inclusion of nursing expertise in therapeutic interventions. As healthcare systems adapt to address such transformations, the development of interdisciplinary collaborations will enable practitioners to deliver patient-centered care that maintains patient dignity and outcomes (Bloor et al., 2009). Lastly, the process to achieve optimal therapeutic endoscopy targets a multidisciplinary approach that integrates technological evolution, continuing education, and patient-centered care concepts. As the complexity of gastrointestinal disease increases to demand treatment protocols of various dimensions, the position of therapeutic endoscopy is going to be increasingly important. Additional research and development in this field need to target creating techniques that enhance procedure efficacy and patient satisfaction. Also, giving healthcare professionals the right tools and knowledge will not only improve therapeutic modalities but also make endoscopy a hub of modern gastrointestinal medicine. Last but not least, embracing these technologies and maximizing our techniques will keep therapeutic endoscopy on the vanguard of effective patient care (Bloor et al., 2009; Corleto et al., 2016).

In therapeutic endoscopy, recent studies have paid a lot of attention to the role of trained personnel to perform endoscopic interventions effectively. A large-scale trial in 23 hospitals across the United Kingdom compared the efficiency of physicians versus nurses in performing gastrointestinal endoscopies. The findings showed no substantial differences in clinical results between the two groups, with implications that nurses can successfully perform diagnostic endoscopies with similar safety and effectiveness as physicians. It is interesting to note that patients showed greater satisfaction rates when they were followed by nurses immediately after the procedure, whereas nurses showed a more extensive examination of the stomach and esophagus. This finding is notable in the way that it emphasizes the potential for expanding the role of nurses in therapeutic endoscopy, effectively improving patient care delivery in most clinical settings (Bloor et al., 2009). Therapeutic endoscopy's use goes beyond simple general diagnostics, especially in the management of inflammatory bowel diseases (IBD) , such as ulcerative colitis and Crohn's disease. The importance of endoscopic evaluation has been established, but the problem of adequate reporting of endoscopic activity remains. Several endoscopic scores have been proposed for this purpose, but are not yet well validated, and their use is chiefly limited to clinical trials. These situations illustrate a clear need for an interdisciplinary standardization of the measurement of endoscopic activity in IBD. With increased interest in mucosal healing as a treatment goal, a better definition and measurement of endoscopic activity are crucial. The overcoming of these hurdles will ensure therapeutic endoscopy continues to be an essential tool for the effective management of IBD (Corleto et al., 2016). Advances in therapeutic endoscopy demonstrate an expanded trend toward patient-centered and holistic management. Stringent evaluation of procedures, operator satisfaction, and therapeutic success is closely linked with patient outcomes. Since the health systems will strive to maximize quality control, evidence synthesis from comparison studies of operator performance—, such as the trial between physicians and nurses, is crucial. Similarly, with more focus on disease activity measurement in IBD, focus on stable endoscopic scoring systems must be high on the agenda. These advancements indicate not only the evolution of therapeutic endoscopy in procedural methods but also the broadening of its parameters to encompass a wider range of patient needs and outcomes. These are trends reflective of the dynamic nature of healthcare, where continuous improvement in methodologies guarantees therapeutic endoscopy is always one step ahead when it comes to efficient patient management (Bloor et al., 2009; Corleto et al., 2016).

CLOSER LOOK

AUTO FLUORESCENCE IMAGING (AFI):

Auto fluorescence imaging (AFI) is an advanced endoscopic technique that enhances the visualization of tissue abnormalities by exploiting the natural fluorescence properties of biological tissues. Certain cellular components, including collagen, elastin, and flavins, emit light when excited by specific wavelengths. AFI captures these signals to differentiate normal tissues from pathological changes, providing a non-invasive, real-time method to detect early lesions that may be difficult to identify under standard white-light endoscopy.

AFI is widely applied in gastroenterology, pulmonology, and otolaryngology. In the gastrointestinal tract, it is particularly valuable for detecting dysplasia, early-stage cancers, and precancerous lesions in organs such as the esophagus, stomach, and colon. Under AFI, healthy tissue typically emits a green fluorescence due to abundant collagen and elastin, whereas abnormal or neoplastic tissues appear magenta or purple due to altered fluorophore composition and structural changes. This color contrast allows clinicians to identify suspicious areas that may require biopsy or further intervention. The technique is often used in combination with conventional white-light endoscopy or other imaging modalities such as narrow-band imaging (NBI) and confocal laser endomicroscopy to improve diagnostic accuracy. AFI enhances sensitivity in detecting lesions, particularly flat or subtle abnormalities, although specificity can be lower due to false-positive signals from inflammation, scarring, or vascular changes. Therefore, AFI is generally considered a complementary tool rather than a standalone diagnostic method.

AFI has also been explored in pulmonary medicine for detecting early lung cancer and premalignant lesions during bronchoscopy. Similar principles apply: abnormal tissues demonstrate altered fluorescence patterns compared to normal bronchial mucosa. In otolaryngology, AFI aids in identifying head and neck tumors, helping surgeons delineate tumor margins more precisely during resection. Despite its advantages, AFI has limitations. Fluorescence signals can be affected by mucus, blood, or lighting conditions, and interpretation requires training and experience. Technological improvements, including optimized filters and real-time image processing, continue to enhance AFI performance.

In conclusion, auto fluorescence imaging represents a significant advancement in diagnostic endoscopy, offering a non-invasive, real-time method to detect early tissue changes. By highlighting subtle differences between normal and abnormal tissues, AFI supports early diagnosis, targeted biopsy, and improved treatment outcomes. Its integration with other imaging techniques continues to expand its clinical utility across multiple medical specialties.

REFERENCES

1. Tringali, A., Thomson, M., Dumonceau, J. M., Tavares, M., Tabbers, M. M., Furlano, R., Spaander, M., Hassan, C., Tzvinikos, C., Ijsselstijn, H., Viala, J., Dall'Oglio, L., Benninga, M., Orel, R., Vandenplas, Y., Keil, R., Romano, C., Brownstone, E., Hlava, Š., Gerner, P., ... Zambelli, A. (2017). Pediatric gastrointestinal endoscopy: European Society of Gastrointestinal Endoscopy (ESGE) and European Society for Paediatric Gastroenterology Hepatology and Nutrition (ESPGHAN) Guideline Executive summary. *Endoscopy*, *49*(1), 83–91. https://doi.org/10.1055/s-0042-111002(accessed on 15th July 2025).
2. Abdullah, M., Daldiyono, D., Fauzi, A., Makmun, D., et al. (2017). *National consensus on the use of sedation drugs in the gastrointestinal endoscopic procedures.* https://media.neliti.com/media/publications/238028-national-consensus-on-the-use-of-sedatio-8d053ad4.pdf (accessed on 15th July 2025).
3. Ahmad, O. F., Stassen, P., & Webster, G. J. (2021). *Artificial intelligence in biliopancreatic endoscopy: Is there any role?* https://core.ac.uk/download/384445568.pdf (accessed on 15th July 2025).
4. Wizenty J, Schumann T, Theil D, Stockmann M, Pratschke J, Tacke F, Aigner F, Wuensch T. Recent Advances and the Potential for Clinical Use of Autofluorescence Detection of Extra-Ophthalmic Tissues. Molecules. 2020; 25(9):2095. https://doi.org/10.3390/molecules25092095 (accessed on 15th July 2025).
5. Albéniz-Arbizu, E., Cabrera Chamorro, C., Caro, L., Carvalho, R., De Groot, N. L., Fry, L. C., Hagel, A. F., et al. (2016). *Performance measures for upper gastrointestinal endoscopy: A European Society of Gastrointestinal Endoscopy (ESGE) quality improvement initiative.* https://core.ac.uk/download/228145464.pdf (accessed on 15th July 2025).
6. Hausmann J, Albert JG (2011) Detecting and Managing Small Bowel Crohn's Disease – Capsule Endoscopy Becoming a First Line Diagnostic Method? J Gastroint Dig Syst S1:002. doi:10.4172/2161-069X.S1-002(accessed on 15th July 2025).
7. Albert, J. G., Bechstein, W. O., Friedrich-Rust, M., Sarrazin, C., et al. (2013). *SEMS vs cSEMS in duodenal and small bowel obstruction: High risk of migration in the covered stent group.* https://core.ac.uk/download/18137371.pdf (accessed on 15th July 2025).
8. M. Turan et al., "Unsupervised Odometry and Depth Learning for Endoscopic Capsule Robots," 2018 IEEE/RSJ International Conference on Intelligent Robots and Systems (IROS), Madrid, Spain, 2018, pp. 1801-1807, doi: 10.1109/IROS.2018.8593623.(accessed on 15th July 2025).
9. Alomair, O. A. (2024). *New trends in management of vascular lower GI bleeding between endoscopy and angiography: Literature review.* https://core.ac.uk/download/640070005.pdf (accessed on 15th July 2025).
10. Andrade, L. C. B. A., Costa, I. D. S., Filho, F. S. M., Filho, R. R. M., et al. (2025). *Technological advances and the evolution of endoscopic procedures in the treatment of upper urinary tract tumors: Clinical impact and future perspectives.* https://core.ac.uk/download/654540037.pdf (accessed on 15th July 2025).
11. Annibale, B., Carabotti, M., Corleto, V. D., DI GIULIO, E., et al. (2019). *Occurrence of acute oesophageal necrosis (black oesophagus) in a single tertiary center.* https://core.ac.uk/download/231749434.pdf (accessed on 15th July 2025).

12. Antonucci, E., Arezzo, A., Caruso, A., Conigliaro, R., et al. (2016). *Over-the-scope clips in the treatment of gastrointestinal tract iatrogenic perforation: A multicenter retrospective study and a classification of gastrointestinal tract perforations.* https://core.ac.uk/download/pdf/154857220.pdf (accessed on 15th July 2025).

13. Ciuti, G., Caliò, R., Camboni, D., Neri, L., Bianchi, F., Arezzo, A., Koulaouzidis, A., Schostek, S., Stoyanov, D., Oddo, C. M., Magnani, B., Menciassi, A., Morino, M., Schurr, M. O., & Dario, P. (2016). Frontiers of robotic endoscopic capsules: a review. *Journal of micro-bio robotics, 11*(1), 1–18. https://doi.org/10.1007/s12213-016-0087-x(accessed on 15th July 2025).

14. Atimati, A. O., Ewah-Odiase, R. O., & Irowa, O. O. (2022). *Pediatric gastrointestinal endoscopy in a Nigerian tertiary hospital.* https://core.ac.uk/download/552647883.pdf (accessed on 15th July 2025).

15. Azab, M., Bharadwaj, S., Hong, A. S., Jayaraj, M., et al. (2019). *Safety of endoscopic retrograde cholangiopancreatography (ERCP) in pregnancy: A systematic review and meta-analysis.* https://core.ac.uk/download/286611719.pdf (accessed on 15th July 2025).

16. Azi, C. I., Carsrud, N. D. V., DelGiodice, M. J., Egli, D., et al. (2024). *The multisystem impact of pseudoxanthoma elasticum (PXE): Systemic manifestations, multidisciplinary management, and diagnostic and* therapeutic advances. https://core.ac.uk/download/621451766.pdf (accessed on 15th July 2025).

17. Banu, P., Constantin, V. D., Nistor, M. F., Popa, I., et al. (2016). Perforated small intestine in a patient with T-cell lymphoma: A rare cause of peritonitis. https://core.ac.uk/download/144552420.pdf (accessed on 15th July 2025).

18. Beekley, A., Davis, K. A., Johnson, D. C., Lim, J., et al. (2018). Early and late complications of bariatric operation. https://core.ac.uk/download/213444927.pdf (accessed on 15th July 2025).

19. DA, Lord & Bell, Geoffrey & A, Gray & A, Quine & J, Bowles & A, Reynolds. (2006). Sedation for Gastrointestinal Endoscopic Procedures in the Elderly: Getting Safer but Still Not Nearly Safe Enough. Br Soc Gastroenterol. (accessed on 15th July 2025).

20. Bijnen, A. B., van Rijn, A. F., Briggs, A. H., Depla, A. C. T. M., Mentges, B., Weusten, B. L. A. M., Cocilovo, C., et al. (2009). Transanal endoscopic microsurgery versus endoscopic mucosal resection for large rectal adenomas (TREND-study). https://core.ac.uk/download/19187030.pdf (accessed on 15th July 2025).

21. Bloor, K., Cheung, W. Y., Coulton, S., Durai, R., et al. (2009). Effectiveness of nurse delivered endoscopy: Findings from randomized multi-institution nurse endoscopy trial (MINuET). https://core.ac.uk/download/50820.pdf (accessed on 15th July 2025).

22. Böbel, Ingo & Martis, Amrita, 2009. "Value Creation in Health Care: The Case of the Princesse Grace Hospital (CHPG) Monaco," MPRA Paper 19689, University Library of Munich, Germany. (accessed on 15th July 2025).

23. van der Stap, N., van der Heijden, F., & Broeders, I. A. (2013). Towards automated visual flexible endoscope navigation. Surgical endoscopy, 27(10), 3539–3547. https://doi.org/10.1007/s00464-013-3003-7(accessed on 15th July 2025).

24. Meng, Q. T., Cao, C., Liu, H. M., Xia, Z. Y., Li, W., Tang, L. H., Chen, R., Jiang, M., Wu, Y., Leng, Y., & Lee, C. C. (2016). Safety and efficacy of etomidate and propofol anesthesia in elderly patients undergoing gastroscopy: A double-blind randomized clinical study. *Experimental and*

therapeutic medicine, 12(3), 1515–1524. https://doi.org/10.3892/etm.2016.3475 (accessed on 15th July 2025).

25. Chang, H. W., Ko, P. J., Liu, H. P., Liu, Y. C., et al. (2011). *Natural orifice transluminal endoscopic surgery: A transtracheal approach for the thoracic cavity in a live canine model.* https://core.ac.uk/download/pdf/82556624.pdf (accessed on 15th July 2025).
26. Chang, W. H., & Lei, W. Y. (2007). *Endoscopic retrograde cholangiopancreatography in elderly patients.* https://core.ac.uk/download/pdf/82371991.pdf (accessed on 15th July 2025).
27. Cinnor, B., Das, A., Early, D. S., Edmundowicz, S., et al. (2017). *Recurrence of intestinal metaplasia and early neoplasia after endoscopic eradication therapy for Barrett's esophagus: A systematic review and meta-analysis.* https://core.ac.uk/download/129069578.pdf (accessed on 15th July 2025).
28. Ciorbagiu, M. C., Mirea, C. S., Moraru, E., Obleaga, A., et al. (2016). *Helicobacter pylori: Types of diseases, diagnosis, treatment and causes of therapeutic failure.* https://core.ac.uk/download/144552985.pdf (accessed on 15th July 2025).
29. Corleto, V. D., Delle Fave, G., Desideri, F., DI GIULIO, E., et al. (2016). *Endoscopic scores for inflammatory bowel disease in the era of 'mucosal healing': Old problem, new perspectives.* https://core.ac.uk/download/74319420.pdf (accessed on 15th July 2025).
30. Deesomsak, M., Aswakul, P., Leelakusolvong, S., & Prachayakul, V. (2013). *The utility of single-balloon enteroscopy for the diagnosis and management of small bowel disorders according to their clinical manifestations: A retrospective review.* https://core.ac.uk/download/pdf/81725137.pdf (accessed on 15th July 2025).
31. Eke, C. B. (2021). *Advances in gastrointestinal endoscopy: Shaping diagnosis and therapy of gastrointestinal disorders in children.* https://core.ac.uk/download/478304720.pdf (accessed on 15th July 2025).
32. Frang, D., Jako, G. J., & Repassy, D. L. (2011). *Minimal and Direct Access Surgery in Urology.* https://core.ac.uk/download/142040468.pdf (accessed on 15th July 2025).
33. Fu, C. Y., Lau, W. K. O., Olivo, M., Raghavan, S., et al. (2011). *New frontier in hypericin-mediated diagnosis of cancer with current optical technologies.* https://core.ac.uk/download/pdf/8683640.pdf (accessed on 15th July 2025).
34. Garcia, J., Gross, S. A., Lahr, R., Rex, D. K., et al. (2019). *Endocuff Vision reduces inspection time without decreasing lesion detection in a randomized colonoscopy trial.* https://core.ac.uk/download/187423803.pdf (accessed on 15th July 2025).
35. Kazimierczak, K. A., & Skea, Z. C. (2015). *"I've used the word cancer but it's actually good news": Discursive performativity of cancer and the identity of urological cancer services.* https://core.ac.uk/download/42130404.pdf (accessed on 15th July 2025).
36. Alali, A. A., & Barkun, A. N. (2023). An update on the management of non-variceal upper gastrointestinal bleeding. *Gastroenterology report, 11*, goad011. https://doi.org/10.1093/gastro/goad011(accessed on 15th July 2025).
37. Slawinski, P. R., Obstein, K. L., & Valdastri, P. (2015). Capsule endoscopy of the future: What's on the horizon?. *World journal of gastroenterology, 21*(37), 10528–10541. https://doi.org/10.3748/wjg.v21.i37.10528 (accessed on 15th July 2025).

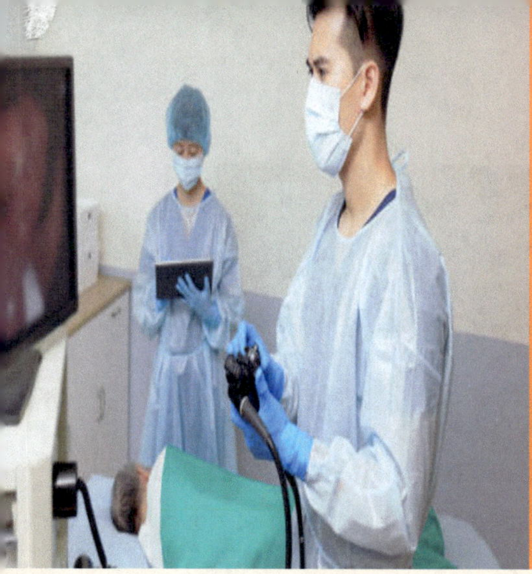

Chapter 12

ADVANCED IMAGING IN ENDOSCOPY

Contents

Introduction....341
12.1. Historical Background of Endoscopy....345
12.2. Types of Advanced Imaging Techniques....348
12.3. Benefits of Advanced Imaging in Endoscopy....352
12.4. Applications of Advanced Imaging in Various Medical Fields....355
12.5. Challenges and Limitations....359
12.6. Future Trends in Endoscopic Imaging....362
Summary....367
References....370

Introduction

Endoscopy has experienced tremendous development over the last decades, and imaging procedures have played a pivotal role in broadening the role of minimally invasive procedures. Advanced imaging methods are used comprehensively, enabling high-definition visualization of anatomical structures, which is indispensable in precise diagnostics and therapeutic interventions. The integration of advanced technology, such as optical imaging and three-dimensional reconstruction, has allowed clinicians to gain better anatomical relationships and pathology insights intra-operatively during endoscopic procedures. This technology has been of particular significance in the delineation of soft tissue morphology, an important consideration for passage through complicated areas of anatomy and improving surgical success. The recent developments in this area suggest revolutionary possibilities for endoscopy, and thus the requirement for further studies and clinical application of these new imaging modalities. Furthermore, the introduction of optical reconstruction methods into endoscopy overcomes some of the inherent limitations of traditional imaging modalities. Not only do they enhance visualization, but they also permit dynamic assessment of soft tissue anatomy during surgery. As recognized in contemporary debate, the move toward minimizing invasiveness in surgical intervention underscores the importance of accurate intraoperative imaging techniques. For instance, computer-assisted surgical systems are designed to enhance a surgeon's navigational ability and thus overcoming technical hurdles of real-time soft-tissue morphology assessment during interventions is crucial. Through the promise of optical imaging, health care professionals can view beyond tissue surfaces, thus improving surgery and ensuring better patient care. The ensuing exploration of such potential is offered, and it creates a powerful story that illustrates the integration of medicine and technology. As the thrilling advances in imaging technologies march on, issues remain, particularly with the design and operation of endoscopes themselves. Historically, the fundamental design of flexible endoscopes has not been extensively altered, and this is a limitation to their application for high-level therapeutic procedures. This standstill has necessitated researchers to evaluate the navigation systems employed in these devices. Automation of endoscope navigation is a potential solution that will enhance usability and procedural efficiency. Research has shown that image-based navigation systems, more and more reliant on visual information, are a good area through which endoscope maneuverability can be improved. The new field of automated systems holds immense promise in breaking through cost and applicability challenges, which ultimately leads the way towards creating solid algorithms required for real-time steering. All these new technologies provide an opportunity to revolutionize endoscopic practice and bridge the gaps in current systems, giving priority to more research on advanced imaging in endoscopy (Figure 12.1).

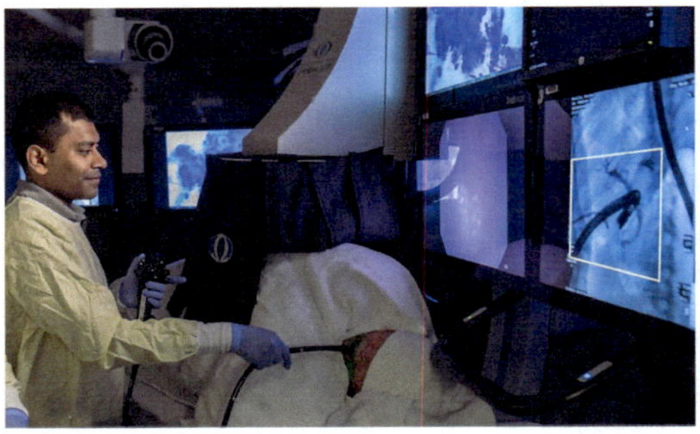

Figure 12.1. Advanced imaging in endoscopy.

Source: https://www.omegamedicalimaging.com/wp-content/uploads/2021/10/Advanced-Endoscopy-1280x772.jpg.

Definition of Endoscopy

Endoscopy is a sophisticated diagnostic as well as therapeutic method that provides direct visual inspection of the body's internal structures through natural openings. It employs a slender, flexible tube known as an endoscope, which is fitted with a camera and light, to transfer high-definition images onto outside monitors. It's a minimally invasive process that makes it possible for both the treatment and diagnosis of numerous gastrointestinal conditions, enabling medical personnel to see organs , including the esophagus, stomach, and colon. The development of endoscopes technologically, from basic fiber optics to current video endoscopes, has significantly enhanced image resolution, allowing practitioners to observe mucosal surfaces and lesions clearly. As such, the definition of endoscopy not only identifies the procedural dynamics but also stipulates the groundbreaking impact that endoscopy has had in patient management in gastroenterology and common medicine and thus highlights its relevance in today's healthcare practice. Technological advances in imaging have further increased the potential of endoscopy, allowing for greater diagnostic yield and intervention. High-definition and optical chromoendoscopy are two modalities that are especially important developments, allowing endoscopists to see early mucosal alterations that would otherwise go unnoticed. These technologies utilize sophisticated light manipulation and image processing to improve visualization, thus making endoscopic interventions more effective. The efficacy of endoscopic treatments can also be significantly improved by web-based training materials to boost the proficiency of practitioners, which has been underscored in recent literature. Through extending the boundaries of lesion detection and characterization with such cutting-edge techniques, the significance of endoscopy is constantly evolving, affirming its very important role in guaranteeing high levels of safety for the patient and clinical outcomes in various medical settings (van der Sommen et al., 2018).

In addition to improving diagnostic performance, endoscopy provides an entry point to various therapeutic procedures that further treat patients. Techniques , such as submucosal dissection and endoscopic mucosal resection highlight the dual role of endoscopy as not only a diagnostic but also a therapeutic intervention. Such advanced procedures, facilitated by newer imaging technology and equipment, are now standard in the treatment of conditions , such as early cancers or complex polyps, directly reducing the need for their more invasive surgical equivalents. Moreover, computer-aided detection has emerged as a vital ancillary tool in the interpretation of the vast visual data generated during endoscopic examination, providing endoscopists with real-time, unbiased second opinions to minimize observer variability. Through the incorporation of advanced imaging technologies into routine endoscopy, the application of this diagnostic modality is being extended ever further, reasserting its position in the advancement of patient-centered care and clinical outcomes in surgical practice (Alam & Matava, 2022).

Role of Imaging in Endoscopic Procedures

The role of imaging in endoscopic surgery has evolved a great deal, enhancing the accuracy and efficiency of minimally invasive surgery. New techniques of imaging allow for real-time visualization of internal structures, which is extremely critical for navigating complex anatomical regions. For example, the use of three-dimensional imaging provides the surgeon with an unrivaled perspective, enabling them to assess morphological changes in soft tissues and perform delicate manipulations. This shift toward better visualization not only decreases the likelihood of complications but also supports well-equipped decision-making during the process of surgery. The seamless interfacing of imaging technology with endoscopic equipment gives a natural and efficient surgical process, minimizing the risk of ergonomic problems commonly associated with traditional methods, as reiterated by more recent studies underlining the effectiveness of mechanized systems in the ergonomic aspect of surgical practice (Bauwens et al., 2020). The integration of sophisticated imaging modalities in endoscopic procedures also puts surgeons in a position to take advantage of computer-assisted surgery (CAS) technologies. These technologies are especially useful in coping with the unpredictable morphological dynamics of soft tissues in the operating field. Advanced imaging systems allow surgeons to have detailed real-time information on tissue structure and motion, improve navigational functions, and provide more information than surface observation alone. The significance of this innovation cannot be overemphasized, since the accomplishment of successful advancement through deformable and dynamic anatomical zones is crucial for successful results in surgery. While new optical techniques for *in vivo* three-dimensional reconstruction are in development, their potential for clinical use in laparoscopic surgery holds promising prospects for the integration of sophisticated technologies into practice (Maier-Hein et al., 2013). Furthermore, the use of advanced imaging within endoscopy is not only a technology update but also a groundbreaking way to treat patients. Enhanced imaging results in more accurate diagnoses, fewer procedure complications, and ultimately faster recovery rates for patients. As more surgeons migrate toward the current trend of minimally invasive surgical procedures, imaging becomes even more paramount. The convenience and efficiency resulting from technological advancements in imaging functionality also make it achievable to improve training and skill development for would-be surgeons. Witnessed with recent technology, the synergy between human proficiency and technological innovation in the field of endoscopic imaging lies at the nucleus of improved surgical accuracy and safety for patients, representing a more holistic advance in medical science (Figure 12.2).

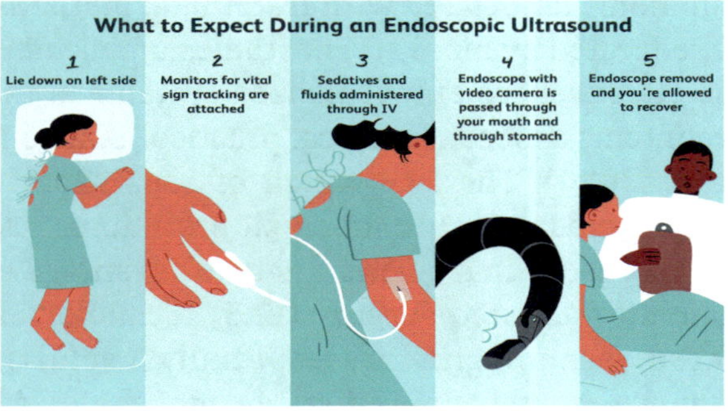

Figure 12.2. Importance of imaging in endoscopic procedures.

Source: https://www.verywellhealth.com/thmb/JZcTuFZZKgn6BEkSf_zIsh_Zok4=/6000x4000/filters:no_upscale():max_bytes(150000):strip_icc()/endoscopic-ultrasound-uses-side-effects-procedure-results-4176265_color1-5c05a05e46e0fb00010588a2.png.

Overview of Advancements in Imaging Technology

Imaging technology in endoscopy has witnessed significant developments that greatly enhance diagnostic accuracy and procedural efficacy. One outstanding development is the availability of actively steerable capsule endoscopes, which make basic passive devices into active robots that can talk to the gastrointestinal tract with precision. The capability allows for more natural disease detection as well as targeted interventions compared to conventional methods. Multi-view pose estimation and single-view depth estimation networks have been integrated into these devices, resulting in real-time motion estimation and depth recovery that greatly enhances the endoscopic experience for both clinicians and patients. The development is a paradigm shift that not only improves visualization but also facilitates the possibility of more advanced therapeutic interventions within the minimally invasive setting (Turan et al., 2018). Yet another vital innovation in imaging technology is the inclusion of 3D imaging capabilities in endoscopic procedures. The technology has been instrumental in enhancing the visual perception of the surgeons, particularly in complicated anatomical regions. Evidence supports the fact that the addition of 3D imaging devices to endoscopic systems can surpass the discomfort traditionally associated with minimally invasive operations. Notably, a new one-handed operated endoscope positioner instrument has been developed, where the endoscope is effectively controlled by the surgeon without cumbersome assembly. This has contributed significantly to the reduction of setup time as well as total surgical time, thereby boosting the efficiency of the procedure and comfort for healthcare practitioners (Bauwens et al., 2020). This synergistic approach not only optimizes the control of the operator but also optimizes the outcomes of the patient, emphasizing the effectiveness of a pairing of advanced imaging technology in surgery. The future of endoscopy imaging technology will be revolutionized with further innovations, particularly in the domain of artificial intelligence and machine learning. These technologies aim to optimize the precision of image analysis and automate several phases of the endoscopic procedure. For instance, advanced algorithms can rapidly process real-time imaging data to identify abnormalities so that on-the-fly decision-making can be made during interventions. As these technologies improve, they may release diagnostic pressure from clinicians while advancing the speed and accuracy of patient care. Moreover, advancing the imaging modalities may soon allow for real-time multimodal imaging data fusion that provides whole-gastrointestinal views of health. These developments point to a drug of sorts, with the excitement and potential of new imaging in endoscopy, for a transformative impact on medical practice and patient management (Figure 12.3).

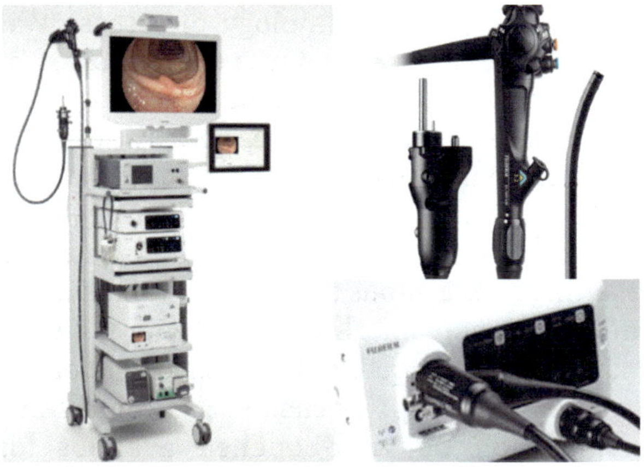

Figure 12.3. Overview of advancements in imaging technology in endoscopy.

Source: https://envisionnext.net/wp-content/uploads/2023/09/2-1024x660.png.

12.1. Historical Background of Endoscopy

Endoscopy has developed to a great extent in medical treatment and diagnosis, evolving from crude observation techniques. Early physicians used primitive instruments to offer a restricted vision of internal situations. The progression started in the 19th century when a German physician came up with the first gastric endoscope, marking a new direction in internal examination. These early devices took advantage of light and mirrors to enhance visibility. The first major endoscopy breakthrough was in 1868 with the creation of the flexible endoscope, allowing for the more flexible inspection of human anatomy. This invention paved the way for centuries of refinement, inspiring research into methods of internal visualization that have stood the test of time, evolving to meet the demands of increasingly complex and advanced medical procedures. With the advent of the 20th century, endoscopy significantly developed with the integration of advanced technologies, thus revolutionizing its use in clinical practice. The development of fiber optic technology during the 1950s transformed endoscopy by offering more illumination and enhanced visualization of inner surfaces. With this change, less invasive and safer procedures were created, and these eventually paved the way for colonoscopy and gastroscopy to become routine diagnostic procedures. Soon, researchers realized the use of endoscopy not only as a diagnostic device but also as a therapeutic agent, such as to perform polypectomies and biopsies. Realization of endoscopys' role in both diagnosis and treatment made the realization of ongoing research towards imaging technologies inevitable. Up to now, endoscopy remains at the center of gastroenterology, combining clinical practice with technological progress as illustrated in research into the crucial role of polypectomy for the avoidance of colorectal cancer (Kaltenbach et al., 2020). The next several decades saw an era of fineness and specialization of endoscopic technique, driven by technology as well as by clinical outcomes. Prolonged development in imaging modalities, such as high-definition cameras and narrow-band imaging, has enhanced accuracy in identifying and characterizing lesions. These features are critical in enhancing patient outcomes, particularly in colorectal cancer surveillance through studies that underscore the role of efficient techniques in polypectomy (Kaltenbach et al., 2020). Additionally, integration of advanced imaging systems has enhanced gastrointestinal pathophysiology knowledge and optimized procedural safety. As technology and equipment evolve, endoscopy's historical context emphasizes its remarkable evolution from rudimentary methods to an advanced discipline that not only aids diagnosis but also shapes therapeutic planning, testament to an ethos of furthering patient care through ongoing innovation.

12.1.1. Early Techniques and Limitations

The technique of endoscopy has also changed significantly since its introduction, with the initial techniques having significant shortcomings that influenced therapeutic and diagnostic outcomes. Endoscopy initially predominantly employed rigid tools, with restricted access and movement within the gastrointestinal tract. Early devices had poor visualization, with the utilization of ambient light sources that were insufficient for complete examination. Therefore, these types of complications like perforation were not uncommon, and precise diagnosis of states was severely compromised. Early attempts at improving the quality of images often proved ineffectual; whereas some advances, like the implementation of general lighting systems, improved structures more, overall resolutions remained too low. Thus, clinicians faced a twofold dilemma of patient safety and the achievement of consistent diagnostic results, which led them to hesitate in employing endoscopic techniques for complex cases, particularly when there was a strong suspicion of serious pathology (Northup et al., 2020). Furthermore, technical shortcomings of initial endoscopic devices hindered their widespread use in clinical applications. The lack of flexible instruments closely restricted the range of procedures that could be performed by endoscopists, particularly in organs like the esophagus and colon, where anatomy and bending cause problems. Early endoscopes, combined with extremely limited vision methods, created issues with the accurate locating of lesions, particularly in the early stages of malignancy. Without advanced imaging modalities to distinguish between minor differences in tissue types, misdiagnosis was the rule. In addition, the interchangeability of early equipment with new diagnostic techniques, such as biopsy devices, was generally not acceptable. As a result, procedures intended to obtain tissue samples were hazardous, undermining the overall reliability of endoscopic procedures at the time (Keswani et al., 2020). For conditions of the gastrointestinal system, constraints in early techniques underscored the necessity for new imaging and instrumentation innovations. As the pathology of disease was better understood, so too was the necessity for more sophisticated endoscopic tools that would offer greater safety and efficacy. This necessity spawned an investigation into the development of new technologies, such as flexible video endoscopes and digital imaging technologies, resulting in enormous advances in visualization and patient outcome. Lastly, limitations of early endoscopic techniques not only shed light on the need for better approaches in gastrointestinal examination but also opened avenues for revolutionary changes in endoscopic practice, thus leading to the advanced imaging modalities employed today (Northup et al., 2020).

12.1.2. Development of Fiber-Optic Technology

The development of fiber-optic technology has been the hub of revolution in endoscopic imaging techniques, significantly enhancing diagnostic precision and procedural efficacy. Traditional endoscopes, where the application of rigid metal tubes limited anatomical intricacy for maneuverability, therefore limited sight for use in adequate diagnosis. The advent of flexible fiber-optic endoscopes allowed for convenient access to areas of concern. Technology has been marked by a significant advancement in light transmission, achieving slimmer and sharper images of inner tissues. Incorporation of multifiber bundles has enabled the transmission of both light and image information at the same time, which has completely changed surveillance and therapeutic use in clinical settings. Apart from this, breakthroughs in fiber-optic technology involve combining advanced imaging modalities , such as autofluorescence and Brillouin spectroscopy, for improving the diagnostic quality of endoscopic investigations. Autofluorescence imaging, for example, utilizes particular wavelengths of excitation to bring out the distinctive fluorescence patterns offered by different tissues. A clinical analysis of endoscopic biopsy samples from the colon revealed striking autofluorescence lifetime contrasts in neoplastic and normal tissues, highlighting the potential of the technique to differentiate malignancies (Chorvat et al., 2013). This enhanced imaging capability not only facilitates early detection of neoplastic changes but also justifies decision-making processes during interventions. Later advancements introduced the incorporation of fiber-based devices to enable non-contact and label-free measurements of tissue properties. Brillouin spectroscopy, in its non-destructive approach, shows how optical sciences converge to assist medical diagnostics. Its application to the development of a miniature fiber-optic Brillouin probe for spatially mapping mechanical properties shows the versatility of fiber technology in clinical applications (Basirun et al., 2020). The potential for revolution in the extent to which one can measure disease conditions in real time is significant and may change therapeutic strategies through greater insights into tissue mechanics. Cumulatively, these developments illustrate the preeminence of fiber-optic technology in modern endoscopic imaging and its central role in the ongoing quest for improved patient outcomes (Figure 12.4).

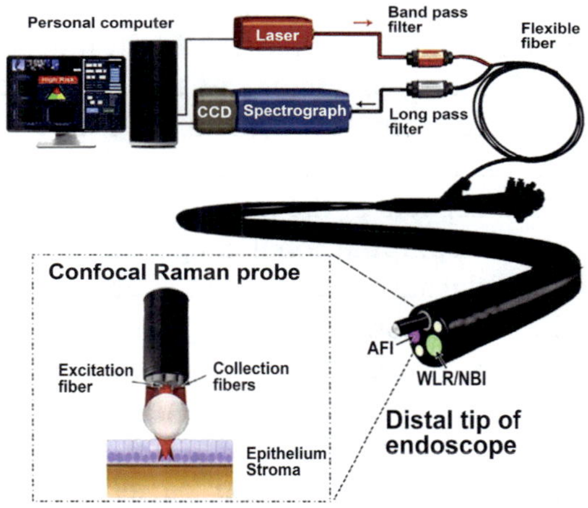

Figure 12.4. Development of fiber-optic technology.

Source: https://onlinelibrary.wiley.com/cms/asset/c7b3f939-c2a1-4f9a-82a1-af60b4e65291/tbio202000018-fig-0001-m.jpg.

12.1.3. Milestones in Imaging Advancements

Throughout the evolution of endoscopic technology, some remarkable milestones in imaging advances have immensely enhanced the detection and identification of gastrointestinal lesions. One of these milestones has been the development of hyperspectral imaging (HSI), which offers a dramatic improvement over traditional optical methods. Traditional endoscopy exploits white light excitation and RGB detectors, which limit the distinction between flat and small neoplastic lesions and the surrounding mucosa. HSI addresses this challenge by imaging a wide band of wavelengths, creating a high-dimensional hypercube that leads to large contrast enhancement of subtle tissue contrasts. This technology is critical, most notably in the detection of early colorectal neoplasia, where lesions are typically less than 10 mm and potentially could be missed. The addition of HSI to endoscopy demonstrates a quantum leap in diagnostic capability with the potential to lead to improved patient outcomes by enabling earlier intervention in patients with colorectal cancer. Another important milestone has been the development of next-generation imaging technologies, which have not only focused on image resolution but also on the functional aspects of the imaging process itself. Advances in computational imaging and the use of multimodal strategies have revolutionized the future of diagnostic endoscopy. An example is the most recent technologies, namely optical coherence tomography (OCT) and narrowband imaging (NBI), both of which aim at maximizing the identification of vascular patterns as well as microstructural changes in tissues.

These technologies are a reaction to having improved optical diagnostics, particularly in addressing complex cases where lesions are not easily visible. By combining sophisticated imaging algorithms with sophisticated illumination sources, these technologies enable clinicians to make more comprehensive and detailed assessments of tissue properties and thus assist clinicians in making improved clinical choices. Further, educational initiatives closely related to these technological advances have encouraged increased interdisciplinarity interaction, further advancing the frontiers of endoscopic imaging. Curricula aimed at infusing biomedical physical principles with clinical practice emphasize the critical need for educating the next generation of healthcare providers in a high-level understanding of these technologies. For instance, infusing hands-on training and research experience within academic environments enables students to work actively with state-of-the-art imaging technologies, enabling them to face challenges in medical practice. As noted, the collaboration between clinical scientists and physicists not only promotes future technology but also supports the function of pushing the boundaries of traditional endoscopic procedures to sophisticated diagnostics and therapeutic methods. Imaging milestones, thus, reflect a blend of technological innovation and commitment to education that informs the future of endoscopic therapy (Ness et al., 2012; Browning, 2022) (Figure 12.5).

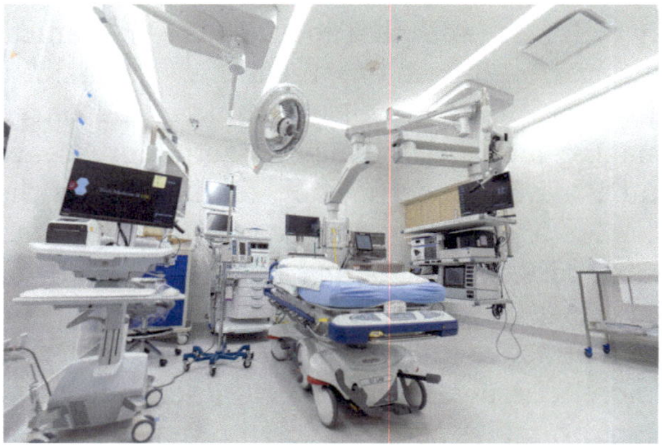

Figure 12.5. Milestones in imaging advancements.

Source: https://www.keckmedicine.org/wp-content/uploads/2023/05/2022.08.12_-Endoscopy-Clinic-Dress-Rehearsal_002-1024x683.jpg.

12.2. Types of Advanced Imaging Techniques

The technology of endoscopic imaging has been greatly improved with developments in technology, allowing for the production of various advanced imaging techniques. Of them, HSI has emerged as a strong modality enhancing the visualization of tissues on endoscopy. HSI employs a technique that captures images at various wavelengths, providing a complete spectral profile of the scanned area. This multi-dimensional approach facilitates enhanced discrimination between malignant and benign tissues. Another recent study encouraged the use of hyperspectral data integrated with machine learning algorithms to improve the accuracy of endoscopy diagnosis. Specifically, the study demonstrated that integration of deep learning architectures with hyperspectral datacubes was able to achieve up to 90% classification accuracy, thus paving the way for more precise and efficient diagnostics in real-world applications (Zhang et al., 2024). These innovations lead the way towards further advanced imaging technologies that have tremendous potential to enhance patient outcomes. Yet another advanced technology in advanced imaging is chromoendoscopy, which increases mucosal visualization and detection of neoplastic lesions with the application of contrast agents during endoscopy. Utilizing specific dyes that stain abnormal tissue selectively, chromoendoscopy allows for closer examination of the gastrointestinal tract. This technique significantly increases the visualization of precancerous lesions, such as adenomatous polyps, which can be excised early in case they are identified to prevent development towards cancer. The effectiveness of chromoendoscopy is further enhanced with the help of NBI, in addition to it, which employs chosen wavelengths of light to enhance the visibility contrast of cancer and normal tissues. Together, these methodologies have revolutionized gastrointestinal procedures by refining early intervention strategies with dramatic improvements in survival rates of gastrointestinal neoplasm patients (Nijjar et al., 2024). As the integration of these imaging modalities evolves further, they hold promise for improved diagnostic capability in endoscopic procedures. Finally, the incorporation of artificial intelligence (AI) into endoscopy has introduced revolutionary strides in diagnostic efficacy and accuracy. AI systems, particularly those that incorporate deep learning algorithms, can be capable of sifting through enormous data generated in the course of endoscopic examinations, finding patterns and abnormalities that could be imperceptible to the naked eye. This capability not only upgrades the diagnostic expertise of the endoscopists but also streamlines the decision-making process for subsequent therapeutic interventions. As AI technologies continue evolving, they are also likely to enhance the accuracy of histological predictions and aid in classifying lesions more accurately. However, the application of AI in the clinical environment is not without challenges, as data standardization, training requirements, and workflow integration are some of the issues that must be addressed (Nijjar et al., 2024). Yet, the potential of the impact of AI on high-tech imaging in endoscopy foretell well for better care and outcomes for patients and present an area of focus for future investigation and development.

12.2.1. High-Definition Endoscopy

High-definition endoscopy has been a revolution in gastrointestinal imaging, significantly enhancing diagnostic capability and therapeutic intervention. This technology enhances the quality of images by increasing resolution, leading to a clearer visualization of mucosal layers and structures. Such quality imaging is particularly crucial in inflammatory bowel diseases (IBDs), where accurate identification of mucosal inflammation is essential for proper management and monitoring. High-definition capability enables clinicians to identify minute dysplasia and lesions that could otherwise have gone unnoticed with conventional endoscopic techniques. In addition, the integration of high-definition endoscopy with molecular imaging techniques has broadened its field of use to enable clinicians not only to diagnose but also to evaluate the treatment response in patients, thereby having a positive impact on clinical outcomes (Tontini et al., 2016). The integration of advanced imaging techniques, such as high-definition endoscopy, has enormously enhanced cellular pathology and morphology visualization. With the greater demand for precise assessment of the gastrointestinal tract, high-definition systems enable the close observation necessary to properly grade such conditions as ulcerative colitis and Crohn's disease. They provide an improved perception of mucosal healing, which correlates directly with the ability to predict long-term outcome in the patient with IBD. High-definition endoscopy enables better assessment of mucosal integrity and overall disease activity for clinicians. Apart from that, their application enables a greater understanding of the disease processes and, ultimately, targeted therapeutic treatments (Tontini et al., 2016). Apart from high-definition endoscopy, autofluorescence imaging (AFI) represents an emerging field in advanced endoscopic technology. Originally based on ophthalmology, AFI is being re-engineered in most fields of medicine, providing promising potential for real-time non-invasive tissue characterization. The autofluorescence characteristics of native biomolecules give clinicians the power to visualize tissue content without the need for exogenous contrast agents. Because of the increasing use of AFI in dermatology and surgery, its possible utility in malignancy identification and discrimination between healthy and diseased tissue is becoming a reality. This paradigm change points to the importance of ongoing research and standardization in the specialty to facilitate maximum clinical benefits, as seen by new studies on AF techniques (Figure 12.6).

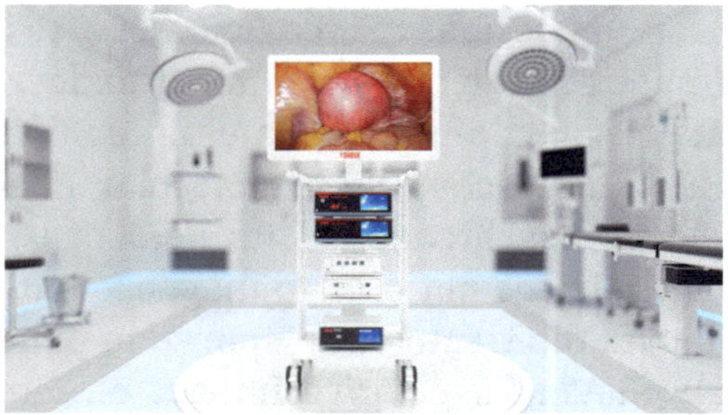

Figure 12.6. High-definition endoscopy.

Source: https://external-content.duckduckgo.com/iu/?u=https%3A%2F%2Flookaside.fbsbx.com%2Flookaside%2Fcrawler%2Fmedia%2F%3Fmedia_id%3D557634253133718%26get_thumbnail%3D1&f=1&nofb=1&ipt=380b3b0c9f12a495cc59e4f15453dd802d37afe42fcc2ab7f6ebf6fdcbe68a73.

12.2.2. Narrow-Band Imaging (NBI)

The advent of NBI has significantly changed the practice of endoscopic procedures, particularly early detection and assessment of gastrointestinal lesions. The NBI technology utilizes specific wavelengths of light to improve visualization of mucosal patterns and vascular architecture not visible by WLE. The imaging modality creates enhanced contrast between the normal tissue and the diseased tissue, which simplifies the premalignant conditions for diagnosis. Enhanced visualization helps practitioners make more informed decisions on biopsy and treatment modalities, which is critical in the appropriate patient management of endoscopic clinics. The ability of NBI to improve lesion detection rate makes it an important tool in advanced imaging in endoscopy, thus leading to improved clinical outcomes and patient outcomes. Evidence based on recent studies favors the superiority of NBI over the standard WLE in the detection of premalignant gastric lesions , such as intestinal metaplasia (IM) and dysplasia. A comparative analysis proved the detection of more lesions by NBI, as well as improved sensitivity, specificity, and predictive values for the identification of such lesions. In a total of 43 patients, NBI diagnosed extensive gastric IM cases and other dysplastic lesions that were not detected by WLE, highlighting its role in diagnosis. The outcomes suggest that the addition of NBI to routine endoscopic investigation can boost the diagnostic yield, enabling early intervention in the case of high-risk lesions for cancer progression. The ability of NBI to upgrade endoscopic diagnostic accuracy is a valuable milestone in the evolution of gastrointestinal endoscopy. With future advancements in clinical gastroenterology, utilization of NBI in clinical work has the potential to make an impact in patient management. The application of this newer technology is particularly beneficial for surveillance recommendations in established premalignant disease. By improving identification of suspicious lesions, NBI can also justify the decision-making process in terms of intervention techniques , such as endoscopic mucosal resection. The efficiency gains through NBI not only add to an improved diagnostic process but may even reduce rates of missed diagnosis. Future research will likely focus on optimizing the application of NBI in various forms of gastrointestinal illness, further cementing its role in the ongoing advancement of endoscopic imaging technology (Lassen et al., 2010; Smith et al., 2019) (Figure 12.7).

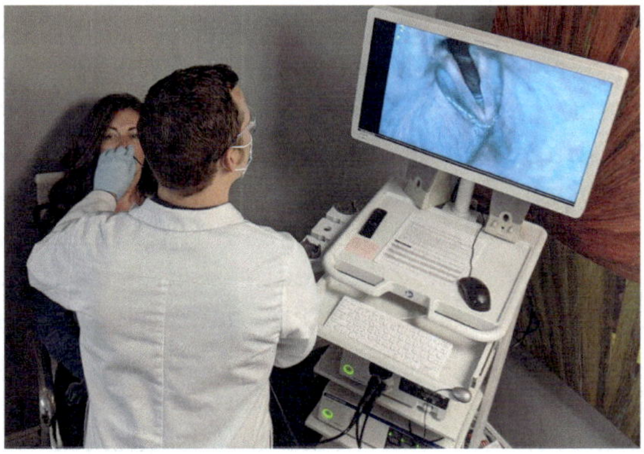

Figure 12.7. Narrow-band imaging (NBI).

Source: https://sa1s3optim.patientpop.com/assets/docs/187408.jpg.

12.2.3. Confocal Laser Endomicroscopy (CLE)

CLE is a significant advance in endoscopic imaging that permits real-time imaging of micro-anatomical structures beneath the mucosal layer. This process, utilizing laser-induced fluorescence for high-resolution imaging, allows the clinician to visualize cellular detail that is often beyond the capability of standard endoscopy. Depth-specific imaging functionality allows clinicians to diagnose conditions that manifest on the microscopic level, such as cancer and inflammatory disease. For instance, recent research highlights the effectiveness of CLE in the diagnosis of oral squamous cell carcinoma (OSCC), which is usually diagnosed late due to the limitations of conventional screening methods. By performing *in vivo* assessments of cellular morphology, CLE greatly enhances OSCC detection in the early stages, leading to improved patient outcomes and reduced recurrence rates after surgery (Aubreville et al., 2017). Beyond oncology, CLE has also shown great promise in gastroenterology and has found use for the diagnosis of IBD, like Crohn's and ulcerative colitis. Endoscopic investigations have traditionally been challenged in providing the cellular detail necessary for the identification of minute lesions or dysplastic change. The union of CLE with standard endoscopy has been proposed as a revolutionary concept, delivering in-depth views of mucosal structure with minimal invasiveness. By enabling clinicians to observe the histopathological features of the gut in real time, CLE can guide treatment decisions and improve monitoring strategies in IBD patients. The combination of surface information from routine endoscopy with cellular-level resolution provided by CLE addresses the acute need for enhanced specificity in gastrointestinal diagnostics (Arranz et al., 2015). As the technology continues to progress, the incorporation of advanced imaging modalities , such as CLE, into routine endoscopic practice holds great promise for enhanced diagnostic yield and therapeutic management. Development of computerized image analysis through artificial intelligence and deep learning algorithms further augments the ability of CLE with improved speed and accuracy in image interpretation. Studies of deep learning for images have presented excellent performance indicators, with better diagnostic accuracy for OSCC than traditional machine learning. This is a demonstration of the incorporation of state-of-the-art computational techniques into CLE, indicating the evolution of CLE from a diagnostic tool to an integral component of precision medicine in endoscopy. Through embracing these technological innovations, the field can contribute to timely interventions, leading to enhanced patient health outcomes (Aubreville et al., 2017) (Figure 12.8).

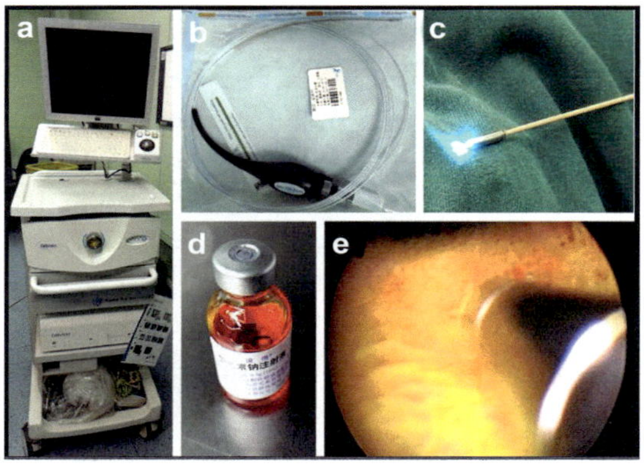

Figure 12.8. Confocal laser endomicroscopy (CLE).

Source: https://www.researchgate.net/publication/333846689/figure/fig1/AS:962201481408513@1606418118069/System-of-confocal-laser-endomicroscopy-a-Clinical-grade-CLE-system-Cellvizio-from.jpg.

12.3. Benefits of Advanced Imaging in Endoscopy

The introduction of high-tech imaging modalities in endoscopy has brought about a revolutionary shift in diagnostic and treatment abilities in the practice of medicine. Modalities , such as AFI are now available to facilitate label-free assessment of cells and tissues. The technique offers enhanced visualization, leading to more precise identification of pathological conditions. For instance, AFI has shown promise of use in surgical specialties, such as thyroid surgery, where it aids inexperienced surgeons in differentiating thyroid from parathyroid tissues. This capacity not only enables the surgery but also enhances patient safety, thereby placing in the spotlight clinical advantages brought about by high-tech imaging instruments in endoscopy (Wizenty et al., 2020). As AFI evolves further, it has the potential to standardize imaging protocols across medical specialties, hence making the benefits of advanced imaging more accessible. Another significant benefit of advanced imaging in endoscopy is associated with its impact on treatment accuracy and efficacy. Recent technological advancements have facilitated the development of steerable endoscopic capsule robots, which enhance navigation inside the gastrointestinal tract. These robotic systems have the potential to provide real-time feedback and allow targeted interventions , such as drug delivery and biopsies, capable of greatly improving patient treatment. Experiments demonstrated the effectiveness of employing unsupervised odometry and depth learning in such capsule robots, pointing towards a promising path towards entirely autonomous diagnostic treatments. As technology continues to evolve, it will work towards further enhancing minimally invasive procedures, thus reducing recovery time as well as total patient experience (Turan et al., 2018). All these developments serve to prove that advanced imaging is not merely for diagnosis but is increasingly being applied to therapeutic methodologies too. Also, the wide availability of advanced imaging modalities has affected the provision of care on a multidisciplinary platform, which in turn has promoted increased interaction among specialists in different disciplines. By being able to visualize complex physiological architectures in real time, physicians can be a part of more informed decision-making. As a case in point, dermatologists utilizing advanced fluorescence imaging to assess skin disorders may work closely with endocrinologists to better understand the relevance of blood glucose levels to patients, for instance. Such cross-specialty discussion is valuable, especially considering the reality that imaging procedures developed for one specialty are likely to yield information in another. Increased reliance on sophisticated imaging enhances individual practitioner skills but also underpins a global understanding of disease mechanisms, a paradigm shift in the practice of medicine (Wizenty et al., 2020).

12.3.1. Enhanced Visualization of Tissues

Advances in imaging modalities in endoscopy have significantly enhanced tissue visualization, allowing medical practitioners to have better diagnostic capability. Advanced visualization allows more accurate inspection of tissue structure, and this is particularly useful in identifying abnormalities , such as tumors or inflammation. AFI, for example, takes advantage of the inherent fluorescence properties of living tissues to discriminate between health and disease without the need for chemical labels. This technique has been particularly encouraging outside ophthalmology, extending to areas like dermatology and surgery, where it serves to identify malignancies or significant structures, such as parathyroid glands during thyroid operations. The translation of these techniques to the clinic represents a pivotal shift towards less invasive diagnostic approaches and has revolutionized the outcome of therapy, as the body of literature attesting to AF's utility in the clinical environment (Wizenty et al., 2020) would affirm. Aside from AFI, the application of optical techniques for 3D reconstruction of soft tissues during the duration of endoscopic procedures has been revolutionary. By stimulating visualization through advanced imaging modalities, surgeons are then capable of gaining accurate anatomical information, encouraging better navigation and decision-making during minimally invasive procedures. The technologies of computer-assisted surgery (CAS) enable tissue morphology-guided and motion-tracking in real-time, essential for accurate surgical navigation. Through these technologies, surgeons can see beyond the immediate tissue surface and learn about structures deep below that are normally concealed in routine endoscopic views. As the field of minimally invasive surgery keeps evolving, the integration of optical imaging with 3D reconstruction techniques is a critical milestone toward improved surgical precision and patient healing amidst continuously changing anatomical configurations (Maier-Hein et al., 2013). The future of tissue visualization using enhanced vision in endoscopy lies with future research and emerging technology. While recent advances have realized significant gains, there remain challenges, most specifically in standardizing imaging protocols and analysis across clinical applications. The key to making findings reproducible and leveraging the full potential of AFI and 3D imaging technologies will be to close the loop between laboratory research and clinical practice. Moreover, with advances in artificial intelligence and machine learning being integrated into imaging techniques, such technologies will have the capability to further elevate endoscopy's capabilities. Through enhanced tissue visualization and computer-assisted detection of pathological changes, such technologies potentially hold the capability to transform the scene of diagnosis, and ultimately lead to earlier diagnosis and improved disease management. Continuous interdisciplinary synergies will be responsible for unlocking the greatest potential of advanced visualization technology in endoscopic use (Figure 12.9).

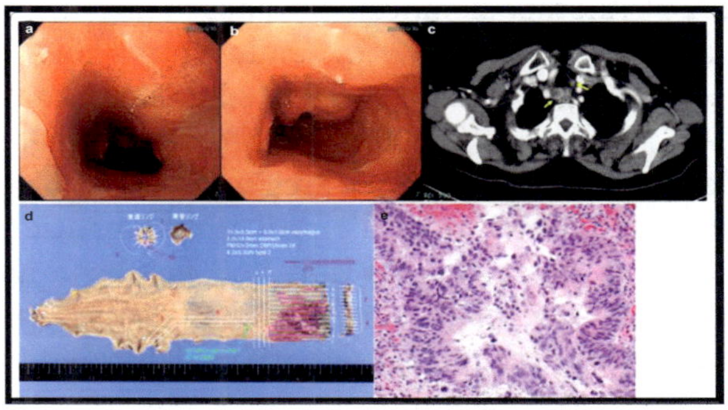

Figure 12.9. Enhanced visualization of tissues in endoscopy.

Source: https://www.researchgate.net/publication/344614870/figure/fig2/AS:983223261724672@1611430101145/Endoscopy-computed-tomography-and-histopathological-findings-for-case-2-a-b-Endoscopy.png.

12.3.2. Improved Diagnostic Accuracy

Redevelopment of endoscopic approaches by advanced imaging modalities has significantly improved diagnostic accuracy, particularly for the identification of malignancies. Routine endoscopic techniques previously employed tended to rely on white light endoscopy (WLE), which can fail to detect subtle tissue aberrations. The development of AFI has brought on board a groundbreaking method for visualization of cellular and structural changes before disease. This is achieved through several applications, where AFI has been capable of supporting clinicians in early neoplasia detection, increasing their diagnostic confidence as they decrease the possibility of false-negative lesions. Evidence supports the fact that AFI is not just effective in dermatology, but it also holds promise for other areas of medicine with its emphasis on enhancing early detection across every anatomical site. Although greater standardization of protocols and techniques is needed, the clinical advancement in AFI speaks well of its critical role in the advancement of diagnostic accuracy in endoscopy (Wizenty et al., 2020). Another significant advance in increasing diagnostic accuracy in endoscopy is the integration of volumetric laser endomicroscopy (VLE). VLE uses OCT to create real-time, high-definition images of tissue architecture to enable microscopic visualization of abnormalities. Research demonstrates that VLE has been an essential tool in the management of Barretts esophagus, which may potentially develop into esophageal cancer. In a total of 1,000 patients, VLE identified suspicious areas not visible to WLE in 59% of the procedures and also helped in the treatment for over half the procedures. Such capabilities not only enhance the yield of biopsies but also significantly enhance neoplastic alteration detection rates, thereby illustrating the impact of the technology on patient outcomes. This adaptability and precision underscore its role as a complementary tool in endoscopy practice to ensure maximized diagnostic accuracy (Smith et al., 2019). The incessant evolution of imaging technology within endoscopy promises a primary trend: the merging of technology and clinical practice towards improved patient outcomes through increased diagnostic accuracy. With more health professionals adopting newer imaging modalities , such as AFI and VLE, there lies an increasing potential for early intervention. Improved diagnostic equipment not only provides a greater scope of tissue visualization but also results in more informed patient care decisions. Obstacles on the horizon are in the form of more standardized training and guidelines to efficiently use these technologies in various healthcare setups. There must be continued research into implementing these new modalities to further optimize their integration into routine practice, ultimately resulting in a more accurate and efficient diagnostic process. With additional refinement of these technologies, they can transform the use of endoscopic diagnostics (Smith et al., 2019; Wizenty et al., 2020).

12.3.3. Reduction in Unnecessary Biopsies

The arrival of high-end imaging technology within endoscopy has brought a revolutionary change to the field of gastrointestinal diagnostics to an unprecedented degree, primarily by reducing the number of unwanted biopsies. Traditional biopsy procedures had been invasive and also tended to yield inconclusive results. By integrating technologies , such as probe-based confocal laser endomicroscopy (pCLE), physicians are now able to conduct real-time, high-definition imaging of the gastrointestinal tract at the cellular level. This capacity also allows for more precise identification of abnormal tissues. As a result, biopsies that are not necessary can be avoided, sparing patients discomfort and costs and making clinical practice more effective and patient care better. In addition, a well-organized system of classification , such as the Miami classification, can also further aid in avoiding unnecessary biopsies by establishing uniform criteria for the diagnostic evaluation of gastrointestinal lesions. This sort of system can classify normal and pathologic conditions by consensus among endoscopists utilizing advanced imaging modalities. Using such established criteria, practitioners would be able to enhance their ability to make accurate diagnoses and reserve biopsies for only where they are really needed. The efficacy of such a strategy is corroborated by evidence suggesting a large difference in autofluorescence lifetime between normal and neoplastic tissue, underscoring the potential of advanced imaging to enhance diagnostic discrimination and avoid unnecessary interventions (Chorvat et al., 2013).

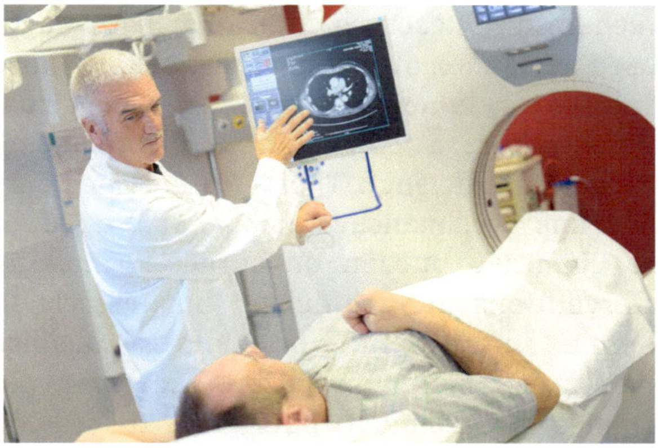

Figure 12.10. Reduction in unnecessary biopsies.

Source: https://cdn.sanity.io/images/0vv8moc6/ajmc/daf65efbaf12c8fdab62955b99dd99f51fec3677-6866x4582.jpg?fit=crop&auto=format.

Ultimately, the impact of reducing unnecessary biopsies extends beyond individual patient outcomes; it contributes as well to overall healthcare efficiencies. By minimizing the need for invasive tissue sampling, healthcare facilities are able to more effectively ration resources, shifting focus to genuinely required procedures. Furthermore, the use of more sophisticated imaging technology not only increases the precision of diagnosis but could also enhance the general quality of the healthcare experience by reducing the physical and mental burden on patients. With constant progress in standard imaging protocol implementation, the future of gastrointestinal diagnosis will experience a fundamental change, leading to significant improvements in patient outcomes and resource utilization (Figure 12.10) (Chen et al., 2014).

12.4. Applications of Advanced Imaging in Various Medical Fields

The integration of advanced imaging techniques in endoscopy has significantly transformed the landscape of various medical fields, enhancing diagnostic accuracy and therapeutic capabilities. One of the prominent applications is in the realm of gastrointestinal endoscopy, where high-definition imaging and fluorescence techniques allow for the detailed visualization of mucosal surfaces. This advancement facilitates the detection of early-stage neoplasms and other pathologies that may otherwise go unnoticed. Furthermore, autofluorescence imaging (AFI) provides a non-invasive approach to assess tissue health, which has shown promising applications in other fields , such as dermatology and surgery. The ability to visualize tissue at a cellular level enhances clinicians' capacity to make informed decisions during procedures, demonstrating that advanced imaging techniques are paramount in driving improvements in patient outcomes across multiple disciplines (Wizenty et al., 2020). In addition to improving diagnostic practices, advanced imaging technologies are revolutionizing therapeutic procedures within endoscopy. A relevant example is the application of automated navigation systems in flexible endoscopes, which addresses the inherent limitations of traditional steering mechanisms. Research indicates that image-based navigation algorithms, particularly those utilizing lumen centralization and visual odometry, are at the forefront of enhancing procedural efficacy. These systems not only improve maneuverability but also reduce the cognitive load on surgeons, allowing for more streamlined interventions, especially in complex intraluminal procedures. Although commercial solutions are still in development, the potential for automated navigation to improve patient safety and procedural success is significant, emphasizing the need for continued research and innovation in this area (Van der Stap et al., 2013). The expansion of advanced imaging applications also underscores the importance of interdisciplinary collaboration in medicine. The convergence of technologies from fields , such as engineering, informatics, and imaging sciences enhances the potential for breakthroughs in endoscopic practices. For instance, the integration of machine learning algorithms with advanced imaging enables the development of sophisticated diagnostic tools capable of real-time analysis of endoscopic images. Such innovations not only aid in the rapid identification of ailments but also pave the way for personalized treatment strategies that can be tailored to individual patient needs. As research progresses, there is a growing recognition of the critical role that advanced imaging plays in not just improving the technical skills of medical professionals but in promoting holistic approaches to patient care across various medical fields (Wizenty et al., 2020).

12.4.1. Gastroenterology

The introduction of advanced imaging technologies into endoscopy has fundamentally altered the standing of numerous medical areas by enhancing accuracy in diagnosis and therapy. One of the key applications is in gastrointestinal endoscopy, where fluorescence and high-definition imaging allow for extensive visualization of mucosal surfaces. This technology allows for the detection of neoplasms in their initial stages, as well as other pathologies, which otherwise remain occult. Moreover, AFI is a non-invasive technique for quantifying the health of tissue, which has proven to have useful applications in dermatology and surgery, too. The ability to visualize tissue at a cellular level enhances clinicians' informed decision-making during procedures, demonstrating that innovative imaging technologies are key to driving patient outcome improvements in numerous specialties (Wizenty et al., 2020). Beyond diagnostic improvements, advanced imaging technologies are revolutionizing therapeutic interventions in endoscopy. One relevant example is the application of computerized navigation systems in flexible endoscopes, addressing inherent flaws in standard steering mechanisms. Research indicates that image-based navigation algorithms, particularly those centered on lumen centralization and visual odometry, are at the forefront of enhancing procedural efficiency. These systems not only allow improved maneuverability but also reduce the cognitive burden on surgeons, making interventions more efficient, particularly in complex intraluminal procedures. Despite ongoing commercial solutions, however, the promise of automated navigation to provide patient safety and procedure success is vast, and emphasis on continued research and development in this area is essential (Van der Stap et al., 2013). Increasing applications of advanced imaging also underscore the need for multidisciplinary cooperation in medicine. The convergence of technologies from across disciplines , such as engineering, informatics, and imaging sciences, enhances the likelihood of advances in endoscopic practice. For instance, integration of machine learning algorithms with high-level imaging enables the manufacture of sophisticated diagnostic devices that can process endoscopic images in real time. These technologies not only enable the fast diagnosis of diseases but also result in treatment regimens tailored to the individual that can be modified to suit the special needs of patients. With ongoing research, the value of imaging is not only in improving the technical expertise of doctors but also in promoting holistic approaches to the care of patients in all areas of medicine is increasingly realized (Wizenty et al., 2020). Gastroenterology has made significant advances due to the introduction of advanced imaging techniques into endoscopic procedures. These developments go beyond improving diagnostic functions to therapeutic measures as well. For instance, developments in OCT and multimodal imaging technologies have revolutionized gastrointestinal disease assessment. Among these innovations, techniques , such as narrow-band imaging and high-definition endoscopy allow better visualization of mucosal structures and vasculature, facilitating earlier visualization of lesions. Such precision is crucial in the field of gastrointestinal oncology, where early detection of malignancy can potentially drastically improve patient outcomes. The ability to assess the histological characteristics of lesions in real-time during endoscopy is paving the way for more personalized treatment approaches in gastroenterology with individually optimized surgical procedures and a diminished need for subsequent invasive biopsies. AI in gastroenterology is transforming the clinician's approach to diagnostic issues, particularly in endoscopy. By utilizing advanced algorithms , such as convolutional neural networks, AI has the capacity to enhance adenoma detection rates during colonoscopies and more accurately characterize detected lesions. Studies demonstrate that AI-augmented analysis can reduce procedural variability, leading to more consistent diagnostic outcomes and ultimately to the optimization of patient care. Specifically, AI use in cross-sectional imaging modalities , such as computed tomography and magnetic resonance imaging, holds tremendous potential. The capacity of AI systems to identify complex conditions—, such as pancreatic ductal adenocarcinoma—reflects the untold potential of such technologies for early diagnosis and personalized planning of treatment. With rising innovation in AI, the application of AI in gastroenterology will have an expanding horizon, further enhancing the effectiveness of endoscopic testing and treatments (Robles-Medranda et al., 2025).

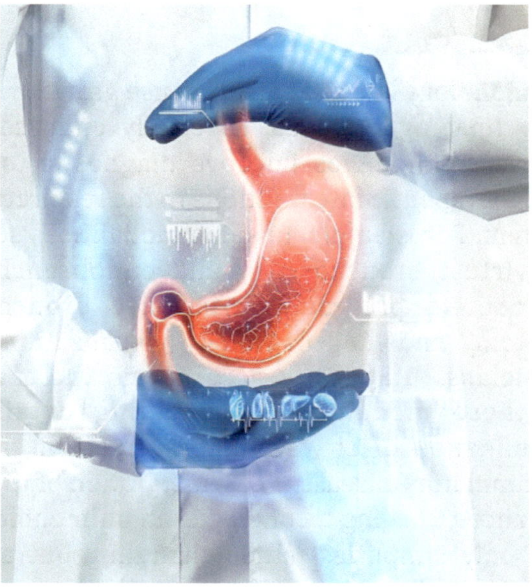

Figure 12.11. Gastroenterology.

Source: https://bighospitals.in/assets/img/service/medical-gastroenterology-img.jpg.

Also, as the gastroenterological landscape evolves with technology, emphasis on procedural optimization and improved diagnostics remains critical. Studies have indicated a growing interest in more advanced endoscopic procedures, such as digital single-operator cholangioscopy, that allow for improved anatomical identification and lesion typing. Imaging's role in biliopancreatic disease evaluation has become increasingly significant, especially given the potential that AI can make such processes automated. Application in biliopancreatic endoscopy—, such as recognition of biliary stenosis and dysplastic precursor lesion grading, demonstrates the requirement for change at a systemic level. This evolution of imaging not only enhances the clinician's ability to make informed decisions but also promotes the implementation of standardized protocols to enhance patient care. Ongoing research and development of these imaging methods will play a critical role in the progress of gastroenterology in the future (Scognamiglio et al., 2025) (Figure 12.11).

12.4.2. Pulmonology

Pulmonology has seen an immense growth with new imaging methods, especially endoscopy. These technologies improve diagnostic tools and therapeutic interventions in the respiratory system. For example, imaging modalities , such as virtual bronchoscopy and endobronchial ultrasound provide non-invasive bronchial anatomy and lung pathology visualization to clinicians. Diagnostic accuracy is increased in these modalities by enabling detailed examination of airway tumors, infection, and inflammatory disease. Thus, integration of these advanced imaging technologies in pulmonology not only simplifies patient handling but also optimizes therapy success through the correct localization of pathology. Education in such advanced imaging methods are crucial to pulmonary professionals, with the intensity of procedure bearing the promise of an extremely high level of technical competence. The newest advancement in simulation.õ education, particularly by use of virtual reality machines, has become a new teaching tool in this context. Training modalities simulate real conditions in practice, and this allows for trainees to practice skills at.õ zero risk to patients. The use of 3D printing of airways also facilitates enhanced understanding and preparation for clinical procedures. As per recent reviews, the importance of obtaining expertise in flexible bronchoscopy and lung isolation techniques underscores the need for innovative training solutions in thoracic anesthesia and pulmonology practice (Casso et al., 2024). Other than that, implications of advanced imaging include therapeutic applications, such as bronchial thermoplasty for the treatment of asthma, which indicates the intersection of pulmonology with interventional techniques. The technique is aided by detailed anatomical visualization from endoscopic methods to allow for precision when intervening. Pulmonologists should gain a deeper understanding of these interventional procedures, particularly considering the rapid evolution of technology in this field. As can be observed from literature, ongoing research and advances in areas like pulmonary hypertension and circulation keep raising the standard of care, pushing the boundaries of possibility in pulmonology (N/A, 2021). Thus, embracing these advancements is crucial for enhanced patient outcomes and advancing the practice (Figure 12.12).

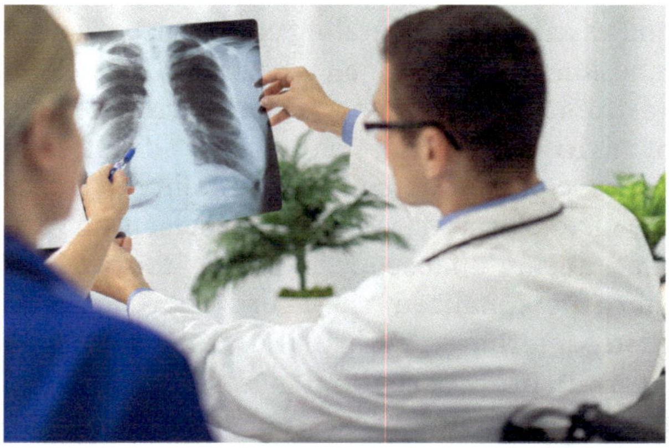

Figure 12.12. Pulmonology.

Source: https://mcr.health/wp-content/uploads/2021/12/Pulmonology-Blog-Image-scaled.jpeg.

12.4.3. Urology

The field of urology has made huge strides with the advent of sophisticated imaging techniques in endoscopy, enhancing therapeutic success and diagnostic precision. Urological disorders typically demand precise visual inspections, and therefore, efficient imaging plays a very critical role. With technological advancements in techniques , such as narrow-band imaging and high-definition endoscopy, urologists are now able to view the urinary tract more clearly than ever before. These developments not only enable detection of malignancy but also aid in the assessment of benign disease, i.e., strictures and stones. Imaging modalities have transformed urology, enabling more individualized intervention that enhances therapeutic impact with reduced invasiveness. Consequently, the evolution of such imaging technologies has been directly aligned with improved patient outcomes and has had a significant impact on clinical practice and management trends in urology, reflecting an unmistakable shift towards more complicated, patient-centered care. AI technology use within urology is indicative of these advanced imaging technologies, offering a multi-faceted approach to enhance diagnostic performance and procedural success. Artificial intelligence platforms can process significant amounts of imaging data and identify patterns and anomalies that the human eye may not detect. This significantly reduces the workload of urologists to allow them to focus on major decision-making tasks. Furthermore, AI is integrable with imaging technologies, and real-time analysis can be performed during endoscopy. This integration enhances preoperative planning, intraoperative navigation, and postoperative assessment, ultimately translating to better outcomes in surgery. As seen in recent appraisals, the incorporation of AI into the clinical environment has transformed traditional practices to be more efficient and productive (Liu et al., 2021). Such a new phenomenon symbolizes a turning point in urologic practice with a glimpse of the future in minimally invasive treatment. Besides, recent advancements in urological robotic surgery have utilized improved imaging for further improvement of surgery. With the advent of robot-assisted surgeries, there has been an added degree of precision and control introduced in urological surgeries. Robots with enhanced imaging can provide surgeons with a superior view, allowing them to perform more complex and delicate procedures. As seen in recent studies, the autonomy levels of surgical robots have vastly enhanced, from basic assistance to complete autonomy in executing operations (Attanasio et al., 2020). This transformation not only minimizes the likelihood of human mistakes but also optimizes surgical procedures, subsequently reducing recovery times and potential complications. The convergence of high-tech imaging and robotics represents a revolutionary era of urology, resulting in more cohesive and effective patient care models and creating new standards in practice.

12.5. Challenges and Limitations

The development of imaging methods in endoscopy brings with it a range of challenges that need to be overcome to maximize their clinical value. One of the major limitations is the slow transfer of new technologies into standard clinical practice. Despite modalities like VLE having been proven to enhance diagnostics, including a 55% rise in neoplasia diagnostic yield, most clinicians remain reluctant to integrate these technologies into their standard practices due to factors like training expense and perceived complexity. The specialized hardware and software that may be required also provide financial barriers for small health facilities. Such hesitation nullifies the worth of complete imaging systems and limits the sharing of best practices in endoscopic procedures, ultimately impacting the trajectory of patient care (Smith et al., 2019). In addition, the technical imperfections of current endoscopic technology represent a significant obstacle in stretching towards better imaging. Despite the potential of visualization-enhancing technologies like optical coherence tomography, the underlying dynamics of flexible endoscopes have remained largely unchanged in the past half-century. The resultant ergonomic inefficiencies see operators struggling with unintuitive steerage systems that make it difficult for them to manage challenging anatomical pathways (Van der Stap et al., 2013). To this end, the lack of commercially supported automated systems determines the challenges of designing solid steering algorithms that can be used in real-time environments. In the face of improving endoscopic imaging, software and hardware innovations are essential to allow clinicians to utilize new imaging technologies optimally. Finally, the addition of advanced imaging to endoscopic procedures necessitates a paradigm shift not only at the training level but also at the level of clinical procedures. The emphasis on conventional means tends to anchor the quest for newer, better means, creating a culture where obsolescence is the rule even as better imaging technologies are created. As with VLE, appropriate identification of the invisible areas of concern using traditional white light endoscopy has the potential to revolutionize diagnostic accuracy and benefit to patients. But without systemic change to promote education on such modalities and reward systems that promote their use, the potential of modern imaging in endoscopy will go unrealized. Resolution of these multisegmented challenges is critical to advance the field and ensure innovations get applied in improved healthcare service delivery (Smith et al., 2019).

12.5.1. Cost and Accessibility of Advanced Imaging Technologies

Within the umbrella of advanced imaging technologies utilized in endoscopy, a heavy assessment of cost and availability is required to understand their broader implications in clinical applications. More advanced imaging technologies , such as magnetic resonance imaging (MRI) and high-resolution ultrasound machines, are usually coupled with extremely high prices that can limit their applications. Hospitals and healthcare centers are also frequently faced with budgeting and reimbursement constraints that can limit the number of advanced imaging devices they can acquire and maintain. These financial barriers could hinder access, especially for patients from resource-poor settings where such technologies may not be readily available, thereby further perpetuating health inequities. The routine use of augmented imaging techniques would typically rely on the availability of sufficient resources, which consequently determines the success of the patient and the efficacy of treatment during endoscopic procedures (Crouser et al., 2020). In addition, the disparity in applying advanced imaging methods can be attributed to variation in training and experience between health care professionals. Studies have proven that ideal use of advanced imaging for endoscopy involves specialized training, which is not equally available across all medical centers. For instance, professionals in certain regions of the nation might not be skilled enough to utilize high-level transvaginal ultrasound (TVS) techniques in diagnosing conditions like endometriosis, which has been established through recent surveys indicating technological underuse (Leonardi et al., 2020). Such training gaps will lead to false negatives and poor surgical planning, which in turn contribute to the issue of technological lag. Thus, the healthcare practitioners must be adequately trained in the use of these new imaging methods to further enhance their real-world use and overall patient care. Finally, the cost-effectiveness of new imaging methods also needs to be weighed against diagnostic precision and corresponding patient outcomes. Even if the initial investment in expensive imaging machines may be out of reach, their capacity for increased accuracy in diagnosis can pay back the healthcare system in the long term. For example, high-grade imaging reduces the incidence of exploratory procedures by being able to accurately assess conditions , such as endometriomas of the ovary and deep endometriosis. This not only saves health costs but also decreases the risk involved with invasive procedures. Moreover, organizational guidelines , such as those by the National Institute for Health and Care

Excellence suggest adding advanced imaging to routine assessment due to its clinical utility, more evidence for its implementation in the face of initial costs (Crouser et al., 2020). Shifting the financial dimensions to complementals of intended benefits is required to promote policies enhancing the availability and use of advanced imaging in endoscopic procedures (Figure 12.13).

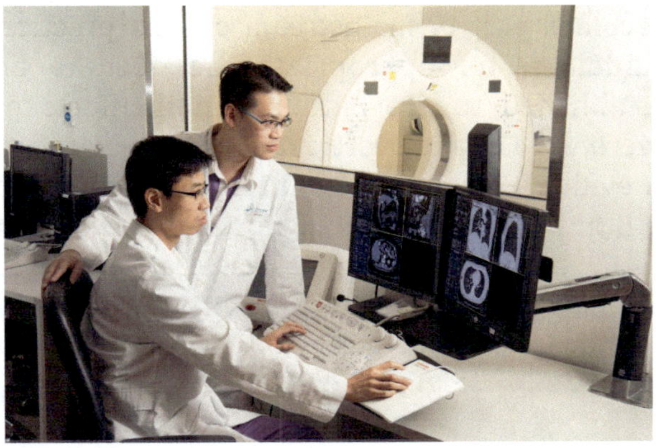

Figure 12.13. Cost and accessibility of advanced imaging technologies.

Source: https://gleneagles.hk/images/20230623_HK01_Radiology_low.jpg.

12.5.2. Training and Expertise Required for Practitioners

Sophistication that is attributed to cutting-edge imaging technology applied in endoscopy necessitates advanced levels of training and expertise among practitioners. As such, imaging technologies, e.g., high-definition endoscopic ultrasound and digital chromoendoscopy, become even more advanced, it is essential that gastroenterologists and interventional surgeons master technology as much as clinical application. This involves mastering the finer aspects of anatomical visualization, disease detection, and the technical conduct of procedures. Continuing professional development is essential; therefore, medical professionals should be subjected to extensive training programs that include theoretical knowledge as well as hands-on exposure. Training to such an extent enables the practitioner to make the correct decisions in real time while carrying out the diagnostic and therapeutic procedures, which translates to improved patient outcomes as well as reduces the risk. The best advancement in training the practitioners has been through the utilization of simulation technologies. Virtual reality (VR) simulations are increasingly becoming useful tools for team training for endovascular procedures and the transition to a multidisciplinary age in healthcare. Virtual reality simulations allow practitioners to practice in simulated settings without exposing patients to unnecessary risks. Enhanced simulation capacity also facilitates better understanding of complex situations, enabling practitioners to hone their technical and nontechnical skills in sophisticated imaging applications. As observed, simulation training achieves a structured practice setting, bridging the gap between emerging endovascular technologies and clinical proficiency, required to ensure high standards of patient care in endoscopy (Cheshire et al., 2015). For the specialty of natural orifice transluminal endoscopic surgery (NOTES), the training issues are still at the center, as the specialty continues to develop. Effective training programs for surgeons and gastroenterologists who are conducting these new procedures include adapting existing practices to involve new techniques that breach mucosal barriers. Simulation training options, including interactive workshops and online websites, are necessary to equip practitioners with the skill set required to successfully perform these intricate procedures. With the shift from first-generation to novel NOTES procedures, so also does the need for extensive educational modalities by which practitioners can become well-acquainted with the subtleties of these novel-generation techniques (Ahn et al., 2016). The ongoing evolution in this specialized field still further accentuates the dynamic linkage between systematic education and procedural expertise.

12.5.3. Potential for Overdiagnosis and Overtreatment

The integration of advanced imaging technologies into endoscopy has introduced new frontiers in diagnostic precision; however, in the process, it has raised severe concerns about overdiagnosis and overtreatment. The capacity of these imaging technologies to identify abnormality at an early stage can result indirectly in the detection of clinically unimportant conditions. One of the best illustrations of this is in lung cancer screening, where the detection of suspicious nodules has the potential to initiate a chain of invasive diagnostic tests and subsequent interventions. Recent expert analysis anticipated that higher diagnostic testing associated with lung cancer screening would overwhelm already stretched healthcare systems with resource deficits, potentially calling into question the necessity and appropriateness of each intervention (Chalela et al., 2024). The overdiagnosis risk does not just strain the healthcare system but also exposes patients to the unnecessary risks of treatment. Overdiagnosis has also become more common in gynecological practice due to the application of high-level imaging classifications. The switch from the American Society for Reproductive Medicine (ASRM) classification to the ESHRE–ESGE criteria markedly increased the diagnosis rate of a septate uterus, typically without clinical necessity. This transition indicates a growing fear of the clinical usefulness of advanced imaging; the guidelines intended to prevent subjectivity have the flip side risk of creating treatment for conditions that don't really pose threats to patient health. What research has indicated is that such overdiagnosis can lead to unnecessary surgeries that offer no actual gain for the patient but drive healthcare costs and procedural damage (Ludwin & Ludwin, 2014). As a result, the diagnostic system must be scrutinized critically in an attempt to prevent misdiagnosis, influencing treatment directions that are not helpful or, worse, detrimental. The implications of overdiagnosis extend beyond immediate health issues and into social realms, namely, healthcare policy and patient autonomy. Patients diagnosed with conditions resulting in aggressive treatment become more anxious, and this is aggravated by cumulative decision-making regarding their care. The danger of overtreatment can lead to erosion of confidence in the healthcare system, as patients are confronted with the outcomes of unnecessary interventions. Secondly, as high-tech imaging becomes part of mainstream clinical practice, guidelines for appropriate use need to be established to prevent unwanted effects of overdiagnosis and overtreatment. Incorporation of evidence-based models in imaging protocols will not only enhance diagnostic precision but also ascertain responsible healthcare resource utilization with both patient safety and healthcare system integrity assured (Chalela et al., 2024) (Figure 12.14).

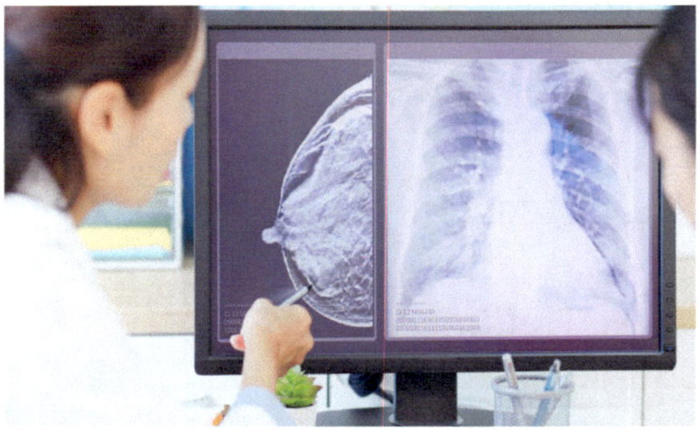

Figure 12.14. Potential for overdiagnosis and overtreatment.

Source: https://www.thewisdomstudy.org/wp-content/uploads/2023/10/Overdiagnosis-blog-banner.png.

12.6. Future Trends in Endoscopic Imaging

With the ongoing advancement of endoscopic imaging technology, the integration of next-generation technologies , such as AI and machine learning will drive the diagnostic and therapeutic phases into a new era. These enable large amounts of imaging data to be processed, hence facilitating improved decision-making, particularly in real time. Some of the newer developments include the use of neural networks to create three-dimensional images of anatomical structures, and these can improve the accuracy of endoscopic procedures by a considerable margin. Techniques , such as ENS are perfect examples, where intraoperative 3D models of brain tumors are constructed. Such a feature not only improves visualization but also assists surgeons in navigating complex anatomical spaces better, thus improving patient success rates and reducing surgical complications. Continued evolution of such AI-driven approaches emphasizes the coming age of precision medicine becoming ever more feasible, especially in highly technical areas , such as neurosurgery (Serna & Prieto, 2017). Further, the introduction of robotics in conjunction with advanced imaging also portends great advances in the field of endoscopy. Computerized surgical systems that possess the capacity to execute intricate operations within a sub-millimeter margin will revolutionize the practice of performing minimally invasive procedures. These robot systems, complemented by sophisticated imaging modalities, will allow for more precise operations and real-time modification guided by biosignals. Not only do automated systems enhance the efficiency of surgery, but they also overcome the limitations of human dexterity and repeatability. As these robots come to a point where they can carry out tasks that were previously deemed too complicated even for seasoned surgeons, they open up possibilities for more complicated procedures to be conducted at greater levels of success, further expanding endoscopic imaging capabilities (Das et al., 2017). Looking ahead, utilizing augmented reality (AR) combined with endoscopic imaging is another promising field for enhancing surgical technique. AR can overlay key information onto the sight of the surgeon, providing contextualization of the anatomical structures during the process of an endoscopy. With a mixture of real-time imaging and computer-added data, surgeons can derive highly valuable information about the spatial nature of their environment. Not only does this fusion of imaging improve the control of the surgeon, but it also maximizes training for those entering into this slim profession. In addition, as AR is becoming more embedded in medical practice, it is also applicable in immersive simulations, which would train the next generation of surgeons in handling complex endoscopic scenarios, thereby improving overall competence and patient safety during operations. The integration of AR with endoscopy imaging will surely shape the future of surgical interventions (Serna & Prieto, 2017).

12.6.1. Integration of Artificial Intelligence (AI)

The use of AI in advanced imaging in endoscopy is a paradigm shift in gastroenterology diagnostic and treatment processes. AI technologies are founded on sophisticated algorithms that have the ability to read massive amounts of imaging data and significantly enhance the ability to detect abnormalities , such as polyps, lesions, or any other pathological changes in the gastrointestinal tract. In the process, AI not only enables disease diagnosis like cancer at an early stage but also increases the effectiveness of therapeutic intervention by making the imaging more precise. As recognized by existing studies, the continuous advancements in imaging informatics have begun revealing hidden patterns that would otherwise not be visible to the naked eye, showing how the integration of AI can lead to noticeable improvements in patient care and diagnostic accuracy, according to research efforts aimed at optimizing imaging techniques in clinical settings (Hsu et al., 2019). Besides this, the potential of AI applications to introduce a more holistic framework within endoscopy is more apparent now. The concept of an endo-histo-omics approach, the amalgamation of endoscopic images, histology, and genomic information, shows how AI can facilitate a whole-picture understanding of conditions , such as IBD. This convergence supports precision medicine initiatives by enabling customization of treatment plans based on comprehensive patient data, thereby enhancing therapy personalization. Standardization of scoring systems enabled by AI further assists in enhancing more standardized measurement of disease activity, which in turn further supports clinical decision-making (Chaudhari et al., 2024).

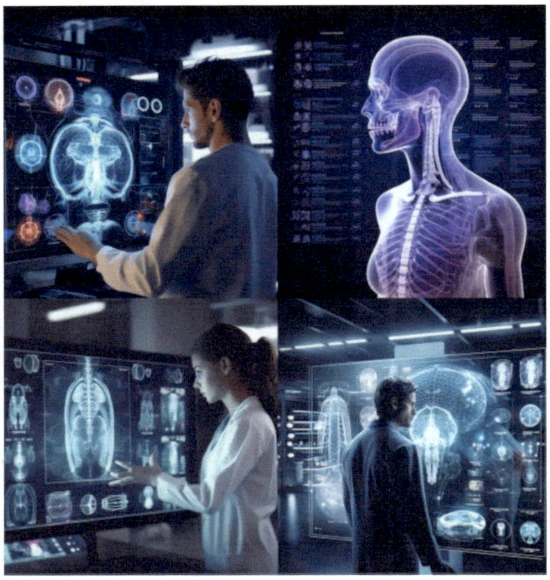

Figure 12.15. Integration of artificial intelligence (AI).

Source: https://theacademic.com/wp-content/uploads/2023/09/neliti_artificial_intelligence_application_in_radiology_4K_5b90bf02-3146-4b31-80e0-2c251f560d56.png.

With the improvement in the capabilities of AI, practitioners must familiarize themselves with such improvements so that they can optimize the use of such sophisticated systems in routine practice. In the context of the role of AI in endoscopy, several challenges must be addressed to successfully implement it. An essential consideration here is the issue of data quality and standardization since the performance of AI algorithms is highly dependent on high-quality representative data. Additionally, issues of reproducibility and a scarcity of randomized controlled trials pose threats to the generalizability of results in AI. Ethical concerns are also involved, which bring about the argument for legal exposures and regulatory procedures that the discipline might need for clinical application. Standardized development of guidelines, complemented by robust interdisciplinary collaboration among clinicians, policymakers, and regulatory bodies, is critical in meeting these challenges and optimizing the use of AI capabilities in practice for advanced imaging and endoscopy (Figure 12.15) (Chaudhari et al., 2024).

12.6.2. Development of Portable Imaging Devices

The evolution of portable imaging devices has changed the practice of endoscopy, which allows for improved diagnostics and unparalleled convenience. Prior methods of endoscopic testing are typically time-consuming to prepare and can cause patient pain, causing patients to resist necessary procedures. Improvements in technologies , such as wireless capsule endoscopy (WCE) are a significant improvement in this regard. WCE, developed in 2000 by Given Imaging Ltd., enables non-invasive examination of the gastrointestinal (GI) tract to facilitate patient compliance and mass screening programs. The innovations not only save healthcare systems but also enhance the quality of care provided to patients, particularly in societies confronted by an aging population and the subsequent rise in digestive disease (Ciuti et al., 2016). This model of innovation emphasizes additional research and development in the field of portable imaging technologies since they possess the potential to introduce strong improvements in diagnostic quality and patient satisfaction. Moreover, the incorporation of microrobotics capabilities into portable imaging devices is a remarkable advancement in their operational functionality. Future capsule endoscopes will probably feature active locomotion and therapeutic module functionality, pushing their uses even more in the clinical setting. This direction aligns with the overall trend toward minimally invasive surgery, where these devices enable more thorough evaluation of soft tissue without the complicating factors of traditional endoscopy. The ongoing development of these devices not only enhances imaging precision but also heralds a revolution in gastrointestinal diagnosis and therapy, focusing on overall patient comfort and engagement in health care practice. With innovations still underway, the future looks bright for portable imaging devices to become an integral part of the medical toolkit (Ciuti et al., 2016). In addition to the development of gastrointestinal imaging, portable imaging technologies are also playing a rapidly more central role in CAS. The reality that three-dimensional models of soft-tissue structures may be replicated in real time during minimally invasive procedures presents unique challenges with the dynamic character of such anatomical regions. Recent information demonstrates an evolving reliance on optical techniques for real-time imaging; these technology options can revolutionize the navigational capability of surgeons by providing a more precise understanding of tissue morphology and motion. Due to this, the integration of advanced optical imaging in portable devices holds tremendous promise to advance outcomes in complex surgical scenarios. The recent innovation of optical intra-operative 3D reconstruction covers not just existing technology hurdles but further presents the clinical application of CAS to a new level of precision and effectiveness. With the evolution of these technologies, they will certainly improve the level of advanced imaging in endoscopy and related surgery areas.

12.6.3. Innovations in Imaging Software and Analysis

The field of endoscopy imaging software and analysis has undergone a revolutionary change, most remarkably encouraged by technological advancements that enhance the accuracy of diagnosis. Enhancement in AFI is a point in evidence demonstrating how enhanced software features advance visualization of tissue and cellular dynamics without the need for exogenous contrast agents. AFI exploits the natural fluorescence of tissue autofluorescence fluorophores to identify pathologies in various organs, beyond the ophthalmic application into dermatology and internal medicine. AFI approaches have been standardized and validated, yet inconsistencies in their application among studies have raised issues regarding standardization and comparability. However, the potential of AFI to act as a substitute for crucial clinical indicators, like diabetology's blood glucose levels, highlights its ability to revolutionize tissue evaluation during endoscopic interventions and enhance patient treatment and outcomes (Wizenty et al., 2020). The integration of sophisticated imaging software not only increases diagnostic potential but also enables optimization of treatment methods through the application of 3D printing technology. 3D printing is emerging to be an efficient means of making personalized medical devices, such as biliary stents tailored to the specific anatomical requirements. Rapid prototyping can be achieved using bio-compatible materials , such as crosslinked polyvinyl alcohol (XL-PVA), which can be seeded with stem cells and cholangiocytes to enhance function in actual clinical situations. By enabling the fabrication of stents that can be configured to patient-specific anatomies, this technology also minimizes complications due to traditional stents. As a result, the collaboration of imaging evaluation and 3D printing may be a revolutionary approach to stent placement that can enhance procedural success and minimize the occurrence of complications for endoscopic procedures (Alexander et al., 2019). Also, ongoing developments in imaging software will enhance data analysis during endoscopy in a significant manner. With the application of AI and machine learning technology, sophisticated imaging data sets can be analyzed to detect subtle abnormalities that may not be recognizable with the naked eye. With the aid of algorithms that have learned from large datasets, such technology can provide real-time feedback during procedure to improve diagnostic accuracy and the likelihood of early detection of disease. As with recent research into the potential of autofluorescence imaging, the integration of advanced analysis techniques is essential to pushing beyond existing limitations and achieving greatest clinical benefits. Lastly, with the development of imaging software to harbor advanced analytical and computational capabilities, it will transform the face of endoscopic interventions by streamlining workflows as well as maximizing overall patient outcomes (Wizenty et al., 2020; Alexander et al., 2019) (Figure 12.16).

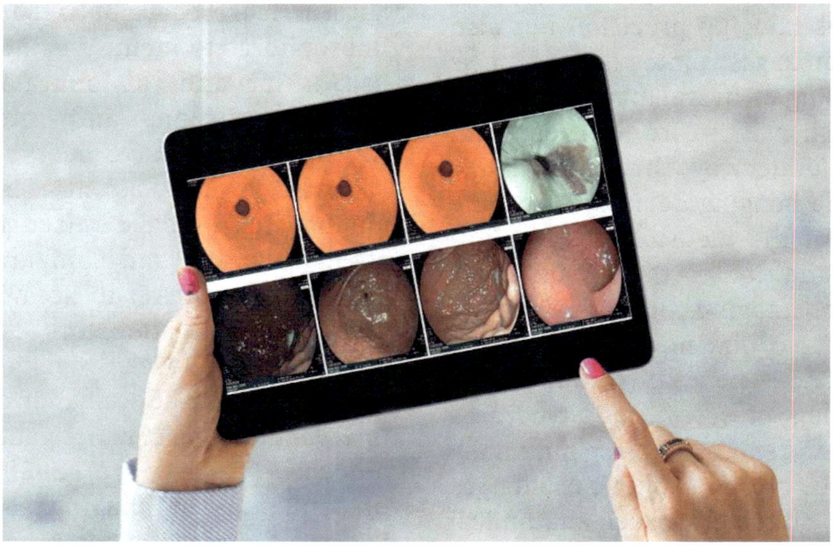

Figure 12.16. Innovations in imaging software and analysis.

Source: https://envisionnext.net/wp-content/uploads/2024/05/endoscopy-image-analysis.jpeg.

SUMMARY

Lastly, the inclusion of emerging imaging technology within endoscopy has undergone a radical shift in transforming the face of diagnostic and therapeutic procedures. These developments have aided to enabled improved visualization of lesions, that have enabled improved differentiation between benign and malignant lesions more accurately. For instance, the application of advanced modalities, such as elastography and contrast-enhanced ultrasound, has demonstrated promise for characterizing pleural diseases that otherwise were not easy to identify with accuracy without intervention. With these advanced imaging techniques, healthcare professionals can make more informed decisions regarding patient care, thus optimizing diagnostic workflows and outcomes. This move towards minimally invasive treatments is in line with shifting healthcare priorities towards patient-focused care and reducing the morbidity of invasive diagnostic techniques. Not to be lost, nevertheless, is the effect of AI alongside advanced imaging. AI-based algorithms have proved to be remarkably good at detecting abnormalities and quantifying pleural fluid volumes, streamlining the diagnostic process with highly accurate results while being very precise. Machine learning algorithms in such systems are capable of interpreting complex imaging data that is very elusive even for experienced professionals, thus improving diagnostic performance. Along with this, the integration of AI with genomic and molecular data also holds immense potential for the development of individualized therapeutic strategies, holding out the vision of personalized medicine's supremacy in the future. Therefore, continued research and experimentation with these technologies are needed to address issues of data privacy and algorithmic transparency to further bring them on board in clinical practice. Finally, the advancement that was yielded from better imaging in endoscopy emphasizes the need for ongoing research and devising clear clinical guidelines. While existing literature shows promising results, larger prospective trials play a crucial part in validating the effectiveness as well as the repeatability of these imaging modalities. As validated by cardiovascular screening research, where the newer imaging technologies, such as CCTA, improved predictive value, it is crucial to replicate such breakthroughs in other fields of medicine, such as gastrointestinal and pulmonary disease management. As progress is made in the discipline, longitudinal evaluations integrating the new imaging technologies with traditional diagnostic technologies will be essential in guiding future recommendations and practice in clinical medicine, and thus enhancing patient outcomes and care in endoscopy and beyond.

The integration of newer imaging technologies into endoscopic procedures has significantly improved the practice of minimally invasive surgery (MIS). One of the primary advances has been the use of optical approaches for *in vivo* 3D reconstruction, where surgeons can visualize soft-tissue structures with a high level of resolution. Such advances simplify surgical navigation, with improved patient-specific, multi-modal data registration during procedures. As outlined in discussions of the topic, high-resolution imaging not only improves preoperative planning but also intraoperative decision-making, therefore increasing the quality of care in advanced surgical procedures. The ongoing evolution of optical imaging methods emphasizes the need for an integrated realization of their applications and technical specifications, a decisive transformation in the surgical interventions that necessitates additional studies and evidence in clinical settings (Maier-Hein et al., 2013). The advancement in high-speed scanning laser systems is another driving force in imaging technologies that ensures more precision and efficiency in endoscopic interventions.

Traditional laser scanners have been plagued by their comparatively slow-scanning capacity, which used to create suboptimal data acquisition and reduced diagnostic precision. Technological advances in the recent past have yielded laser scanners capable of scanning at speeds greater than 1,000 times faster than traditional scanners. Such a capability to quickly scan increases the potential for real-time imaging, allowing for dynamic monitoring of anatomic structures during procedures. These technical developments in lasers not only widen the scope of applications in endoscopy but also raise great questions regarding their integration into routine clinical practice and their implications on patient outcomes and procedural efficiencies (Adam et al., 2012). Finally, the future of sophisticated imaging in endoscopy is likely to be based upon the interdisciplinary approach integrating concepts from engineering, medicine, and computational science to address existing problems. With new imaging modalities continuously emerging, an association between technological innovations and their applications in real-time surgery must be forged. To address this challenge posed by the dynamic nature of soft tissues as well as the anatomical variability inherent in patients, researchers should focus on improving registration and interpretation of advanced imaging data in real-time intraoperatively. As more and more practitioners are aware of these cutting-edge technologies, training and education programs will be needed to enable them to use the maximum benefits of these technologies, ultimately leading to improved surgical results and patient protection (Adam et al., 2012; Maier-Hein et al., 2013).

CLOSER LOOK

CLINICAL ENVIRONMENT:

The clinical environment encompasses the physical, social, and organizational settings in which healthcare is delivered. It plays a pivotal role in patient care, staff performance, and overall healthcare outcomes. A well-structured clinical environment not only facilitates safe and effective medical interventions but also supports patient comfort, staff efficiency, and adherence to professional standards.

Physically, the clinical environment includes hospitals, clinics, outpatient facilities, and specialized units such as intensive care or surgical suites. The layout, equipment, lighting, hygiene, and accessibility of these spaces directly affect the quality of care. Proper design ensures smooth workflow, minimizes cross-contamination, and allows rapid access to emergency resources. For example, clearly marked zones, organized storage of supplies, and ergonomically designed workstations reduce errors and fatigue among healthcare professionals. Infection control measures, including appropriate ventilation, hand hygiene stations, and surface disinfection protocols, are integral to maintaining a safe environment for both patients and staff.

Beyond physical infrastructure, the clinical environment encompasses organizational culture and social interactions. Effective communication, teamwork, and a supportive atmosphere are essential for patient safety and staff satisfaction. Healthcare teams rely on clear protocols, structured handovers, and interdisciplinary collaboration to coordinate care efficiently. A positive clinical culture encourages reporting of errors, continuous learning, and adherence to ethical and professional standards.

Patient-centered considerations are central to the clinical environment. Factors such as privacy, noise reduction, lighting, and patient education contribute to comfort, trust, and engagement in care. A welcoming and responsive environment can reduce anxiety, improve adherence to treatment plans, and enhance overall patient satisfaction. Furthermore, the environment must accommodate diverse patient needs, including cultural, linguistic, and accessibility considerations.

The clinical environment is also influenced by technology and digital integration. Electronic health records, monitoring systems, telemedicine platforms, and imaging devices enhance diagnostic accuracy, streamline documentation, and improve coordination. However, reliance on technology requires adequate staff training, cybersecurity measures, and ergonomic planning to prevent workflow disruption or user fatigue.

In conclusion, the clinical environment is a multifaceted setting where physical infrastructure, organizational culture, social interactions, and technological integration converge to influence healthcare delivery. Optimizing these factors is essential for patient safety, staff efficiency, and quality outcomes. By fostering a safe, supportive, and well-equipped environment, healthcare organizations can promote better clinical performance, enhance patient experiences, and ultimately improve health outcomes across diverse care settings.

REFERENCES

1. Adam, J., Ayazi, A., Brown, R., Chen, Y., et al. (2012). *Hybrid Dispersion Laser Scanner.* https://core.ac.uk/download/323077511.pdf (accessed on 15th July 2025).
2. Ahn, W., De, S., Gromski, M. A., Matthes, K., et al. (2016). *Pre-clinical training for new NOTES procedures: From ex-vivo models to virtual reality simulators.* https://core.ac.uk/download/84831131.pdf (accessed on 15th July 2025).
3. Wizenty J, Schumann T, Theil D, Stockmann M, Pratschke J, Tacke F, Aigner F, Wuensch T. Recent Advances and the Potential for Clinical Use of Autofluorescence Detection of Extra-Ophthalmic Tissues. Molecules. 2020; 25(9):2095. https://doi.org/10.3390/molecules25092095(accessed on 15th July 2025).
4. Alam, F., & Matava, C. (2022). A new virtual world? The future of immersive environments in anesthesiology. *Anesthesia & Analgesia, 135*, 230–238. https://doi.org/10.1213/ane.0000000000006118 (accessed on 15th July 2025).
5. Alexander, J. S., Ballard, D., Boktor, M., et al. (2019). *3D Printing for Bio-Synthetic Biliary Stents.* https://core.ac.uk/download/212867687.pdf (accessed on 15th July 2025).
6. M. Turan et al., "Unsupervised Odometry and Depth Learning for Endoscopic Capsule Robots," 2018 IEEE/RSJ International Conference on Intelligent Robots and Systems (IROS), Madrid, Spain, 2018, pp. 1801-1807, doi: 10.1109/IROS.2018.8593623.(accessed on 15th July 2025).
7. Ciuti, G., Caliò, R., Camboni, D., Neri, L., Bianchi, F., Arezzo, A., Koulaouzidis, A., Schostek, S., Stoyanov, D., Oddo, C. M., Magnani, B., Menciassi, A., Morino, M., Schurr, M. O., & Dario, P. (2016). Frontiers of robotic endoscopic capsules: a review. *Journal of micro-bio robotics, 11*(1), 1–18. https://doi.org/10.1007/s12213-016-0087-x(accessed on 15th July 2025).
8. Arranz, A., Desco Menéndez, M., Fresno, M., Gómez García, J., et al. (2015). *Fluorescence multi-scale endoscopy and its applications in the study and diagnosis of gastrointestinal diseases: Set-up design and software implementation.* https://core.ac.uk/download/30047495.pdf (accessed on 15th July 2025).
9. Attanasio, A., Scaglioni, B., De Momi, E., Fiorini, P., & Valdastri, P. (2020). Autonomy in surgical robotics. *Annual Review of Control Robotics and Autonomous Systems, 4*, 651–679. https://doi.org/10.1146/annurev-control-062420-090543 (accessed on 15th July 2025).
10. Aubreville, M., Bohr, C., Denzler, J., Jaremenko, C., et al. (2017). *Automatic classification of cancerous tissue in laser endomicroscopy images of the oral cavity using deep learning.* https://core.ac.uk/download/618224174.pdf (accessed on 15th July 2025).
11. Maier-Hein, L., Mountney, P., Bartoli, A., Elhawary, H., Elson, D., Groch, A., Kolb, A., Rodrigues, M., Sorger, J., Speidel, S., & Stoyanov, D. (2013). Optical techniques for 3D surface reconstruction in computer-assisted laparoscopic surgery. *Medical image analysis, 17*(8), 974–996. https://doi.org/10.1016/j.media.2013.04.003(accessed on 15th July 2025).
12. Basirun, C., Chou, J., Gao, S., Kabakova, I., et al. (2020). *Background-free fiber optic Brillouin probe for remote mapping of micromechanics.* http://arxiv.org/abs/2005.12266 (accessed on 15th July 2025).

13. Hsu, W., Baumgartner, C., Deserno, T., & Section Editors for the IMIA Yearbook Section on Sensors, Signals, and Imaging Informatics (2019). Advancing Artificial Intelligence in Sensors, Signals, and Imaging Informatics. *Yearbook of medical informatics*, *28*(1), 115–117. https://doi.org/10.1055/s-0039-1677943(accessed on 15th July 2025).

14. Bauwens, K., Blanckaert, B., De Pauw, T., Dewaele, T., et al. (2020). *A novel hybrid 3D endoscope zooming and repositioning system: Design and feasibility study.* https://core.ac.uk/download/286549295.pdf (accessed on 15th July 2025).

15. Smith, M. S., Cash, B., Konda, V., Trindade, A. J., Gordon, S., DeMeester, S., Joshi, V., Diehl, D., Ganguly, E., Mashimo, H., Singh, S., Jobe, B., McKinley, M., Wallace, M., Komatsu, Y., Thakkar, S., Schnoll-Sussman, F., Sharaiha, R., Kahaleh, M., Tarnasky, P., ... Chang, K. (2019). Volumetric laser endomicroscopy and its application to Barrett's esophagus: results from a 1,000 patient registry. *Diseases of the esophagus : official journal of the International Society for Diseases of the Esophagus*, *32*(9), doz029. https://doi.org/10.1093/dote/doz029(accessed on 15th July 2025).

16. van der Stap, N., van der Heijden, F., & Broeders, I. A. (2013). Towards automated visual flexible endoscope navigation. *Surgical endoscopy*, *27*(10), 3539–3547. https://doi.org/10.1007/s00464-013-3003-7(accessed on 15th July 2025).

17. Browning, C. M. (2022). *Seeing the big picture: System architecture trends in endoscopy and LED-based hyperspectral subsystem integration.* https://core.ac.uk/download/551575723.pdf (accessed on 15th July 2025).

18. Casso, G., Grandjean, C., Granell Gil, M., Noirez, P., et al. (2024). *Innovations to improve lung isolation training for thoracic anesthesia: A narrative review.* https://core.ac.uk/download/611830239.pdf (accessed on 15th July 2025).

19. Chalela, R., de Koning, H. J., Frille, A., Hardavella, G., et al. (2024). *How will lung cancer screening and lung nodule management change the diagnostic and surgical lung cancer landscape?* https://core.ac.uk/download/613697847.pdf (accessed on 15th July 2025).

20. Chaudhari, U., Danese, S., et al. (2024). *Artificial intelligence and Endo-Histo-OMICs: New dimensions of precision endoscopy and histology in inflammatory bowel disease.* https://core.ac.uk/download/610641563.docx (accessed on 15th July 2025).

21. Chen, Y., Dekker, E., Fockens, P., Lauwers, G. Y., et al. (2014). *Miami classification for probe-based confocal laser endomicroscopy.* https://core.ac.uk/download/28949274.pdf (accessed on 15th July 2025).

22. Cheshire, N. J. W., Desender, L., Rudarakanchana, N., Van Herzeele, I., et al. (2015). *Virtual reality simulation for the optimization of endovascular procedures: Current perspectives.* https://core.ac.uk/download/55765307.pdf (accessed on 15th July 2025).

23. Chorvat, D., Chwirot, B., Cothren, R. M., Cross, S., Curvers, W. L., et al. (2013). *Fluorescence lifetime spectroscopy of tissue autofluorescence in normal and diseased colon measured ex vivo using a fiber-optic probe.*

24. Crouser, E. D., Maier, L. A., Wilson, K. C., Bonham, C. A., Morgenthau, A. S., Patterson, K., Abston, E., et al. (2020). Diagnosis and detection of sarcoidosis: An official American Thoracic Society clinical practice guideline. *American Journal of Respiratory and Critical Care Medicine, 201*, e26–e51. https://doi.org/10.1164/rccm.202002-0251st (accessed on 15th July 2025).

25. Das, N., & Yip, M. (2017). *Robot Autonomy for Surgery.* http://arxiv.org/abs/1707.03080 (accessed on 15th July 2025).

26. Euclid Collaboration, Scognamiglio, D., Schrabback, T., Tewes, M., Gillis, B., Hoekstra, H., Huff, E., Marggraf, O., et al. (2025). *Euclid preparation LX: The use of HST images as input for weak-lensing image simulations.* https://www.semanticscholar.org/paper/aab36fa0857315e56921ad1b7b8be1a93af05981 (accessed on 15th July 2025).

27. Kaltenbach, T., Anderson, J. C., Burke, C. A., Dominitz, J. A., Gupta, S., Lieberman, D. A., Robertson, D. J., et al. (2020). *Endoscopic removal of colorectal lesions: Recommendations by the US Multi-Society Task Force on Colorectal Cancer. The American Journal of Gastroenterology, 115*, 435–464. https://doi.org/10.14309/ajg.0000000000000555 (accessed on 15th July 2025).

28. Keswani, R. N., Sethi, A., Repici, A., Messmann, H., & Chiu, P. W. Y. (2020). *How to maximize trainee education during the Coronavirus Disease-2019 pandemic: Perspectives from around the world. Gastroenterology, 159*, 26–29. https://doi.org/10.1053/j.gastro.2020.05.012 (accessed on 15th July 2025).

29. Lassen, A., Ohashi, A., de Vries, A. C., Mayinger, B., et al. (2010). *Narrow band imaging for the detection of gastric intestinal metaplasia and dysplasia during surveillance endoscopy.* https://core.ac.uk/download/18519586.pdf (accessed on 15th July 2025).

30. Leonardi, M., Robledo, K., Goldstein, S. R., Benacerraf, B. R., & Condous, G. (2020). *International survey finds majority of gynecologists are not aware of and do not utilize ultrasound techniques to diagnose and map endometriosis. Ultrasound in Obstetrics and Gynecology, 56*, 324–328. https://doi.org/10.1002/uog.21996 (accessed on 15th July 2025).

31. Liu, P., Lu, L., Zhang, J., Huo, T., Liu, S., & Ye, Z. (2021). *Application of artificial intelligence in medicine: An overview. Current Medical Science, 41*, 1105–1115. https://doi.org/10.1007/s11596-021-2474-3 (accessed on 15th July 2025).

32. Ludwin, A., & Ludwin, I. (2014). *Comparison of the ESHRE-ESGE and ASRM classifications of Müllerian duct anomalies in everyday practice.* https://core.ac.uk/download/286323237.pdf (accessed on 15th July 2025).

33. Mahmood, A., El Eraky, E., Virk, G. S., Chaudhry, M. B., Bhinder, M. A., Saleem, A., Sajawal, M., et al. (2024). The role of advanced imaging techniques in predicting cardiovascular outcomes in asymptomatic individuals: A systematic review and meta-analysis. *Journal of Advances in Medicine and Medical Research.* https://www.semanticscholar.org/paper/70e852d0d623d32c42cdaa207c0fdc17e1e7b8da (accessed on 15th July 2025).

34. Marchi, G., Mercier, M., Cefalo, J., Salerni, C., Ferioli, M., Candoli, P., Gori, L., et al. (2025). *Advanced imaging techniques and artificial intelligence in pleural diseases: A narrative review. European Respiratory Review, 34.* https://www.semanticscholar.org/paper/05f5945f0d70069ced4e332f762dfed8066a9637 (accessed on 15th July 2025).

35. Nijjar, G. S., Aulakh, S. K., Singh, R., & Chandi, S. K. (2024). *Emerging technologies in endoscopy for gastrointestinal neoplasms: A comprehensive overview. Cureus, 16.* https://www.semanticscholar.org/paper/626d6cc18681abd436bbe47d771267a89e611c42 (accessed on 15th July 2025).

36. Northup, P. G., García-Pagán, J. C., García-Tsao, G., Intagliata, N. M., Superina, R., Roberts, L. N., Lisman, T., et al. (2020). *Vascular liver disorders, portal vein thrombosis, and procedural bleeding in patients with liver disease: 2020 practice guidance by the American Association*

for the Study of Liver Diseases. Hepatology, 73, 366–413. https://doi.org/10.1002/hep.31646 (accessed on 15th July 2025).

37. Serna, A. ., & Prieto, F (2017). *Hacia el modelado 3D de tumores cerebrales mediante endoneurosonografía y redes neuronales.* Towards a 3D modeling of brain tumors by using endoneurosonography and neural networks*

38. Revista Ingenierías Universidad de Medellín, vol. 16, no. 30, pp. 129-148, 2017 (accessed on 15th July 2025).

39. Robles-Medranda, C., Verpalen, I., Schulz, D., & Spadaccini, M. (2025). *Artificial intelligence in biliopancreatic disorders: Applications in cross-imaging and endoscopy. Gastroenterology.* https://www.semanticscholar.org/paper/7cb1ac77dd384794e6b1763af4012e6c028dd7f5 (accessed on 15th July 2025).

40. Tontini, G., Neumann, H., & Rath, T. (2016). *Advanced gastrointestinal endoscopic imaging for inflammatory bowel diseases.* https://core.ac.uk/download/237177058.pdf (accessed on 15th July 2025).

41. van der Sommen, F., Curvers, W. L., & Nagengast, W. B. (2018). Novel developments in endoscopic mucosal imaging. *Gastroenterology, 154*, 1876–1886. https://doi.org/10.1053/j.gastro.2018.01.070 (accessed on 15th July 2025).

42. Van Ness, G., & Widenhorn, R. (2012). *Engaging the community through an undergraduate biomedical physics course.* https://core.ac.uk/download/37772889.pdf (accessed on 15th July 2025).

43. Zhang, S., Liu, Y., Liao, W., Tan, R. R. Z., Bi, R., & Olivo, M. (2024). *Ex vivo tissue classification using broadband hyperspectral imaging endoscopy and artificial intelligence: A pilot study. IEEE Sensors Journal, 24*, 24737–24749. https://www.semanticscholar.org/paper/1f637894b909d33e7ee09ba1b8bc5c675dd38def (accessed on 15th July 2025).

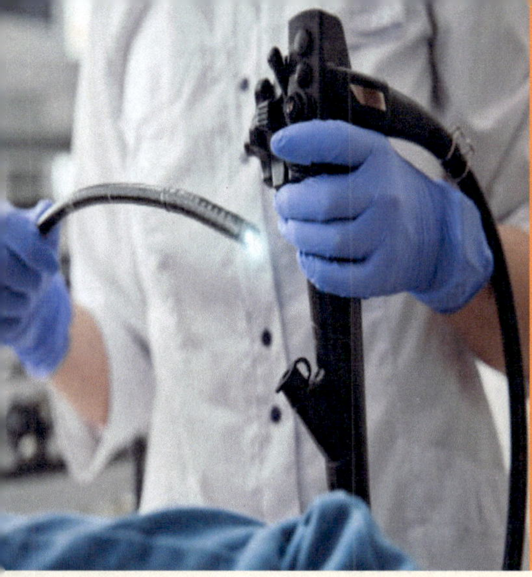

Chapter 13

PEDIATRIC ENDOSCOPY

Contents

Introduction....375
13.1. Historical Background....378
13.2. Types of Pediatric Endoscopy....381
13.3. Indications for Pediatric Endoscopy....385
13.4. Preparation for Pediatric Endoscopy....388
13.5. Risks and Complications....391
13.6. Advances in Pediatric Endoscopy....394
Summary....399
References....402

Introduction

Pediatric endoscopy is now a standard part of modern pediatric medicine, providing minimally invasive methods for the diagnosis and treatment of many gastrointestinal diseases in children. In addition to minimizing the bodily trauma normally incurred with traditional surgical interventions, it also enables quicker recovery times and shorter hospital stays. As more is known about children's unique anatomical and physiological differences, the need for advanced endoscopic techniques for this specific age group becomes increasingly necessary. Pediatric endoscopy covers the whole range of procedures, including but not limited to, esophagogastroduodenoscopy, colonoscopy, and endoscopic retrograde cholangiopancreatography, each for particular clinical problems and with the highest consideration for the safety and comfort of pediatric patients. The evolution of pediatric endoscopy has been strongly facilitated by cross-disciplinary collaboration and technological advancements. Innovations , such as high-definition imaging, flexible scopes, and improved sedation techniques have transformed the landscape of gastrointestinal diagnosis and treatment among children. Moreover, increased emphasis on human-centered design in health systems acknowledges the importance of understanding the special needs and experiences of pediatric patients and their families. This is not only intended to improve procedural efficiency but also to develop a supportive environment that addresses emotional as well as psychological dimensions pertaining to medical procedures. For this to be effective, stakeholders must be engaged from the beginning, bringing clinical practice into congruence with the multifaceted stressors that pediatric populations experience, thus promoting improved patient outcomes and satisfaction (Melles et al., 2020).

A second critical realm for pediatric endoscopy is its role within the broader framework of precision medicine. Since the last decade, precision medicine has developed as a significant paradigm for tailoring healthcare to the unique biological and clinical characteristics of the patient. Such tailoring is particularly pertinent in the treatment of inflammatory bowel diseases (IBD), which is more and more of a concern in children. Knowledge of the various presentations of IBD in children requires an astute understanding of disease trajectory, susceptibility, and treatment response, thus validating research and clinical needs. Using prospective cohort studies to identify precision markers and the integration of multi-omics data, pediatric endoscopy can help contribute to more effective, tailored interventions that hold potential for improved health outcomes in this vulnerable population (Denson et al., 2019). These advances are not only technological in nature but also reflect a paradigm shift towards improved and more empathetic child healthcare (Figure 13.1).

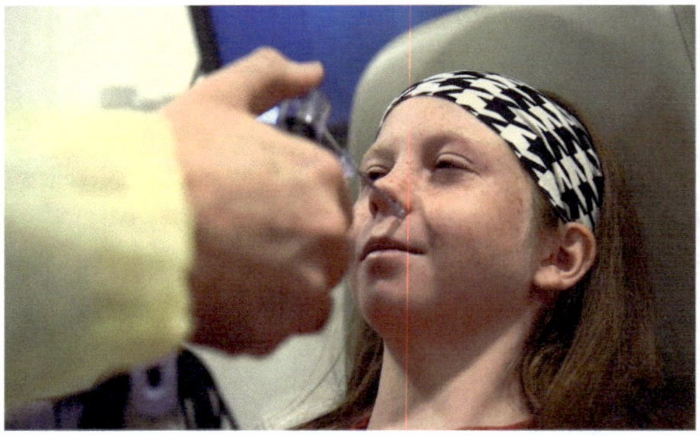

Figure 13.1. Pediatric endoscopy.

Source: https://i1.ytimg.com/vi/3EgwrpV8ygg/maxresdefault.jpg.

Definition of Pediatric Endoscopy

Pediatric endoscopy is a sub-specialist medical intervention that involves the use of an endoscope to investigate and intervene in the gastrointestinal and respiratory tree of children. This technique is worth its weight in gold in the diagnosis of a host of conditions, from gastrointestinal illness to respiratory irregularity. The term pediatric endoscopy encompasses more than mere visualization; therapeutic interventions that may be done in conjunction with such an evaluation, like biopsies, dilations, and removals of foreign bodies, are all included. The rising prevalence of conditions requiring such procedures accentuates the need for understanding the procedural nuances of pediatric endoscopy in light of children's and adults' differing anatomy and physiology. Pediatric endoscopy is therefore not merely a definitive investigative tool but also utilized as a focused therapy for various conditions in children. Following the multidisciplinary care principles, pediatric endoscopy is useful for conditions that are multifaceted in nature, such as in specialized clinics called aerodigestive clinics. Aerodigestive clinics are a coordinated strategy where different medical and surgical teams work in unison to provide total assessments and treatments. For instance, in a 2021 Israeli study, it was determined that a large number of pediatric patients presenting at an aerodigestive clinic underwent extensive testing using triple endoscopy, flexible bronchoscopy and gastroscopy which were combined to manage associated pulmonary and gastrointestinal disorders (Gendler et al., 2021). This combined approach recognizes the imperative of multifaceted care models in pediatric endoscopy, accepting that children with aerodigestive illness can benefit immensely from coordinated care pathways, which ultimately translate to better patient outcomes and parental satisfaction. In addition to therapeutic and diagnostic purposes, an important aspect of pediatric endoscopy is the careful preparation required to guarantee optimal outcomes and comfort for the patient. Bowel preparation, though, is most significant, as good bowel cleansing significantly enhances visualization and reduces contamination hazards during the procedure. Research has established that the use of care bundles can improve the quality of bowel preparation, lowering anxiety in patients and improving family satisfaction with the hospital process (Abd-Elmageed et al., 2020). This is to highlight that pediatric endoscopy does not merely entail technical proficiency at the time of procedure but requires taking into account before factors influencing overall patient experience and outcome. Hence, the definition of pediatric endoscopy must cover both the procedural and preparatory components to appreciate its place in pediatric care.

Importance in Pediatric Medicine

The significance of pediatric medicine is found in its unique challenges and demands, which are significantly different from those of adults, particularly those involving gastrointestinal disease in need of pediatric endoscopy. Unlike adult patients, children tend to have a myriad of disorders that can be best treated with specialized care and diagnostic examinations. Pediatric endoscopy provides an important tool for diagnosing diseases such as gastrointestinal bleeding, malabsorption, and inflammatory bowel disease. With minimally invasive techniques, they significantly enhance the safety and efficacy of diagnosis in pediatric patients. Ultimately, the unique training of medical professionals in this area is required to treat the subtle physiological variations that present in children to ensure better outcomes. Through continuous development of pediatric endoscopy, its use becomes increasingly important in bridging the gap in complete care for young patients who suffer from gastrointestinal pathology. Besides, pediatric endoscopy is a significant diagnostic modality for early diagnosis of conditions that, if left to be diagnosed later on, can lead to severe health complications. For instance, timely intervention for gastrointestinal bleeding prevents severe anemia and other resultant conditions from arising, significantly improving the quality of life of a child. Another equally valuable role is in the surveillance of children at risk of having malignancies, allowing for effective management interventions. The adoption of cutting-edge methods like video capsule endoscopy into pediatric facilities is an example of the devotion to enhancing diagnostic powers. Pediatric gastroenterologists must undergo thorough training in these practices, particularly as innovations and technologies surge forward. To lead the way in these practices is not only to advance individual care but to further the entire field of pediatric medicine. By setting higher standards and raising expectations, the medical world advances. Finally, the worth of pediatric endoscopy is also amplified in terms of the emotional and developmental character of child care. Medical procedure dread and anxiety can be particularly challenging for young patients, and therefore the efforts of compassionate medical caregivers are critical. Pediatric endoscopists must not only be technically proficient but also in creating a reassuring environment for kids and their families. This calls for knowledge of child psychology and good communication with both young patients and their guardians. Additionally, training courses need to emphasize emotional intelligence and the art of communication in addition to procedural skills to support well-rounded patient care. In this context, the act of pediatric endoscopy is not merely a technical practice; it is a promise to understand and fulfill children's diverse requirements within the medical setting for healthy healthcare outcomes (Figure 13.2).

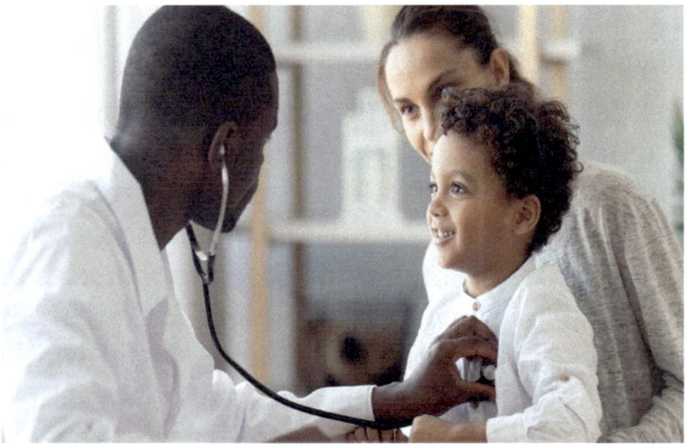

Figure 13.2. Importance in pediatric medicine.

Source: https://www.waldenu.edu/media/5390/seo-2158-bs-african-american-pediatrician-353293868-1200x675.

13.1. Historical Background

The history of pediatric endoscopy has followed a sequence of technological advancements and the refinement of clinical skills. The earliest history of endoscopic therapy can be traced to the middle of the 20th century, when physicians first began exploring the gastrointestinal tract with crude devices. These initial efforts provided the background for subsequent innovation towards flexible endoscopes, which became widely available in the 1970s. The realization that these devices could be adapted for use among children transformed the discipline, as pediatric patients most commonly require diverse considerations due to their unique anatomical and physiological characteristics. Pediatric endoscopes were specifically then became developed, and this was a breakthrough method in diagnosing as well as treating gastrointestinal ailments among children, thus forming the basis on which modern pediatric endoscopy is established. Greater availability of advanced imaging technology has propelled pediatric endoscopy practice even further. Advances in imaging modalities , such as high-definition visualization and the development of miniature scopes, have increased the precision of procedures. Not only did these advances enhance diagnostic accuracy, but procedure-related risks were also minimized, generating a safer operating environment for both practitioners and patients. Along with the creation of sedation techniques tailored specifically to pediatric populations, physicians are now in a position to perform complex procedures with increased comfort and safety for the child. This convergence of technology and pharmacologic advancement is part of a larger pattern seen in pediatrics, as ongoing research contributes to best practice daily, representing a commitment to providing effective and safe care to children. As we look into the future of pediatric endoscopy, it is increasingly important to view the larger landscape of data science and machine learning in this subspecialty. The emergence of Surgical Data Science (SDS) has begun revolutionizing how surgical procedures, such as endoscopic procedures, are performed. With an eye to data capture, organization, and analysis, SDS is intended to enhance the quality of interventional care by facilitating informed decision-making and outcomes. Translational success has been limited to date in surgical applications, although attempts to continue developing data analytics and standardizing protocols hold out the potential for greater incorporation of these technologies into practice. As the field evolves further, it is likely to provide vital data on pediatric endoscopy to inform advancements that enhance procedural efficacy and patient safety through evidence-based measures informed by empirical data (Hein et al., 2021; Hoang et al., 2022).

13.1.1. Development of Endoscopic Techniques

The development of endoscopic techniques has transformed the practice of pediatric medicine in such a way that there are minimally invasive procedures that enhance diagnostic and therapeutic capabilities. Classically, operations tended to be with large incisions and prolonged convalescence, particularly in children, who have alternate physiology and anatomy to adults. Endoscopic technology has permitted a shift toward more refined techniques, less physical trauma, and attendant postoperative complications. Technologies , such as VATS and flexible endoscopes have enhanced procedures , such as bronchoscopies, gastrointestinal evaluations, and laparoscopic surgeries, to be more efficient and safer for children. In addition to upgrading clinical outcomes, such technologies also make the family and patient experience better by reducing hospitalization and anxiety. New technologies keep upgrading endoscopic procedures to unlock new fields of use in pediatric medicine. For instance, capsule endoscopy (CE) has dramatically changed the evaluation of the gastrointestinal tract, particularly for the detection of conditions , such as Crohn's disease and gastrointestinal bleeding. Developed in 2000, CE employs a swallowable pill with a camera that photographs as it travels through the gastrointestinal tract, especially useful in pediatric patients who may not be compliant with traditional endoscopic examination. This non-invasive method offers anesthetic-free options without the use of anesthesia, minimizing patient discomfort. Additionally, with ongoing developments in CE technology, like increased image resolution and battery longevity, more complete evaluations of gastrointestinal ailments can be achieved. More innovation is required to transcend its limitations, like the inability to take biopsies, thereby further streamlining the diagnostic process and firming its place in pediatric endoscopy. The integration of artificial intelligence (AI) into endoscopic practice is a promising advance that can facilitate diagnostic accuracy and procedural success. AI software can be employed to assist with image analysis, providing real-time assistance in endoscopy by identifying abnormalities more effectively than current practice. The technology is particularly valuable for pediatric endoscopy since the early identification of disease can substantially determine the outcome of treatment and the patient's general health. In addition, AI can further be tapped to improve procedural training, i.e., visualization and navigation can be simpler in complex situations. With ongoing developments in pediatric endoscopy, the interaction of newer technology with established techniques is bound to lead to significant improvements in safety and efficiency, ultimately favoring pediatric patients and expanding the extent of endoscopic applications in this vital area of healthcare.

13.1.2. Milestones in Pediatric Endoscopy

The history of pediatric endoscopy stands as the pinnacle of deeper technological developments in medical interventions, particularly in minimal access surgery (MAS). New technologies that entail the development of specialized instruments and techniques exclusively tailored for pediatric patients now allow physicians to have less intervention with shorter recovery times and little post-operative pain. Miniaturization of the equipment and robot-assisted surgery have revolutionized pediatric surgery to make complex procedures that were once deemed too risky for children possible. Encouraging the multidisciplinary approach that unites pediatric surgeons, anesthesiologists, and new technologies, the specialty has made use of the latest technologies in anesthesia monitoring to ensure increased patient safety and successful outcomes of procedures. The continuous development of these technologies will be the impetus for greater optimization of MAS and pediatric endoscopy, hence translating to improved outcomes in vulnerable populations (Pelizzo et al., 2024). Besides, point-of-care (POC) technologies have been indispensable allies in the progression of diagnostic capability in pediatric endoscopy. The integration of microneedle sensors that facilitate non-invasive access to an enormous set of biomarkers illustrates the power of advanced engineering in helping personalize medicine for pediatric patients. They provide real-time feedback during diagnosis and minimize the pain felt by child patients, thus enhancing their overall clinical experience. Lab-on-a-microneedle platforms that utilize varied sensing techniques represent a leap towards faster and more accurate diagnostics for pediatric care. This paradigm shift not only allows physicians to optimize treatment strategies but also produces innovations in non-invasive monitoring essential to the care of chronic child diseases. The future of pediatric endoscopy will largely rely on such technologies, bringing together precision medicine and enhanced procedural techniques (Hu et al., 2024). The turning points in pediatric endoscopy do not involve merely the advancement in surgical techniques but the necessity of continuing research and the establishment of dedicated equipment. Recognizing the reality that the majority of pediatric diseases are peculiar and often complex, there is an increasing necessity for specialized devices that are made to be safe and effective in endoscopic procedures. This need is emphasized by challenges in developing orphan devices that are necessary for rare childhood diseases, but are rendered complicated by regulatory and financial constraints. As noted, optimization of pediatric anesthesia is equally important, as enhancing monitoring technologies makes a significant contribution towards overall operation safety. It is through collaborative efforts by clinicians, researchers, and engineers that such shortcomings ought to be addressed so that not only technically, pediatric endoscopy improves, but also in a manner that takes into account the uniqueness of children as patients so that improved health outcomes are enhanced (Pelizzo et al., 2024) (Figure 13.3).

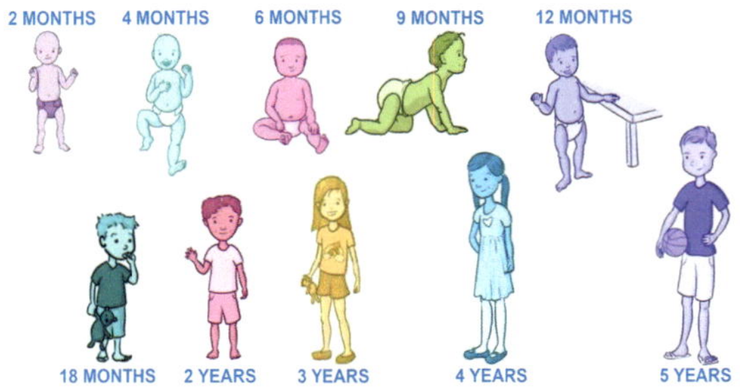

Figure 13.3. Milestones in pediatric endoscopy.

Source: https://d16qt3wv6xm098.cloudfront.net/VpdWLjRCRIirBEr7cARbM4QsQKiugNA_/_.jpg.

13.1.3. Evolution of Equipment and Technology

The evolution of technology and equipment in pediatric endoscopy has revolutionized the landscape of gastrointestinal diagnosis and treatment. With evolutionary improvements in high-definition imaging and pediatric-specific equipment, the potential to evaluate and treat a wide array of gastrointestinal diseases in children has been significantly enhanced. These advances are particularly significant in the context of the complexity of pediatric anatomy and physiology. The development of non-invasive technologies, such as the wireless capsule endoscopy, has also enhanced the approach towards managing gastrointestinal diseases like Crohn's disease and ulcerative colitis. Mucosal healing, the perfect result, is now made more possible with the use of the new device that allows detailed visualization of the gut, making the entire management easier and pediatric endoscopy a safer option (Sara et al., 2024). In addition, implementation of unsedated transnasal endoscopy is another advancement emphasizing both safety and efficiency in the management of children. With this state-of-the-art approach gaining traction, it has numerous benefits over traditional sedation-based techniques, including reduced risk from anesthesia, particularly in younger patients requiring more than one procedure. Both adult and pediatric success with sedation-free endoscopy is proven by a structured system of specialty training and integration of emerging technologies.

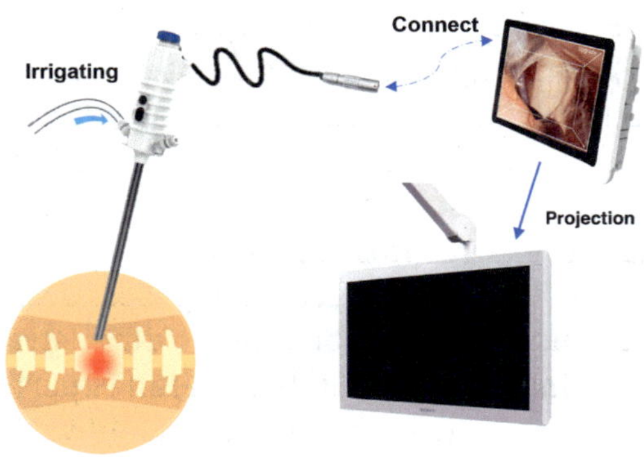

Figure 13.4. Evolution of equipment and technology.

Source: https://pub.mdpi-res.com/bioengineering/bioengineering-11-00099/article_deploy/html/images/bioengineering-11-00099-g001.png?1705892588.

These techniques, along with distraction interventions like Virtual Reality Systems, are employed to developmentally prepare children and make them at ease during procedures. With the solution of the special requirements of pediatric patients, unsedated endoscopy is paving the way for more accessible and secure diagnostic techniques (Friedlander et al., 2024). Further, the relentless innovation of endoscopic equipment not only targets diagnostic purposes but also places great emphasis on improving treatment methods for gastrointestinal disease complications. Therapeutic endoscopy has now progressed to where strictures and potential malignancies of inflammatory bowel diseases can now be treated effectively in pediatric patients. High-definition endoscopic equipment and methods , such as chromoendoscopy, significantly enhance dysplasia detection, allowing clinicians to make more accurate decisions regarding management of the patient. As pediatric endoscopy evolves alongside technical innovation, these innovations are an extension of the horizon for therapeutic options, ultimately translating to improvement in global health outcomes in children with complex gastrointestinal disease (Sara et al., 2024) (Figure 13.4).

13.2. Types of Pediatric Endoscopy

Pediatric endoscopy encompasses a variety of minimally invasive medical interventions to look at and treat illnesses of the internal systems of children. Some of the most common methods used are gastrointestinal, respiratory, and urinary endoscopies. Gastrointestinal endoscopy in the shape of esophagogastroduodenoscopy (EGD) and colonoscopy allows direct visualization of the esophagus, stomach, and intestines, which makes diagnosis and therapeutic interventions possible for gastroesophageal reflux disease or inflammatory bowel disease. These procedures have seen numerous advances as technology improves, having enhanced efficacy and safety in children. The addition of audiovisual distraction techniques, including virtual reality and animated videos, has positively influenced the experience of the procedure by reducing anxiety and pain (Ramdhanie et al., 2024). Therefore, the benefits of pediatric endoscopy extend beyond the diagnostic value, as it also improves the overall care experience, particularly for children who are more sensitive to medical interventions. Another significant type of pediatric endoscopy is airway endoscopy, which has a critical role in the assessment and management of laryngeal airway diseases. Abnormalities of the larynx , such as congenital defects, infections, or tumors, may significantly affect a child's ability to breathe freely. Techniques , such as flexible laryngoscopy enable direct evaluation of airway obstruction and symptomatology evaluation in a clinical setting. Rigid bronchoscopy can be used when a more accurate evaluation is needed, enabling practitioners to classify conditions , such as laryngeal clefts accordingly (Xu, 2023). These diagnostic methods are not just of considerable utility in establishing a correct diagnosis, but can also be employed to guide treatment protocols that may entail nonoperative care or endoscopic surgical repair, based on the extent of findings. Such advances in pediatric airway management significantly improve postoperative outcomes and quality of life in such patients. Lastly, the urologic endoscopy plays a vital role in the management of pediatric urinary tract disorders. Ureteroscopy and cystoscopy are common procedures performed to assess for recurrent urinary tract infection or anatomical abnormalities. With these procedures, the ureters and bladder may be visualized and targeted interventions like stone fragmentation or tumor resection can be done. As with airway and gastrointestinal endoscopy, pediatric urologic endoscopy has also focused on maximizing safety and minimizing discomfort. Miniaturized equipment, as well as the use of sedation protocols tailored for children, are central to an improved procedural experience (Ramdhanie et al., 2024). Together, these various types of pediatric endoscopy point to the importance of minimally invasive techniques in the diagnosis and treatment of a wide variety of conditions and ultimately in the improvement of children's health outcomes in much of medicine.

13.2.1. Gastrointestinal Endoscopy

Gastrointestinal tests, when considered in terms of pediatric endoscopy, have progressed significantly over the past several decades. As pointed out, in Korea, pediatric patients have undergone gastrointestinal and colonic endoscopy procedures for over 30 years, and there exists an aggregation of abundant knowledge and experience in the field (Lee, 2022). Difficulty still exists, however, in breaking through the misperception among patients and guardians regarding what exactly endoscopic procedures are. The majority of individuals perceive endoscopy as an uncommon and dangerous intervention, which can result in delaying diagnosis and treatment. This conservatism is further exaggerated in the context of more invasive interventions, such as percutaneous endoscopic gastrostomy (PEG), making educational outreach even more imperative for enhanced appreciation of gastrointestinal endoscope role in pediatrics. Sedation practices form an integral part of pediatric gastrointestinal endoscopy, with a direct bearing on the success of procedures and on patients' comfort. Sedation administration plays an immense role in the overall experience for kids since they have variable physiology and psychological demands compared to adults. Practice now suggests two general approaches: the need for an anesthesiologist while using general anesthesia and procedural sedation, which can be administered by a gastroenterologist (Lightdale, 2013). The selection of the most appropriate method of sedation is based on a fine balance between patient protection, maximizing procedural efficacy, and preserving cost-effectiveness. With continued developments in research, it is essential to assess the associated risks and benefits of child-specific sedation protocols for gastrointestinal endoscopy to maximize overall results. The application of pediatric gastrointestinal endoscopy not only allows for diagnosis but also therapeutic uses, thus changing the face of pediatric gastroenterology. The more the value of the procedures becomes appreciated, the faster there is a tendency towards implementing endoscopic techniques into general pediatric care. This is a detailed understanding of the procedural indications, techniques, and situational context in which these treatments are performed, as seen in the Korean experience (Lee, 2022). This harmonization must be multi-disciplinary in nature, including not just gastroenterologists but also surgeons and anesthesiologists, to develop an integrated program that does all it can to cater to the patients' well-being. Through optimizing collaborative practice and medical education, healthcare practitioners can also increase the availability of gastrointestinal endoscopy, eventually increasing diagnostic and therapeutic effectiveness in children (Figure 13.5).

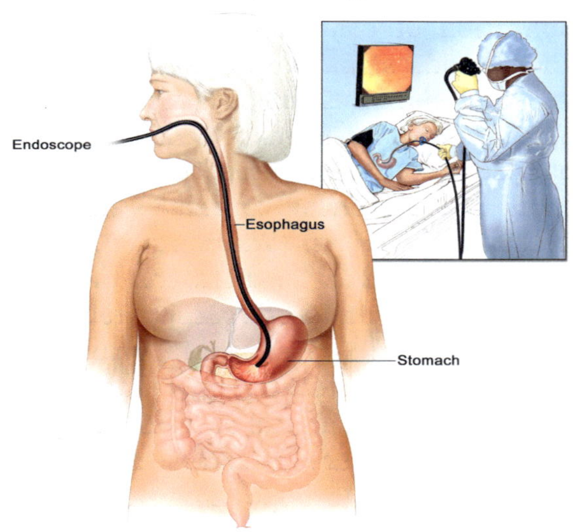

Figure 13.5. Gastrointestinal endoscopy.

Source: https://nci-media.cancer.gov/pdq/media/images/433287.jpg.

13.2.2. Bronchoscopy

Bronchoscopy is a key procedure in pediatric endoscopy practice, applied primarily to diagnose and treat various airway conditions in children. The technique gives direct visualization of the tracheobronchial tree and allows for identification of pathology like foreign bodies, strictures, or congenital anomalies. In children, particularly those with preexisting respiratory disease, bronchoscopy is a critical intervention for the removal of aspirated foreign bodies and the relief of airway obstruction that, in this vulnerable group, can be fatal. Moreover, the role of bronchoscopy is not limited to immediate therapy; it plays a similar critical role in preoperative assessment to enable appropriate preparation of children for other operations. With advancements in technology, bronchoscopy has been enhanced with enhanced visualization and treatment modalities utilized during the procedure. The significant role of bronchoscopy in the treatment of tracheobronchial anomalies is even more vital in managing patients with tracheobronchial anomalies. For example, children with left pulmonary artery sling (PAS) usually present with significant tracheal stenosis that is a challenge to surgical treatment. Here, bronchoscopy provides invaluable information on the anatomy and physiology of the airway. This information guides surgical planning and, hence, subsequent interventions. As noted, bronchoscopy is vital in the follow-up of congenitally abnormal heart and tracheobronchial involvement, as they tend to have complications that require serial endoscopy. The interprofessional care of such patients highlights the synergy between endoscopic and surgical experts with a focus on the roles of bronchoscopy in maximizing outcomes in pediatric patients with airway difficulty (Porcedda et al., 2019). Moreover, the fact that bronchoscopy can now be developed and used as an initial treatment for children reinforces the need for expertise in training and generating guidelines addressing the anatomical and physiological characteristics of children. The revised practice guidelines emphasize proper management of the challenging airway of children and project potential challenges for practitioners in conducting bronchoscopy. Application of more advanced techniques , such as balloon dilation and stent placement, indicates the progress of bronchoscopy as a versatile tool in airway management. As bronchoscopy keeps expanding its applications in pediatric care, ongoing research and collaboration among specialists are essential to further optimize best practices and patient outcomes and safety (Apfelbaum et al., 2021). These advances ensure that bronchoscopy is not just a diagnostic procedure, but also an essential component of advanced pediatric endoscopy (Figure 13.6).

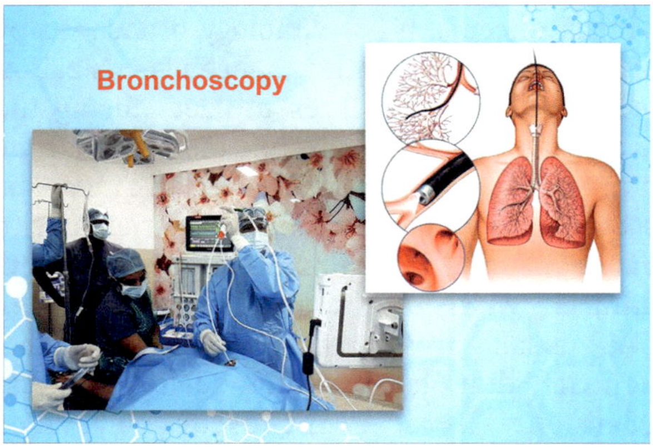

Figure 13.6. Bronchoscopy is an essential procedure.

Source: https://www.srijayamchestclinic.com/images/services/bronchoscopy.jpg.

13.2.3. Ureteroscopy

Ureteroscopy has emerged as an essential intervention in the management of urological disorders of children, particularly stone disease and obstructions of the ureters. The procedure allows for direct visualization of the ureter and renal pelvis and facilitates diagnosis as well as removal of too-large stones that cannot be dealt with conservatively. Compared to older methods like ESWL, ureteroscopy is a more focused intervention, one significant in children who could have unique anatomy to account for. The need for productive modalities of treatment is brought to attention by the increasing incidence of pediatric nephrolithiasis, and it is at this juncture that clinicians seek efficient ways of eliminating hospitalization and ensuring recovery. Through adopting ureteroscopy, healthcare practitioners can facilitate minimal invasiveness and fewer postoperative complications, in tandem with the overall goals of pediatric endoscopy for ensuring safe and effective solutions for younger patients. Although it has its advantages, pediatric ureteroscopy is not without difficulty and risk that need to be considered in detail. Postprocedural complications of ureteral injury, infection, and obstruction are particularly significant concerns, given children's anatomical and physiological differences from adults. Recent evidence indicates that, although complications following modern ureteroscopy are normally low, careful preoperative workup is crucial to minimize risks. Outcome determinants consist of stone size and location, as well as the surgical technique used. There is evidence that the application of contemporary ureteroscopes and methods significantly enhances success rates and minimizes complications. Therefore, ongoing research remains to be done to further optimize ureteroscopy practice so that it still adapts to the evolving context of endoscopic treatment in children (Wagenius et al., 2021; Matos et al., 2023). Furthermore, there have been advances in ureteroscopy technology with resultant more advanced visualization and instrument technology that directly impacts pediatric surgical success. Integration of flexible ureteroscopes and laser lithotripsy gives surgeons the opportunity to carefully perform procedures with higher precision, resulting in radically enhanced stone-free rates among children. These advances are particularly relevant given the multidisciplinary presentation typical in pediatric cases, where successful application entails interventional cooperation between urologists, anesthesiologists, and pediatricians. The increasing application of ureteroscopy is a testament to the transition towards more individualized medicine, with treatments specially tailored for child patients. Continuous monitoring of technique and outcome will be essential in propelling advancements in pediatric ureteroscopy, establishing its place as an integral component of pediatric endoscopy (Wagenius et al., 2021; Matos et al., 2023).

13.3. Indications for Pediatric Endoscopy

The indications for endoscopy in children have gained more attention, particularly due to the complexity of conditions in children. Obstructive sleep apnea (OSA) is one of the primary conditions requiring endoscopy in children because it greatly impairs a child's quality of life. Drug-induced sleep endoscopy (DISE) has emerged as a critical diagnostic modality in this context as a way whereby physicians can dynamically visualize airway obstruction. A notable trend is increased focus on the pediatric application of DISE, prompted by the development of specialized sedation protocols that ensure patient safety and procedural efficiency. Increased accuracy in these techniques maximizes diagnostic capability, facilitating improved treatment protocols while minimizing potential complications arising from airway management in children. With growing evidence for the use of DISE, pediatric endoscopy is also indicative of the move toward more individualized, personalized approaches to the treatment of airway disease (Xiao et al., 2025). Besides OSA, another highly significant indication for pediatric endoscopy is the evaluation of children with craniofacial deformities or congenital conditions , such as Down syndrome. These children tend to have upper airway obstructions due to anatomical distortions. With endoscopic procedures, physicians can identify specific areas of collapse and thus direct what future surgical corrections can be performed. In particular, DISE has been essential in assessing those complex patients with unique airway problems, establishing a template for subsequent surgical corrections that can substantially maximize respiratory function. Global opinion of sleep apnea experts online reflected an excellent level of agreement regarding the utility of DISE in the respective patient group, with the vast majority deeming it a first-line diagnostic tool following adenotonsillectomy in the presence of residual OSA symptoms. The sanctions emphasize the importance of individualizing endoscopic examinations to the respective needs of pediatric patients with different anatomical parameters (Iannella et al., 2024). Finally, pediatric endoscopy is a significant diagnostic and therapeutic option for gastrointestinal pathology, especially in those children presenting with chronic abdominal pain or gastrointestinal hemorrhage. Endoscopic examination in these patients may diagnose conditions , such as inflammatory bowel disease, structural defects, or even malignancy. By direct visualization of the gastrointestinal tract, diagnostic yield is enhanced and therapy is directed. As new endoscopic technology becomes available, such as the possibility of conducting therapeutic interventions in the same session, the potential for pediatric endoscopy grows. The routine integration of endoscopy into pediatric care not only stresses its diagnostic importance but also underscores its ability to successfully treat numerous gastrointestinal diseases. Therefore, as more pediatricians are utilizing endoscopic techniques, implications for patient outcomes and patient care are becoming progressively profound (Xiao et al., 2025) (Figure 13.7).

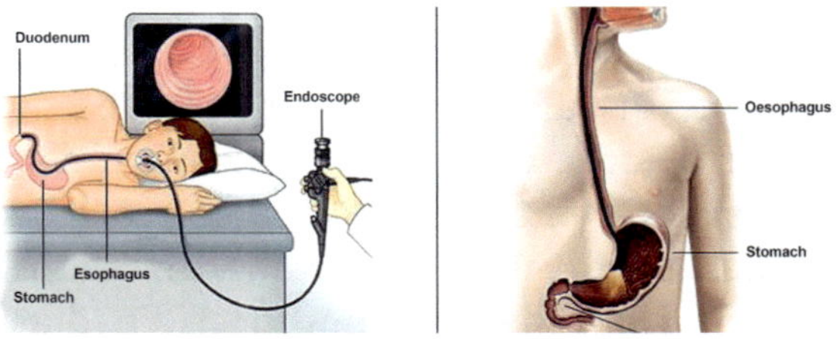

Figure 13.7. Indications for pediatric endoscopy have garnered increased attention.

Source: https://drsamitjain.com/images/services/pediatric-endoscopy1.jpg.

13.3.1. Diagnostic Purposes

Pediatric endoscopy plays a critical role in diagnostic applications, particularly in diagnosing gastrointestinal conditions that can adversely affect a child's health. Children's intricate anatomy and unique physiological responses demand precise diagnostic equipment to assess symptoms and inherent conditions accurately. For instance, gastrointestinal illnesses , such as chronic intestinal pseudo-obstruction (CIPO) possess non-specific symptoms that are apt to be delayed, leading to sudden health complications. As seen in recent works, an integrated process that involves radiology, endoscopy, and lab tests allows for improved diagnosis of CIPO and other gastrointestinal conditions. This pluralistic diagnostic procedure recognizes the role of pediatric endoscopy as not only elucidating the etiology of the signs but also pointing clinicians towards effective therapeutic interventions. Also, pediatric endoscopy serves as a vital diagnostic tool for OSA when conventional management fails. The role of DISE in the diagnosis of tongue-base obstruction, a frequent complication after adenoidectomy and tonsillectomy in children, has now been highlighted by a systematic review. By mimicking a sleep state, DISE provides irreplaceable information on sites of obstruction, and it is feasible to carry out targeted surgical interventions. The reliability of DISE in identifying and mapping obstructions underscores its crucial position in refining diagnoses and tailoring management plans for children with chronic OSA. With the rising popularity of surgical treatment of conditions like tongue-base obstruction, the specificity of diagnosis presented by endoscopic procedures becomes even more important. In addition to diagnosing specific conditions, pediatric endoscopy facilitates disease monitoring and observing reactions to therapy. The visualization of the gastrointestinal tract allows for real-time assessment and strategic modification of therapeutic protocols. In the case of CIPO, where understanding of gastrointestinal motility is optimal, endoscopic evaluation is capable of determining the effectiveness of medical treatment and surgery. This adaptability of diagnosis and treatment is representative of the unifying role that endoscopy plays in managing complex pediatric conditions. In conclusion, pediatric endoscopy is an important device in the diagnostic arsenal, complementing clinicians' capacity to provide comprehensive care that is tailor-made for each child, thereby maximizing overall health outcomes.

13.3.2. Therapeutic Interventions

Therapeutic interventions in pediatric endoscopy are progressively becoming of vital importance in the treatment of gastrointestinal pathology, particularly in children with multisystem disorders. The use of endoscopic techniques extends beyond the limits of mere diagnostics; they are therapeutic measures with the potential to greatly enhance a child's quality of life. Therapies , such as polypectomy in the child with familial adenomatous polyposis or balloon dilation of strictures can be performed effectively with endoscopy. Such procedures not only minimize the need for open operations but also allow for quicker recovery and lower risks associated with general anesthesia. Advanced procedural techniques and pediatric-specific equipment ensure the effectiveness and safety of such interventions, ensuring good results in an age group with its own unique set of physiological differences from adults. Another consideration to hold in mind in endoscopic therapeutic interventions is the multidisciplinary character with mutual collaboration among specialists like pediatric gastroenterologists, surgeons, and anesthesiologists. Such collaboration is required in creating individualized treatment plans, considering the unique anatomical and physiological considerations of children. Particularly, endoscopic retrograde cholangiopancreatography (ERCP) is one of the procedures that requires special skill due to variation in disease presentation, as biliary atresia does not present similarly in children and adults. The meeting point of specialties sees risks minimized and the child gets concentrated care focused on his or her specific condition.

Continuous technological improvements and skill development, combined with increased pediatric education, further underscore the importance of a multidisciplinary approach to achieving therapeutic benefit. Psychological and social factors also play significant roles in the therapeutic interventions associated with pediatric endoscopy. Children presenting for gastrointestinal procedures are often stressed and apprehensive, further complicating treatment adherence and recovery. Resolution of such psychological problems in the form of pre-procedure advice and counseling may maximize the procedural process for patient and family. Additionally, open communication regarding the procedures and probable outcomes maximizes post-procedure adherence and satisfaction with medical care generally. As pediatric medicine increasingly becomes interwoven with an understanding of the psychosocial milieu, it is clear that successful therapeutic practice will need to be holistic. Such an approach not only assaults physical well-being but also seeks to foster emotional health in children with challenges related to gastrointestinal illness, thereby offering a more integrated approach to patient management in pediatric endoscopy.

13.3.3. Management of Congenital Anomalies

Management of congenital anomalies in children needs a multi-pronged approach that tackles early detection, family-focused treatment, and access to expert care. Congenital malformations, like those seen in genital and circulatory systems, typically require early treatment to minimize the health and quality-of-life impact over many years. In pediatric endoscopy, endoscopic interventions or laparoscopies can be pivotal diagnostic and therapeutic procedures in managing symptomatic malformations. For instance, early diagnosis through endoscopic measures can improve overall treatment for conditions like Hirschsprung disease or congenital heart defects and, ultimately, lead to better outcomes following surgery. Moreover, the research conducted by Dr. Doris Sylvanus General Regional Hospital emphasizes demographic distribution of congenital anomalies and confirms the need for particular management strategies in various populations, particularly in urban cities like Palangka Raya, where incidence rates are comparatively higher (Hayati & Thaihutu, 2025). The socioeconomic status implications on the management of congenital anomalies cannot be overemphasized, particularly regarding access and quality of care provided. In regions where the resources for healthcare are limited, such as in some low- and middle-income nations, children with the congenital heart disease may experience extended delays in diagnosis and treatment. A study conducted in Pakistan indicated that children from rural origins were diagnosed later than children from urban origins, illustrating the disparity in healthcare access (Marhaba et al., 2025). This indicates the requirement of certain interventions, like awareness among people and better health infrastructure, to allow equal opportunities for the development of congenital anomalies in children. Moreover, closure of these gaps has the potential to enhance the timeliness of treatment and enhance health outcomes across various demographic strata. Pediatric endoscopy is an established mode in the management of congenital defects, particularly with its role in advancing minimally invasive surgical techniques that reduce complications and recovery time. With improving healthcare systems, the use of endoscopic interventions as part of the standard care for congenital malformations is increasingly relevant. For instance, of the spectrum of congenital anomalies, those that need to be treated surgically can be best managed with endoscopic interventions, which are less invasive compared to traditional surgery. Additionally, as has been observed from research on congenital heart diseases, early intervention not only assists with alleviating acute medical issues but also enhances the long-term outcome for children so affected.

Therefore, healthcare professionals must be careful in developing pediatric endoscopy facilities to address the rising demand for proper management interventions of congenital anomalies, so that all children are provided with access to essential specialist care (Hayati & Thaihutu, 2025; Marhaba et al., 2025) (Figure 13.8).

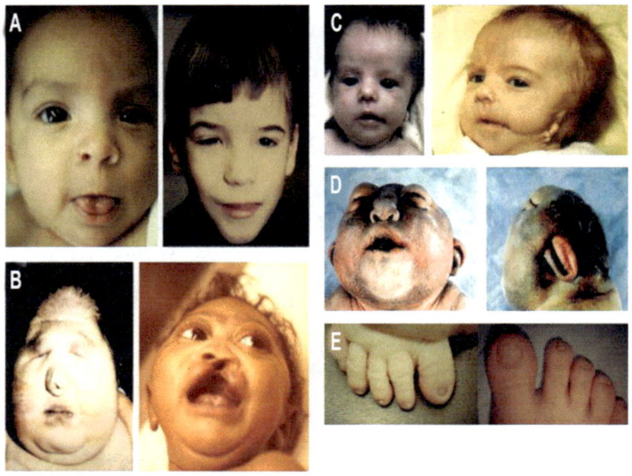

Figure 13.8. Management of congenital anomalies.

Source: https://s3.amazonaws.com/HMP/c360/imported/transfer/Screen_Shot_2016-08-23_at_12.17.20_PM.png.

13.4. Preparation for Pediatric Endoscopy

Preparation for pediatric endoscopy is critical in guaranteeing success in the process and lowering the incidence of complications. The process begins with high preoperative assessment, during which professionals are supposed to take thorough medical histories, such as prior gastrointestinal disorders and currently existing comorbidities that could influence the endoscopic process. Pediatric patients have differential reactions to sedation and anesthesia; therefore, the medical staff must inform guardians of potential risks involved along with procedural protocols. Further, there might be some dietary restrictions advised close to immediately before the procedure, which helps reduce the risk of aspiration in addition to enhancing visualization for the procedure. Preparation in itself is not enough. There has to be adequate preparation because that is what would enable smooth functioning and also provide a comfortable environment for the child to minimize anxiety and ensure cooperation during endoscopy. In addition to dietary restrictions and medical history, psychological preparation also should not be left out. Children become anxious about medical procedures, and that can manifest as anxiety or emotional distress. To this end, medical practitioners may implement steps to familiarize pediatric patients with the endoscopic process. This may involve pre-procedure tours of the facility as well as the provision of age-appropriate informational materials, all meant to depersonalize the environment and remove fear. Caregivers are also important in dispelling the fear of a child by providing emotional support and explaining the procedure. The development of effective communication between healthcare providers, patients, and families is at the core of ensuring a comfortable preparatory experience. Such practices make a significant contribution to the emotional stability and compliance of the child during the procedure. Clinical preparation also involves the application of dietary management, and this is of particular importance when planning for underlying gastrointestinal disorders in children. Conditions , such as inflammatory bowel disease (IBD) may influence both the choice of preparations and the potential consequences of endoscopic procedures. Symptomatic treatment and nutritional management are, in fact particularly important in preventing complications from sedation and endoscopy itself. According to current recommendations established by medical associations, endoscopic treatment in IBD patients must be performed with pre-procedure care and routine preparations aimed at preventing complications and precision of diagnosis and treatment (Matsuoka et al., 2018). Along with this, breath tests can also be an additional diagnostic tool before endoscopy to detect functional gastrointestinal symptoms and assess the extent of intervention required (Rezaie et al., 2017). These strategic insertions into the preparation phase operate to highlight the necessity for a multifaceted strategy to pediatric endoscopy that ultimately reduces patient outcomes and satisfaction issues.

13.4.1. Pre-Procedure Assessments

The importance of pre-procedure assessments in pediatric endoscopy cannot be overstated, as they play a key role in maintaining patient safety and optimizing procedural results. Thorough assessment allows health care professionals to examine the child's history of illness, such as previous ailments that might complicate the anesthesia or the procedure itself. These assessments typically include a thorough examination of the patient's airway, cardiovascular stability, and overall health to identify any risks for anesthesia or sedation. Specifically, guidelines formulated by some anesthesiology organizations emphasize the need to assess children with difficult airway histories to inform the anesthetic strategy (Apfelbaum et al., 2021). By knowing the problems in advance, healthcare workers have a better chance of implementing practices that minimize risks and therefore lead to more effective procedures as well as improved safety for the child patient. In addition to evaluating physical well-being, pre-procedure screening also serves the essential function of educating patients and parents regarding what needs to be done during endoscopy. There is a potential to minimize stress and establish a welcoming environment where parents are informed of the reasons for procedures, potential risks, and the anticipated outcome. Family education is central to preparing the child for the experience itself, particularly in explaining the reason for sedation and the need to fast beforehand. Furthermore, open discussion allows healthcare staff to allay any fears that will inevitably be there in the family, and this can make a significant contribution to enhancing the experience for both the child and the parents. The extent of these discussions assists in establishing trust, which is critical in pediatric care, especially in intimidating procedures (Schneider et al., 2021). Lastly, the assessment process also comprises diagnostic considerations, such as laboratory testing or imaging tests, that can provide essential information about the child's underlying health status.

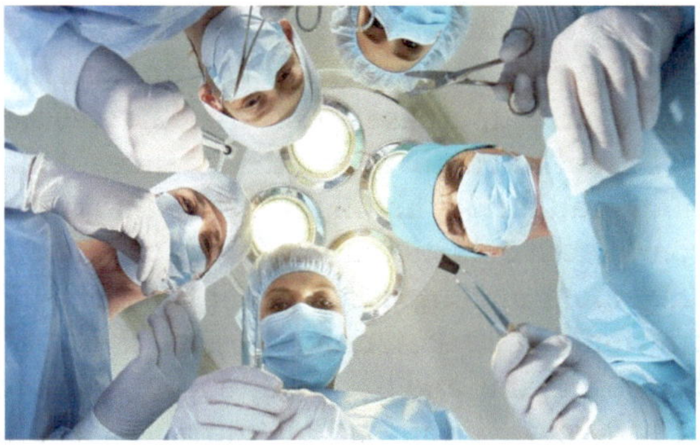

Figure 13.9. Pre-procedure assessments.

Source: https://sa1s3optim.patientpop.com/assets/images/provider/photos/2349512.jpg.

For instance, laboratory tests may uncover disorders of coagulopathy or infection that warrant pre-endoscopy assessment. Furthermore, the tests enable practitioners to implement a tailored approach to each child's anesthetic plan, allowing for adjustment on an individualized patient-by-patient basis. Pediatric endoscopy is a subspecialty that requires a variety of professionals , including anesthesiologists, gastroenterologists, and nurses, to collaborate in a way that enables planning and implementation of diagnostic and treatment care as appropriately suited to diagnostic and treatment intervention. This hybrid approach, developed through judicious pre-procedure assessments, not only optimizes pediatric endoscopy safety and effectiveness but also enables the cultivation of an integrated understanding of each patient's individualized care pathway (Figure 13.9).

13.4.2. Parental Involvement and Education

Parental involvement plays a critical role in determining educational attainment for children, influencing the academic performance and development of children. Many studies have reaffirmed that where parents are involved in education for their children, there is likely to be markedly enhanced performance across various measures, including grades and graduation rates. For instance, increased parental involvement has been linked to a greater chance of high school graduation, highlighting the importance given to active participation in education. Such engagement encompasses a range of behaviors from homework assistance to participation in school programs and has an extensive impact on students' motivation and attitudes to learning, particularly in difficult topics like pediatric health care training, where understanding may be critical to the management of conditions requiring interventions , such as endoscopy (Kantova, 2024). Moreover, the advent of technology and social networking systems has also changed the face of parental engagement in education. As educational institutions continue to integrate digital platforms into curricula, openings for parents to become involved in their children's learning have increased. Social networking sites (SNSs) have the potential to facilitate parental involvement by enabling communication and cooperation between teachers and parents. Nevertheless, research indicates that while the application of SNSs will augment motivation and attitude towards learning, it can also complicate findings in regards to parental participation. Parents need to be able to navigate these online environments well to assist with children's learning without overloading them, particularly in specialized fields, like comprehending the intricacies of pediatric endoscopy, which can frequently be difficult for young students (Yu, 2024). To utilize parental engagement in a child's learning to the fullest, especially in specialized subjects, it is important to create organized support systems. Such systems can include workshops that educate parents about their role in making a difference and assets that provide instructional support in how to engage interactively with their children's learning environments. Schools can also help by playing a role as an agent of change in bringing parents into the process through communication channels and cooperation, with parents being told about their children's progress. This co-curricular approach not only enhances performance academically but also fosters a supportive learning environment, which is useful in complex subject matters that require delicate handling, such as pediatric endoscopy. Ultimately, establishing effective bridges between home and school can result in monumental educational benefits for children (Kantova, 2024) (Figure 13.10).

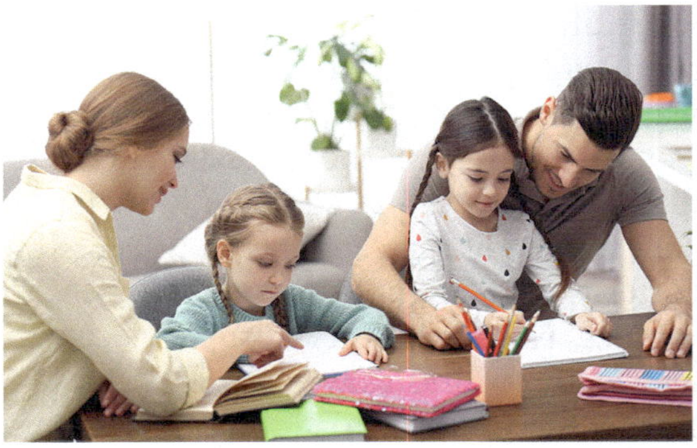

Figure 13.10. Parental involvement role in shaping educational outcomes for children.

Source: https://www.dynamics.edu.sg/images/resources/img-parents-supporting-childs-education.jpg.

13.4.3. Anesthesia Considerations

In deciding on pediatric endoscopy anesthesia, it is crucial to identify the unique physiological and psychological characteristics of children. Children differ from adults in their susceptibility to anesthetic drugs and exhibit significant variability based on their developmental stage, weight, and health. Administration of anesthesia necessitates a scrupulous preoperative assessment that includes examination of medical history, surveillance of prior anesthetic history, and inquiry of parental concerns. Ethical dilemmas are frequent, particularly when children complain about induction of anesthesia. Anesthesia care professionals are faced with the pragmatic dilemma of whether to honor the denial of the child or proceed with the procedure while attempting to meet an interplay of legal and ethical standards for pediatric care. In this respect, the recognition of the importance of consent, both of guardians and of that of the child, lends the platform to ethical decision-making in pediatric anesthesia (Haltom & Martin, 2024). In pediatric endoscopy, anesthesia administration should be carefully choreographed to consider the special needs of the patient as well as the procedures in question. For instance, airway procedures need closer examination, particularly when foreign body aspiration is in question, as underscored by instances of misdiagnosis leading to unwarranted suffering. Delay in addressing respiratory distress among children might necessitate emergency interventions, such as rigid bronchoscopy with general anesthesia, which can seriously alter the clinical course and prognosis in such patients (Goulioumis et al., 2023). Second, good communication with the parents and child regarding anesthesia procedures can decrease anxiety and enhance cooperation, thereby resulting in a smoother induction and a more successful procedure. Anesthesia implications extend beyond the actual immediate perioperative environment, such as postoperative care and risk of complications. Close observation for any indication of anesthetic side effects, most notably respiratory and cardiovascular, must be done in light of the fact that children as patients may present some unique difficulties depending on their size and physiological requirements. Pain control techniques should also be adjusted by the degree of child development, since techniques applied to adults may not apply as such. Maintaining that anesthesia plan with a focus on safe recovery from sedation is essential to stage interventions timely in the event of complications. Lastly, continued education and training in pediatric anesthesia techniques remain critical for practitioners, which helps them effectively and ethically address the subtle demands of this population (Figure 13.11).

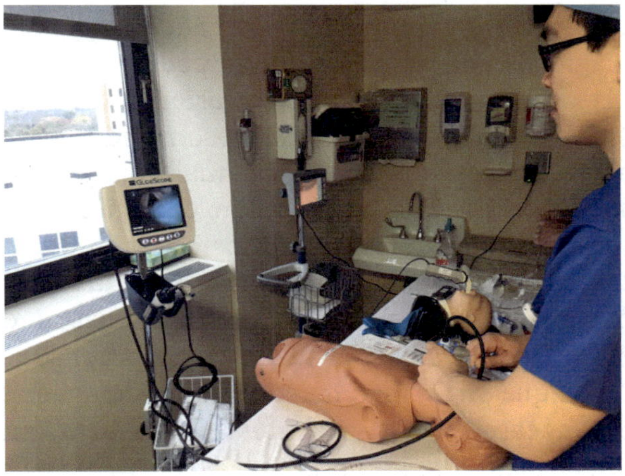

Figure 13.11. Anesthesia considerations.

Source: https://www.mcw.edu/departments/anesthesiology/fellowships/-/media/684B5BC1D570401FB932AF71B97604B0.ashx?anchor= middlecenter&scale= both&mode= crop&hash=BD1B5D124D9CA13A4AD40AB2DA357607.

13.5. Risks and Complications

Pediatric endoscopy, while invaluable in the diagnosis and management of gastrointestinal illness, is not complication-free and risk-free. One very much-noted risk is that of complications during the procedure, from superficial irritations to potentially life-threatening ones like bleeding or perforation. Children and adolescents with preoperative illnesses , such as EA-TEF are more prone to such complications. Anastomotic stricture, dysphagia, and gastroesophageal reflux are established complications, in which TNE is of choice because it is minimally invasive. This strategy avoids some of the risks associated with general anesthesia, providing a robust alternative for routine monitoring and modifications of medical management, thereby enabling clinicians to navigate through the complexities of pediatric practice more safely (Joseph et al., 2024). Through the analysis of the specific complications of endoscopy, the diagnosis and management of pediatric celiac disease is a case in point. Historically, the gold standard for diagnosis has been endoscopic duodenal biopsy, which is potentially dangerous, such as infection or sedation complications. Although less invasive serological tests exist, these generally position themselves at the center of contentious debates regarding specificity and sensitivity. The cost of taking out a diagnostic technique with risks must be weighed against the necessity of early intervention to avoid long-term consequences, e.g., profound macronutrient deficiencies. Indeed, employing endoscopic methods on children who are suspected of having celiac disease should be undertaken cautiously to balance efficacy with safety so that risks do not exceed the hoped-for benefit of earlier diagnosis (Bashir et al., 2022). Complicating further the pediatric endoscopy setting are the late complications of the anatomical alterations that may occur as a result of previous interventions. Procedures like those that repair EA-TEF can have severe alterations in gut function, leading to many endoscopic interventions over the course of decades. Serial endoscopies accumulate risk, including complications from sedation and the mechanical burden of repeated intervention over time. As children grow up, the need for ongoing monitoring becomes crucial, but this underscores the importance of the development of risk reduction strategies. The use of less invasive techniques, such as unsedated TNE, points to a trend to enhance these procedures, hopefully making the involved risks lower while achieving long-term effective management (Joseph et al., 2024).

13.5.1. Common Risks Associated with Procedures

There is a particular kind of risk for pediatric endoscopy that is associated with anatomical and physiological variation in children. The operations, typically minimally invasive forms of open operation, can prove to be quite problematic in and of themselves. A critical risk is involved with complications developing after the operation. Children, with their small body anatomical dimensions, are particularly susceptible to operative complication, including respiratory and gastrointestinal complications. The success of endoscopic management of such complications has been well documented, with high success and negligible mortality rates. But care providers need to be vigilant, since the potential for complications means there should be specialized precautions for endoscopy procedures, maximizing patient gains while reducing risks (Hoerning et al., 2025). Another risk factor is introduced by applying anesthesia to child patients who are candidates for endoscopic procedures. A comparison study evaluating the incidence of complications related to anesthetic techniques in pediatric endoscopy reported that respiratory complications were most prevalent. Certain risk factors significantly raised the risk of undesirable outcomes, including younger age, lower body weight, and underlying conditions. Crucially, the study identifies the imperative for vigilant pre-procedure assessments and preparations under pediatric anesthesia since coupling bronchoscopic procedures with gastrointestinal procedures did not represent an additional risk but nevertheless carried the possibility of harm (Schneck et al., 2024). Thus, awareness of such risks allows medical practitioners to implement corresponding mitigation strategies, safeguarding children's welfare during endoscopic procedures. Other than surgical and anesthesia complications, psychosocial factors of endoscopic procedures offer a second layer of concern. The procedure can prove particularly daunting to children and their families, with the tendency to heighten stress and anxiety.

These responses can inadvertently impact physiological parameters, which can result in complications during the procedure. Health care providers must highlight thorough pre-procedure counseling to educate families on what to expect, with the hope of minimizing anxiety and maximizing overall outcomes. By addressing the physical and psychological risks of pediatric endoscopy, healthcare practitioners will enhance the quality of care to make the medical procedures not only effective in treating physical ailments but also friendly to the emotional equilibrium of the child, ultimately making a balanced dimension to pediatric care.

13.5.2. Long-term Complications

The late morbidity of pediatric endoscopy is significant, and particularly in those with congenital abnormalities , such as EA and TEF. Despite better survival of children with these conditions, many cases suffer from chronic morbidities that can significantly impair their quality of life. In a retrospective report of patients with EA/TEF, it was found that 61.1% of them developed gastroesophageal reflux disease (GERD) that often required repeated surgical intervention and long-term proton pump inhibitor therapy. Of the patients diagnosed with GERD, only 13.4% were able to be weaned off the medication without relapse, reflecting the chronic nature of this illness in children. In addition to that, the requirement for repeated endoscopic evaluation further strengthens the necessity of observing and controlling such complications in the long term, meaning that follow-up in the long term is essential in management (Bashir et al., 2024). Another significant long-term complication secondary to pediatric endoscopy is esophageal strictures, which have been observed in a large majority of patients with EA/TEF.

The study had revealed that 77.6% of the children evaluated required esophageal dilation due to stricture, and most of them were diagnosed at 24 months of age. Stricture can lead to recurrent hospitalization and recurrent surgery, whose total adds up to create a multifaceted matrix of health needs as the children grow up. Eosinophilic esophagitis (EoE), an additional complication detailed in roughly 20% of patients, necessitates a sequence of escalating treatments, highlighting the level of complexity involved in managing such co-morbidities. The pathology behind these complications underscores the significance of meticulous surveillance strategies to address evolving clinical profiles of such pediatric patients (Bashir et al., 2024).

Long-term complications are of major interest in the context of operations, such as intraperitoneal onlay mesh (IPOM) ventral hernia repair, when they relate to pediatric operations. Although it has been discovered in studies that mesh complication is seen with relatively low frequency—about 0.62%—across longer follow-ups, their impact is determinant. Proper evaluation of reoperation and chronic pain rates due to mesh use ensures that surgeons remain conscious of potential adverse outcomes that can arise many years following a procedure. In addition, the distinction between complications arising directly from surgical interventions and those ensuing from pre-existing conditions must be established in future research for further refinement in the overall quality of pediatric care (Figure 13.12).

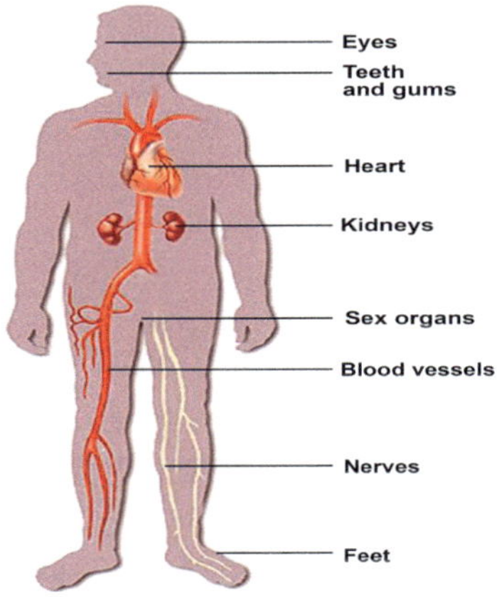

Figure 13.12. Long-term complications.

Source: https://www.diabetes-care.wales/wp-content/uploads/2022/09/13-Long-Term-Complications-of-Diabetes-Image.jpg.

13.5.3. Strategies for Risk Mitigation

In pediatric endoscopy, sound risk reduction practices are not only essential to ensure patient safety but also to achieve optimal overall procedural success. One fundamental approach is the careful selection and preparation of children for the procedure. This involves a careful history of the child's medical illness, dietary restrictions, and any underlying conditions that may impact anesthesia safety or procedural risk. Pre-procedure evaluation also includes psychological preparation, most important in children who may experience apprehension regarding invasive procedures. With the use of detailed pre-assessment protocols and communication based upon age, health care providers can significantly reduce anxiety and facilitate compliance, ultimately leading to more uneventful endoscopic procedures. The inclusion of these preparatory measures follows a trend towards greater recognition that the success of pediatric endoscopy relies most on minimizing inherent risks of the procedure and the patient population (Chhibber et al., 2021). Furthermore, the utilization of new technologies and guidelines plays a critical role in maximizing safety in pediatric endoscopic procedures. Individual training programs for the unique anatomy and physiological responses of children ensure that clinicians are well trained to handle frequent and rare complications. Incorporation of pediatric protocols utilizing less invasive techniques can also decrease trauma and the incidence of complications. Moreover, collaborative models incorporating multidisciplinary teams facilitate an interdisciplinary approach to patient care. These teams usually involve pediatric gastroenterologists, anesthesiologists, and nurses together, making plans against the possible complications and hence making the process easier with reduced risk. All these improvements, along with evidence-based medicine guidelines, heavily contribute towards risk prevention in pediatric endoscopy (Abbott & Ayres 2014). In addition to procedural techniques, continuous monitoring and outcome assessment are fundamental aspects of pediatric endoscopic risk prevention. Post-procedure treatment entails vigilant monitoring for complications, with evidence-based recovery pathways tailored to the pediatric age group. A collection of adverse event data with subsequent analysis can inform the revision of future guidelines and optimize current practice. An open culture of transparency and improvement allows healthcare professionals to identify risk factors and patterns for pediatric endoscopy best. This proactive approach not only enhances safety but also guarantees enhanced patient outcomes and family satisfaction. Thus, the inclusion of a robust evaluation framework within the risk management plan is crucial in guaranteeing the efficacy and safety of pediatric endoscopic procedures, consistent with the overall goal of child health improvement (Chhibber et al., 2021).

13.6. Advances in Pediatric Endoscopy

Pediatric endoscopy has witnessed revolutionary advances in the last few years, primarily in the therapeutic and diagnostic management of gastrointestinal disease (GID) in children. Increased realization that mucosal healing is a crucial treatment endpoint in pediatric IBD has driven advances in endoscopic technologies. Technologies , such as high-definition endoscopes and non-surgical methods like wireless capsule endoscopy are revolutionizing the diagnosis of the gastrointestinal system. These technologies enable pediatric gastroenterologists to better diagnose diseases , such as Crohn's disease and ulcerative colitis, resulting in targeted interventions that decrease hospital stays and avoid more invasive surgical procedures. Routine application of endoscopic scoring systems also contributes to the potential of comprehensive assessments, facilitating better management of disease progression and therapeutic responses and thus coming in line with contemporary treatment models to optimize pediatric patient outcomes (Isoldi et al., 2024). Besides diagnostic purposes, pediatric endoscopy also now includes a variety of interventional procedures to manage complications of gastrointestinal diseases. Cases of stenosis and strictures, the procedure for which involves surgery in the majority of cases, can be treated effectively by endoscopic balloon dilation or stenting at times. These less invasive interventions reduce the extent of open surgery, with a quick recovery and maintain patient safety. In addition, the advancement in anesthesia techniques, especially for children, has facilitated the possibility of having a safer endoscopy setup where procedures could be performed with less discomfort and stress. A growing emphasis on preserving gastrointestinal function through endoscopic management is a fine reflection of the movement towards less invasive intervention in pediatric health, where preserving quality of life is paramount (Isoldi et al., 2024). Pediatric endoscopy encompasses more than mere evaluation and intervention; it also includes active measures for prevention of potential complications of infection, including those from viral agents. In pediatric solid organ recipients, for instance, Epstein–Barr virus (EBV) is highly pathogenic for the development of posttransplant lymphoproliferative disorder (PTLD). Through timely monitoring of EBV viral loads with endoscopy, clinicians are able to identify and manage such complications before they become problematic. This proactive approach, coupled with the implementation of guidelines for immunosuppressive therapy, shows how advances in endoscopy can enhance patient outcomes in high-risk cases. Evolution of these practices continues to reinforce the importance of multidisciplinary collaboration to improve health outcomes for vulnerable pediatric patients (Figure 13.13).

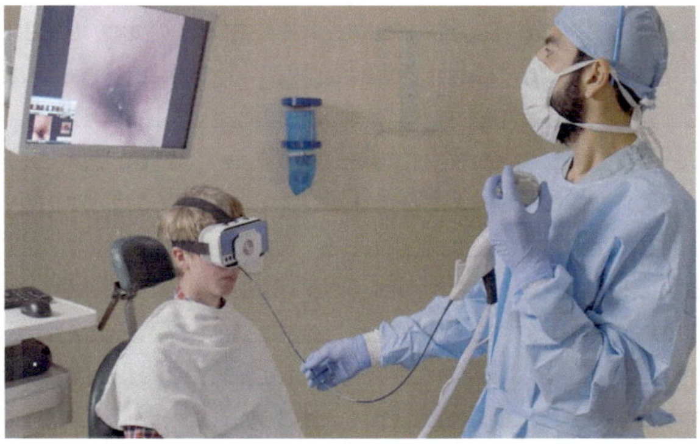

Figure 13.13. Advances in pediatric endoscopy.

Source: https://scopeforward.com/wp-content/uploads/2024/02/Transnasal-Endoscopy.jpg.

13.6.1. Technological Innovations

The advancement of pediatric endoscopy has also utilized technological advances that enhance precision and reduce invasiveness. Among them is the incorporation of robotic surgery intervention, which offers a significant advancement in surgical techniques. Utilizing technologies , such as the Da Vinci Surgical System allows pediatric surgeons to perform complex procedures with more dexterity and accuracy than manual techniques. Enhanced visual feedback through three-dimensional imaging has improved depth perception, particularly useful when operating on delicate anatomical structures in children. With the profession increasingly embracing these advances, robot-assisted surgeries not only improve the success rate of surgical interventions but also decrease postoperative complications, rendering them a preferred option to cure most conditions in children (Rivero-Moreno et al., 2023). Capsule endoscopy has been another game-changing technology within pediatric gastroenterology, revolutionizing small-bowel disorder diagnosis. It is a non-sedating method that allows the entire gastrointestinal tract to be visualized completely without sedation, particularly valuable in a pediatric environment. ESGE recommendations always favor small-bowel capsule endoscopy as a first-line investigation of small-bowel bleeding due to its superior safety profile and increased patient tolerance (Pennazio et al., 2022). In addition, the detection of lesions that are not visible using conventional endoscopy improves diagnostic potential and can prompt early intervention. The implementation of capsule endoscopy in the clinic demonstrates a paradigm shift from being institution-oriented to patient-focused care in pediatric endoscopy. In addition to robotic platforms and capsule technology, machine learning will also get its time to play the revolutionary game in future pediatric endoscopy. By employing algorithms that can observe and learn surgeons' techniques, this technology promises to create personalized training programs to improve surgical skills. There is fresh evidence that machine learning can provide *in-vivo* feedback in real-time intra-procedure, enabling surgeons to adjust their techniques in real-time and optimize patient outcomes (Rivero-Moreno et al., 2023). Also, the application of automated performance metrics could bring an era of surgical training based on adaptive teaching tools, with novice surgeons being taught by adaptive teaching tools. As these technological innovations continue to unfold, they promise to transform the future of pediatric endoscopy and ultimately improve both the diagnostic and therapeutic approaches in the field (Figure 13.14).

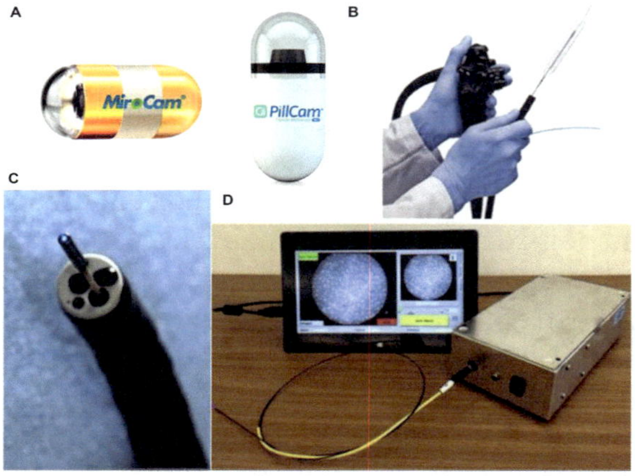

Figure 13.14. Technological innovations.

Source: https://febs.onlinelibrary.wiley.com/cms/asset/854d79af-e2e3-4967-ab7d-bb0edd7a0fbf/mol212792-fig-0002-m.jpg.

13.6.2. Minimally Invasive Techniques

Growth in pediatric endoscopy has been significantly impacted by the adoption of minimally invasive techniques, which entail several advantages over traditional surgical methods. These approaches highlight decreased incisions and less tissue trauma, hence reduced recovery time and postoperative pain in children. With continued advancements in technology, the application of minimally invasive technology has demonstrated enhanced diagnostic performance and therapeutic intervention. Specifically, the integration of flexible endoscopy with laparoscopic surgery has been vital in identifying intraoperative complications to enable remediation to be made at an urgent pace. This interaction maximizes operating outcomes with the added benefit of providing a safer environment to perform complex procedures on children, who inherently possess differing anatomical and physiological characteristics. Thus, the application of minimally invasive techniques within pediatric endoscopy is a field that brings enhanced effectiveness and safety to interventions. Percutaneous internal ring suturing (PIRS) application is among the benefits of minimally invasive procedures in children, particularly for herniotomy. Laparoscopic procedures become achievable with fewer visibility problems in employing this technique because it can be performed using a single incision at the umbilicus. Five years of studies on PIRS application reported high success with fewer complications, which illustrates how efficient PIRS is in children. The low intraoperative rates of tissue damage and the low postoperative complication rates indicate the safety of the procedure. Secondly, the shorter hospital stay associated with PIRS allows for quicker discharge, further boosting patient satisfaction and keeping healthcare costs low. Therefore, PIRS offers a benchmark for future pediatric operating procedure development, showing the paradigm-shifting effect of minimally invasive interventions on the treatment of common pediatric conditions. Also, the co-effect of intraoperative endoscopy with minimally invasive surgery has been shown to increase the effectiveness of pediatric surgery by providing immediate scrutiny of internal organs. Research indicates that incorporating endoscopy in laparoscopic operations can potentially enhance anatomical patient profiling, thereby enabling more precise procedures. The method has been proved to play a central role in the treatment of extensive gastrointestinal pathologies, such as achalasia and peptic stenosis in children, for which the correct identification of organs is essential. Endoscopy application for 83 children undergoing minimally invasive surgery is the focus of the retrospective analysis that supports the technique's role in avoiding severe complications and ensuring surgical anastomoses. By providing immediate diagnosis and intervention, intraoperative endoscopy is a useful instrument in minimally invasive surgery, establishing a new standard of care that guarantees safety and efficacy in pediatric endoscopic procedures (Pogorelić et al., 2020; García-Hernández et al., 2021).

13.6.3. Future Directions in Research

With the progress in the pediatric endoscopy area, future research directions must reflect the intertwined nature of surgical care delivery and patient outcomes, especially in light of the recent global health emergencies that have hit the world, such as the COVID-19 pandemic. The pandemic has reflected unprecedented disturbances in surgical services worldwide, limiting access to essential procedures among children. These disturbances emphasize the need for thorough evaluation of surgical care pathways to make sure that they are not weakened in the context of disturbances. Continued research efforts must be aimed at creating strong contingency plans that incorporate surgical services into national health strategies to make sure that children with surgical requirements get timely and proper treatment, irrespective of outside pressures. Such studies can guide health policymakers on what to do in terms of creating policies not only to efficiently manage pandemics but also to maximize the provision of pediatric surgical care in routine practice (Søreide et al., 2020). Apart from solving issues at a system level, future pediatric endoscopy studies should also explore new technological advancements to enhance diagnostic and therapeutic interventions. These could involve the integration of new-generation imaging modalities and minimally invasive tools into routine practice, a move toward precision medicine. Research studies could involve preclinical and clinical trials to evaluate the safety and effectiveness of new endoscopic tools and methods specifically for use in pediatrics. Facilitating multidisciplinary collaboration between engineers, pediatric gastroenterologists, and other clinicians could accelerate such technologies in development. Such advancements are important because they can lead to improved results in children who undergo advanced gastrointestinal procedures, providing them with the best possible treatments with less danger (Clancy et al., 2018). Additionally, as pediatric gastrointestinal illnesses continue to be better understood, future research should work on the implications of genetic and molecular understanding in the context of pediatric endoscopy. Investigating the role of specific genetic mutations seen in pediatric gastrointestinal conditions, such as cystic fibrosis, may allow for the construction of targeted therapeutic interventions. New avenues of research here may include the evaluation of CFTR modulator treatments and their potential application to pediatric populations with such orphan conditions. With the help of preclinical models for the testing of the efficacy of such treatment, researchers are in a position to guide clinical practice by informing therapeutic protocols that are tailored to the individual needs of young patients. Such a focus on personalized medical therapies has the potential to enhance the effectiveness of treatments provided by endoscopic procedures and would significantly improve long-term outcomes in afflicted children (Clancy et al., 2018) (Figure 13.15).

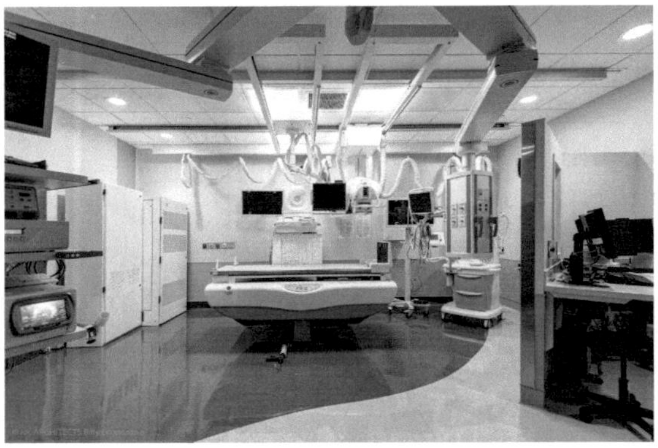

Figure 13.15. Future directions in research.

Source: https://www.rwjbh.org/images/endoscopy-Suite-1.jpeg.

SUMMARY

In conclusion, pediatric endoscopy has proven to be a highly effective modality for the diagnosis and treatment of numerous gastrointestinal disorders in children. Its relative lesser invasiveness allows for direct intervention and visualization inside the gastrointestinal tract, thus enabling improved patient outcomes. The effectiveness of treatments , such as vedolizumab (VDZ) in the management of IBD serves to illustrate the efficacy and benefits of endoscopic procedures. Studies indicate that VDZ achieves good mucosal healing rates even in kids who have previously been exposed to anti-tumor necrosis factor (TNF) agents, a state that in no way diminishes its efficacy in promoting gastrointestinal health (Jossen et al., 2019). This highlights the need for ongoing study into how best to maximize endoscopic procedures for the sole use of the pediatric patient group, which remains safe and effective. In addition, the diagnostic value of pediatric endoscopy is further optimized, as indicated by a study that compared the utility of the use of duodenal bulb biopsies in diagnosing celiac disease. Through systematic reviews and meta-analyses, evidence indicates that celiac disease's diagnostic yield in children is significantly enhanced by performing biopsies from the duodenal bulb (McCarty et al., 2018). This finding is priceless as it guides clinical practice towards the optimal sites for biopsy within endoscopy. Better diagnostic findings result in earlier interventions, which can have a profound impact on the management direction of disease among children. These advancements are the ongoing advancement of pediatric endoscopy and moving further towards a better quality of care and healthier long-term outcomes for adolescent patients with gastroenterological disorders. Lastly, the implications of pediatric endoscopy extend far beyond mere diagnostics and therapeutic interventions; it also has profound psychosocial connotations for families and patients. Relief from symptoms and the promise of curative intervention may dramatically enhance the quality of life in children with chronic gastrointestinal disease. With changing knowledge and technology in this domain, there is a necessity to focus on the holistic aspect of treatment involving mental and emotional health as well as physical. Constant investment in acquiring skills and research will ensure pediatric endoscopy remains one of the cornerstones of pediatric gastroenterology, eventually resulting in a holistic solution to children's ailments. Second, there will be rigorous training and adherence to ethical standards to ensure new practices are in the best interest of young patients and their families.

In pediatric endoscopy, awareness of technological improvements and methods is critical in a bid to improve diagnostic and therapeutic outcomes. Augmented reality (AR) is one such innovative tool, whereby digital information is overlaid onto the real world. With the assistance of AR, physicians can create enhanced surgical planning ability and increase the accuracy of procedures. Not only does this new technology make the procedural process flow easier, but it also serves to enlighten patients and their families about complex medical scenarios. The application of AR to pediatric endoscopy is a wonderful advancement, creating a three-dimensional approach to medicine that promotes greater understanding, minimizes complications, and ultimately results in improved patient outcomes. These developments highlight the need for ongoing change in clinical practice to ensure pediatric patients are not only treated effectively but also compassionately and educatively (Eckert et al., 2019). Clinical practices' partnership with laboratory capacity is also central to pediatric endoscopy, specifically in diagnosing infectious diseases. The microbiology lab is crucial, offering key insights that guide clinical decisions. An exhaustive understanding of tests and their history is crucial to practitioners since the success of pediatric endoscopic procedures can hinge on accurate pre-operative assessment of potential infections. The interface of healthcare experts and microbiologists is of paramount significance, producing a platform on which correct diagnoses can lead to early interventions. For instance, appreciation of optimal sampling and transport may have a high impact on treatment outcomes. Protocols that have been laid down by experts demand a scientific focus to this interaction, primarily concentrating on those tests that are most useful for pediatric patients undergoing endoscopic examination (Goulioumis et al., 2023). Also, the unique needs of the pediatric patient demand special attention under the endoscopic system. With procedures becoming more complex, specimen management and interpretation become challenging. Emphasis on pediatric concerns ensures that uniform practices are modified to fulfill the unique physiological and psychological needs of children. For instance, heightened sensitivity in specimen management protocols must be observed to avoid complications arising from improper handling. Training material, including comprehensive manuals summarizing main points regarding specimen tests and management, is crucial for clinicians. These guidelines not only provide the major areas to be emphasized while diagnosing but also foster an integrated method of managing and understanding pediatric infectious diseases. Given priority to these areas, the field of pediatric endoscopy could become more efficient, indirectly leading to a more robust approach towards patient care (Goulioumis et al., 2023).

CLOSER LOOK

CONGENITAL MALFORMATIONS:

Congenital malformations, also known as birth defects, are structural or functional anomalies present at birth that can affect virtually any part of the body. They arise during embryonic or fetal development and may result from genetic factors, environmental influences, or a combination of both. These anomalies vary widely in severity, ranging from minor cosmetic differences to life-threatening conditions, and can impact physical, cognitive, and social development.

The causes of congenital malformations are multifactorial. Genetic factors include chromosomal abnormalities, such as trisomy 21 (Down syndrome), and single-gene mutations, which can lead to conditions like cystic fibrosis or phenylketonuria. Environmental influences during pregnancy, including maternal infections, exposure to teratogenic drugs, alcohol, or radiation, also contribute to the development of malformations. Nutritional deficiencies, particularly folic acid deficiency, are strongly linked to neural tube defects, such as spina bifida and anencephaly. In many cases, the exact cause remains unidentified, highlighting the complex interplay of genetics and environment.

Congenital malformations can affect various organ systems. Cardiovascular anomalies, such as ventricular septal defects or tetralogy of Fallot, are among the most common and often require surgical intervention. Musculoskeletal defects include clubfoot or limb reductions, while craniofacial anomalies encompass cleft lip and palate. Neural tube defects and central nervous system malformations can lead to significant neurological impairment, affecting motor and cognitive functions. Some congenital malformations, such as certain kidney or gastrointestinal anomalies, may remain asymptomatic until later in life.

Early detection and diagnosis are crucial for effective management. Prenatal screening, including ultrasound, genetic testing, and maternal serum markers, enables early identification of many malformations, allowing for timely interventions or informed decision-making. Postnatal evaluation by pediatricians, geneticists, or specialized surgeons ensures appropriate treatment and support. Management strategies vary depending on the type and severity of the malformation and may include surgical correction, medical therapy, rehabilitation, and long-term monitoring.

The impact of congenital malformations extends beyond physical health. Families may face psychological, social, and financial challenges, emphasizing the need for comprehensive care that includes counseling, education, and support services. Public health measures, such as maternal nutrition programs, vaccination, and avoidance of teratogens, play an important role in prevention.

In conclusion, congenital malformations are complex conditions arising from genetic and environmental factors. Early detection, individualized management, and multidisciplinary care are essential to optimize outcomes and enhance quality of life. Awareness and preventive strategies remain key components in reducing the burden of these conditions on individuals and society.

REFERENCES

1. Ryan Abbott & Ian Ayres, Evidence and Extrapolation: Mechanisms for Regulating Off-Label Uses of Drugs and Devices, 64 *Duke Law Journal* 377-435 (2014) Available at: https://scholarship.law.duke.edu/dlj/vol64/iss3/1(accessed on 15th July 2025).
2. Abd-Elmageed, F. N. M., Hashad, R. E. S., Eldemery, N. I., & Badawy, G. G. (2020). Evaluating the applicability of a bowel preparation care bundle protocol for pediatric endoscopic surgery: Randomized controlled trial. *Egyptian Journal of Health Care, 11*(1), 1211–1214. https://journals.ekb.eg/article_252380_f749136495c2893b6b0d90e305dc1324.pdf (accessed on 15th July 2025).
3. Ajani, J. A., D'Amico, T. A., Bentrem, D. J., Chao, J., Cooke, D. T., Corvera, C. U., Das, P., et al. (2022). *Gastric cancer, Version 2.2022, NCCN clinical practice guidelines in oncology. Journal of the National Comprehensive Cancer Network, 20*, 167–192. https://doi.org/10.6004/jnccn.2022.0008 (accessed on 15th July 2025).
4. Apfelbaum, J. L., Hagberg, C. A., Connis, R. T., Abdelmalak, B., Agarkar, M., Dutton, R. P., Fiadjoe, J. E., et al. (2021). *2022 American Society of Anesthesiologists practice guidelines for management of the difficult airway. Anesthesiology, 136*, 31–81. https://doi.org/10.1097/aln.0000000000004002 (accessed on 15th July 2025).
5. Chhibber, A., Kharat, A., Kneale, D., Welch, V., Bangpan, M., & Chaiyakunapruk, N. (2021). Assessment of health equity consideration in masking/PPE policies to contain COVID-19 using PROGRESS-plus framework: a systematic review. *BMC public health, 21*(1), 1682. https://doi.org/10.1186/s12889-021-11688-7(accessed on 15th July 2025).
6. Bashir, A., Krasaelap, A., Lal, D. R., Gourlay, D., Pan, A. Y., Jan, N., McCord, S., et al. (2024). Esophagitis, treatment outcomes, and long-term follow-up in children with esophageal atresia. *Journal of Pediatric Gastroenterology and Nutrition.* https://www.semanticscholar.org/paper/441a3f6420287061b5bf4ab4bce20a5f1c2dbc54 (accessed on 15th July 2025).
7. Bashir, B., Soomro, T., Qureshi, R., Zaki, M., Chandio, B., & Bouk, M. A. (2022). Diagnostic accuracy of serum anti-tissue transglutaminase antibody in diagnosis of pediatric celiac disease. *Pakistan Journal of Medical and Health Sciences.* https://www.semanticscholar.org/paper/bd718cf66db2b99bbf19976d01cdd46efd8a5c52 (accessed on 15th July 2025).
8. Clancy, J. P., Cotton, C. U., Donaldson, S. H., Solomon, G. M., VanDevanter, D. R., Boyle, M., Gentzsch, M., et al. (2018). *CFTR modulator theratyping: Current status, gaps and future directions. Journal of Cystic Fibrosis, 18*, 22–34. https://doi.org/10.1016/j.jcf.2018.05.004 (accessed on 15th July 2025).
9. Denson, L. A., Curran, M., McGovern, D., Koltun, W. A., Duerr, R. H., Kim, S. C., Sartor, R. B., et al. (2019). *Challenges in IBD research: Precision medicine. Inflammatory Bowel Diseases, 25*, S31–S39. https://doi.org/10.1093/ibd/izz078 (accessed on 15th July 2025).
10. Di Nardo, G., Di Lorenzo, C., Lauro, A., Stanghellini, V., Thapar, N., Karunaratne, T. B., Volta, U., et al. (2016). *Chronic intestinal pseudo-obstruction in children and adults: Diagnosis and therapeutic options. Neurogastroenterology & Motility, 29.* https://doi.org/10.1111/nmo.12945 (accessed on 15th July 2025).
11. Eckert, M., Volmerg, J. S., & Friedrich, C. M. (2019). *Augmented reality in medicine: Systematic and bibliographic review. JMIR Mhealth and Uhealth, 7*, e10967–e10967. https://doi.org/10.2196/10967 (accessed on 15th July 2025).

12. El Choueiri, J., Pellicanò, F., Caimi, E., Laurelli, F., Di Cosmo, L., Rada, A. D., Cernigoi, D., et al. (2025). *Advancements in spinal endoscopic surgery: Comprehensive techniques and pathologies addressed by full endoscopy beyond lumbar disc herniation. Journal of Clinical Medicine, 14.* https://www.semanticscholar.org/paper/ca78ae3677bedfc5bcdb400d52bf1b2b11054ab0 (accessed on 15th July 2025).

13. Friedlander, J. A., Leinwand, K., Bhardwaj, V., & Nguyen, N. (2024). *A guide on transnasal endoscopy: Setting up a pediatric unsedated endoscopy program. Frontiers in Pediatrics, 11.* https://www.semanticscholar.org/paper/eea5a5fe7bbaeacd60eda87ea2ae0442493ab3f2 (accessed on 15th July 2025).

14. García-Hernández, C., Carvajal-Figueroa, L., Archivaldo-García, C., Landa-Juárez, S., & Izundegui-Ordóñez, G. (2021). Intraoperative endoscopy as an adjuvant to minimally invasive surgery in pediatrics. *Journal of Laparoendoscopic & Advanced Surgical Techniques: Part A.* https://www.semanticscholar.org/paper/57f9c93848dcc83da0a265839173b018d95bbee5 (accessed on 15th July 2025).

15. Gendler, Y., Seguier-Lipszyc, E., Silbermintz, A., Hain, M., Stern, Y., Kravarusic, D., Politi, K., et al. (2021). *Aerodigestive clinics as emerging pediatric care model: The first 100 patients in Israel. IMAJ, 23*(9), 569–575. http://ima-files.s3.amazonaws.com/305485_1665cab5-4d96-4125-9d1b-46d1d3a2440b.pdf (accessed on 15th July 2025).

16. Goulioumis, A., Peridis, S., Koudmnakis, E., & Athanasopoulos, I. (2023). A foreign body lodged in the glottis of a toddler for a prolonged time: Anatomical considerations and review of the literature. *Cureus, 15.* https://www.semanticscholar.org/paper/45f8a75ec588fd38b9094f7f1e150eb0e43819e7 (accessed on 15th July 2025).

17. Haltom, J. P., & Martin, A. S. (2024). *Ethical and practical considerations of pediatric refusal in clinical anesthesia: An educational review. Pediatric Anesthesia, 34,* 689–696. https://www.semanticscholar.org/paper/4cd79cb6d57b718889ac442b5d3e339fb8b52f29 (accessed on 15th July 2025).

18. Hayati, R., & Thaihutu, Y. (2025). *Pattern of congenital anomalies in pediatric patients at Dr. Doris Sylvanus General Regional Hospital: A one-year retrospective study. The International Journal of Medical Science and Health Research.* https://www.semanticscholar.org/paper/678d19b2d1a58652207e84c1e41fa65d7cb7d2ad (accessed on 15th July 2025).

19. Hoang, D. M., Pham, P. T., Bach, T. Q., Ngo, A. T., Nguyen, Q. T., Phan, T. K. T., Nguyễn, H. G., et al. (2022). Stem cell-based therapy for human diseases. *Signal Transduction and Targeted Therapy, 7.* https://doi.org/10.1038/s41392-022-01134-4 (accessed on 15th July 2025).

20. Hoerning, A., Seitz, G., Schluckebier, D., & de Laffolie, J. (2025). Therapeutic intervention in pediatric endoscopy – management of post-surgical complications and bleeding. *Visceral Medicine.* https://www.semanticscholar.org/paper/10b244072a3916b9e1b4b29cdc4c19b1d3cbb302 (accessed on 15th July 2025).

21. Hu, Y., Chatzilakou, E., Pan, Z., Traverso, G., & Yetisen, A. K. (2024). *Microneedle sensors for point-of-care diagnostics. Advanced Science, 11.* https://doi.org/10.1002/advs.202306560 (accessed on 15th July 2025).

22. Iannella, G., Magliulo, G., Greco, A., De Virgilio, A., Maniaci, A., Lechien, J., Calvo-Henríquez, C., et al. (2024). Clinical application of pediatric sleep endoscopy: An international survey. *Children, 11.* https://www.semanticscholar.org/paper/158a85bc01a82b999a88147b66da3db5ab1e4cf0 (accessed on 15th July 2025).

23. Ishman, S. L., Chang, K. W., & Kennedy, A. A. (2018). *Techniques for evaluation and management of tongue-base obstruction in pediatric obstructive sleep apnea. Current Opinion in Otolaryngology & Head & Neck Surgery, 26*, 409–416. https://doi.org/10.1097/moo.0000000000000489 (accessed on 15th July 2025).

24. Isoldi, S., Mallardo, S., Quitadamo, P., Leter, B., & Cucchiara, S. (2024). *Review on advances in pediatric endoscopy in the management of inflammatory bowel disease. Current Pediatric Reviews, 20.* https://www.semanticscholar.org/paper/5c94c2080c48284ae00602ee4443921e00dbe434; https://doi.org/10.2174/0115733963268547231128101929 (accessed on 15th July 2025).

25. Joseph, M., Corrado, M. M., Odiase, E., Friedlander, J. A., Smith, C., & Nguyen, N. (2024). *Sedation-free transnasal esophagoscopy to evaluate and monitor esophageal diseases in children with esophageal atresia-tracheoesophageal fistula. JPGN Reports, 5*, 166–169. https://www.semanticscholar.org/paper/82410e19c73830c052c510381d4da0bcb83a233f (accessed on 15th July 2025).

26. Jossen, J., Kiernan, B. D., Pittman, N., & Dubinsky, M. C. (2019). *Anti-tumor necrosis factor-alpha exposure impacts vedolizumab mucosal healing rates in pediatric inflammatory bowel disease. Journal of Pediatric Gastroenterology and Nutrition, 70*, 304–309. https://doi.org/10.1097/mpg.0000000000002556 (accessed on 15th July 2025).

27. Kantova, K. (2024). *Parental involvement and education outcomes of their children. Applied Economics, 56*, 5683–5698. https://www.semanticscholar.org/paper/33979f5ada8164b9b664bd895dc37d22d63f3edf (accessed on 15th July 2025).

28. Lee, Y. (2022). *Pediatric percutaneous endoscopic gastrostomy in Korea – When? By whom? How? Journal of Korean Medical Science, 37.* https://www.semanticscholar.org/paper/07b3c241b1d1a6a2677afc627d1cd46d7777bac4 (accessed on 15th July 2025).

29. Lightdale, J. (2013). *Techniques in Gastrointestinal Endoscopy.* https://www.semanticscholar.org/paper/75398cadf6b621c8a73202e483a945972582e589 (accessed on 15th July 2025).

30. Maier-Hein, L., Eisenmann, M., Sarıkaya, D., März, K., Collins, T., Malpani, A., Fallert, J., et al. (2021). *Surgical data science – From concepts toward clinical translation. Medical Image Analysis, 76*, 102306–102306. https://doi.org/10.1016/j.media.2021.102306 (accessed on 15th July 2025).

31. Marhaba, A. A., Gul, J., Jan, M. A., Karim, S. A., Waqas, M., & Ikram, M. (2025). *Prevalence and management of congenital heart diseases in Pakistan: A comprehensive cross-sectional study. Journal of Health, Wellness and Community Research.* https://www.semanticscholar.org/paper/741b3fd6c7928a9675f3187a8ba53483f7a9a1fc (accessed on 15th July 2025).

32. Maskal, S., Ellis, R., Mali, O., Lau, B., Messer, N., Zheng, X., Miller, B., et al. (2024). *Long-term mesh-related complications from minimally invasive intraperitoneal onlay mesh for small to medium-sized ventral hernias. Surgical Endoscopy, 38*, 2019–2026. https://www.semanticscholar.org/paper/6271e1bf838a38736a6f35a2a1a9074eb69e8c25 (accessed on 15th July 2025).

33. Matsuoka, K., Kobayashi, T., Ueno, F., Matsui, T., Hirai, F., Inoue, N., Kato, J., et al. (2018). *Evidence-based clinical practice guidelines for inflammatory bowel disease. Journal of Gastroenterology, 53*, 305–353. https://doi.org/10.1007/s00535-018-1439-1 (accessed on 15th July 2025).

34. McCarty, T. R., O'Brien, C., Gremida, A., Ling, C., & Rustagi, T. (2018). *Efficacy of duodenal bulb biopsy for diagnosis of celiac disease: A systematic review and meta-analysis. Endoscopy International Open, 6*, E1369–E1378. https://doi.org/10.1055/a-0732-5060 (accessed on 15th July 2025).

35. Melles, M., Albayrak, A., & Goossens, R. (2020). *Innovating health care: Key characteristics of human-centered design. International Journal for Quality in Health Care, 33*, 37–44. https://doi.org/10.1093/intqhc/mzaa127 (accessed on 15th July 2025).

36. Miller, J. M., Binnicker, M. J., Campbell, S., Carroll, K. C., Chapin, K. C., Gilligan, P. H., Gonzalez, M. D., et al. (2018). *A guide to utilization of the microbiology laboratory for diagnosis of infectious diseases: 2018 update by the Infectious Diseases Society of America and the American Society for Microbiology. Clinical Infectious Diseases, 67*, e1–e94. https://doi.org/10.1093/cid/ciy381 (accessed on 15th July 2025).

37. Palomeque Matos, M. (2023). *Urinary lithiasis and extracorporeal shock wave lithotripsy: New approachments.* https://core.ac.uk/download/590213801.pdf (accessed on 15th July 2025).

38. Pelizzo, G., Destro, F., Pierucci, U. M., Costanzo, S., Camporesi, A., Diotto, V., Calcaterra, V., et al. (2024). *Minimal access in pediatric surgery: An overview on progress towards dedicated instrument developments and anesthesiologic advances to enhance safe completion of procedures. Children, 11*, 679–679. https://doi.org/10.3390/children11060679 (accessed on 15th July 2025).

39. Pennazio, M., Rondonotti, E., Despott, E. J., Dray, X., Keuchel, M., Moreels, T. G., Sanders, D. S., et al. (2022). *Small-bowel capsule endoscopy and device-assisted enteroscopy for diagnosis and treatment of small-bowel disorders: European Society of Gastrointestinal Endoscopy (ESGE) Guideline – Update 2022. Endoscopy, 55*, 58–95. https://doi.org/10.1055/a-1973-3796 (accessed on 15th July 2025).

40. Pogorelić, Z., Čohadžić, T., Jukić, M., & Nevešćanin Biliškov, A. (2020). *Percutaneous internal ring suturing for the minimal invasive treatment of pediatric inguinal hernia: A 5-year single surgeon experience. Surgical Laparoscopy, Endoscopy & Percutaneous Techniques.* https://www.semanticscholar.org/paper/2bf8d6225c4f6342a0068d007babee62681f7017 (accessed on 15th July 2025).

41. Porcedda, G., Brambilla, A., Favilli, S., Murzi, B., Mirabile, L., Baggi, R., & Arcieri, L. (2019). *Combined surgical and endoscopic approach for ring–sling complex. The Thoracic and Cardiovascular Surgeon, 68*, 051–058. https://doi.org/10.1055/s-0039-1678670 (accessed on 15th July 2025).

42. Ramdhanie, G. G., Nurrohmah, A., Mulya, A. P., Mediani, H., Sumarni, N., Mulyana, A., & Hasanul, H. M. (2024). *A scoping review of audiovisual distraction techniques among children in reducing invasive procedure pain. Journal of Multidisciplinary Healthcare, 17*, 4363–4372. https://www.semanticscholar.org/paper/c512cc09ef6019c0fa14fb4fce0917e96453abd5 (accessed on 15th July 2025).

43. Rezaie, A., Buresi, M., Lembo, A., Lin, H. C., McCallum, R. W., Rao, S. S. C., Schmulson, M. J., et al. (2017). Hydrogen and methane-based breath testing in gastrointestinal disorders: The North American consensus. *The American Journal of Gastroenterology, 112*, 775–784. https://doi.org/10.1038/ajg.2017.46 (accessed on 15th July 2025).

44. Rivero-Moreno, Y., Echevarria, S., Vidal-Valderrama, C., Stefano-Pianetti, L., Cordova-Guilarte, J., Navarro-Gonzalez, J., Acevedo-Rodriguez, J. E., et al. (2023). *Robotic surgery: A comprehensive review of the literature and current trends. Cureus.* https://doi.org/10.7759/cureus.42370 (accessed on 15th July 2025).

45. Schneck, E., Knittel, F., Markmann, M., Balzer, F., Rubarth, K., Zajonz, T., Schreiner, A., et al. (2024). Assessment of risk factors for adverse events in analgosedation for pediatric endoscopy: A 10-year retrospective analysis. *Journal of Pediatric Gastroenterology and Nutrition.* https://www.semanticscholar.org/paper/70b776148887c5172341e6ec7227e1ba1cae68f3 (accessed on 15th July 2025).

46. Schneider, B. J., Naidoo, J., Santomasso, B., Lacchetti, C., Adkins, S., Anadkat, M. J., Atkins, M. B., et al. (2021). Management of immune-related adverse events in patients treated with immune checkpoint inhibitor therapy: ASCO guideline update. *Journal of Clinical Oncology, 39*, 4073–4126. https://doi.org/10.1200/jco.21.01440 (accessed on 15th July 2025).

47. Siau, K., Iacucci, M., Dunckley, P., Penman, I., Pawlak, K. M., Král, J., Khan, R., et al. (2020). *The impact of COVID-19 on gastrointestinal endoscopy training in the United Kingdom. Gastroenterology, 159*, 1582–1585.e3. https://doi.org/10.1053/j.gastro.2020.06.015 (accessed on 15th July 2025).

48. Søreide, K., Hallet, J., Matthews, J. B., Schnitzbauer, A. A., Line, P. D., Lai, P. B. S., Gestal Otero, J. J., et al. (2020). *Immediate and long-term impact of the COVID-19 pandemic on delivery of surgical services. British Journal of Surgery, 107*, 1250–1261. https://doi.org/10.1002/bjs.11670 (accessed on 15th July 2025).

49. Squires, R. H., Ng, V. L., Romero, R., Ekong, U. D., Hardikar, W., Emre, S., & Mazariegos, G. (2014). *Evaluation of the pediatric patient for liver transplantation: 2014 practice guideline by the American Association for the Study of Liver Diseases, American Society of Transplantation and the North American Society for Pediatric Gastroenterology, Hepatology. Hepatology, 60*, 362–398. https://doi.org/10.1002/hep.27191 (accessed on 15th July 2025).

50. Su, C. C., Chou, C. K., Mukundan, A., Karmakar, R., Sanbatcha, B. F., Huang, C. W., Weng, W. C., et al. (2025). Capsule endoscopy: Current trends, technological advancements, and future perspectives in gastrointestinal diagnostics. *Bioengineering.* https://www.semanticscholar.org/paper/573a9f6fa99d1c1688470cd9ad55b7ed4e4cfd65 (accessed on 15th July 2025).

51. Von Hoff, D. D., Ervin, T. J., Arena, F. P., Chiorean, E. G., Infante, J. R., Moore, M. J., Seay, T. E., et al. (2013). Increased survival in pancreatic cancer with nab-paclitaxel plus gemcitabine. *New England Journal of Medicine, 369*, 1691–1703. https://doi.org/10.1056/nejmoa1304369 (accessed on 15th July 2025).

52. Wagenius, M. (2021). *Complications and Treatment Aspects of Urological Stone Surgery.* https://core.ac.uk/download/479542435.pdf (accessed on 15th July 2025).

53. Xiao, Z., Li, X., Zhou, L., Long, X., Tian, L., & Li, W. (2025). *Drug-induced sleep endoscopy and its recent clinical applications in combination with other procedures in children: A narrative review. Nature and Science of Sleep, 17*, 1067–1077. https://www.semanticscholar.org/paper/95699805fe6339ecc214fca0ef2bb5ee420d8c29 (accessed on 15th July 2025).

54. Xu, Z. C. (2023). *[Diagnosis and treatment of disorders of laryngeal airway in children and prospect]. Lin chuang er bi yan hou tou jing wai ke za zhi = Journal of Clinical Otorhinolaryngology, Head, and Neck Surgery, 37*(12), 939–942. https://www.semanticscholar.org/paper/55319

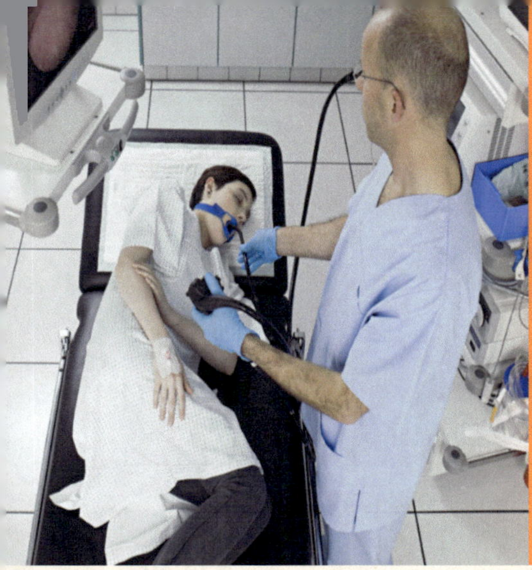

Chapter 14

COMPLICATIONS OF ENDOSCOPY

Contents

Introduction....407
14.1. Types of Endoscopic Procedures....411
14.2. Common Complications....414
14.3. Patient-Related Factors....417
14.4. Technical Factors....421
14.5. Prevention Strategies....424
14.6. Management of Complications....428
Summary....432
References....435

Introduction

The complexity associated with endoscopy extends beyond its diagnostic and therapeutic advantages, requiring careful examination of potential complications. As the procedure has become an integral aspect of modern medical practice, it is important that health workers and patients realize the advantages and disadvantages associated with endoscopy. Complications can range from relatively superficial, such as mucosal irritation, to critical, such as perforation of internal organs or gross infection. Detection of these complications not only decreases their incidence but also enhances the overall efficacy of endoscopic procedures. Moreover, the variety of clinical environments in which endoscopy is practiced—gastroenterology and oncology, for instance—mandates that practitioners remain vigilant and sensitive to specific risks inherent in conditions being treated. Therefore, an overall review of endoscopic complications is necessary to ensure maximum patient safety and outcomes. New developments , such as prehabilitation, demonstrate the dynamic relationship between endoscopic interventions and strategies for patient preparation. Prehabilitation has been proven to significantly enhance the physical condition and quality of life of patients who are undergoing procedures , such as oesophagogastric cancer procedures, eventually resulting in fewer surgical complications. Given the heterogeneity in the availability of and definitions of prehabilitation services among healthcare centers, it is evident that there is still room for improvement in applying these supportive interventions across the board. A collection of survey results confirms the agreement that integrating prehabilitation should be regarded as routine care for patients on curative pathways to improve their resilience during endoscopic procedures. By virtue of uniting preoperative treatment with endoscopic technology, healthcare providers can significantly improve the clinical success of patients, highlighting the importance of interpreting and reacting to both risks and benefits of such new medical technology (Barman et al., 2024). Additionally, endoscopic innovations, such as ERAT, illustrate how enhanced techniques can redefine traditional reactions to surgical complications. This minimally invasive technique offers a worthy option to traditional appendectomy by addressing appendiceal obstructions directly through endoscopic management. Without bypassing surgery, ERAT is less likely to result in complications and encourages a quicker recovery for the right patient population, especially those with other comorbidities. The technical progress in endoscopic techniques, such as application of microbubble contrast media and the mother-baby endoscopic system, also further solidifies the potential of this technology to decrease the complication rate associated with surgical diabetes. As we proceed into the technical aspects of endoscopic treatment and the associated risks, it is increasingly evident that the technological advances must be paired with robust risk mitigation practices (Zhang et al., 2024) (Figure 14.1).

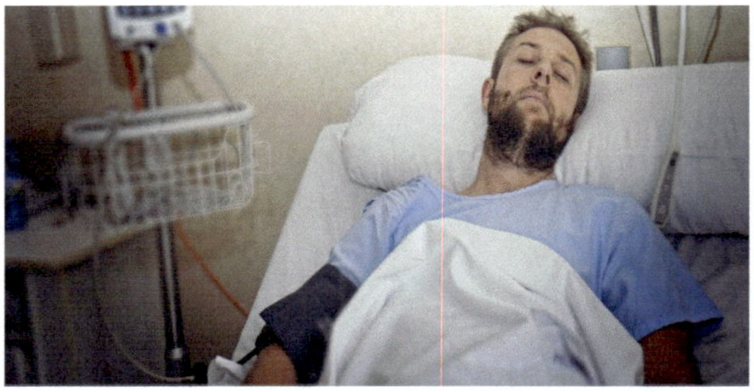

Figure 14.1. Complications of endoscopy.

Source: https://clinicbooking.com/uploads/users/33/articles/blog-single-1728923775-shutterstock_297047780.jpg.

Definition of Endoscopy

Endoscopy is a medical procedure that allows medical practitioners to view the internal organs of a patient's body, particularly the gastrointestinal tract, by employing the services of a flexible tube fitted with a camera and light source. The minimally invasive procedure offers diagnosis and treatment of diseases without the necessity of extensive surgical intervention, reducing recovery time and associated risks. Endoscopic procedures can be applied to an array of indications, including biopsies, foreign body extraction, and hemostasis or stricture management. Use of endoscopy is also feasible in some specialized areas like bariatric surgery, which demands full awareness of related complications and the mechanism to avert them. A proper definition of endoscopy, therefore, not only explains its technical excellence but also explains its uppermost status in current medical practice. The evolution of endoscopic techniques has greatly enhanced their effectiveness, particularly in the management of complications in the course of therapeutic interventions. Innovative techniques , such as the Unilateral Biportal Endoscopy (UBE) Interlaminar Approach, show how technology has made spinal operations less invasive while providing improved anatomical visualization. This particular technique utilizes two portals to access the interlaminar space, allowing for controlled decompression of neural structures with minimal disturbance of surrounding tissues and hence decreased risk of complications. Such innovations highlight the ongoing need for training, study, and experience on the part of endoscopists so that they can effectively handle potential complications that may arise within the clinical setting, facilitating better patient outcomes in the process (Gonçalo Januário, 2025). Endoscopists must also be acutely sensitive to endoscopic procedure complications when working. With the growing incidence of obesity-related disorders, the need for effective bariatric endoscopy has emerged. The European Society of Gastrointestinal Endoscopy (ESGE) has emphasized the need for specialized training to deal with the multiple complications that can occur during the procedure and necessitate comprehensive knowledge of obesity and obesity-related complications. This includes being cognizant of the higher prevalence of gastrointestinal diseases in obese patients and being competent to work in a multidisciplinary environment. By completing proven training and gaining hands-on practice in tertiary referral centers, endoscopists can attain proficiency in managing bariatric endoscopy and surgical procedure complications, finally ensuring patient safety and improved therapeutic efficacy (Boškoski et al., 2023) (Figure 14.2).

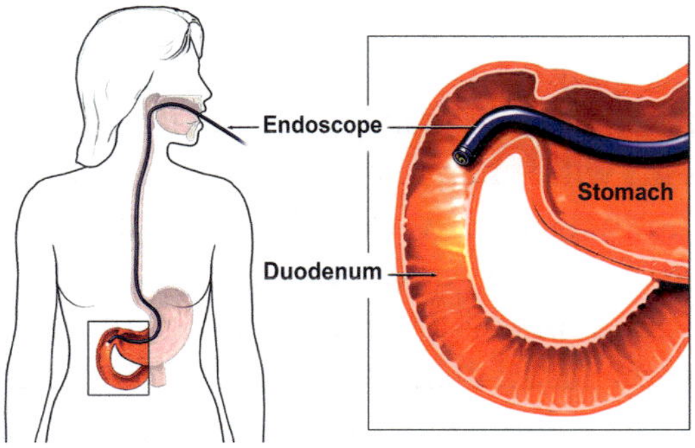

Figure 14.2. Endoscopy.

Source: https://assets.nhs.uk/prod/images/ADTYWB.2e16d0ba.fill-920x613.jpg.

Significance of Endoscopy in Medical Diagnostics

Endoscopy has emerged as a significant technique in medical diagnostics, particularly in the visualization of internal structures and organs that are otherwise not accessible. The ability to conduct minimally invasive examinations allows direct visualization, and this is interpreted to be more accurate diagnoses than through the use of traditional imaging modalities. Pathologies , such as tumors, polyps, and inflammatory conditions can be identified through the use of endoscopic procedures and provide vital information that can guide further treatment. For instance, endoscopic ultrasound (EUS) application has significantly revolutionized the diagnosis of gastric duplication cysts (GDCs), an uncommon congenital anomaly. Ultrasound and EUS, in an interesting case, diagnosed a large GDC that caused segmental portal hypertension, highlighting the significant role of EUS in diagnosing unusual but clinically significant diseases (Boicean et al., 2024). Hence, endoscopy not only enhances diagnostic precision but also allows therapeutic intervention, being a pillar for contemporary medical practice. In addition, endoscopy is of critical significance in cancer prevention and screening, especially in colorectal cancer (CRC). The American Cancer Society highlights the importance of screening among individuals aged 45 and above, citing that it can significantly reduce incidence and mortality in CRC. Many endoscopic treatments, among them colonoscopy, facilitate the early detection and removal of adenomatous polyps and other precancerous lesions and, therefore, prevent cancer formation (Wolf et al., 2018). Screening not only identifies existing anomalies but is also a preventive intervention in public health, which allows for timely interventions and improvement of patient outcomes. Hence, endoscopy is an important procedure in the diagnosis and prevention of cancer at the initial stage, thus making it indispensable as a part of the wider scope of medical diagnostics.

Endoscopy is not risk-free, however, and for this reason alone, an intimate understanding of its dangers is required. Complications of endoscopic procedures range from minor, such as gastrointestinal upset, to disastrous effects like perforation or hemorrhage. These risks emphasize the importance of operator skill, patient choice, and the adoption of appropriate techniques.

For example, management of complications arising from colorectal screening can pose further diagnostic issues and necessitate further interventions, therefore complicating patient care. It is, thus, although endoscopy forms an essential component of diagnostics and treatment, ongoing education and adherence to precautions are vital in preventing complications and improving patient care. Continuous monitoring of post-endoscopic procedure adverse events is required to improve practice quality and ensure patient safety for this important diagnostic method.

Overview of Potential Complications

The potential complications of endoscopy procedures are a wide range of risks that can be highly variable based on the type of procedure. Bleeding, perforation, and infections are some of the most common complications that are often encountered. Bleeding is possible during polypectomies or biopsies, and it is a risk factor, especially for patients who are receiving anticoagulant therapy. Perforation, though uncommon, is a severe complication with significant morbidity; GI tract integrity must be preserved, and any compromise will lead to peritonitis and will require immediate surgical intervention. Infections may occur due to the infusion of foreign substances through the endoscope, and there is a risk of contamination and it is challenging to maintain aseptic technique throughout the procedure. Thus, clinicians will be obligated to take seriously the benefits of endoscopic procedures against these complications risks to get the best patient outcomes. Complications due to endoscopy could be serious and demand multi-disciplinary management. For instance, perforation cases might entail not only surgical closure but intensive post-surgical care to prevent secondary complications like sepsis. Hence, early diagnosis and intervention are important in preventing bad outcomes. In addition, endoscopy may overlay risk on patients' underlying medical conditions, such as cardiovascular disease. Extensive pre-procedure assessment to identify patients at risk for complications is important. Patients with established thrombocytopenia, for instance, would require platelet transfusion before highly manipulative procedures. Incorporation of patient history in detail and meticulous procedure planning will minimize risks and enhance safety in endoscopic practice. In consideration of the ongoing pandemic burden of COVID-19, the delivery of surgical care, including endoscopy, has been significantly impacted. Patients are experiencing delayed access to necessary interventions, which ultimately leads to worsening of their conditions and development of secondary complications, as identified in recent literature.

The pandemic has raised awareness of the importance of proper handling of permissions for surgical and endoscopic interventions. Stakeholders are now more clearly acknowledging the necessity of having contingency plans in place to handle unexpected events that may disrupt care delivery so that patients with emergent endoscopic requirements are not neglected. With the healthcare systems developing to address these challenges, prioritization of endoscopy procedures must be incorporated in national health planning agendas as fundamental to maintaining patient general well-being and averting potential complications arising from delay in treatment (Søreide et al., 2020) (Figure 14.3).

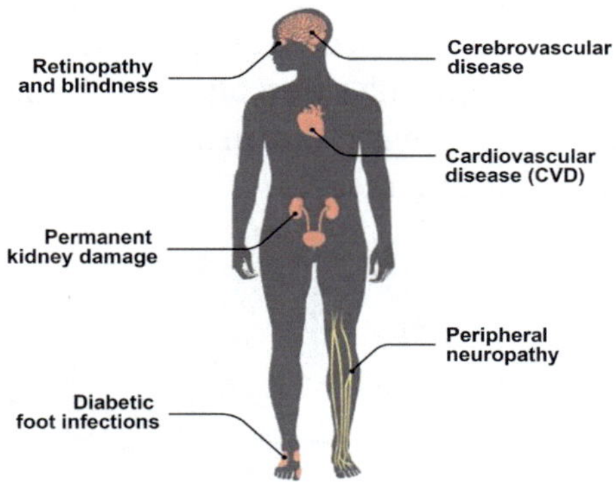

Figure 14.3. Overview of potential complications.

Source: https://post.medicalnewstoday.com/wp-content/uploads/sites/3/2022/01/1552759-Type-2-Diabetes-Mellitus-Complications_Header-Body_1296x728.png.

14.1. Types of Endoscopic Procedures

Endoscopic procedures are diverse, created to examine various regions of the human body as well as body diseases. Among the most common ones are upper GI endoscopies, which consist of esophagogastroduodenoscopy (EGD). The procedure is instrumental in diagnosing conditions , such as gastritis, peptic ulceration, and esophageal varices. Through the utilization of a flexible endoscope introduced orally, physicians can visualize the upper gastrointestinal tract, biopsy, or even establish therapeutic interventions. The ability to address issues in real-time enhances the diagnostic yield and therapeutic efficacy. Though complications , such as perforation, bleeding, and infection, while unusual, do necessitate careful patient selection and preparation, as discussed more exhaustively in the literature regarding the subtlety of endoscopic procedures (Cook et al., 1999). Other than upper GI endoscopy, colonoscopy is today an important procedure in colorectal cancer screening and management. With this procedure, not only is it possible to examine the colon, but polyps can also be removed to prevent malignant transformation. In a study of adenomatous polyps, it is established that a high percentage of malignant lesions are caused by missed or inadequately treated polyps on colonoscopy (Moldovan et al., 2017). Standardization of the procedure has improved rates of early detection, with markedly better patient outcomes. The procedure is risky, though, with perforation of the bowel and huge bleeding being complications encountered, albeit statistically rare. Awareness of risk makes it easier to plan discussions with patients regarding the relative benefit versus complications of screening regularly. Flexible bronchoscopy is another important endoscopic procedure, particularly in pulmonary medicine. Such an approach facilitates direct visualization of the airways and lungs and enables the diagnosis and treatment of various respiratory disorders like infections, tumors, and foreign body aspiration. The procedure can also facilitate bronchoalveolar lavage with the ability to have microbiological analysis and cytological studies. Bronchoscopy, though useful, has some risk, since pneumothorax and airway trauma are possible complications that require skilled operators and diligent patient evaluation before the procedure. Like any other endoscopic procedure, the benefits must be weighed against the potential complication risk so that patients may get the most informed management. In general, one must have a good understanding of types and corresponding risks of endoscopic procedures to enhance patient care in all medical disciplines.

14.1.1. Gastrointestinal Endoscopy

Gastrointestinal endoscopy has become a pivotal tool in the diagnosis and management of a host of gastrointestinal diseases, including gastroesophageal reflux disease (GERD) and peptic ulcers. The procedure, however, is not free from complications that impact patient outcomes in a significant way. Of these, bleeding and perforation are most concerning. Bleeding secondary to biopsies and polypectomies occasionally may necessitate blood transfusion and surgery in patients with coagulopathies or on anticoagulants. Perforation is a rare but dangerous complication that may lead to peritonitis and immediate surgical intervention. Incidence and prevalence of such complications warrant careful scrutiny of indications for endoscopy and the methods employed, especially in resource-poor countries where resources may not always be accessible and competency is uneven (Hunt et al., 2017). With the potential complications that may come from gastrointestinal endoscopy, a lot of emphasis must be laid on the right patient selection and preparation. Strict examination of patients' histories, including previous gastrointestinal interventions and current drug intake, can also be able to minimize risks. In addition, patient education concerning the risk for complications before the procedure may enable them to be ready for any adverse outcomes. Clinical procedures have come to suggest risk stratification based on patients' individual profiles, which can enhance the safety of endoscopic procedures. By better training and increased standardization of protocols, the rate of complications can be decreased, further highlighting the necessity of continuing education within the medical profession regarding best practice in endoscopy (García-Tsao et al., 2016). Gastrointestinal endoscopy complications highlight the necessity of continued surveillance and research into rates of complications and management strategies. The application of complication reporting and review protocols will assist in the observation of trends and areas of improvement. For instance, institutions can adopt protocols calling for post-procedure follow-up assessment to determine complications early. Application of multicenter trials in establishing national standards for complication rates will assist clinicians in making more informed choices concerning patient care. The importance of multidisciplinary management of endoscopic patients cannot be overstated; coordination of gastroenterologist, surgeon, and anesthesiologist services is necessary to optimize outcomes and minimize risks associated with the procedure (Hunt et al., 2017) (Figure 14.4).

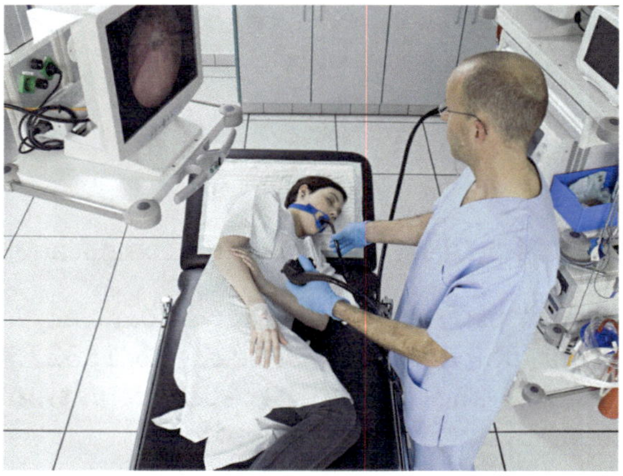

Figure 14.4. Gastrointestinal endoscopy.

Source: https://www.higherlevelhealthcare.com/wp-content/uploads/2016/02/Knowing-About-Endoscopy.jpg.

14.1.2. Bronchoscopy

The application of bronchoscopy, although an indispensable part of pulmonary disease evaluation and management, is not complication-free. More common risks that are most frequently implicated include bleeding, infection, and pneumothorax, but less common complications can sometimes arise, such as pneumomediastinum or pneumoperitoneum. These are typically from barotrauma by lung overinflation or alveolar rupture during the procedure. The Macklin effect refers to how air can dissect interstitial tissues following such rupture and lead to complications that complicate clinical examinations. Early detection and diagnosis of such conditions are central to avoiding severe consequences, and imaging methods , such as computed tomography (CT) can be a breakthrough in detecting and evaluating such rare events after bronchoscopy is completed (Chaimae et al., 2025). Apart from routine risks associated with bronchoscopy, there may also be complications related to particular procedures, such as bronchoplastic surgery. With these procedures, anastomotic site is particularly at risk for complications that may occur during the early postoperative period. In monitoring with bronchoscopy, doctors can detect anastomotic complications, which are fistulas and stenosis, that are vital in patient healing. Endoscopic examination following bronchoplasty was studied, where observations , such as circular slough and mucosal coloration change can reliably predict these complications. This has been noted to emphasize the significance of early bronchoscopy in establishing minor changes at the anastomotic site, thus allowing for early intervention measures and improved patient outcomes (Fukui et al., 2024).

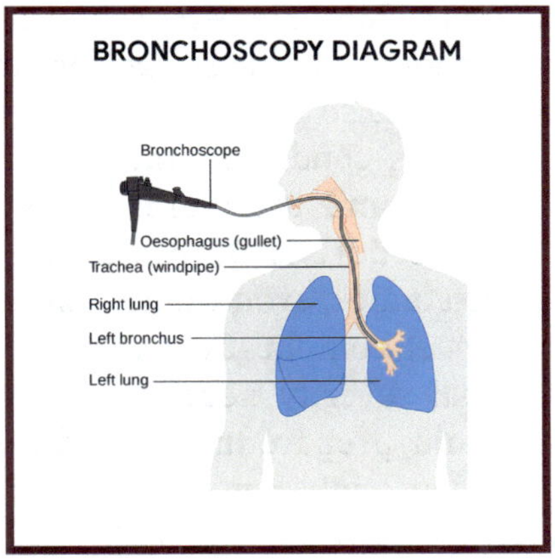

Figure 14.5. Bronchoscopy.

Source: https://nurseslabs.com/wp-content/uploads/2018/10/BRONCHOSCOPY-DIAGRAMBronchoscopy.jpg.

Ultimately, the value of bronchoscopy goes beyond diagnostic purposes as a tool for the proactive treatment of complications in various clinical contexts. The ability to identify serious complications at a pre-emptive level is essential for the procurement of appropriate patient care. Identification of prospective risks associated with bronchoscopy, including those associated with surgical procedures , such as bronchoplasty, enables health care providers to initiate proper follow-up interventions, thereby enhancing patient surveillance and management. By having a better understanding of complexities and utilizing advanced imaging techniques for assessment, the health environment can facilitate the response to complications, thereby fostering better patient outcomes and reducing morbidity from bronchoscopy procedures (Figure 14.5).

14.1.3. Urological Endoscopy

Urological endoscopy is among the advances of major significance in the management of urological disease, particularly urolithiasis, which has increasingly become prevalent among patients. This less-invasive technique allows for immediate visualization and therapy of stones in the various segments of the urinary tract, i.e., the kidneys, ureters, bladder, and urethra. Before the advent of endoscopic techniques, surgical therapy of stones had been largely based on open surgical operations like ureterolithotomy and nephrolithotomy, which in most instances were associated with prolonged convalescence and higher morbidity rates. Introduction of endoscopy has brought improved patient outcomes, with comparable efficacy at a lower rate of complications when compared to traditional surgery. As the technology continues to advance, familiarity with the various endoscopic techniques and how they connect to surgical management becomes increasingly significant in terms of improving patient quality of life and surgical outcome (Kim, 2020). Among the significant problems that relate to any form of endoscopic procedure, like urological endoscopy, is the risk of developing complications throughout and after the intervention. Though these interventions are designed to inflict a minimal amount of damage, possible risks of infection, bleeding, and rupture of neighboring tissues must be thoroughly researched. The Clavien-Dindo grading is a significant tool for assessing and grading the severity of postoperative complication to enable healthcare workers to address complications pre-emptively and minimize risks substantially. By analyzing patient outcome data following urological endoscopy, healthcare providers are able to determine trends in complication rates, thereby enhancing surgical performance and patient care. The role of preoperative examinations, especially in risk populations , such as the elderly, cannot be overstated since examinations determine surgical procedures that can diminish the risk of post-procedure complications (Serretta et al., 2019). Further, the integration of new technologies and improved endoscopic instrumentation expanded the range of treatment options but at the same time necessitates ongoing education and training for urological surgeons. As less invasive techniques become increasingly prevalent, the skills to control possible complications must keep up with these advances. Surgical teams must be proficient not just in performing the operations but also in recognizing and properly controlling complications in case they do occur. Greater attention is being given to interdisciplinary care, particularly for the patient at higher risk for complications due to comorbid illness or advanced age.

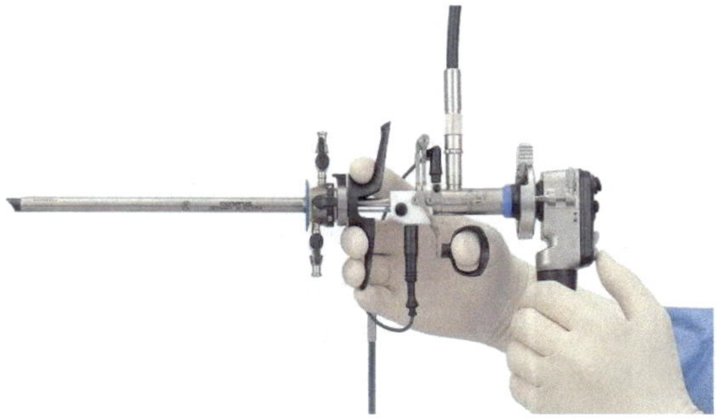

Figure 14.6. Urological endoscopy.

Source: https://www.massdevice.com/wp-content/uploads/2024/09/Olympus-4K-camera-head-CH-S700-08-LB.jpg.

This is even more so given that nearly 25% of the urological population is above 75 years of age, and so there has to be a balance of finesse with respect to the safety of urological endoscopy and controlling its risks (Serretta et al., 2019) (Figure 14.6).

14.2. Common Complications

Endoscopy, beneficial as it is in diagnosis and treatment, has complications of its own. Two of the most frequent complications are bleeding and perforation. These can happen due to the invasive nature of the procedure and the potential disruption of the gastrointestinal tract or adjacent anatomical integrity. For instance, with techniques like endoscopic retrograde cholangiopancreatography (ERCP), manipulations required in penetrating bile ducts can lead to hemorrhage or tissue perforation. Such complications are also increased in those patients with pre-existing conditions that may weaken tissue integrity, and therefore, more caution during the procedure is warranted. As quoted in numerous studies, even though the absolute incidence of such complications is relatively low, their potential severity necessitates thorough knowledge and preparedness on the part of medical professionals performing endoscopic procedures (Azab et al., 2019). Apart from bleeding and perforation, infection is a dangerous complication following endoscopic procedures. Endoscopic interventions, particularly when biopsies or drainage are done, can seed pathogens into normally non-contaminated body regions, leading to postoperative infections. The risk is also heightened in immunocompromised patients or in the event of underlying infections. In some of these endoscopic interventions, the administration of prophylactic antibiotics is required to be administered as part of a risk reduction process, and thus, proper prophylaxis measures become highly relevant. Complications , such as cholangitis, an infection of the bile duct, may arise from ERCP, particularly if stones are being dislodged within the bile duct and retained. This is why proper post-procedure observation and patient education regarding signs of infection are required so that any problem can be rectified promptly, with overall improved patient outcomes (Azab et al., 2019). Finally, another serious domain of complications of endoscopy is the risk of drug and anesthesia-related complications. Patients undergoing endoscopy tend to receive sedation or general anesthesia, each carrying inherent risks. Adverse reactions may present in the form of respiratory complications, cardiovascular instability, or allergic reactions, thereby making recovery after the surgery more difficult. Also, vigilant selection and monitoring of the anesthetic drugs are most critical, particularly in those with higher risk, e.g., elderly patients or comorbidities. The requirement continues to achieve a balance between satisfactorily sedating to satisfy the patient's comfort and preventing such anergic reactions. Thus, a thorough pre-procedure assessment and consent interview is of utmost significance to be able to manage such risks effectively so that patients are well-informed while undergoing endoscopic procedures

14.2.1. Perforation of Organs

Organ perforation risk during endoscopic procedure is one of the serious complications which predominantly is restricted to gastrointestinal intervention. This may occur when there is undue force or anatomical distortion with pathology. Perforation can lead to leakage of gastrointestinal contents into the peritoneum, which causes potentially lethal diseases like peritonitis or sepsis that may necessitate urgent surgery. Awareness of such a complication underscores the need for attentiveness and careful pre-procedure planning. There are risk factors that researchers have identified to contribute to increased perforation susceptibility, including the patient's predisposition and procedure complexity itself, highlighting the importance of adequate patient evaluation before endoscopy (Alkhazal'eh, 2023). Additionally, there are certain endoscopic procedures that are predisposed to cause perforation more than others. Dilation or extraction of obstructive lesions, for example, exposes adjacent organs to risk. Particularly, therapeutic ERCP can involve manipulation in the area where duodenal perforation or bile duct perforation is at risk. Statistical reports of complications have shown varying rates of perforation, with some procedures more frequent than others. Such complications can lead to prolonged hospitalization, extra healthcare costs, and potential adverse patient outcomes, further reinforcing the imperative for training and acquaintance with endoscopic practice (Tang et al., 2023). Lastly, perforation management following endoscopy demands an understanding of both short-term and long-term impacts on patient care. Early recognition and intervention are fundamental to preventing the consequences of perforation because immediate surgical intervention can minimize morbidity and mortality from this complication.

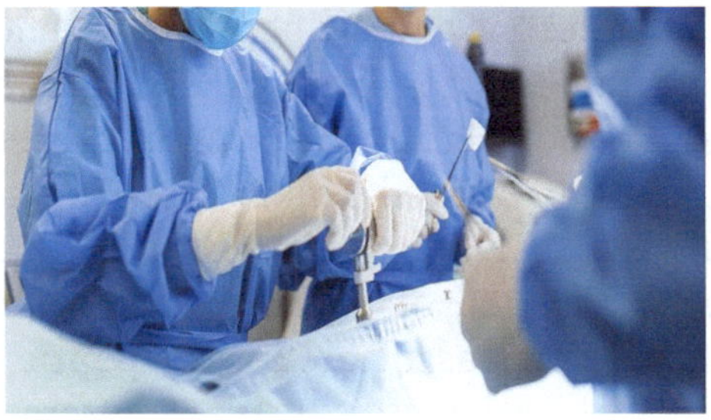

Figure 14.7. Perforation of organs.

Source: https://eprk6hywmdt.exactdn.com/wp-content/uploads/IVC-Filters-Causing-Perforation-of-Veins-and-Organs-Featured-Image.webp.

Decision for treatment can otherwise be determined based on perforation location and extent and also the patient's general health status. Initiation of monitoring and post-procedure protocols can substantially minimize risk and maximize outcomes for patients. Finally, recognizing and taking control of the risk for perforation in the context of endoscopy is crucial to improving procedural safety and promoting the best patient recovery (Sana'a Alkhazal'eh, 2023) (Figure 14.7).

14.2.2. Infection Risks

Within the context of endoscopic procedures, risks of infection are an ongoing relevant issue that needs vigilant attention from health care providers. There is a risk of infectious complications in the form of bacteremia and cholangitis due to the invasive nature of the procedure. Specifically, during processes like ERCP, there is a reported risk of inoculation of bacteria into the bloodstream, particularly among those patients who already have weakened immune systems. In studies, it has been demonstrated that antibiotic prophylaxis is beneficial in reducing the risk of post-ERCP bacteremia among high-risk groups of patients. But it is crucial that such prophylaxis selection and timing are individualized according to patient profiles since the effectiveness of antibiotics varies in different patient populations and also in some underlying diseases and guidelines should be perfected with further research (Kowalski & Przybyłkowski, 2024). Another crucial point in infection risk in endoscopy is the prevalence of *Helicobacter pylori*, an organism highly associated with peptic ulcer disease. This pathogen is also asymptomatic in the majority of its infected patients until they present with complications, which could make the clinical presentation more complicated for gastroenterologists. In a study among patients who have been exposed to upper gastrointestinal endoscopy, there has been a disconcerting rate of about 49.66% of *H. pylori* infection, particularly in the elderly and those with a history of NSAIDs usage (Calori et al., 2024). These findings emphasize preoperative screening and potential treatment of *H. pylori* infection in anticipation of elective endoscopic procedures, particularly in patients with relevant symptoms or risk factors. Screening and preemption of such infections will prevent endoscopic procedure-related postoperative complications. Infection control practice during endoscopic procedures cannot be overemphasized. Appropriate disinfection of endoscopes and adherence to sterilization protocols are needed to minimize the risk of healthcare-associated infection. Despite advances in techniques of sterilization, endoscopic equipment-borne infection has been observed to result in outbreaks, highlighting vulnerabilities in current practice (Kowalski & Przybyłkowski, 2024). Environmental factors within healthcare settings, such as hospital cleanliness and adherence of staff to infection prevention measures, are significant determinants of infection transmission risk. Lastly, strict infection control measures and pre-procedure infection screening for diseases like *H. pylori* can greatly reduce overall infection risk with endoscopy. As endoscopy develops, however, ongoing education and vigilance in these areas will be essential to safeguard patient well-being and optimize clinical outcomes.

14.2.3. Bleeding During or After the Procedure

Bleeding during or after endoscopy is a significant complication that results in severe patient morbidity. Many factors predispose to this risk, particularly in patients with pre-existing conditions , such as liver disease. The hemostatic mechanism in the case of liver cirrhosis is greatly altered and is characterized by decreased coagulation factors and thrombocytopenia. As such, such patients are bound to present with a multifaceted coagulation profile that complicates assessment of procedural bleeding risk. The usual prothrombin time and INR tests are likely to fall short of reflecting the hemostatic function in such patients and cause clinicians to underestimate bleeding risk. With this understanding, utilization of more integrated hemostatic tests becomes crucial, remembering that the interaction between prohemostatic and antihemostatic mechanisms significantly impacts bleeding results. Impressive procedural planning with thorough patient assessment will avoid bleeding complications in such at-risk populations (Northup et al., 2020). The environment of endoscopic procedures, particularly for esophageal and gastrointestinal procedures, places additional significance on extremes of bleeding complication variability. For instance, post-endoscopic submucosal dissection bleeding (PEB) is among the challenging outcomes to predict, particularly because the bleeding can be early or late after the intervention. In studies, early PEB has been associated with lesion diameter, procedure time, and consumption of antiplatelet medications like clopidogrel.

The prevalence of early bleeding has been reported at 2.4%, making it necessary to establish risk factors to implement early intervention. Conversely, late PEB can present without an antecedent symptom, and close monitoring during the healing phase is essential. Endoscopists also need to keep a keen eye on ulcer characteristics that indicate a higher risk of bleeding and take active steps in such patients to improve outcomes (Nam et al., 2019). Treatment strategies in high-risk patients for procedural bleeding must consider preparation and response strategies. For those found to have greater than one risk factor for early PEB, alternatives , such as selective second-look endoscopy can be beneficial for early treatment and diagnosis. The use of pre-procedure testing in the form of imaging and laboratory work to risk-stratify can improve patient safety. Following high-risk procedures, protocols for monitoring should exist to diagnose and treat early manifestations of bleeding. The physician must balance prophylactic therapy risks against the likelihood of bleeding events, and only in the light of a knowledge of the complexities of each patient's circumstances should decisions be made. Overall, control of endoscopy bleeding complications needs a multidimensional approach with risk stratification, attentiveness in the procedure, and adequate follow-up measures (Northup et al., 2020) (Figure 14.8).

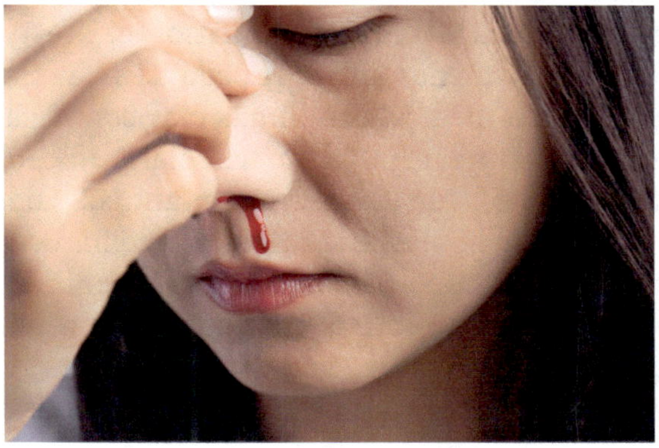

Figure 14.8. Bleeding during or after the procedure.

Source: https://www.verywellhealth.com/thmb/kyQpHdG_CSQUmsm0d6lUkKbTNRk=/5520x3684/filters:no_upscale():max_bytes(150000):strip_icc()/close-up-of-woman-with-bleeding-nose-1180586363-a44410be16484bd3b4f10fbc4a04078a.jpg.

14.3. Patient-Related Factors

Factors related to the patient are relevant in endoscopy both for the decision regarding the necessity of the procedure and its complications. GERD is probably the most frequent illness for which endoscopic treatment is performed and affects a high proportion of adults in industrialized countries. Those presenting with common symptoms of GERD can require endoscopy to assess potential complications like esophagitis or strictures (Maret-Ouda et al., 2020). In addition, age, sex, and BMI also play a significant role in outcomes because older patients or patients with higher levels of obesity are at increased risk for gastrointestinal complications. Minimization of such risks necessitates judicious evaluation of the clinical history of each patient as well as a deep understanding of their symptomatology, thereby substantiating the imperative for customized care and determination of lifestyle factors before endoscopic procedures. Further, concomitant medical conditions may complicate endoscopic interventions, particularly in those with chronic liver disease or on anticoagulant therapy. The hemostatic imbalances shared by cirrhotic patients, i.e., thrombocytopenia and coagulopathy, profoundly influence procedure outcomes. Risk of bleeding remains an overarching issue, with traditional coagulation tests like INR being unable to effectively predict hemostatic function in such patients (Northup et al., 2020). Clinicians should carefully evaluate every patient's liver function and healthy status worthy of recommendation, considering the implications of their comorbidities to prepare appropriately for the potential complications of endoscopy. Therefore, a general evaluation directed towards individual patient factors not only decides the timing and urgency of the procedure but also guides perioperative management measures to prevent risks. Patient adherence and pre-procedure preparation are also critical predictors of endoscopy-related complications. Adherent patients, following pre-procedure advice , such as dietary restrictions and medication adjustment, are more likely to experience effective results with fewer complications. Non-adherence can lead to inadequate bowel preparation or increased procedural risks, thus highlighting the importance of patient education and active involvement in their care pathway. Clarity of communication regarding the requirement for lifestyle modifications, specifically for patients having GERD or who require anticoagulation, is likely to have a favorable impact on procedural experience and outcome (Maret-Ouda et al., 2020; Northup et al., 2020). Finally, tailoring endoscopic practice to specific patients based on these patient-specific factors is likely to improve safety and efficacy and reduce the frequency of procedure-related complications.

14.3.1. Pre-Existing Medical Conditions

The presence of concurrent medical conditions is an essential factor for endoscopic procedure success rates, with a tendency to increase the risk of complications. Some studies emphasize that patients with chronic medical conditions , such as cardiovascular disease, diabetes, and COPD, are more susceptible to post-endoscopy complications. For instance, cardiovascular complications can complicate the process of sedation procedures and recovery, with risks of adverse events , such as arrhythmias or hypotension. Moreover, studies revealed that diabetic patients may experience impaired healing of wounds and susceptibility to infections because of a compromised immune system and vascular disorders. Therefore, assessing a patient's medical history becomes inevitable in deciding to proceed with endoscopy and adapting certain preparatory and intra-procedural steps to avert risks associated with these pre-existing conditions. The complexity of managing patients with existing medical illnesses during endoscopy necessitates a multidisciplinary process in the evaluation and perioperative care of patients. Preprocedure screening should include proper evaluations of a patient's chronic disease, which can inform the healthcare team regarding the anticipated risks as well as any necessary modifications of customary endoscopic methods. Techniques , such as intensified monitoring of vital signs and altered sedation techniques can be implemented to ensure stability throughout the procedure. Proper integration of anesthetic techniques and closely monitored intra-procedural treatment becomes crucial in patients with severe comorbid conditions. A proper understanding of how concomitant diseases influence the endoscopic process is therefore critical towards maximizing patient safety and outcomes. Patient outcomes following endoscopy may also be dictated by the medical team's understanding of how specific pre-existing medical conditions influence recovery. For instance, patients with liver disease may have impaired drug metabolism and, as such, careful agent choice and dosing of anesthetic agents must be performed to avoid postoperative complications. Furthermore, the presence of conditions , such as obesity and sleep apnea can lead to additional airway management challenges and potential respiratory complications during sedation. One study that came out some time ago underscored the value of follow-up and monitoring after procedures in relation to the patient's overall state of health, particularly in patients with chronic medical illness, since they may require extended observation and supportive management. Such considerations not only help reduce short-term procedural risk but also promote longer-term recovery and satisfaction. Addressing these multifactorial factors is crucial to optimize the peri-endoscopic care continuum in patients with pre-existing medical conditions (Figure 14.9).

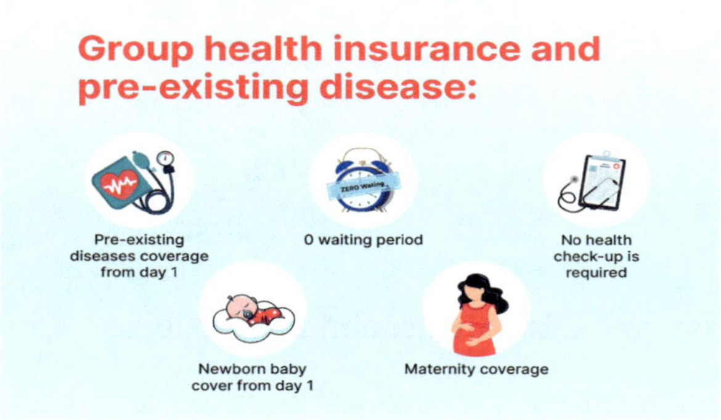

Figure 14.9. Pre-existing medical conditions.

Source: https://assets-global.website-files.com/6145f7156a1337613524d548/62419fd8c16fe585927601d0_Pre-existing_Infographic02-01.jpg.

14.3.2. Age and Overall Health

The relationship between age and general health lies at the heart of grasping the complexities in relation to endoscopy procedures. As age progresses, the individual is likely to experience a loss of physiological reserves and consequently become more vulnerable to different health issues. Geriatric patients are often associated with comorbidities , such as hypertension, diabetes, or cardiovascular disease, which may add to the risks of endoscopic procedures. Furthermore, physiological alteration with age can influence not only the success of procedures but also recovery times. For instance, decreased renal function and alterations in drug metabolism may complicate anesthetic and sedation plans, necessitating customized approaches to ensure patient safety. According to these issues, a keen assessment of the health condition of the older patient is essential before the scheduling of endoscopic procedures to avoid the risk of adverse events. The specific importance of gastrointestinal disorders, which are prevalent among the elderly, further complicates the management of endoscopic procedures. Conditions , such as *Helicobacter pylori* infection and inflammatory bowel disease, for example, ulcerative colitis and Crohn's disease, illustrate the intersection of health complexity and age. The Maastricht/Florence 2021 Consensus Report emphasizes that the rising antibiotic resistance with *H. pylori* necessitates cautionary treatment strategies, especially for older patients, who may respond differently to standard therapies (Malfertheiner et al., 2022). Additionally, the variations in inflammatory load experienced in chronic gastrointestinal illness emphasize the importance of an endoscopic treatment approach in a multidisciplinary plan for older patients. With specific application of treatment and prevention approaches, health care providers can optimize the outcome in these vulnerable individuals. In the practice of gastrointestinal illness, the influence of the age factor not only on presentation of illness but also on management and therapeutic response needs to be considered. Third, holistic care with an expert team should be included in optimizing treatment models for very old inflammatory bowel disease patients. The report of a recent guideline by medical specialty stakeholders cites the need for individually tailored pharmacological and non-pharmacological treatments that consider the unique health profiles of patients over 16 years (Lamb et al., 2019). This multi-disciplinary approach facilitates the explanation of patient needs better and enhances inter-setting communication towards the ultimate aim of endoscopic procedure complication reduction. It is thus important to know the particular health concerns of older adults from the perspective of maximizing endoscopic practice and enhancing patient outcomes.

14.3.3. Medication Interactions

Drug interactions pose significant hazards during endoscopic intervention, particularly in patients on long-term therapy for chronic conditions. The above reaction of sedatives used for endoscopy and home medication taken by the patient is capable of creating very risky complications. For instance, the use of opioids for post-procedure pain can lead to dangerous interactions, particularly when there is concomitant use of antidepressants. The combination of these drug classes can lead to unwanted side effects , such as serotonin syndrome, which can manifest with severe clinical features and necessitate close observation and management. Historically underemphasized in endoscopy, awareness of these drug interactions is critical for healthcare professionals to mitigate risks of compound medication regimens. The occurrence underscores the need for full medication reconciliation before and following endoscopic interventions to prevent complications and ensure patient safety. Apart from opioids and antidepressants, other medication classes can equally be culpable for negative interactions during endoscopic interventions. The advent of newer forms of therapy in endoscopy, such as endoscopic ultrasound (EUS) and ERCP, has opened up newer fields of therapy for biliopancreatic disease. However, new techniques necessitate us understanding the concurrent medication regimens of patients better, as inconsistencies lead to issues , such as pancreatitis, which occurs most commonly with ERCP procedures. The clinicians must also consider the pharmacokinetics and potential interactions with gastroenteric medications, anticoagulants, or antiplatelet drugs that are prescribed to patients. The risk of adverse drug effects is thus still a significant consideration as endoscopic technology continues to expand in advancement, requiring meticulous medication management in the outpatient setting. Furthermore, the heightened risk of medication interaction complications for endoscopy extends to the wider area of biliopancreatic disease management.

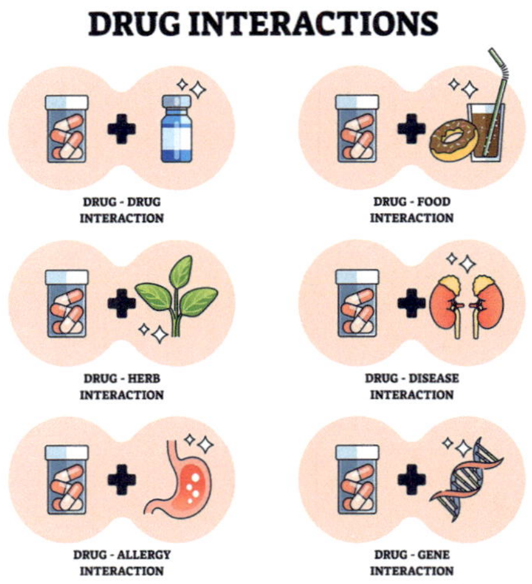

Figure 14.10. Medication interactions.

Source: https://www.docseducation.com/sites/default/files/inline-images/bl_ex_2.jpg.

As endoscopy procedures are performed increasingly, a multi-disciplinary approach becomes necessary in identifying and managing risks related to medication. Procedures like diligent pre-procedure screening, obtaining patient medication histories, and ongoing education on the healthcare team all serve as backbone functions in avoiding the enumerated risks. The complexities of drug interactions underscore the necessity for an integrated model of care, with gastroenterologists working in close conjunction with primary care physicians and pharmacists. By improved communication and interprofessional care, the medical teams can manage the complexity of the patients' medication regimens more effectively, ultimately reducing the rate of complications during and after endoscopy, as evidenced in the relevant literature (Maluf-Filho et al., 2012; Gaffney et al., 2015) (Figure 14.10).

14.4. Technical Factors

Technical factors that may lead to challenges both during and after procedures to a large extent shape the complexity of endoscopic procedures. Foremost among these are the skill levels of the surgeons and the complexity of the apparatus employed. Such high technologies as robot systems enable precision but come with their own set of complicating factors in terms of requiring specialized training to operate them and even equipment failure. Literature indicates that the level of procedural difficulty, particularly in cases like robot-assisted pancreaticoduodenectomy, affects patient results, with increased rates of complications due to specific technical difficulties and patient-related factors, e.g., the PD-ROBOSCORE, which quantifies the complexity of surgery performed (González-Abós et al., 2025). Accordingly, without the right surgical experience and skill with the technology, postoperative pancreatic fistulas are one complication that can occur, highlighting the need for technical competence in manipulation during endoscopic procedures. Another crucial technical consideration is the selection of appropriate procedural strategies among high-risk patients, particularly those undergoing ERCP. The incidence of pancreatitis associated with ERCP emphasizes the importance of proper planning and execution in the case of such patients. Technical proficiency in the identification and prevention of risk factors, such as patient characteristics and specific intervention-related qualities, is significant in the prevention of complications (Pal et al., 2025). Therefore, the use of preventive measures, such as specific pharmacological interventions , such as ulinastatin, can enhance patient outcomes through lowering the incidence of post-ERCP pancreatitis and its complications. Such an anticipatory approach requires a clear technical application and acquaintance with the patient's individual health data to optimize the surgery experience and minimize unwanted results. Additionally, the technical parameters determining endoscopic interventions are more than just the immediate skill and limitation of the surgeon and the chosen devices. Endoscopic equipment technology and its operation are intrinsic characteristics that could determine the success of the procedure and safety. Technological advances are focused on enhancing visualization and maneuverability, but must be extensively tested and validated to prevent negative outcomes. Misdesign of suboptimal instruments, for instance, can lead to trauma and misdiagnosis, adding to the complexity of patient care. Clinical staff must remain current with advancements in endoscopic technology and monitor their impact on patient safety continually. Through accepting robust training and adhering to evidence-based practice, healthcare professionals can navigate the complex terrain of technical considerations, therefore mitigating complications and maximizing the success of endoscopic procedures.

14.4.1. Equipment Malfunction

The advanced nature of endoscopic equipment presents serious concerns regarding equipment failure as one of the major complications of endoscopic procedures. Sophisticated endoscopic equipment, designed to be accurate and effective, is not exempt from failure. The sophisticated engineering is normally intertwined with user operation and device capability and is thus subject to instances where both user error and device design can result in malfunction. Based on a study, the majority of failures occur when the device's primary functions are being executed, such as tissue securing and transecting. This observation illustrates the stark need for extensive training among medical professionals to counter the dangers of these advanced devices, thereby sharing with producers and medical personnel alike the responsibility of countering this ongoing problem (Riggs, 2017). Assessment of the impact of equipment malfunction in endoscopy would also involve quantifying the adverse consequences resulting from such a malfunction. The fact that there is a correlation between the complexity of devices and the gravity of consequences shows that the more complicated the devices are, the greater the potential for severe complications. Specifically, where failure occurs during treatment, the impact can range from simple inconvenience to extreme patient damage. Notably, endoscopy failure mode can lead to complications that not only prolong medical procedures but also require subsequent surgeries to rectify problems caused by machine malfunctions. Research describes that the greatest severity of adverse effects is generally linked with process operations where critical tasks are performed, thereby highlighting the significance of proactive prevention mechanisms in the entire surgical process (Dao et al., 2020). In light of endoscopic device failure issues, there is an utmost need for ongoing innovation and improvement in medical device design. There should be collaboration among surgeons and engineers because collective efforts can lead to more reliable equipment that prioritizes safety and efficiency. Incorporating rigorous testing procedures before coming up with the equipment available for market release has the potential to reveal failure points and address them proactively. In addition, encouraging ongoing communication between manufacturers and users can facilitate enhancing device design to accommodate actual operating room settings. Lastly, encouraging a culture of inclusive risk assessment and education can work significantly in rendering endoscopic procedures safer, eradicating the root causes of equipment malfunction and resulting complications (Riggs, 2017) (Figure 14.11).

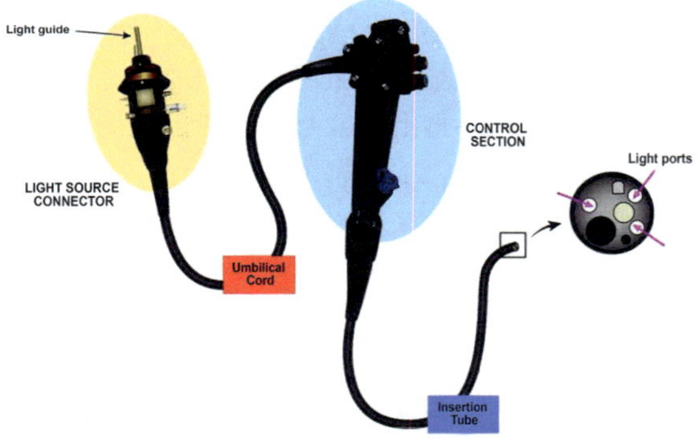

Figure 14.11. Equipment malfunction.

Source: https://i.ytimg.com/vi/kHONXxQK3iE/maxresdefault.jpg.

14.4.2. Operator Skill and Experience

The competence and experience of the operator directly influence the outcome and complications after endoscopic procedures. Trained endoscopists are important in enhancing diagnostic yield and minimizing complications. Through research, it is proven that operators who perform procedures are often more capable of diagnosing conditions, such as malignancies, and managing complex situations during endoscopy. This ability is particularly critical in risk prevention from interventions like colonic stenting, which requires some technical competence and decision-making capabilities. The European Society of Gastrointestinal Endoscopy underscores that colonic stenting should be done or directly supervised by an individual who can demonstrate proficiency in both colonoscopy and fluoroscopic techniques and one who regularly performs colonic stenting (van Hooft et al., 2020). These standards highlight the requirement of ongoing training and skill assessment to ensure patient safety during endoscopic procedures. Over the past few years, there has been ongoing improvement through technological development in aiding operator skill and experience with the incorporation of artificial intelligence (AI) in endoscopic procedures. Computer-aided polyp detection systems have also been shown to hold promise in raising adenoma detection rates (ADRs), especially where operators are not as experienced. Evidence hints towards the integration of AI technologies being a significant contributor to ADR, with results documenting the increase from 20.3%–29.1% in a randomized trial (Wang et al., 2019). Such outcomes indicate the manner in which increased technological assistance can compensate for inadequacies in the experience of the operator, generally affecting the final outcome for patients. Nevertheless, it is important to recognize that the dependence on technology should not be at the expense of the requirement for skilled operators, but instead as a support tool meant to complement and augment their capability and proficiency during the procedures. In addition, the operator skill implications are also realized in the management of patients and the likelihood of complications during endoscopy. Less skilled or poorly trained operators may inadvertently increase the risk for bad events, e.g., perforation or bleeding, particularly in those needing technical sophistication. Complications may precipitate the need for reoperation, leading to patient morbidity and increased healthcare costs. Evidently, strict training packages and assurance systems are paramount to validating operator proficiency and competence with endoscopic techniques. By placing emphasis on education and confirmation of skill in endoscopy, the medical field can establish a climate of excellence that not only minimizes complications but also improves the overall effectiveness of endoscopic procedures for better patient care results.

14.4.3. Procedure Complexity

Endoscopic procedure complications are generally intimately related to the complexity of the methods employed. Though processes , such as the development of transjugular intrahepatic portosystemic shunt (TIPS) or higher levels of endosonographic application become increasingly complicated, the expertise required of physicians increases geometrically. For instance, TIPS, intended for the treatment of portal hypertension, has been both in technique and devices, with stent-graft placement covered by polytetrafluoroethylene (PTFE), involving increased expertise in handling complex vascular anatomy and preventing complications like intraperitoneal hemorrhage or shunt malfunction. These advances reflect the dynamic nature of endovascular intervention and underscore the need for special training in their execution. Lee et al. (2023) highlights the evolution and risk elements of these complex interventions, once more highlighting the requirement for effective training systems to prevent endoscopic procedure complications. To boot, the challenge in achieving competence with advanced endoscopic techniques is significant. Training courses in many European countries illustrate superb inconsistency in the availability and organization of proper educational experiences. This lack of standardization can lead to inconsistency of skill development among trainees and in their readiness to perform advanced procedures independently. Most of the programs do not have systematic access to simulation models or complete curricula, thereby giving trainees minimal hands-on experience time for procedures like ERCP and EUS. Lekkerkerkerker & Voermans (2023) illustrates the need for standardized training, since it is said that the absence of uniform frameworks leads to unequal levels of procedural competency and the subsequent impacts on patient outcomes and complication rates incurred during advanced endoscopy. With the complexity involved in such processes, it is necessary to test trainees' performance against standardized competency assessment tools. Successful training should shift away from just volume-based towards a focus on outcome and proficiency in procedural skills. Continuous evaluation by metrics like complication rates and procedure success can better determine a trainee's readiness for independent practice. Integration of instruments like the Direct Observation of Procedural Skills (DOPS) or the EUS and ERCP Skills Assessment Tool (TEESAT) can facilitate this shift by offering formal performance feedback. Such frameworks not only enhance trainees' skills but may also reduce the incidence of procedure-related complications. Finally, placing priority on overall training methodologies in challenging endoscopic procedures is a means to increase safety and efficacy, thereby reducing the complication rate of these intricate procedures.

14.5. Prevention Strategies

With endoscopy complications in mind, prevention has to be brought about through effective measures and their actualization to mitigate risk, particularly where there are pre-existing conditions , such as liver disease. Pre-procedure risk evaluation is one vital area of prevention and entails the evaluation of patient hemostasis and overall health. The opinion of experts is that patients suffering from cirrhosis have complex hemostatic changes that are difficult to assess in terms of bleeding risk. Uncertain conventional tests , such as INR or platelet count, may fail to comment on procedural bleeding risk precisely. Therefore, practitioners need to utilize global hemostasis tests , such as thromboelastography (TEG), in an effort to better measure hemostatic function and consequently tailor their procedural strategy appropriately to ensure that sufficient interventions are ready for any ensuing complications from endoscopy (Northup et al., 2020). In addition to thorough risk assessments, procedural techniques should also be optimized in a manner that decreases the risk of complications. For instance, the use of imaging guidance with ultrasound for invasive procedures can significantly reduce the risks of vessel puncture and perforation. Such interventions not only enhance safety but also enable clinicians to exert greater control over the procedure. Furthermore, customized pre-procedure treatment can optimize patient outcomes. Allocation of personalized care to higher-risk patients, such as modified anticoagulation regimens or targeted transfusions, may be vital in reducing complications.

This comprehensive strategy aligns with guidelines that emphasize the importance of addressing patient-specific causes of bleeding and thrombotic complications, per procedure-related risks literature in patients with cirrhosis (Chen et al., 2020). Finally, repeated education and training for health professionals who undertake endoscopy procedures are critical in the prevention of complications. Physician experience and familiarity with complicated endoscopic procedures are some of the most important aspects of successful outcomes. Examples of continuous medical education programs , such as workshops and simulations in the care of complex patients, can make practitioners proficient in procedural techniques and management of complications. Furthermore, interdisciplinary collaboration between the specialists, including anesthesiologists and hepatologists, presents a concerted approach to caring for the patient, including control of all potential complications that may occur during endoscopy. Through integration of risk evaluation, procedure optimization, and education of health practitioners, healthcare systems can ensure safer endoscopic practice and minimize complications associated with these unavoidable diagnostic and therapeutic interventions (Northup et al., 2020) (Figure 14.12).

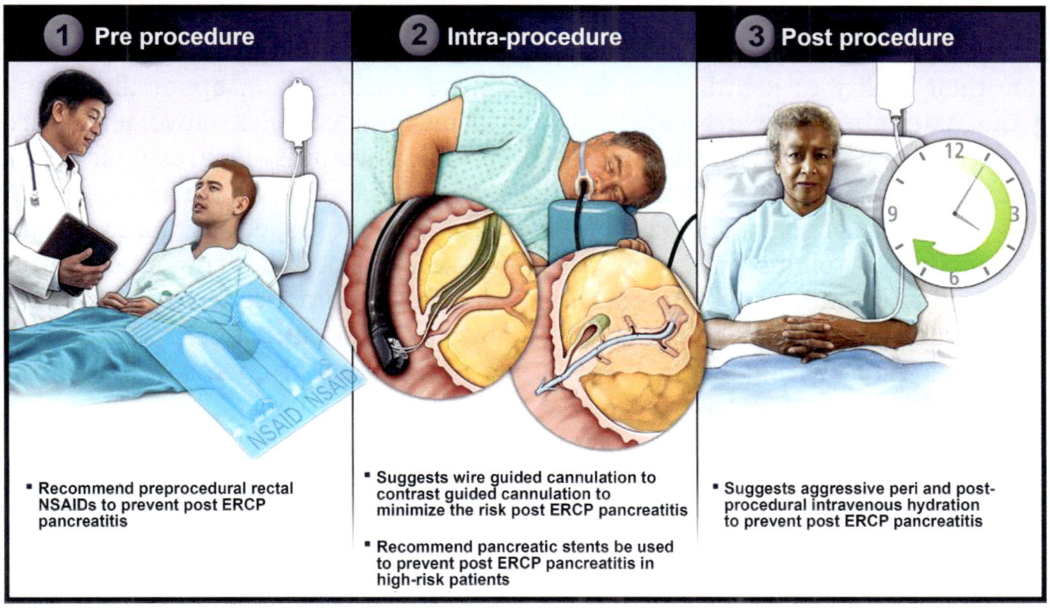

Figure 14.12. Prevention strategies.

Source: https://www.giejournal.org/cms/attachment/6aa607c6-9676-4952-93ee-a504a8864448/fx1_lrg.jpg.

14.5.1. Pre-Procedural Assessments

The importance of pre-procedural evaluations in endoscopy cannot be overstated as they significantly help in minimizing procedure-related complications. Appropriate evaluation of patients before any endoscopic treatment helps in the identification of potential risks that can happen during or post-procedure. Major aspects of this assessment are taking a complete history, becoming sensitive to current medications of the patients, and noting any complications from previous surgery. This is important, as it allows the health care team to tailor the procedure to suit the individual's needs, thus reducing the potential for adverse outcomes. In addition, as Campos et al. emphasize, the absence of standardized training and evaluation procedures across Europe further underpins the need for structured pre-procedure testing; standardization has the potential to enhance patient safety and procedure efficacy across varied healthcare settings (Lekkerkerker & Voermans, 2023). Extensive tests are likewise most crucial in subspecialty fields , such as bariatric endoscopy, where the complexity of procedures requires an integrated approach to patient evaluation. The blending of bariatric training with gastroenterology emphasizes the necessity for specialist attention to pre-procedure assessment, such as exhaustive medical and surgical history, medications, and prior attempts at weight reduction. Such in-depth investigations enable gastroenterologists and surgeons to more adequately prepare for the unique issues with these patients. As an illustration, the evaluation of sleep apnea or cardiovascular illness can radically alter procedural safety and success. Incorporating , such assessments within training programs not only better equips health professionals but also improves augmented patient vigilance and alertness during endoscopic procedures (de Moura et al., 2022). The function of pre-procedural testing ultimately transcends information gathering; it actually determines the quality of care delivered in endoscopic practice. A robust evaluation protocol can also serve as a predictive marker for potential complications, and preventive actions may be taken. Through the establishment of a culture of careful assessments, medical practitioners can enhance their ability to identify red flags indicating that patients are at a greater risk for poor outcomes. Standardized testing that incorporates competency assessment of practitioners can produce better quality training outcomes, ensuring that endoscopists possess the capabilities to handle complex cases. Noted through the requirement of advanced-level training programs within Europe, with the focus on the indication for pre-procedure evaluation being required to guarantee patient safety and reduce complications in endoscopy (Lekkerkerker & Voermans, 2023).

14.5.2. Use of Advanced Technology

The evolution of technology in endoscopy has significantly transformed diagnostic and therapeutic procedures, making procedures safer and more effective. Among the advances is the development of self-expanding metal stents (SEMS) used in treating obstructive gastrointestinal tract conditions. Recent studies have shown an evident difference in complications between uncovered SEMS and covered SEMS (cSEMS). In particular, data indicates that while cSEMS has some advantages, it is more prone to migration than its uncased counterpart, with a whopping 56% of the cSEMS migrating and not a single SEMS installation having migrated. This discrepancy necessitates careful considerations in the selection of stents in clinical practice, testifying to the need for wise adoption of advanced technology in treatment planning in a bid to minimize complications of endoscopic procedures (Albert et al., 2013). Moreover, advancements like laparoscopic surgery have revolutionized surgical approaches across all specialties, including endoscopy. The advantages of laparoscopic surgery are several and encompass diminished postoperative pain, shorter hospitalization, and reduced infection risks. These benefits hold even in sophisticated procedures , such as liver transplantation (LT), where adoption of laparoscopic skills has immensely improved patient results. With the provision of an opportunity for surgeons to perform complex movements through less invasive wounds, laparoscopic technology is indispensable in modern surgery. With the evolution of the specialty, the combining of skills, e.g., diagnostic and therapeutic laparoscopy into endoscopic practice, testifies to the capability to maximize patient care and prevent routine complications of open surgery (Berloco et al., 2012).

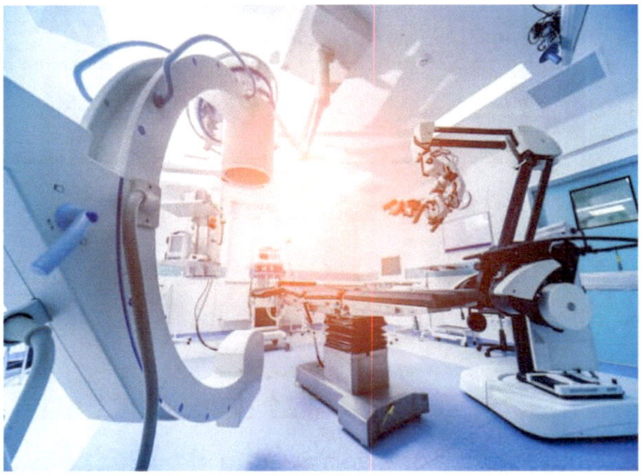

Figure 14.13. Advancement of technology in the field of endoscopy.

Source: https://www.healthcarebusinesstoday.com/wp-content/uploads/2021/02/AdobeStock_269860798-696x464.jpeg.

Moreover, the combination of advanced imaging modalities with endoscopic techniques has also maximized therapeutic efficiency and diagnostic accuracy. Advanced imaging modalities , such as narrow-band imaging and high-definition endoscopy, enable enhanced visualization of mucosal layers that assist in the detection of lesions that might otherwise be missed. All of these advancements empower clinicians to make more informed decisions during procedures and thereby lower the risk of missed diagnosis and improper therapy. As technological innovations find their way into the field of endoscopy, it becomes increasingly clear that integration of such technology not only grants a lift in procedural success but also in complications with the traditional approach. Eventually, the implementation of these technologies is an important step towards realizing greater safety and effectiveness for endoscopic procedures (Figure 14.13).

14.5.3. Training and Certification for Practitioners

The complexities presented in endoscopic procedures make certain that rigorous training and certification mechanisms are necessary for practitioners. Gaining proficiency in endoscopy is not only necessary to perform the procedures in a safe manner, but also to treat inherent complications that may arise. For instance, one study of American Speech-Language-Hearing Association (ASHA)-certified speech-language pathologists (SLPs) found discrepancies between training provided for laryngeal endoscopy and application of topical nasal anesthesia. They reported having strong confidence levels in their procedural knowledge but were hesitant to support their competence. This disparity is indicative of the imperative need to improve training programs that prepare practitioners with a mix of theoretical knowledge and practice to make them competent to cope with varying situations while undergoing endoscopic procedures (Baker-Rush et al., 2024). Moreover, having standard guidelines for training is crucial to enhance the competence of endoscopy providers, as revealed through recent United Kingdom evidence regarding colonoscopy performance. The Joint Advisory Group on Gastrointestinal Endoscopy required trainees to demonstrate particular skills, like knowledge of polypectomy and management of frequent complications. Regardless of this, self-assessment among colonoscopists showed diverse levels of confidence and competence, especially among clinical endoscopists and medically qualified endoscopists. The indecisiveness of some practitioners to perform complex procedures, along with a lack of backup in an event where there are complications, translates to how essential detailed certification procedures that take these challenges into account and solidify skill acquisition among learners are (Rankin et al., 2024).

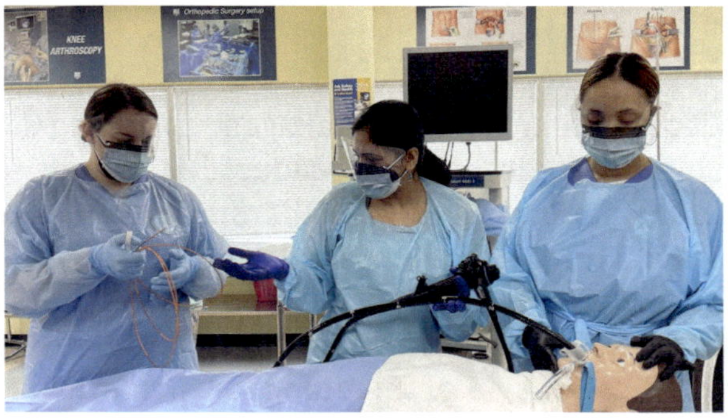

Figure 14.14. Training and certification for practitioners.

Source: https://storage.googleapis.com/aims-edu/images/000/001/614/fullscreen/Endoscopy%20Tech%20Training%208.jpg.

Furthermore, the effects of substandard training and certification extend far beyond practitioner confidence; they directly affect patient safety, as well as care outcomes. Training for endoscopic procedures is evolving, with a requirement for an interprofessional education model under which collaboration between specialisms can enhance learning and competence, for example. Building rapport between established practitioners and less experienced practitioners by utilizing mentorship can significantly improve the learning experience. This collaborative model not only encourages hands-on skill development but also provides a forum for practitioners to learn and coordinate with respect to potential complications. By integrating such practices into training programs, healthcare facilities can make sure that practitioners are not only skilled but also adequately prepared to deal with the complexities inherent in endoscopy, thereby maximizing patient safety and procedure success (Baker-Rush et al., 2024; Rankin et al., 2024) (Figure 14.14).

14.6. Management of Complications

Adequate complications management during the course of endoscopic procedures is crucial to ensure patient safety and the final result. The complexity of these procedures necessitates endoscopists to be attentive to potential adverse outcomes, which can range from self-limiting complications, e.g., bleeding or perforation, to potentially life-threatening conditions. A proactive complication management involves careful patient selection and the development of risk profiles before the procedure. High-risk patients can be identified, and in turn, more rigorous monitoring measures and protective strategies can be implemented, improving patient safety. Besides, as set in earlier research, enforcing a safety culture that emphasizes prevention is routine endoscopic practice that ensures complications are dealt with in an orderly fashion and places paramount importance on the well-being of patients (Yamamoto et al., 2023). Incorporation of evidence-based guidelines is also key to proper management and prevention of complications of endoscopy. For instance, in Peutz-Jeghers syndrome (PJS), a relevant but unusual complication that typically necessitates chronic medical management, there are particular clinical guidelines that need to be developed. They are constructed, through multidisciplinary collaboration between specialists, to promote accurate diagnosis and calculated management of the complications associated with hamartomatous polyps. These recommendations must fulfill the varying degrees of complexity of PJS, from gastrointestinal obstruction or risk of intussusception. Through adherence to currently available protocols centered on vigilant monitoring and timely intervention, healthcare practitioners can exert considerable control on the health-related quality of life of patients presenting with such scenarios (Yamamoto et al., 2023). An adequate follow-up scheme following a procedure is important in being able to manage complications effectively. Early diagnosis and treatment are crucial once complications have developed, and open communication with patients and families regarding the potential risks involved is crucial. Highlighting the importance of informed patients in early detection of warning signs for complications instills a culture in which the patients themselves are more likely to seek attention at an early stage. In addition, establishing certain guidelines for managing complications—whether conservative or invasive—enables the healthcare teams to respond quickly and efficiently. Lastly, the incorporation of appropriate risk analysis, continuous education, and commitment to safety will contribute significantly towards the minimization of complications and better patient care in endoscopy (Waddingham et al., 2022) (Figure 14.15).

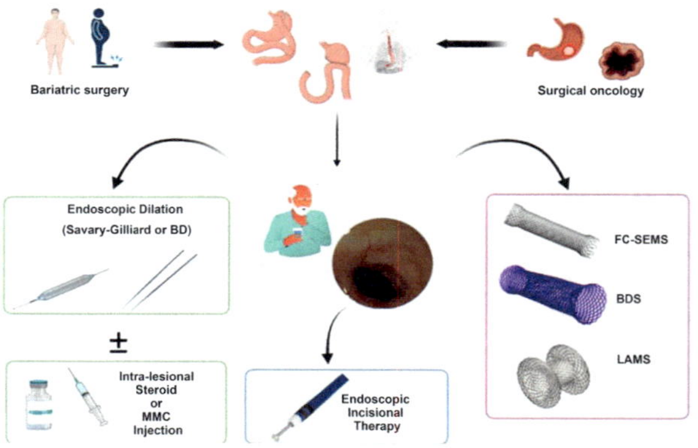

Figure 14.15. Management of complications arising from endoscopic.

Source: https://www.mdpi.com/jpm/jpm-15-00111/article_deploy/html/images/jpm-15-00111-g003.png.

14.6.1. Immediate Response Protocols

There is a need to have immediate response protocols in place to manage the potential complications of endoscopy procedures. The protocols are designed to facilitate easy identification and handling of adverse events that may occur during or after endoscopic interventions, lowering risk to patient safety. Extensive protocols generally include a set of pre-established procedures, such as immediate medical evaluation, interaction with the operating team, and utilization of multidisciplinary support when needed. Through adherence to established guidelines, healthcare professionals can better limit the severity of complications like perforation, hemorrhage, or infection, thereby resulting in improved patient outcomes. Also, ascertaining adherence to such protocols by means of continuous quality improvement programs has been important in ensuring compliance with best practice, the importance of standardization in clinical settings being thus underlined (Tam et al., 2025). Training and preparedness on the part of staff are at the center of the success of immediate response protocols. Healthcare teams need to have knowledge and skills to recognize and respond to complications as quickly as possible, and this requires constant drills and simulations of different adverse situations. This training helps all members of the team, from endoscopists to nursing personnel, understand the critical procedures for identifying complications and perform their own tasks without interruption under pressure. Furthermore, integration of the protocols in electronic health records can enhance compliance, as in prior studies that involved standardized biopsy protocols to reach better clinical compliance (Tam et al., 2025). Integration in this manner not only eases the process of communication but also allows for real-time decision-making based on established protocols, and hence the importance of being prepared and coordinated in acute care situations. Additionally, post-procedure observation is also a critical component of immediate response protocols, particularly for higher-risk patients. Continuous monitoring in the recovery room allows early warning signs of complications , such as excessive bleeding or infection, to be recognized, allowing for early intervention. The utilization of metrics for measuring the rate and severity of complications can assist with evidence-based improvement in protocol efficiency. In addition, building a culture of communication and safety among staff makes a working environment where one can air grievances openly, also improving patient safety. For instance, disaster response structures utilized in other hospital emergencies highlight the significance of having readily available procedures in place to guarantee that collective strategies are in place upon emerging crises, hence serving as an exemplification of the importance of robust instant response systems in the area of endoscopic procedures.

14.6.2. Long-Term Follow-up Care

Long-term follow-up care is an important aspect of complications due to endoscopic procedures. Due to complex procedures, complications may occur at various times after surgery, influencing the patient's condition and pattern of recovery. Follow-up visits are essential to recognize recurrent symptoms, such as those of GERD, which develops in about 20% of adults in high-income countries. Most patients develop health issues due to esophageal complications like strictures or adenocarcinoma that need ongoing assessment and adjustment of their treatments to efficiently avert such complications. By the implementation of a formal follow-up protocol, the practitioner can perform timely intervention, thereby improving patient outcome and quality of life in patients who have been exposed to endoscopy, because routine follow-up can detect underlying complications before they advance into more complex conditions (Maret-Ouda et al., 2020). Beyond the assessment of symptoms and disease progression, long-term follow-up management also plays a key role in ascertaining the effectiveness of treatment interventions. For instance, responders with GERD to proton pump inhibitors (PPIs) may require a re-evaluation of their medication schedule in the long run, particularly with observational studies identifying potential side effects associated with long-term use of PPIs. Follow-up allows clinicians to make adjustments in treatment regimens to circumvent complications from long-term reliance on medication. Integration of lifestyle interventions , such as dietary modification or reduction of body weight, can also be included in the follow-up process because they can reduce the burden of treatment and improve patient compliance (Maret-Ouda et al., 2020). Regular follow-ups provide means for patient education and support and hence for a collaborative care strategy whereby patients are empowered to take active roles in their own recovery. In addition, long-term observation is particularly important in cirrhotic patients with complex comorbidities who may be at greater risk of bleeding from procedures and other complications.

The vascular and hemostatic derangements induced by chronic liver disease mandate an appreciation of the pathogenesis of post-endoscopic complications to be advanced. Follow-up appointments can identify changes in patients' hemostatic balance that are complicated by underlying disease states like portal hypertension or renal failure. Patients should be screened regularly by healthcare providers and follow-up management should be individualized to each of their unique medical histories and disease processes. This individualized approach of long-term follow-up care not only minimizes complications but also safeguards vulnerable groups of patients and emphasizes the necessity for an organized process in the context of endoscopic care (Figure 14.16).

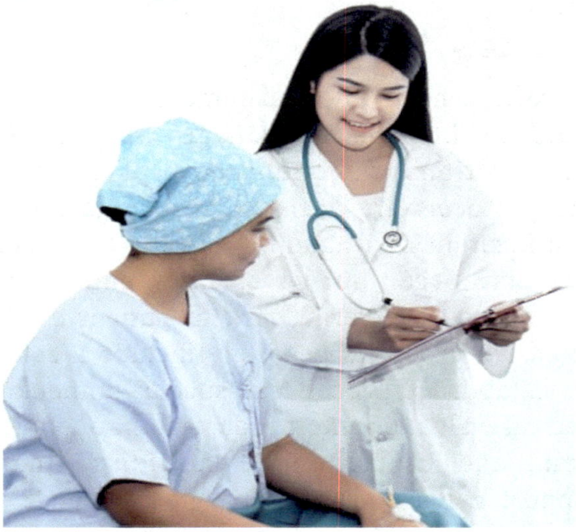

Figure 14.16. Long-term follow-up care.

Source: https://www.hcgoncology.com/uploads/images/follow-up-care-after-your-cancer.jpeg.

14.6.3. Patient Education and Support

Patient education and support are key ingredients in avoiding the endoscopic procedure complications. Having patients feel confident that they are well informed about risks and expected outcome of their procedures is important in improving adherence to post-procedure care and reducing anxiety. Complete education also supports shared decision-making, which enables patients to actively participate in their treatment. By defining potential complications—, such as infection or bleeding—and going through symptom recognition, clinicians can encourage a better comprehension on the part of patients that ultimately leads to earlier intervention and better clinical results. Evidence confirms the reality that correct patient education can eliminate the gap between patients' health literacy and compliance and, consequently, minimize adverse events after endoscopy. Therefore, there is a need to have open communication channels between patients and providers in an effort to enhance the quality of post-endoscopic care. The role of nursing assistance in patient education cannot be overstated, particularly in raising compliance levels for instructed post-operative care. Nurses are uniquely positioned to deliver focused education, which targets specific patient problems and modulates information consistent with individual needs. For instance, studies revealed that structured educational interventions on self-care methods immensely enhanced patient compliance and outcomes among patients with chronic illnesses like diabetes and hypertension (Rostami et al., 2024). Similarly, in endoscopy, nursing support can help in developing an improved understanding of lifestyle modification, to avoid complications. Through motivational interviewing and behavioral methods, nurses are able to develop an environment to promote self-efficacy. This is a crucial practice as, apart from assisting in reducing the risk of complications, it also serves a critical function on the patient's recovery journey as a whole. Having patients' perceptions of healthcare practices will inform education and support interventions. Patient studies have demonstrated how individual experience and education influence adherence to care regimens, such as those after endoscopy (Ju et al., 2024). Patients are likely to seek the advice of others and emotional support based on shared experience, a phenomenon that favors the establishment of peer networks or support groups following an endoscopy procedure. Further, an understanding of what hindrances—e.g., emotional disturbance or physical disability—patients face in adhering to recommendations for care may assist clinicians in tailoring interventions for every patient in accordance with their specific needs. Overall, these results emphasize the importance of an integrated approach incorporating input from patients while offering maximal educational efforts. By addressing the psychological and social components of patient care, medical professionals can help significantly enhance the effectiveness of education programs focusing on prevention of endoscopic procedure complications (Figure 14.17).

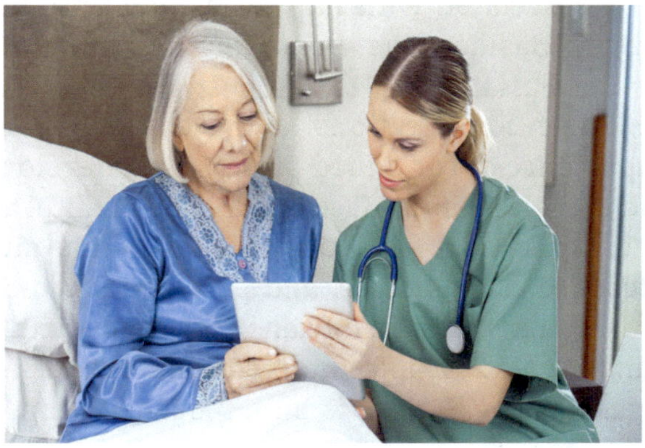

Figure 14.17. Patient education and support.

Source: https://s3.amazonaws.com/utep-uploads/wp-content/uploads/2017/04/22150239/Helping-Patients_Image-1.jpg.

SUMMARY

Lastly, endoscopy complications are multifaceted and are based on what procedure is done. While the majority of endoscopic methods are regarded as minimally invasive with fairly high safety profiles, the risk for complications can never be entirely ruled out. Certain ones, like ERCP, for instance, can be followed by pancreatitis to perforation, highlighting the necessity of meticulous technique and patient selection. The systematic review and meta-analysis of ERCP during pregnancy illustrates the complexity, highlighting that while the procedure can be done safely, the clinician must take note of the heightened risk in pregnancy (Azab et al., 2019). Familiarity with these potential complications is essential for health workers and patients, as it directly affects informed consent and realistic expectations regarding outcomes from endoscopic treatment. Also, the development of new techniques and innovations in current endoscopic procedures can minimize the risk of complications and improve patient safety. For example, new technology , such as non-radiation ERCP technology, is of major importance in being able to mitigate the risk of exposure to susceptible groups, i.e., pregnant women. From current research as shown, such methods have been associated with improved safety profiles, which indicates that research and innovation are crucial. Besides, the trend towards newer methods, like peroral endoscopic myotomy (POEM) for achalasia of the esophagus, provides insight into how endoscopic techniques can evolve to minimize complications at the expense of effectiveness. These evolving practices highlight the importance of continued professional development for endoscopists to embrace safer methodology and technique in the face of intricate medical ailments (Caldaro et al., 2015). Finally, the management of complications of endoscopy involves a multifaceted approach that involves extensive training, advanced technologies, and patient-centric care. By being aware of the dangers and taking steps to minimize them, clinicians can significantly enhance patient outcomes while ensuring that the utility of endoscopic interventions outweighs their harms. The integration of patient education regarding these risks is an important component of this process, allowing individuals to become active participants in their care decisions. The future of endoscopy is not about inventing increasingly high-tech approaches but about building an environment where safety and efficacy are paramount and, ultimately, lead to better patient satisfaction and health outcomes. With continued research illuminating the nuances of endoscopic practice, commitment in education and innovation will be important to bridging these challenges.

The complexities in the practice of endoscopy greatly outweigh the mere act of performing the procedure itself, entailing a spectrum of complications that may present during or after the intervention. Among the salient features of such complications is the fact that superficial GI lesion cases need serious scrutiny and expertise for treating such cases. The European Society of Gastrointestinal Endoscopy (ESGE) recommends that evaluation should be carried out by a competent endoscopist with high-definition white-light and chromoendoscopy, either virtual or dye-based. Failure to adhere to these standards will result in suboptimal outcomes, like inadequate lesion assessment or lost diagnoses, and eventually compromise patient safety and quality of care. The emphasis on the clinician's skill points to the importance attached to rigorous training and competency in endoscopy, which is important in minimizing complications while maximizing diagnostic and therapeutic efficacies in clinical practice (Pimentel-Nunes et al., 2022). Beyond the paramount role of clinician skill, the guidelines set for superficial lesion management underscore the necessity of careful pre-procedure planning. Routine use of advanced imaging modalities, such as endoscopic ultrasonography or computed tomography, before endoscopic resection is not advocated by ESGE, a trend in a more cautious approach. This recommendation is supported by the paramount role of direct visualization methods compared to potentially unnecessary imaging methods in the majority of instances. In addition, the proposal for endoscopic submucosal dissection (ESD) as the preferred treatment option for esophageal and gastric lesions has considerable bearing on the management of patients. Having endoscopists experienced with the techniques of ESD can mean higher complete resection rates and, as a consequence, prevent the development of complications , such as residual disease and need for surgical intervention (Pimentel-Nunes et al., 2022). Lastly, being aware of the consequences of resection results is an important component of endoscopic therapy. ESGE classifies resection results into different levels of risk, which guides further management. Examples of such classifications, such as resection being classified as low-risk or high-risk according to histological results, facilitate individualized follow-up and surveillance planning necessary to maximize patient outcomes. Following a successful curative ESD, the protocol allows active surveillance rather than immediate additional treatments if there are no high-risk criteria. In contrast, the presence of high-severe-risk factors, such as lymphovascular invasion, requires comprehensive post-resection staging and multidisciplinary review to establish an optimal management plan. This systematic process indicates that there is a high degree of awareness of endoscopic procedure complications, ultimately aiming to enhance patient safety and treatment success (Pimentel-Nunes et al., 2022).

A CLOSER LOOK

INTRA-PROCEDURAL TREATMENT

Intra-procedural treatment refers to the interventions and management strategies applied during a medical procedure or surgery to ensure patient safety, optimize outcomes, and address complications in real-time. This phase is critical because it allows clinicians to monitor physiological status, respond to adverse events, and tailor therapeutic interventions according to dynamic patient needs. Effective intra-procedural care requires a coordinated team approach, advanced monitoring tools, and adherence to established clinical protocols.

Monitoring is a cornerstone of intra-procedural treatment. Continuous assessment of vital signs, oxygenation, hemodynamic parameters, and, when necessary, neurological status, allows clinicians to detect early deviations from normal physiology. In surgical or invasive procedures, anesthetic depth, fluid balance, and blood loss are closely tracked. In endoscopic or interventional radiology procedures, real-time imaging guides the precision of therapeutic interventions. This vigilant monitoring enables immediate corrective measures, such as fluid resuscitation, vasopressor administration, or airway management, reducing the risk of complications.

Pharmacological management is another key component. Intra-procedural medications may include anesthetics, analgesics, sedatives, or muscle relaxants, titrated to maintain patient comfort and procedural tolerance. Additionally, anticoagulants, antiarrhythmics, or vasoactive agents may be administered to address specific intraoperative needs. Proper drug selection, dosage, and timing are crucial to balance therapeutic efficacy with the risk of adverse effects.

Procedural interventions themselves are often adjusted in real-time based on intra-procedural findings. For instance, in endoscopic procedures, tissue biopsies, hemostasis, or lesion removal may be performed as indicated. In surgical procedures, intraoperative imaging, navigation, or minimally invasive techniques help guide resections, repairs, or device placements. Surgeons and interventionalists must remain adaptable, modifying the approach according to anatomical variations, unexpected pathology, or patient stability.

Effective intra-procedural treatment also emphasizes teamwork and communication. Anesthesiologists, surgeons, nurses, and technicians collaborate to coordinate monitoring, medication delivery, and procedural steps. Clear communication ensures timely responses to complications, reduces errors, and enhances procedural efficiency.

In conclusion, intra-procedural treatment is a dynamic, multifaceted process that integrates continuous monitoring, pharmacological management, real-time procedural adjustments, and coordinated teamwork. Its goal is to maintain patient stability, manage complications, and optimize procedural outcomes. Mastery of intra-procedural strategies is essential for clinicians, as it directly influences safety, efficacy, and long-term success of medical and surgical interventions.

REFERENCES

1. Ajani, J. A., D'Amico, T. A., Bentrem, D. J., Chao, J., Cooke, D. T., Corvera, C. U., Das, P., et al. (2022). Gastric cancer, version 2.2022, NCCN clinical practice guidelines in oncology. *Journal of the National Comprehensive Cancer Network, 20*, 167–192. https://doi.org/10.6004/jnccn.2022.0008 (accessed on 15th July 2025).
2. Albert, J. G., Bechstein, W. O., Friedrich-Rust, M., Sarrazin, et al. (2013). *SEMS vs cSEMS in duodenal and small bowel obstruction: High risk of migration in the covered stent group.* https://core.ac.uk/download/18137371.pdf (accessed on 15th July 2025).
3. Alecu, L., Nitipir, C., Slavu, I., Stanculeanu, et al. (2019). *Laparoscopic resection of gastric GISTs. Where do we stand now? A single-centered experience.* https://core.ac.uk/download/232440347.pdf (accessed on 15th July 2025).
4. Alkhazal'eh, S. (2023). Anesthesia options for pediatric endoscopy: A review of intravenous sedation and general anesthesia. *Journal of Pediatric Advance Research.* https://www.semanticscholar.org/paper/b98fb935c19c7d555bc5659aeb0efb718a017f32 (accessed on 15th July 2025).
5. Azab, M., Bharadwaj, S., Hong, A. S., Jayaraj, et al. (2019). *Safety of endoscopic retrograde cholangiopancreatography (ERCP) in pregnancy: A systematic review and meta-analysis.* https://core.ac.uk/download/286611719.pdf (accessed on 15th July 2025).
6. Baker-Rush, M. L., Zemsky Dineen, M., & Kaseda, E. T. (2024). Exploring speech-language pathologists' training and use of topical nasal anesthesia during laryngeal endoscopy in the United States. *International Journal of Language & Communication Disorders, 60*(1), e13140. https://www.semanticscholar.org/paper/d38a1bf7065301155dfa51de68d4a5be0618ca92 (accessed on 15th July 2025).
7. Barman, S., Walker, R., Pucher, P., Jack, S., Whyte, G., Grocott, M., West, M., et al. (2024). A national survey of the provision of prehabilitation for oesophagogastric cancer patients in the UK. *Annals of The Royal College of Surgeons of England, 107*, 300–306. https://www.semanticscholar.org/paper/590d6269a1ed8d4886ece6ffba3f28f6f1777483 (accessed on 15th July 2025).
8. Berloco, P. B., Di Laudo, M., Frattaroli, F. M., Guglielmo, et al. (2012). *Laparoscopy in Liver Transplantation: The Future Has Arrived.* https://core.ac.uk/download/154948504.pdf (accessed on 15th July 2025).
9. Boicean, A., Prisca, D., Bratu, D., Băcilă, C., Tănăsescu, C., Chicea, R., Fleacă, R., et al. (2024). Uncommon presentation of gastric duplication cyst with left-sided portal hypertension: A case report and literature review. *Diagnostics, 14*, 675–675. https://doi.org/10.3390/diagnostics14070675 (accessed on 15th July 2025).
10. Boškoski, I., Pontecorvi, V., Ibrahim, M., Huberty, V., Maselli, R., Gölder, S., Kral, J., et al. (2023). Curriculum for bariatric endoscopy and endoscopic treatment of the complications of bariatric surgery: European Society of Gastrointestinal Endoscopy (ESGE) position statement. *Endoscopy, 55*, 276–293. https://www.semanticscholar.org/paper/6fc8e9c2b33a61919de5d9ae7dbc9a2065fcef12 (accessed on 15th July 2025).
11. Caldaro, T., Contini, A. C., Costamagna, G., Cucchiara, et al. (2015). *Treatment of esophageal achalasia in children: Today and tomorrow.* https://core.ac.uk/download/54519265.pdf (accessed on 15th July 2025).

12. Calori, J. D., Temba, N. J., Karoli, P. M., Ng'weshemi, S., Matobogolo, B. M., Mwashambwa, M., Mpondo, B. C. T., et al. (2024). Prevalence and risk factors of Helicobacter pylori infection among patients with peptic ulcer disease undergoing upper gastrointestinal endoscopy at Benjamin Mkapa Hospital, Dodoma, Tanzania. *EAS Journal of Parasitology and Infectious Diseases.* https://www.semanticscholar.org/paper/4b26a41ed716c1fabce304ef8321290a6988ddb5 (accessed on 15th July 2025).

13. Chaimae, A., Samia, B., Rayhana, C. S., Anass, A. R., Mahamoud, C. A. C. A., Nour, A. E., Othman, A., et al. (2025). Unusual and rare manifestations after bronchoscopy: Pneumoperitoneum, pneumoretroperitoneum, and pneumomediastinum—Case report. *Case Reports International.* https://www.semanticscholar.org/paper/02274b6928c281711c26a4adc95275bce12a9745 (accessed on 15th July 2025).

14. Chen, C., Gao, G., Xu, Y., Pu, L., Wang, Q., Wang, L., Wang, W., et al. (2020). SARS-CoV-2–positive sputum and feces after conversion of pharyngeal samples in patients with COVID-19. *Annals of Internal Medicine, 172*, 832–834. https://doi.org/10.7326/m20-0991 (accessed on 15th July 2025).

15. Cook, A., Jenkins, L. M., & Plant, P. (1999). *A casemix analysis of hospital admissions in six specialties for Barking & Havering Health Authority.* https://core.ac.uk/download/10631591.pdf (accessed on 15th July 2025).

16. Dao, T. M. H., Nguyen, T. K. T., & Schirling, D. (2020). *The Future of Robotic-Assisted Laparoscopic surgery.* https://core.ac.uk/download/334494868.pdf (accessed on 15th July 2025).

17. de Moura, D. T. H., Jirapinyo, P., & Thompson, C. C. (2022). *Training in Bariatric Endoscopy.* https://doi.org/10.1002/9781119529675.ch23 (accessed on 15th July 2025).

18. Fukui, M., Suzuki, K., Imashimizu, K., Ichikawa, T., Matsunaga, T., Hattori, A., Tomita, H., et al. (2024). Simple endoscopic estimation to predict anastomotic complications after bronchoplastic procedures. *European Journal of Cardio-Thoracic Surgery.* https://www.semanticscholar.org/paper/4190ca723874148efa00c302cd8e6e560196e012 (accessed on 15th July 2025).

19. Gaffney, R., & Schreibman, I. (2015). Serotonin syndrome in a patient on trazodone and duloxetine who received fentanyl following a percutaneous liver biopsy. *Case Reports in Gastroenterology, 9*, 132–136. https://www.semanticscholar.org/paper/2d34812aca95ecbfd56643758c26b8abf0352e01 (accessed on 15th July 2025).

20. García-Tsao, G., Abraldeș, J. G., Berzigotti, A., & Bosch, J. (2016). Portal hypertensive bleeding in cirrhosis: Risk stratification, diagnosis, and management: 2016 practice guidance by the American Association for the Study of Liver Diseases. *Hepatology, 65*, 310–335. https://doi.org/10.1002/hep.28906 (accessed on 15th July 2025).

21. González-Abós, C., Landi, F., Lorenzo, C., Rey, S., Salgado, F., & Ausania, F. (2025). Is robotic pancreaticoduodenectomy non-inferior to open pancreaticoduodenectomy in patients with high PD-ROBOSCORE? *Surgical Endoscopy, 39*, 2364–2369. https://www.semanticscholar.org/paper/90ec9f667b14d9134b00d63ea281d11a06c071c7 (accessed on 15th July 2025).

22. Hunt, R. H., Armstrong, D., Katelaris, P., Afihene, M., Bane, A., Bhatia, S., Chen, M., et al. (2017). World Gastroenterology Organization global guidelines. *Journal of Clinical Gastroenterology, 51*, 467–478. https://doi.org/10.1097/mcg.0000000000000854 (accessed on 15th July 2025).

23. Januário, G. (2025). Unilateral biportal endoscopy (UBE), recommendations for the interlaminar approach. *Neuroscience and Neurological Surgery.* https://www.semanticscholar.org/paper/2a744359276a50bb3044767438a2adb65ec2c6df (accessed on 15th July 2025).

24. Ju, H. H., Ottosen, M., Alford, J., Jularbal, J., & Johnson, C. (2024). Enhancing foot care education and support strategies in adults with type 2 diabetes. *Journal of the American Association of Nurse Practitioners, 36*, 334–341. https://www.semanticscholar.org/paper/7619a02f288226eca84d130aebf990c19a1b9f95 (accessed on 15th July 2025).

25. Kim, B. (2020). Surgical management of urinary stone. *Journal of The Korean Medical Association, 63*, 677–683. https://www.semanticscholar.org/paper/f95143a3e1054f2db0a2fa18afa845c4f6551cba (accessed on 15th July 2025).

26. Kowalski, M., & Przybyłkowski, A. (2024). Prevention of bacterial infection in biliary and pancreatic endoscopy—A review. *Diagnostics, 14.* https://www.semanticscholar.org/paper/56d610597e2d1ee77341cd4f7061bad22b46b6c7 (accessed on 15th July 2025).

27. Lamb, C. A., Kennedy, N. A., Raine, T., Hendy, P., Smith, P. J., Limdi, J. K., Hayee, B., et al. (2019). British Society of Gastroenterology consensus guidelines on the management of inflammatory bowel disease in adults. *Gut, 68*(Suppl 3), s1–s106. https://doi.org/10.1136/gutjnl-2019-318484 (accessed on 15th July 2025).

28. Lee, E., Eghtesad, B., García-Tsao, G., Haskal, Z. J., Hernández-Gea, V., Jalaeian, H., Kalva, S. P., et al. (2023). AASLD practice guidance on the use of TIPS, variceal embolization, and retrograde transvenous obliteration in the management of variceal hemorrhage. *Hepatology, 79*, 224–250. https://doi.org/10.1097/hep.0000000000000530 (accessed on 15th July 2025).

29. Lekkerkerker, S. J., & Voermans, R. P. (2023). EUS and ERCP training in Europe: Time for simulation, optimization, and standardization. *United European Gastroenterology Journal, 11*, 407–409. https://doi.org/10.1002/ueg2.12399 (accessed on 15th July 2025).

30. Malfertheiner, P., Mégraud, F., Rokkas, T., Gisbert, J. P., Liou, J.-M., Schulz, C., Gasbarrini, A., et al. (2022). Management of Helicobacter pylori infection: The Maastricht VI/Florence consensus report. *Gut, 71*, 1724–1762. https://doi.org/10.1136/gutjnl-2022-327745 (accessed on 15th July 2025).

31. Maluf-Filho, F., de la Mora Levy, J. G., & Micames, C. (2012). Advances in diagnosis and treatment of biliopancreatic diseases. *Gastroenterology Research and Practice, 2012.* https://www.semanticscholar.org/paper/1b68fe621ed1b64e4f06a05faf4655a48580289b (accessed on 15th July 2025).

32. Maret-Ouda, J., Markar, S. R., & Lagergren, J. (2020). Gastroesophageal reflux disease. *JAMA, 324*, 2536–2536. https://doi.org/10.1001/jama.2020.21360 (accessed on 15th July 2025).

33. Moldovan, C. A., Alexandru, S., & Ungureanu, F. D. (2017). *The prevalence of high dysplastic colonic adenomatous polyps in a 3-year endoscopic retrospective study from a single clinical center.* https://core.ac.uk/download/144553184.pdf (accessed on 15th July 2025).

34. Nam, H. S., Choi, C. W., Kim, S. J., Kim, H. W., Kang, D. H., Park, S. B., & Ryu, D. G. (2019). Risk factors for delayed bleeding by onset time after endoscopic submucosal dissection for gastric neoplasm. *Scientific Reports, 9.* https://doi.org/10.1038/s41598-019-39381-1 (accessed on 15th July 2025).

35. Northup, P. G., García-Pagán, J. C., García-Tsao, G., Intagliata, N. M., Superina, R., Roberts, L. N., Lisman, T., et al. (2020). Vascular liver disorders, portal vein thrombosis, and procedural bleeding in patients with liver disease: 2020 practice guidance by the American Association for the Study of Liver Diseases. *Hepatology, 73*, 366–413. https://doi.org/10.1002/hep.31646 (accessed on 15th July 2025).

36. Pal, S., Bhaduri, G., Mohta, S., Panja, S., Mahankali, S., & Bohidar, N. P. (2025). Efficacy of ulinastatin in preventing post-ERCP pancreatitis in high-risk patients: A prospective cohort study. *Journal of Digestive Endoscopy.* https://www.semanticscholar.org/paper/2e1221b0f28482eb1b1cc28e44385adc18f86218 (accessed on 15th July 2025).

37. Pimentel-Nunes, P., Libânio, D., Bastiaansen, B. A. J., Bhandari, P., Bisschops, R., Bourke, M. J., Esposito, G., et al. (2022). Endoscopic submucosal dissection for superficial gastrointestinal lesions: European Society of Gastrointestinal Endoscopy (ESGE) guideline – Update 2022. *Endoscopy, 54*, 591–622. https://doi.org/10.1055/a-1811-7025 (accessed on 15th July 2025).

38. Rankin, M., Hambleton, S. A., Derbyshire, E., O'Toole, P., & Smith, G. (2024). Assessing the state of polypectomy practice: Are we ready for the new colonoscopy training pathway? *Frontline Gastroenterology, 16*, 195–201. https://www.semanticscholar.org/paper/93fe2943db08d55c0738eada9a02b1b7e2a03bd1 (accessed on 15th July 2025).

39. Riggs, M. K. (2017). *A novel approach to assess minimally invasive surgical device failure utilizing adverse event outcome severity and design complexity.* https://core.ac.uk/download/217209854.pdf (accessed on 15th July 2025).

40. Rostami, A., Sabet, H. R., Azarm, E., Kangari, H., Elihaei, Z., Khodadoustan, S. B., & Hosseini, K. P. (2024). Self-care management, patient education, and nursing support in patients with diabetes and hypertension. *Galen Medical Journal.* https://www.semanticscholar.org/paper/8823bb5599d63d07c8331d3cf56dee3944bca262 (accessed on 15th July 2025).

41. Serretta, V., Muffoletto, F., Tulone, G., Dioguardi, S., Guzzardo, C., Billeci, S., Baiamonte, D., et al. (2019). MP10-12 Comparison between the ASA score and the modified frailty index (MFI) in urologic oncological and non-oncological urological interventional procedures. *The Journal of Urology, 201*, e122. https://www.semanticscholar.org/paper/ff4f1b2d9d6e252f050f6f722bbd6cc5fe91c18e (accessed on 15th July 2025).

42. Singhal, K., Azizi, S., Tu, T., Mahdavi, S. S., Lee, J., Chung, H. W., Scales, N., et al. (2023). Large language models encode clinical knowledge. *Nature, 620*, 172–180. https://doi.org/10.1038/s41586-023-06291-2 (accessed on 15th July 2025).

43. Søreide, K., Hallet, J., Matthews, J. B., Schnitzbauer, A. A., Line, P.-D., Lai, P. B. S., Gestal Otero, J. J., et al. (2020). Immediate and long-term impact of the COVID-19 pandemic on delivery of surgical services. *British Journal of Surgery, 107*, 1250–1261. https://doi.org/10.1002/bjs.11670 (accessed on 15th July 2025).

44. Tam, S. S., Williams, B., Kohli, R., & Saeed, S. (2025). Standardized biopsy protocols improve adherence to eosinophilic esophagitis and celiac disease endoscopic biopsy guidelines. *JPGN Reports, 6*, 113–120. https://www.semanticscholar.org/paper/ccc4b523098c66a28b9fd6a37e27f0cd4e559c5e (accessed on 15th July 2025).

45. Tang, P., Ali, K., Khizar, H., Ni, Y., Cheng, Z., Xu, B., Qin, Z., et al. (2023). Endoscopic versus minimally invasive surgical approach for infected necrotizing pancreatitis: A systematic review and meta-analysis of randomized controlled trials. *Annals of Medicine, 55.* https://www.semanticscholar.org/paper/1099e6c6efddaffd34907bc3f762a7c2c866d5ae (accessed on 15th July 2025).

46. van Hooft, J. E., Veld, J., Arnold, D., Beets-Tan, R. G. H., Everett, S., Götz, M., van Halsema, E. E., et al. (2020). Self-expandable metal stents for obstructing colonic and extracolonic cancer:

European Society of Gastrointestinal Endoscopy (ESGE) guideline – update 2020. *Endoscopy, 52*, 389–407. https://doi.org/10.1055/a-1140-3017 (accessed on 15th July 2025).

47. Waddingham, W., Kamran, U., Kumar, B., Trudgill, N., Tsiamoulos, Z., & Banks, M. (2022). Complications of diagnostic upper gastrointestinal endoscopy: Common and rare – recognition, assessment and management. *BMJ Open Gastroenterology, 9.* https://www.semanticscholar.org/paper/302f73c3d0aa66bd3a04ebd3a2d81c7168c22e48 (accessed on 15th July 2025).

48. Wang, P., Berzin, T. M., Glissen Brown, J. R., Bharadwaj, S., Becq, A., Xiao, X., Liu, P., et al. (2019). Real-time automatic detection system increases colonoscopic polyp and adenoma detection rates: A prospective randomized controlled study. *Gut, 68*, 1813–1819. https://doi.org/10.1136/gutjnl-2018-317500 (accessed on 15th July 2025).

49. Wolf, A. M. D., Fontham, E. T. H., Church, T. R., Flowers, C. R., Guerra, C. E., LaMonte, S. J., Etzioni, R., et al. (2018). Colorectal cancer screening for average-risk adults: 2018 guideline update from the American Cancer Society. *CA: A Cancer Journal for Clinicians, 68*, 250–281. https://doi.org/10.3322/caac.21457 (accessed on 15th July 2025).

50. Yamamoto, H., Sakamoto, H., Kumagai, H., Abe, T., Ishiguro, S., Uchida, K., Kawasaki, Y., et al. (2023). Clinical guidelines for diagnosis and management of Peutz-Jeghers syndrome in children and adults. *Digestion, 104*, 335–347. https://www.semanticscholar.org/paper/6cbff3fb75aea2145eab70ca27836f3e6c0e3ec3 (accessed on 15th July 2025).

51. Zhang, A., Fan, N., Zhang, X., Guo, H., Zhou, Y., Zeng, L., Lin, Y., et al. (2024). Endoscopic retrograde appendicitis therapy. *Therapeutic Advances in Gastroenterology, 17.* https://www.semanticscholar.org/paper/51db953d05958a31e1da4d5248d5413a8a043f31 (accessed on 15th July 2025).

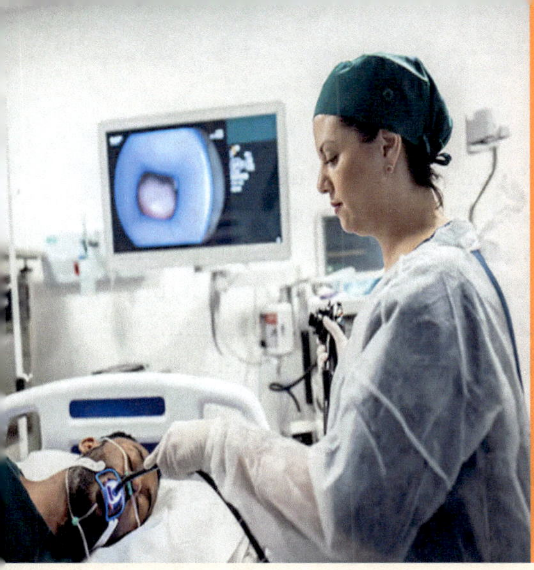

Chapter 15

ENDOSCOPY IN INFLAMMATORY BOWEL DISEASE (IBD)

Contents

Introduction.....441
15.1. Types of Inflammatory Bowel Disease (IBD).....444
15.2. Role of Endoscopy in Diagnosis.....447
15.3. Therapeutic Endoscopy Techniques.....451
15.4. Risks and Complications of Endoscopy.....454
15.5. Advances in Endoscopic Technology.....457
15.6. Patient Perspectives and Experiences.....460
Summary.....465
References.....468

Introduction

Endoscopy's place in the investigation of inflammatory bowel disease (IBD), specifically Crohn's disease and ulcerative colitis, is a paradigm shift. These are chronic illnesses characterized by episodic acute exacerbations and pathologic alterations in gastrointestinal tissue leading to disabling diarrhea, bleeding, and cramping pain. With IBD continuing to affect a significant portion of the world's population, there has been an increased need for improved management. Endoscopy not only serves as a diagnostic tool to evaluate mucosal inflammation but also helps establish disease activity during follow up. Clinicians aim to achieve not only symptom control but also mucosal healing, which has been a key objective in the management of IBD. A proper endoscopic evaluation is thus essential since it influences therapeutic options and ultimately patient outcomes by applying a tailored strategy to each individual's status (Cai et al., 2021). With IBD, pain control is likewise always a significant concern as patients mostly have symptoms that transcend the primary gastrointestinal presentations. Chronic pain in the abdomen, a symptom most commonly used to describe those with IBD, can persist even during periods of remission, pointing towards the complex interaction of pain and inflammation. This symptom resists treatment paradigms that address gut inflammation predominantly but neglect the issue of chronic pain. Initial studies reveal that successful control of endoscopy in IBD is related to positive alterations in pain perception and overall quality of life in the patients. However, there remains a lot of disagreement between mucosal healing as characterized through endoscopic indices and continuing subjective symptoms reported by patients, highlighting the need for further investigation into the mechanisms and related management strategies (Bakshi et al., 2021). The union of endoscopic findings with aggressive pain management interventions is a paradigm shift in the therapy of the multifaceted problems of IBD. Emerging evidence gives precedence to the necessity for enhanced protocols that recognize the role of both gastrointestinal and extrabdominal symptoms and active patient-clinician communication.

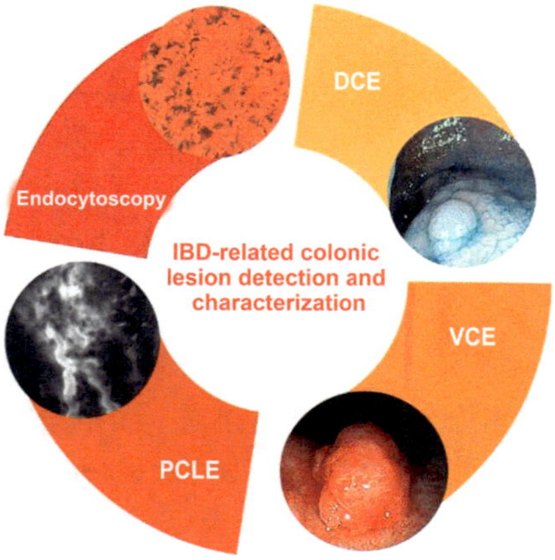

Figure 15.1. Endoscopy in inflammatory bowel disease (IBD).

Source: https://pub.mdpi-res.com/diagnostics/diagnostics-13-02547/article_deploy/html/images/diagnostics-13-02547-g001.png?1690857223.

Evaluation of multiple avenues of therapy, such as medication management and psychosocial interventions, must incorporate endoscopy as a cornerstone of treating IBD. Lastly, a hybrid framework that integrates endoscopic findings with a holistic understanding of patient-reported outcomes will be able to guarantee improved clinical practice and address the severe demand for effective pain relief interventions in IBD patients (Cai et al., 2021) (Figure 15.1).

Definition of Inflammatory Bowel Disease (IBD)

IBD is a chronic inflammatory disease of the gastrointestinal tract, primarily classified into two large categories: Crohn's disease and ulcerative colitis. Both of them share common environmental and genetic determinants and lead to dysregulation of immune response against intestinal microbiota. Crohn's disease affects any part of the gastrointestinal tract with transmural inflammation, whereas ulcerative colitis affects the colonic mucosa and is typically associated with diffuse inflammation. This dichotomy is required for adequate clinical management, since each subtype necessitates different kinds of treatment. As knowledge increases about IBD, increasingly now there is recognition that its etiology, multifactorial in nature, will require a complete definition that will have space for the interplay among genetic predispositions, environmental exposures, and immune dysregulation. Clinical course of IBD can dramatically vary across patients, typically having symptomatic relapses of weight loss, abdominal pain, and diarrhea, hence warranting early diagnosis. Endoscopic assessment is the prime diagnostic technique, with direct visualization of intestinal mucosa and quantification of inflammatory activity. Technology , such as high-definition colonoscopy and chromoendoscopy further enhances detection capability, with increased likelihood of detection of subtle mucosal lesions and dysplasia. The value of these modalities cannot be overstressed, as early and correct diagnosis of IBD is crucial in the management of appropriate treatment regimens. Furthermore, gaining insight into the severity and extent of the illnesses through endoscopy can direct long-term management plans and the need for ongoing surveillance, since the risk of developing colorectal cancer is profoundly increased in IBD patients. The connection to IBD management is underscored by the evolution in imaging technology and scoring indices for better mucosal healing evaluation. The Paddington International virtual ChromoendoScopy ScOreor PICaSSO endoscopic score, for instance, depicts a useful tool for predicting histological outcomes and is gaining popularity in regular clinical practice (Nardone et al., 2022). Such synergy between endoscopic evaluation and histology comforts the clinician of successful treatments and enhances patient care. There is also a need for standard protocols in surveillance monitoring, particularly as a consequence of advancements in visualization technology that can identify lesions not detectable before (Manchanda et al., 2019). As the technologies advance, so does IBD knowledge, rendering endoscopy a fundamental part of the continuous battle to optimize patient outcomes and redefine treatment protocols in this complex disease.

Role of Endoscopy in Diagnosis and Management

Endoscopy plays an important role in the diagnosis and management of IBD, that is, Crohn's disease and ulcerative colitis. This minimally invasive method allows for direct visualization of the gastrointestinal tract so that it is feasible for gastroenterologists to assess mucosal inflammation, ulceration, and other pathological changes. Furthermore, endoscopic techniques enable biopsies to be taken, which are essential for histological analysis and definitive diagnosis. The direct access to tissue from the involved areas enables clinicians to gauge the severity of the disease and differentiate among various types of IBD. The accurate data gathered by endoscopic examinations are extremely useful in outlining the appropriate treatment plan, taking into consideration each patient's condition's unique pathological characteristics. In addition, endoscopy has a key role in IBD patients' ongoing management and surveillance. Regular endoscopic monitoring needs to be performed to measure disease activity, monitor responses to therapies, and screen for complications , such as dysplasia and colorectal cancer. IBD patients have an increased risk of developing colorectal cancer, as the use of surveillance colonoscopies in their routine care has been made particularly important. Surveillance aims at the detection of precancerous lesions early so that patient outcomes are improved by intervention at an early stage. As highlighted in recent studies, the majority of instances of colorectal cancer in IBD patients are likely due to missed opportunities during surveillance. The integration of robust surveillance regimens with advanced endoscopic equipment will enhance detection rates and eventually result in enhanced prevention measures for cancer, enhancing the overall quality of care in this patient population (Saitta & Garg, 2021). Furthermore, artificial intelligence (AI) is being used to supplement endoscopic techniques in transforming the field of IBD treatment. Artificial intelligence technologies, particularly machine learning methods, enhance the diagnostic accuracy by improving lesion detection and characterization during endoscopy. These advances are particularly crucial in gastroenterology, where highly precise lesion recognition can become a direct determinant of treatment. AI is capable of assisting in processing vast amounts of endoscopic information, hence enabling physicians to make more effective decisions regarding patient management. The evolving role of AI in the context of endoscopy not only promises to improve diagnostic precision but also fits into the larger goal of maximizing the care of patients with inflammatory bowel disease as a significant step towards healthcare excellence (Rio et al., 2023) (Figure 15.2).

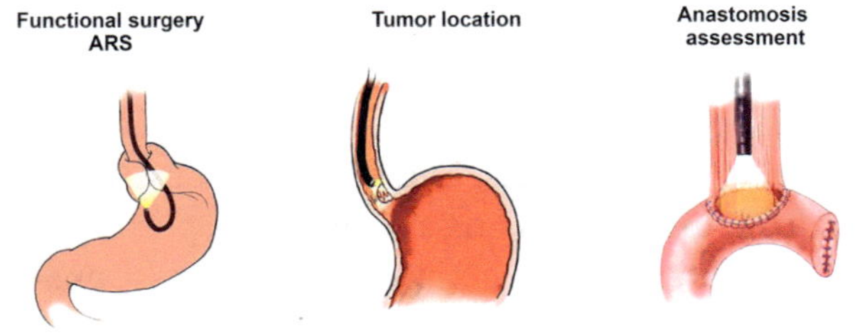

Figure 15.2. Importance of endoscopy in diagnosis and management.

Source: https://www.frontiersin.org/files/Articles/1186945/fgstr-02-1186945-HTML/image_m/fgstr-02-1186945-g001.jpg.

15.1. Types of Inflammatory Bowel Disease (IBD)

IBD comprises primarily two distinct conditions: Crohn's disease and ulcerative colitis. Crohn's disease can affect any region of the gastrointestinal tract, from the mouth to the anus, but most frequently occurs in the ileum and colon. This form of IBD is characterized by transmural inflammation and may lead to complications , such as strictures, fistulas, and abscesses. Conversely, ulcerative colitis occurs only in the colon and rectum and is characterized by chronic superficial inflammation of the mucosal layer.

The anatomical difference mandates specialized treatment methods in a bid to effectively manage symptoms and prevent serious complications about each disease. Endoscopy is key to differential diagnosis among these diseases because their presentations overlap and aids doctors in making a correct diagnosis, thus directing follow-up management in the IBD disease treatment framework. IBD's unpredictable presentation and course in affected individuals attest to its nature. Ulcerative colitis, for instance, could be accompanied by painful, bloody diarrhea and stomach pain, whereas Crohn's disease might be manifested through abdominal cramps and weight loss that vary extremely between patients. This heterogeneity calls for constant monitoring to serve the patients in their best interests through proper interventions. The existing guidelines point to the necessity of a multidisciplinary approach, consolidating the work of gastroenterologists, surgeons, dieticians, and highly specialized nurses in addressing the IBD's etiological multifactorial nature. Continuous communication and coordination between healthcare professionals can optimize patient outcomes, particularly in relation to evolving evidence-based treatment in relation to drug and nondrug therapies for Crohn's disease and ulcerative colitis, as highlighted in recent reviews of the management platform (Lamb et al., 2019). As a rule, having knowledge of the types of inflammatory bowel disease is important for effective clinical management, especially regarding the potential development of colorectal cancer (CRC). Based on evidence, patients with long-standing IBD, and more so those with ulcerative colitis, are at higher risk for CRC and hence in need of regular surveillance and early intervention. Endoscopy not only offers diagnostic potential but also an essential role in dysplasia screening and early cancer detection within the realm of surveillance examination. Timely access to endoscopic evaluation can improve patient outcome by offering early treatment potential at the expense of reduced incidence of advanced disease. Accordingly, a synergistic strategy focused on awareness and early detection of IBD and its sequelae, such as CRC, remains a critical objective in clinical practice and public health initiatives (Md. Hossain et al., 2022) (Figure 15.3).

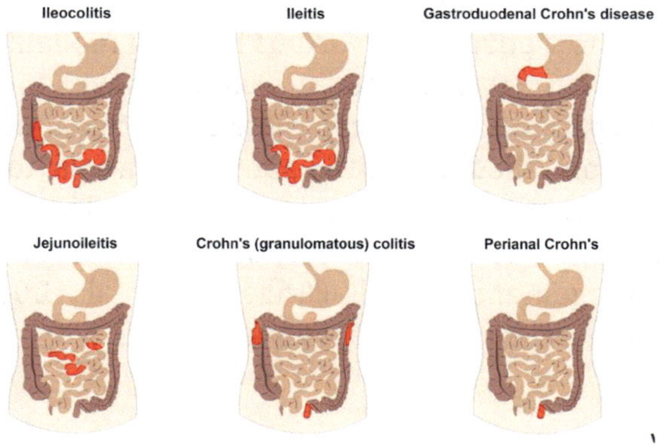

Figure 15.3. Types of inflammatory bowel disease (IBD).

Source: https://www.ibdrelief.com/uploads/files/types20of20Crohn's20social_og_image_135.jpg.

15.1.1. Crohn's Disease

The management of Crohn's disease, a prominent subset of IBD, has dramatically evolved over the past several decades, especially with advancements in endoscopic techniques. Endoscopy is a critical diagnostic and assessment tool for Crohn's disease with direct visualization of the intestinal mucosa and the ability to procure biopsies. These tests not only confirm diagnosis but also serve to define the limit of disease activity, and this is most critical to proper treatment planning. New evidence demonstrates that following the introduction of biologic therapy, there has been a dramatic increase in endoscopic evaluation among patients who were diagnosed with Crohn's disease. This shift emphasizes the expanding role of comprehensive disease assessment in ordinary clinical practice to enhance patient care within a changing therapeutic environment (Young et al., 2025). In addition to traditional endoscopy, the role of non-invasive imaging modalities is progressively recognized in the management of Crohn's disease. Methods , such as magnetic resonance imaging (MRI) and computed tomography (CT) enterography allow for vivid visualization of the gastrointestinal tract without invasive modality. Such modalities can quantify transmural inflammation better than endoscopy itself, with a clear understanding of disease progression. This is particularly helpful in patients who may not be suitable for repeated endoscopic procedures due to complications or intolerance. With the current guidelines emphasizing a treat-to-target strategy, the integration of these non-invasive imaging modalities with conventional endoscopic evaluation is critical in implementing personalized treatment as well as monitoring outcomes for Crohn's disease patients (Kucharzik et al., 2025). Additionally, the integration of advanced endoscopic techniques has proven to have an impressive impact on surgery in patients with Crohn's disease. Conventional surgical resection was previously a compulsory intervention in patients with complications or disease that was refractory. However, more recent data of routine endoscopic assessment included lower surgery rates, as practitioners can initiate specific medical treatment earlier based on endoscopic findings. Endoscopy and advanced imaging allow for phenotyping of Crohn's disease more accurately, leading to better treatment results and fewer complications requiring surgery. Therefore, the progression of endoscopic practice has a crucial role to play not only in the diagnosis and management of Crohn's disease but also in planning long-term care, promoting a multidisciplinary team approach to meet patient needs optimally (Young et al., 2025).

15.1.2. Ulcerative Colitis (UC)

UC is an IBD that is chronic in nature with ulceration and inflammation, primarily of the colon's mucosal lining. Trusted by its uncontrolled remissions and exacerbations, UC is highly difficult to diagnose and treat. The chronic inflammation differentiates UC from Crohn's disease and leads to distinctive endoscopic findings that are both relevant for diagnosis and treatment decision-making. Endoscopy, or ileocolonoscopy, is now the standard of measurement for describing the extent and severity of colonic inflammation because it allows for direct visualization of the mucosa. However, the application of endoscopic evaluation has its limits when considering the severity of the complications and in such patients where standard endoscopy is contraindicated, and it highlights the need for add-on imaging modalities for a better understanding of disease activity and complications (Bhattaru et al., 2024). Inclusion of newer imaging technologies has played an ever more important part in the management of UC, particularly when endoscopy is not possible or yields non-diagnostic results. Non-invasive techniques with magnetic resonance enterography (MRE) and others can gather important information that cannot be obtained via endoscopy. For instance, MRE has been useful for the detection of extramural lesions and quantifying disease chronicity that cannot be identified by endoscopy. Second, MRE can be used as an essential tool for distinguishing between Crohn's disease and ulcerative colitis, especially in refractory conditions or postoperative complications. Imaging, in this case, not only aids in making the diagnosis but also helps in guiding treatment decisions, thus enhancing patient outcome while avoiding the hazards of invasive procedures (Radmard et al., 2024). With the complementary roles of endoscopy and high-technology imaging in the treatment of UC, a multidisciplinary care practice is required. This type of practice enables clinicians to tailor interventions based on the needs of the patient, thereby optimizing management practices. For instance, while endoscopy makes it possible to conduct simultaneous therapeutic interventions , such as biopsies and stricture treatments, imaging modalities can follow disease activity and response to treatment constantly without exposing patients to risk of complications , such as perforation. With each passing time, practice in the management of IBD continues to evolve, and ongoing research into how adequately various imaging modalities complement endoscopic treatment will mean that patients receive complete care. In summary, the combined use of the above diagnostic tools is important to overcome the complexity of ulcerative colitis effectively and improve patient management overall (Bhattaru et al., 2024; Radmard et al., 2024) (Figure 15.4).

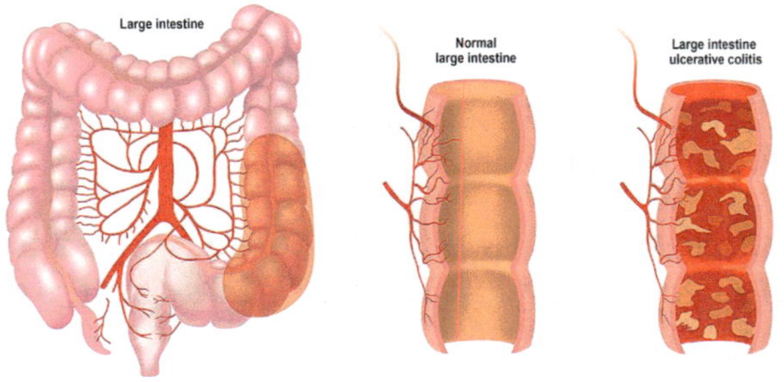

Figure 15.4. Ulcerative colitis (UC) represents a chronic inflammatory bowel disease (IBD).

Source: https://www.cdc.gov/inflammatory-bowel-disease/media/images/2024/06/IBD-UlcerativeColitis-Graphic.jpg.

15.1.3. Indeterminate Colitis (IC)

IC is an individual challenge of the IBD continuum. It is defined by features which do not necessarily put it into the realm of either Crohn's disease or ulcerative colitis on clinical, endoscopic, radiological, and histologic grounds. This lack of certainty can complicate diagnosis and management since both forms of IBD require an individualized therapeutic approach. Endoscopy is critical in the diagnosis of IC, allowing direct visualization of mucosal inflammation and the performance of biopsies that may show histopathological findings distinguishing it from its differentiating relatives. Importantly, the thorough assessment during endoscopy may determine treatment strategies, highlighting the need for experienced interpretation by gastroenterologists with knowledge of IBD pathophysiology. With the increasing recognition of IC, its connection to CRC has become increasingly interesting to the medical community. Current evidence indicates that patients with chronic inflammation, whatever the precise IBD category, are at higher risk of developing CRC over time. The endoscopic surveillance in such patients cannot be overstated. Regular colonoscopic evaluation enables early detection of neoplasia or dysplasia, and this is highly significant in optimizing outcome management.

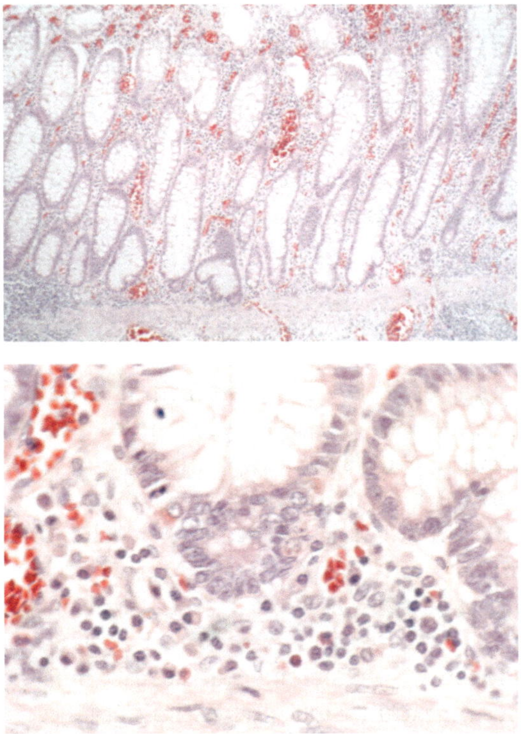

Figure 15.5. Indeterminate colitis (IC).

Source: https://jcp.bmj.com/content/jclinpath/57/12/1233/F2.large.jpg.

With the growing rate of CRC globally, as discussed in its epidemiology, the role of endoscopy in monitoring IC patients becomes even more crucial in building an era where early intervention strategies can create a significant impact on survival (Md. Hossain et al., 2022). Guidelines for the management of diseases that may be imitating IC, such as primary sclerosing cholangitis (PSC), emphasize the importance of individualized treatment in the context of IBD (Chapman et al., 2019). This particularly applies to patients with indeterminate colitis, in which individualized treatment plans are required not just to treat the inflammatory aspects of the disease but also its related co-morbidities. As practitioners make efforts to establish effective management regimens for IC, multidisciplinary coordination among gastroenterologists, hepatologists, and surgeons becomes essential. Through holistic endoscopic assessments, medical professionals can have a deeper understanding of each patient's individual pathology, hence enabling personalized interventions taking into account the inflammatory bowel disease as well as its possible complications, such as PSC and CRC. The evolution of these protocols is an evolutionary advancement towards the integrated management of the patient in the case of IBD (Figure 15.5).

15.2. Role of Endoscopy in Diagnosis

Endoscopy is a central diagnostic and management device in IBD, providing valuable information regarding the mucosal topographies of the gut. Through enabling direct visualization of the intestine, endoscopy assists in differentiating between UC and Crohn's disease (CD), two of the principal forms of IBD that are often imitative of one another. The capability of endoscopic procedures to provide biopsies further enhances diagnostic accuracy so that tissue samples can be analyzed through histology. Histological abnormalities have been found to be present in patients whose endoscopic findings are macroscopically normal, which emphasizes the importance of careful evaluation in diagnosis (Chen et al., 2024). This capability not only allows physicians to diagnose the existence of inflammation but also the character of the inflammatory process, which is essential in tailoring treatment regimens and disease prognosis. Moreover, endoscopy serves a role beyond diagnosis as it is an integral part in the follow-up of the disease course and assessment of the impact of therapy in patients with IBD. In regular endoscopic evaluation, the doctor can quantify the degree of mucosal healing, which has now emerged as a key endpoint in treating these chronic diseases. Mucosal healing is strongly associated with long-term excellent outcomes, like reduced rates of hospitalization and surgery, hence filling in a novel paradigm for managing IBD. Endoscopic assessment of lesion findings , such as inflammation or ulceration can direct the therapeutic adjustment, as evidenced by the relationship between histological and endoscopic markers of disease activity (Mureşan et al., 2024). Endoscopy is therefore not only an important diagnostic tool but also in management and surveillance, justifying its pivotal place in the global care of IBD patients. Advances in endoscopic technology have greatly enhanced diagnostic ability for IBD, leading to more sensitive approaches in managing patients. Technologies , such as balloon-assisted endoscopy and chromoendoscopy better visualize underlying mucosal pathology, which tends to be subtle in nature. These technologies have been of greatest benefit in pediatric patients, whose endoscopic findings can be quite disparate from those of adult patients (Chen et al., 2024). With increasing awareness of the role of upper gastrointestinal tract in children with IBD, endoscopic examination is an essential part of the complete evaluation. Hence, the addition of newer endoscopic modalities not only improves diagnosis but also aids in understanding the disease pathophysiology and thus therapeutic planning. The different functions of endoscopy in IBD thus accentuate its significance in initial diagnosis and chronic management of the group of disorders (Figure 15.6).

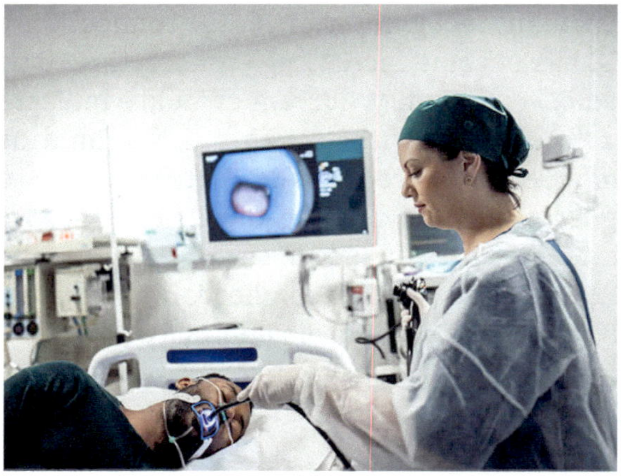

Figure 15.6. Role of endoscopy in diagnosis.

Source: https://media.post.rvohealth.io/wp-content/uploads/2023/10/doctor-patient-endoscopy-medical-procedure-732x549-thumbnail-732x549.jpg.

15.2.1. Visualizing the Gastrointestinal Tract

Imaging of the gastrointestinal tract is a cornerstone in the management of IBD, such as Crohn's disease and ulcerative colitis. The advent of endoscopy has revolutionized the diagnostic and treatment profile of IBD, enabling clinicians to visualize mucosal surfaces directly. Through procedures like esophagogastroduodenoscopy (EGD) and colonoscopy, physicians can assess the extent of inflammation, seek out pathological lesions, and take biopsies—all vital for appropriate diagnosis. Moreover, the visualization of the GI tract facilitates the establishment of an individualized treatment plan, an aspect that is highly relevant for the management of chronic diseases , such as IBD. Advanced imaging modalities not only aid in proper diagnosis but also follow-up on disease activity or remission, making it necessary to include advanced endoscopic methods in contemporary IBD management. Endoscopic evaluation has proved to be valuable in identifying mucosal healing, a critical predictor of the efficacy of therapy in patients with IBD. Mucosal healing is associated with good clinical outcomes, such as more remission, reduced hospitalization and operations, and reduced risk of colorectal cancer. With these strong relationships in mind, endoscopy remains the gold standard to establish IBD activity and severity. Implementing routine endoscopic monitoring facilitates the detection of dysplastic changes at an early stage, thereby benefiting overall management of the condition in the long run. In the same way, the evolving capabilities of endoscopic technology, such as high-definition imaging and chromoendoscopy, indicate visualization use in enhancing diagnostic accuracy and therapeutic interventions and thereby enhancing the long-term outcomes of inflammatory bowel disease patients, as indicated in the literature. Another characteristic of visualizing the GI tract through endoscopy in managing IBD is the ability to provide therapeutic interventions at the same time while diagnosing. New endoscopic techniques have expanded the front line of treatment options for clinicians.

Therapeutic procedures , such as balloon dilation of strictures and endoscopic mucosal resection of neoplastic lesions are now routine procedures in the therapeutic treatment of IBD. Furthermore, the safety of these procedures has also been further confirmed by research that indicates a low incidence of severe adverse events, even in low body mass index (BMI) patients (Al-Hagawi et al., 2024). This is a further reminder of the overriding importance of endoscopic visualization not only as a diagnostic procedure but as a means of successful treatment of IBD-related complications (Núñez et al., 2021). Thus, technological progress of endoscopy will continue to be an integral part in optimizing therapy for IBD patients, as an aspiration is ongoing vigilance for risk reduction coupled with enhanced therapeutic gain (Figure 15.7).

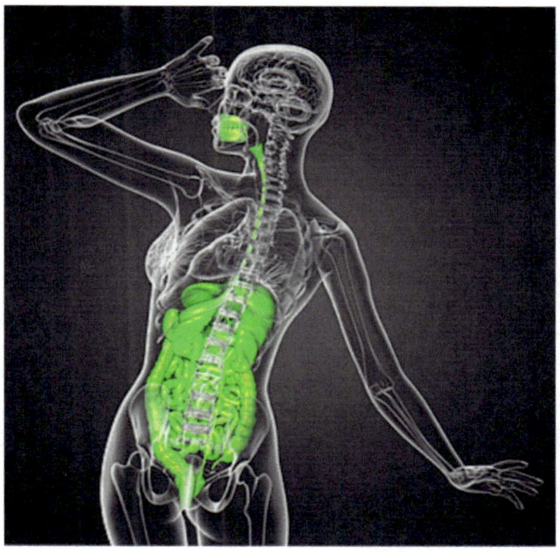

Figure 15.7. Visualizing the gastrointestinal tract.

Source: https://png.pngtree.com/thumb_back/fh260/background/20220220/pngtree-threedimensional-medical-visualization-of-the-human-gastrointestinal-tract-photo-image_16893154.jpg.

15.2.2. Biopsy Collection for Histological Analysis

Biopsy specimen acquisition during endoscopy is pivotal to the histological analysis that is needed for the diagnosis of IBD. The technique allows clinicians to obtain tissue samples from the affected regions of the gastrointestinal tract that are subjected to microscopic examination for signs of inflammation, epithelial damage, or other pathologic changes. Precise biopsies' collection is critically crucial since it directly affects the validity of diagnostic results. In a literature review of diagnostic approaches in IBD, endoscopic visualization along with histological analysis remains central to the effective management of this multi-factorial illness, underscoring the value of efficient biopsy protocols in obtaining representative tissue samples and minimizing mucosal trauma (Foscarini et al., 2025). Endoscopic methods have evolved significantly over time to enable focused procedures against lesions that characterize most IBD patterns. Techniques , such as double-balloon endoscopy (DBE) expand the limits of standard endoscopy, making it possible to access parts of the small intestine previously inaccessible. DBE facilitated biopsy retrieval from the jejunum in a case report involving a canine model, where lymphocytic-plasmacytic jejunitis was diagnosed after initially out-of-range results with standard endoscopy (Ayala et al., 2011). This raises to the forefront the necessity of using sophisticated endoscopic techniques to obtain maximally diagnostic biopsies, ultimately leading to more individualized treatment regimens for IBD patients. Also, not only is histologic examination of biopsy specimens necessary to confirm the presence of IBD, but it also provides us with information regarding the severity, activity, and complications of the disease. This wide-ranging assessment can help guide clinical decision-making, from immunosuppressive medication choice to surgery. With the introduction of new biomarkers, such as extrachromosomal circular DNA, further research may expand the diagnostic toolset for IBD, complementing standard biopsy techniques (Foscarini et al., 2025). Thus, ongoing progress in endoscopic and histological methods holds the key to improved control of IBD to ensure timely and efficient diagnosis and treatment of patients.

15.2.3. Differentiating Between Types of Inflammatory Bowel Diseases (IBD)

IBD, comprised largely of CD and UC, possesses different clinical and pathological presentations that must be differentiated to facilitate appropriate management. CD is characterized by patchy, transmural inflammation of any part of the gastrointestinal tract and is often complicated by the appearance of strictures and fistulas. UC virtually always affects the colonic mucosa in the form of continuous mucosal inflammation confined to the rectum but extending proximally. This focal pattern of UC presents a striking contrast to CD's segmental pattern and underscores the importance of accurate diagnosis through endoscopic studies. Endoscopy is a useful approach for the visualization of the gastrointestinal tract, assessment of mucosal damage, and the taking of biopsies to further identify the nature of the IBD, hence facilitating easy formulation of specific therapeutic interventions for the affected individuals (Seyedian et al., 2019). The diagnostic process in distinguishing between CD and UC not only serves treatment purposes but also the prediction of disease course and complications. Endoscopy plays an important role in disease severity and extent evaluation, with direct visualization of mucosal inflammation. It is particularly helpful for patients with an indeterminate presentation, where characteristic features of ulceration patterns and histological findings may give vital information. For instance, the finding of granulomas on biopsy is indicative of CD, whereas UC biopsies may reveal crypt abscesses and goblet cell depletion. With the newer modalities of chromoendoscopy and high-definition imaging, clinicians can enhance the detection of the subtle mucosal details that help to distinguish these conditions, thereby impacting surveillance practices and patient treatment (Wang et al., 2019). Further, the separation of IBD types has implications beyond both emergent diagnosis and treatment. Understanding the pathophysiological mechanisms specific to CD and UC is of paramount importance in long-term prognosis anticipation, e.g., for the risk of colorectal cancer in UC. Patients with long-standing UC are at more risk, which calls for surveillance colonoscopy to prevent this risk. However, CD patients can be faced with special complications that require surgery to be carried out more frequently. Intelligent endoscopic technology development, particularly the use of artificial intelligence in the detection and characterization of polyps, can further enhance differentiation so that management can be appropriately personalized. Thus, advancement of our knowledge and practice of endoscopic techniques in IBD forms the core of enhanced outcomes in patients and informs future research priorities (Seyedian et al., 2019) (Figure 15.8).

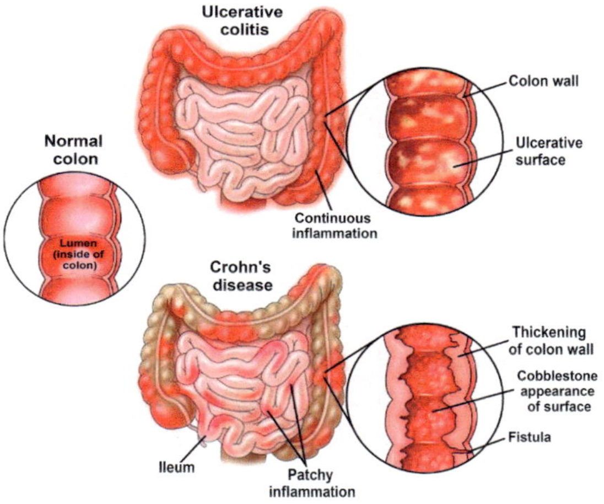

Figure 15.8. Differentiating between types of inflammatory bowel diseases (IBD).

Source: https://patient.gastro.org/wp-content/uploads/2021/07/CGH-Patient-Ed-IBD2.0-2019.jpg.

15.3. Therapeutic Endoscopy Techniques

Therapeutic endoscopy techniques are one of the most important advances in the management of IBD, particularly the optimization of treatment modalities. Therapeutic techniques in endoscopy surpass ordinary diagnostic purposes because they allow intervention that has the potential to alter the course of the disease. Among the most surprising developments are advanced imaging technologies that offer real-time imaging of the intestinal mucosa, which is crucial for the identification of dysplasia and other complications of IBD. Methods , such as endoscopic ultrasound and chromoendoscopy enhance visualization, allowing clinicians to perform targeted biopsies and therapy in real-time. These innovations therefore, contribute a great deal to the achievement of endoscopic remission, which is increasingly being recognized as an absolutely crucial target in the treatment of IBD. Their combination enhances diagnostic accuracy and the effectiveness of decision-making regarding treatment, rendering them invaluable in contemporary gastroenterological practice. Besides, the growing application of artificial intelligence in therapeutic endoscopy is promising more accuracy and standardization in IBD assessment. Interobserver variation in the traditional endoscopic evaluation often leads to variable treatment strategies. AI technology-based approach brings in a very interesting prospect where algorithms can assist clinicians in the evaluation of mucosal healing and inflammatory patterns in a more objective way. The potential for enhanced diagnostic accuracy augments the therapeutic capabilities provided by high-technology endoscopy. Furthermore, developments in emerging endoscopic devices, such as probe-based confocal laser endomicroscopy, allow for *in vivo* histological examination, providing knowledge of intestinal lesion microenvironment. This intersection of technology not only aids in optimal disease assessment but may improve outcomes through the facilitation of early therapeutic intervention (Zammarchi et al., 2023). Finally, IBD treatment is being revolutionized as researchers explore the potential of molecular endoscopy technology. Although still in their infancy, these methods aim to analyze cellular and molecular targets in real time with endoscopes, reporting on mucosal inflammation and response to therapy. As opposed to traditional histologic examination by biopsy, molecular endoscopy has the potential to offer rapid, non-invasive measurements. This is best for patients who may be resistant to repeated biopsy procedures. Current research has validated the application of employing multiple biomarkers simultaneously in an attempt to enhance the accuracy of the assessment of disease activity, moving toward more tailored treatment of IBD. As therapeutic endoscopy continues to develop along with emerging technology, integration of these technologies is set to change patient care and improve long-term outcomes in the management of IBD (Dragoni et al., 2020) (Figure 15.9).

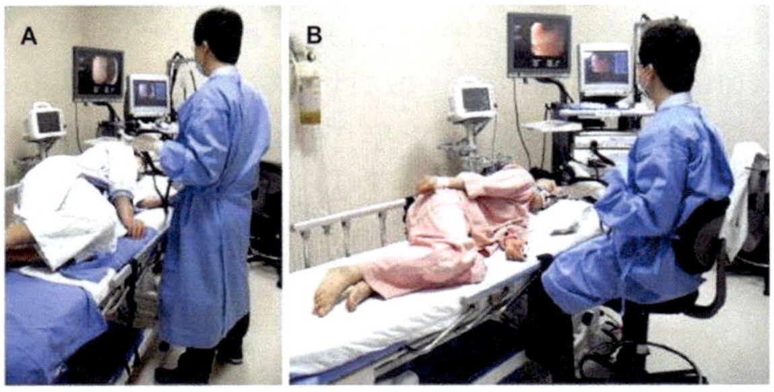

Figure 15.9. Therapeutic endoscopy techniques.

Source: https://f6publishing.blob.core.windows.net/a1481835-b013-4dcd-8a01-48a6d76fb1dd/WJG-21-759-g002.jpg.

15.3.1. Endoscopic Mucosal Resection (EMR)

The employment of EMR is a significant advancement for IBD-related lesion management. EMR is especially useful for resecting HR-CAN, which encompasses several non-polypoid lesions that are notoriously difficult to treat with conventional surgical techniques. Recent evidence shows that this method can be highly effective in obtaining high en bloc resection rates, which are important to guarantee the complete removal of cancer tissue and minimize invasive surgery. Specifically, data show that en bloc and R0 resection rates are greater than 90% in EMR-treated patients with colonic IBD, which indicates its effectiveness as a safe treatment for dysplastic lesions. Hence, EMR not only facilitates targeted therapy but is also an invaluable tool for maintaining mucosal integrity in IBD patients (Maselli et al., 2024). The success of EMR is also augmented through integration with advanced imaging modalities that provide better visual information regarding the mucosa of the gastrointestinal tract. Novel technologies , such as multiphoton excitation-based imaging, chromoendoscopy with dyes, and confocal laser endomicroscopy with probe-based optics, allow for better delineation of dysplasia before resection. These modalities improve endoscopist perception of mucosal changes and inflammation, thereby ultimately aiding in planning the procedure for EMR. Besides, emerging technologies, like artificial intelligence (AI), can potentially predict dysplasia and enable risk stratification, potentially revolutionizing endoscopic management of IBD. Using these innovative imaging technologies, clinicians will be in a position to make evidence-based decisions to optimize the effectiveness of EMR, consequently promoting better patient outcomes while reducing surgery complications (Santacroce et al., 2023). While helpful, EMR in managing IBD comes with its challenges. The occurrence of persistent inflammation may complicate the resection process, which is a cause for concern of local recurrence and metachronous lesions post-procedure. In a retrospective study, recurrence was observed in around 3%, highlighting the need for persistent monitoring and follow-up in patients who have received EMR for HR-CANs. In addition, complications, albeit in most cases manageable, arose in approximately 12.5% of cases, highlighting the need for carrying out these procedures in specialized centers with sufficient expertise and facilities. As IBD remains a major risk factor for colorectal cancer, ongoing studies of how best to optimize EMR methods and determine long-term survival remain important to establishing its position as a gold standard of care for the treatment of dysplastic lesions in this group of patients (Maselli et al., 2024).

15.3.2. Balloon Dilatation for Strictures

Treatment of strictures of IBD has come a long way with advances in endoscopic procedures. Balloon dilatation has been a popular treatment for fibrostenotic strictures, particularly in Crohn's disease. It is a non-invasive procedure where a balloon catheter is placed inside the stricture and inflated to stretch the contracted segment of the bowel. The efficacy of balloon dilatation is indicated by its ability to relieve obstructions and avoid subjecting patients to more invasive surgery. While physicians seek to balance successful treatment with patient quality of life, balloon dilatation is a valuable intervention within the growing corpus of endoscopic treatments for IBD (Clement & Reyes, 2024). Greater support for balloon dilatation is a marker of more extensive information on stricturotomy and the critical role of endoscopic treatment in the overall management of IBD complications. Before its widespread adoption, strictures often needed to be corrected surgically, with high risk and potential for complications. The addition of balloon dilatation to routine care has transformed the management of strictures by making site-specific treatment available with less risk. Repeated dilatation appears, from current literature, to provide sustained symptom relief with minimal requirement for surgical resection and thus optimal patient benefit. Aside from this, combined with other treatments , such as stenting, balloon dilatation is also in line with the trend of providing less invasive solutions for complex IBD presentations (Núñez et al., 2021). Despite its advantages, balloon dilatation is not without limitations and potential complications. Techniques should be taken meticulously so as not to cause bowel perforation or re-emergence of the stricture. With the evolving nature of endoscopic treatment of IBD, there must be ongoing research to delineate more subtle therapeutic interventions and uniform protocols. The intricacy in managing strictures requires an adequate grasp of the pathophysiology of the disease as well as careful patient selection for optimal outcomes. With greater insight into the nuances of balloon dilatation, particularly with advancing technologies, clinicians can further advance its application as a keystone therapy within the course of IBD management (Clement & Reyes, 2024) (Figure 15.10).

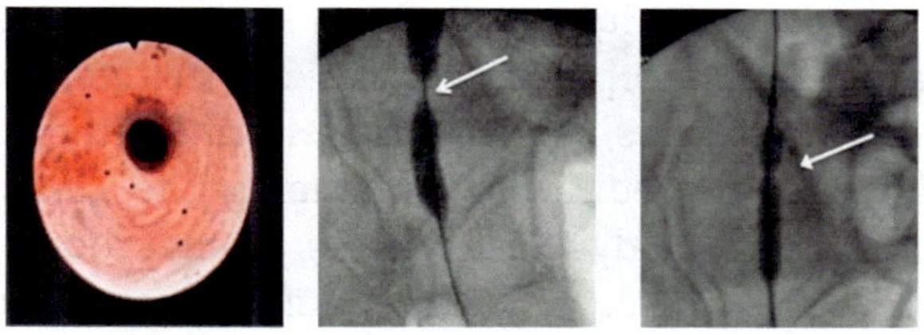

(a) Endoscopic view | (b) Fluoroscopic view of a stricture | (c) Balloon dilatation under fluoroscopic guidance

Figure 15.10. Balloon dilatation for strictures.

Source: https://www.researchgate.net/publication/328428967/figure/fig1/AS:960080434450438@1605912421209/Minimally-invasive-management-of-ureteric-strictures-balloon-dilatation.png.

15.3.3. Endoscopic Submucosal Dissection (ESD)

ESD has emerged as an important technique in IBD patient treatment, particularly for the resection of HR-CAN. It is a paradigm shift from conventionally used resection methods, in which non-polypoid lesions and large non-pedunculated polyps can be removed with high precision, which are usually challenging to remove effectively. In a multicenter retrospective study conducted at various Italian Tertiary Endoscopy Centers, it was demonstrated that ESD was safe and effective and achieved en bloc and R0 resection rates of 95.9% and 85.4%, respectively, in IBD patients with HR-CAN (Maselli et al., 2024). This skill is critical in the treatment of dysplastic lesions because it aims to address the immediate need to lower the increased risk of colorectal cancer present within this patient population. The specific nature of ESD includes the methodical submucosal dissection, allowing for complete resection of lesions with minimal destruction of the surrounding normal tissue. This technique is particularly relevant in the IBD environment, where preserving bowel function and length is crucial because of the chronic and potentially complicated nature of the disease. Advanced imaging techniques, such as dye-enhanced chromoendoscopy and artificial intelligence-enhanced tests, contribute significantly to the ESD procedure by enhancing the visual delineation of dysplastic areas (Santacroce et al., 2023). Moreover, such techniques can also forecast relapse and track inflammation, thereby providing an overall working system for the management of IBD complications with reduced surgical complexity. Considering the promising outcomes that are intrinsic to ESD, further evaluation and optimization of the procedure are crucial to determine its sustainability and safety. The study had a 12.5% rate of adverse events and highlighted the importance of having experienced operators to manage potential complications in an optimal way (Maselli et al., 2024). With mounting research evidence, such as follow-up on long-term outcomes, the role of ESD in permitting a surgery-sparing approach for IBD patients will increase further. The use of sophisticated endoscopic equipment has a lot to offer in the tailoring of bespoke treatment protocols, improving the overall objective of enhanced patient quality of life while reducing the surgical burden in this delicate group of patients (Santacroce et al., 2023).

15.4. Risks and Complications of Endoscopy

Endoscopy is considered to be widely recognized as a valuable diagnostic and therapeutic tool in IBD therapy. However, it is not free from inherent risks and complicating factors. Of these, gastrointestinal bleeding is a significant concern, particularly in those who may already have compromised mucosal integrity to start with, from ulceration or inflammation secondary to IBD. Such patients are at higher risk for either procedural bleeding or post-biopsy bleeding, in which the delicate tissues are insufficiently resilient to undergo instrumental trauma. Moreover, bowel wall perforation is another complication involving the intentional or accidental penetration of the gastrointestinal tract by the endoscopic equipment. The risk of this event can increase in individuals with extensive disease or wide strictures, necessitating precise technique and careful patient selection when performing endoscopy. Aside from bleeding and perforation, patients who are undergoing endoscopy can also have adverse reactions secondary to sedation, which is often used to make the patient more comfortable during the procedure. Sedation has its own risk profile, with the major concern being respiratory depression or cardiovascular events, especially in patients who have underlying conditions. Such risks require meticulous pre-procedure evaluation to determine the safety of the patient. Also, the specific type of IBD can complicate sedation further, as some patients can have their own response to sedation altered by their illness. Hence, a multidisciplinary strategy becomes very crucial with active participation of both gastroenterologists and anesthesiologists to customize the strategy for sedation based on the patient, thereby reducing the risks related to the endoscopic procedure while maximizing the benefit. Finally, the long-term consequences of endoscopic treatment in IBD patients need careful investigation. Research has demonstrated that complications may arise even after the immediate risks associated with the procedure have lapsed. For instance, research has theorized that scar tissue or stricture development may ensue following multiple procedures, rendering subsequent endoscopic or surgical interventions more complex. Moreover, there may be a relationship between the severity of IBD and post-endoscopic complications, such as observed in recent cohort analysis. Specifically, complications related to mesh-associated issues in surgery have been noted among IBD patients, indicating that the nature of the disease can, to a great extent, ascertain outcomes in surgery (Lovén et al., 2025). Lastly, highlighting such risks highlights the importance of ongoing monitoring and a whole-person understanding of the interplay between endoscopy and IBD management, as well as the requirement for maximal precautions that weigh risk avoidance against therapeutic benefit (Younis et al., 2024).

15.4.1. Perforation of the Gastrointestinal Tract

Gastrointestinal perforation is a serious complication in patients with IBD, particularly in those with Crohn's disease. Perforation is typically a result of intense inflammation, thinning of the bowel wall, and eventual rupture. The incidence has been described to be between approximately 1.5% and 16% in patients with Crohn's disease, and the small bowel is most commonly affected. Standard surgical resection of the perforated segment is generally required due to the higher failure rate and high morbidity of primary repair. Early diagnosis and treatment are essential; therefore, endoscopic evaluation plays a significant role in ascertaining the level of inflammation and determining signs of possible perforation. Multidisciplinary team communication between surgeons, gastroenterologists, and radiologists is essential to optimize patient treatment for such emergent conditions. Perforation, in case it happens in colonic Crohn's disease, carries a risk of causing toxic megacolon, which refers to excessive overdistension of the colon. This complication needs urgent intervention due to the risk of septic shock and systemic inflammatory response syndrome. Endoscopy can also be both diagnostic and therapeutic, allowing the checking of mucosal integrity and the identification of strictures or abscesses that predispose to perforation. If medical therapy by other methods, such as with immunosuppressants and steroids, fails, surgery is indicated to prevent further complications. The American Society of Colon and Rectal Surgeons emphasizes the importance of taking into consideration the severity of colitis in such patients and recommends surgical treatment in those who are unresponsive to medical treatment with severe acute colitis, particularly in the event of signs of perforation (Lightner et al., 2020). Furthermore, the long-term consequences of bowel perforation can have a significant effect on the overall management of IBD. While operative therapy can alleviate acute distress, it does not achieve a cure of the underlying disease and, in certain situations, can lead to secondary complications , such as short bowel syndrome. Patients undergoing resection are at higher risk for recurrence of Crohn's disease, and endoscopic surveillance is part of post-operative care. The response to routine endoscopies is also included for those patients with a background history of perforation, offering early diagnosis of recurrent disease activity as well as the potential development of colorectal dysplasia or cancer. For colorectal cancer, even patients with chronic Crohn's colitis must be carefully followed because of their increased risk compared to the general population (Wolf et al., 2018). The complex process of IBD treatment with a history of gastrointestinal perforation demands a comprehensive, interdisciplinary approach to achieve optimal patient outcomes (Figure 15.11).

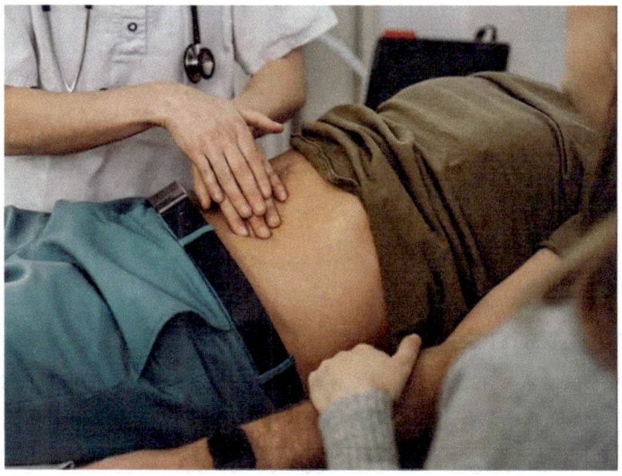

Figure 15.11. Perforation of the gastrointestinal tract.

Source: https://media.post.rvohealth.io/wp-content/uploads/2024/04/doctor-examining-patient-stomach-abdomen-area-for-pain-732x549-thumbnail.jpg.

15.4.2. Infection Risks

The presence of risk for infection in patients being endoscoped for IBD should be investigated thoroughly since such patients are in a compromised status. Patients with IBD are likely to require immunosuppressive medication for their disease, significantly impairing their immune function and leaving them vulnerable to infection. This phenomenon is more significant in postoperative cases, such as in the case of biopsies or interventions that breach the mucosa of the gastrointestinal tract. A study of post-transplant gastrointestinal biopsies revealed that infection-related colitis was present in 26.1% of the patients, emphasizing a direct relationship between compromised immune systems and the occurrence of infection following such interventions (Jaison et al., 2024). Thus, infection risk necessitates rigorous pre-endoscopy screening and scrupulous post-procedure surveillance to avoid complications for IBD patients. Moreover, the variability of infection that can be present renders mitigation strategies during endoscopy in IBD problematic. The infections and IBD flares superimpose on each other, and the patients might present with overlapping symptoms of infection and IBD flare-ups, posing diagnostic difficulties. Biopsy may be suggestive of various infection-related pathologies, so an alert and reactive clinical approach is needed. The necessity of early detection cannot be overestimated since delay in diagnosis leads to a high risk of morbidity. Above all, endoscopic interventions are informative but potentially harmful as well; the key is to detect possible complications within the general course of treatment for IBD patients (Li et al., 2024). Therefore, professionals must use an interdisciplinary strategy, combining gastroenterologists with infectious disease specialists to deliver integrated treatment accounting for infection danger subtleties. As there has been a greater emphasis on improved therapeutic outcomes for IBD in terms of risk for infection, there are some recent advances to be considered in therapeutic intervention. For instance, newer technologies like SGLT2 inhibitors, which are primarily targeted against metabolic derangement, have been reported to be effective in causing mucosal healing in IBD. Just like with any new therapy, however, there remains the potential for infections, for instance, urinary tract infections, particularly highlighted in more recent studies (Li et al., 2024). Such observations require research to be continued to determine new treatment safety profiles and attend to chronic infection risks of IBD therapies. This is an indication of the need for ongoing monitoring of patients and individually adapted therapeutic approaches to maximize treatment efficacy while preventing infectious complications, notably during and after endoscopic evaluation.

15.4.3. Bleeding During or After Procedure

Incidence of endoscopic bleeding during or after endoscopic procedures in IBD patients is a key concern. These procedures, particularly when employing techniques like Balloon-Assisted Endoscopy (BAE), not only become necessary for diagnosis but also for treatment, but they carry inherent risks. Bleeding can be caused by mucosal or submucosal lesions, as was observed in a study where 0.75% of procedures were complicated by such events, necessitating clinical interventions like the application of hemostatic clips. These occurrences not only contribute to the intricacies of patient handling but also require prudence on the part of the clinician in intervening, especially in light of compromised gastrointestinal tract status in IBD. The delicate mucosal lining itself, supplemented as frequently by inflammation, underscores the necessity for advanced modalities that attempt to minimize trauma in such interventions. Also, management of blood loss is crucial in IBD because the patients present with comorbidities and a history of prior gastrointestinal bleeding. The more than 532 BAE procedures' retrospective analysis rightly captures the safety and effectiveness of these procedures despite the risk associated. Among the interventions performed, bleeding that required hemostatic clips was observed in 0.56% of the cases, a sign of the risk of complications as one of the implications of therapeutic endoscopy. High-level practices and careful pre-procedure assessments are essential in determining the risk of complications so that the clinicians are able to take preventive measures, such as using anticoagulants carefully if required, because inappropriate handling would pose more risk of venous thromboembolism in the patients (Jiang et al., 2023).

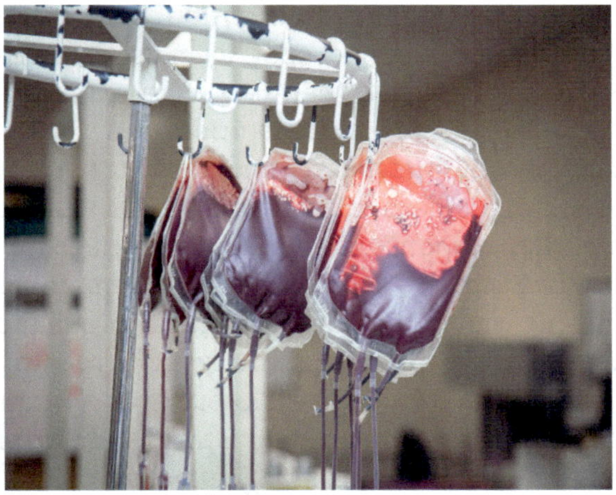

Figure 15.12. Bleeding during or after procedure.

Source: https://www.hamiltonhealthsciences.ca/wp-content/uploads/2022/04/blood-transfusion-bags-in-a-medical-facility-2022-01-22-00-18-57-utc-scaled.jpg.

In light of these considerations, the issue of procedure and post-procedure bleeding becomes paramount to the broader considerations of endoscopic therapy in the care of IBD. The clinician must not only be concerned with the diagnostic and therapeutic efficacy of endoscopy but also prioritize patient safety as a means of avoiding and controlling the risk of bleeding. With such a high rate of patients who have endoscopic procedures experiencing complications , such as strictures and possible hemorrhage, proper follow-up procedures and monitoring of the patient are critical after interventions. Implementing a holistic care strategy that unites respectful observation and professional intervention methodology can significantly enhance IBD patient outcomes presenting for endoscopy, ultimately resulting in better success with fewer rates of related adverse bleeding events, thereby enhancing the safety profile of endoscopic modalities , such as those performed in BAE (Fazal et al., 2025) (Figure 15.12).

15.5. Advances in Endoscopic Technology

Endoscopic technology evolution has introduced significant advances that enhance IBD management. Among them, image-enhanced endoscopy (IEE) technologies, particularly virtual chromoendoscopy (VCE), have taken center stage for playing a central role in disease activity assessment and surveillance colonoscopy in IBD patients. VCE systems facilitate clinicians to better visualize the mucosal surface, allow them to detect quiescent disease activity and identify colorectal neoplasms (CRN) associated with chronic inflammation. Apart from providing greater diagnostic accuracy, such a feature also allows for a more individualized therapeutic approach that addresses each patient with IBD according to their own needs. The use of such advanced endoscopic techniques has the potential to maximize patient outcomes and facilitate earlier detection of complications and thus emphasize their essential role in contemporary gastrointestinal practice (Yang, 2023). In a bid to capitalize on technological progress, VCE has evolved as a revolutionary tool for overall assessment in the management of IBD. Initially confined to the small bowel, its use has been further advanced by improvements to extend to panenteric evaluation to detect lesions that are not reachable through traditional means. Systematic review of VCE application finds its high diagnostic yield, particularly in suspicion of CD, where rates of sensitivity and specificity are significantly high. Moreover, VCE has been found to be able to alter management plans following diagnosis, indicating its application in IBD management. Relative value of VCE over other imaging modalities , such as computed tomography and magnetic resonance enterography, makes it an essential tool in the diagnostic arsenal for patients with IBD (Pal et al., 2023). In addition, the merging of artificial intelligence with endoscopic tools is a turning point that holds promise to accelerate endoscopic evaluations in IBD. Technological progress , such as computerized image analysis supports gastroenterologists in assessing vast quantities of data more quickly, hence reducing the time spent on capsule reading with high sensitivity and specificity.

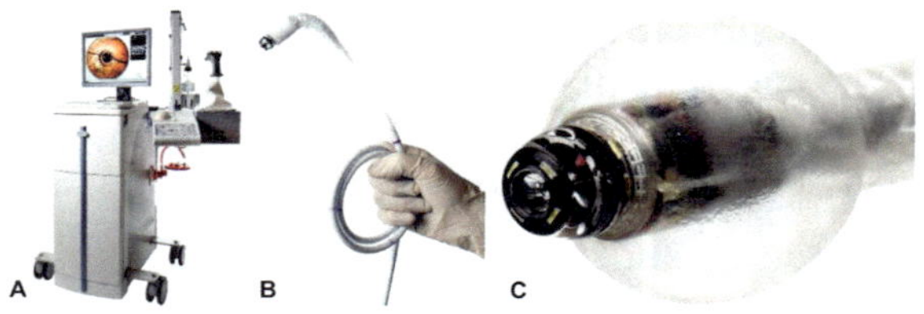

Figure 15.13. Advances in endoscopic technology.

Source: https://pub.mdpi-res.com/applsci/applsci-11-11351/article_deploy/html/images/applsci-11-11351-g007.png?1638279367.

Other IBD-specific scoring systems, such as the Capsule Endoscopy Crohn's Disease Activity Index and Ulcerative Colitis Scoring System, enhance diagnostic accuracy as well. The future of endoscopy for the treatment of inflammatory bowel disease, therefore, rests as much on these technologies as it does on the deployment of artificial intelligence to facilitate a more effective and personalized approach to patient care. And with advancing technologies, they can potentially remake expectations of practice for the treatment of IBD (Pal et al., 2023; Yang, 2023) (Figure 15.13).

15.5.1. High-Definition Imaging

High-definition imaging is a breakthrough in the advancement of endoscopic procedures, particularly in IBD surveillance. Since IBD patients are at higher risk of developing colorectal cancer, the precision in identifying neoplasia is of great importance in managing them. High-definition white light endoscopy (HD-WLE) has been found to be of higher quality than standard-definition procedures, allowing clinicians to spot dysplastic lesions that would not have been seen with traditional methods. This higher resolution is important as it directly affects treatment strategies and patient outcome, and therefore acts to result in an earlier response in the clinical management of IBD. Secondly, HD-WLE is also combinable with high-tech imaging modalities to enhance the specificity and sensitivity of screenings for neoplasia in high-risk patients (Huang et al., 2025). Compared to other endoscopic modalities, HD-WLE is highly effective in terms of neoplasia detection ratio and ranked only after dye-based chromoendoscopy (DCE), but even ahead of certain virtual chromoendoscopy. The network meta-analysis of endoscopic surveillance methods proved that even though DCE dominated enhanced neoplasia detection, HD-WLE offered equal positive predictive value. Of special significance is the fact that this indicates the potential of HD-WLE as a viable alternative to DCE when not feasible due to either patient or procedural issues. The extended withdrawal times of DCE only serve to highlight the efficiency of HD-WLE regarding operations, which can enable the possibility of earlier examination. Effective detection of precancerous lesions thus enables strategic management to reduce cancer risk among the IBD patient population (Huang et al., 2025). Furthermore, the integration of HD-WLE in routine surveillance practice among IBD patients is evidence of the ongoing evolution of endoscopic technology towards improved clinical outcomes. It is imperative for clinicians to stay abreast with the latest developments in imaging modalities to facilitate timely intervention that can radically alter the outcome of disease evolution. Targeted biopsy techniques in the setting of HD-WLE, especially when augmented by further imaging improvements, are significant in a sensitive evaluation of dysplastic changes in the colonic mucosa. While researchers continue to explore new approaches, the focus has to be on maximizing surveillance effectiveness and reducing procedural hassles. This dual action helps ensure patients receive maximum care specific to their own needs, ultimately benefiting in long-term health and well-being in the management of IBD (Huang et al., 2025).

15.5.2. Capsule Endoscopy

The advent of capsule endoscopy has revolutionized the IBD diagnostic pattern, particularly when conventional endoscopic techniques are lacking. The new, non-invasive technique allows for total visualization of the gastrointestinal tract and facilitates the detection of lesions beyond the conventional endoscope's reach. Capsule endoscopy yield in diagnosis of suspected Crohn's disease (CD) is quite broad, ranging from 6%–80%, with sensitivity being remarkably high, ranging from 77%–93%, and specificity being remarkably high, ranging from 80%–89% (Pal et al., 2023). By giving a very clear picture of the small intestine, this technology is especially valuable in diagnosing proximal and superficial lesions that other modalities , such as computed tomography or magnetic resonance enterography, tend to miss. As capsule endoscopy has developed over time in managing IBD, it is no longer utilized for diagnosis alone but also for ongoing management and follow-up of the condition. Studies have found that up to 88% of patients with established CD will have their care changed based on capsule findings (Pal et al., 2023). Capsule endoscopy has also been shown to have greater retention in patients with established disease than in those recently suspected of CD. This is particularly critical in postoperative states, where lesions may arise in areas that are inaccessible by standard ileocolonoscopy. Also, capsule endoscopy has been instrumental in revealing occult CD in individuals with IBD-unclassified (IBD-U) to provide a more accurate diagnosis and suitable therapeutic interventions. Technological improvement, for example, the addition of AI, can enhance the efficacy of capsule endoscopy in treating IBD. AI software is being developed to assist healthcare professionals in analyzing endoscopy images, giving predictive information that can be used to guide treatment. These computerized models are designed to analyze a wide array of variables, potentially refining prognostic understanding and treatment risk stratification for treatment patients. As the potential of capsule endoscopy is underpinned by AI and other technologies, its role in the holistic management of IBD patients is expected to grow, paving the way for more precise and individualized therapeutic strategies (Figure 15.14).

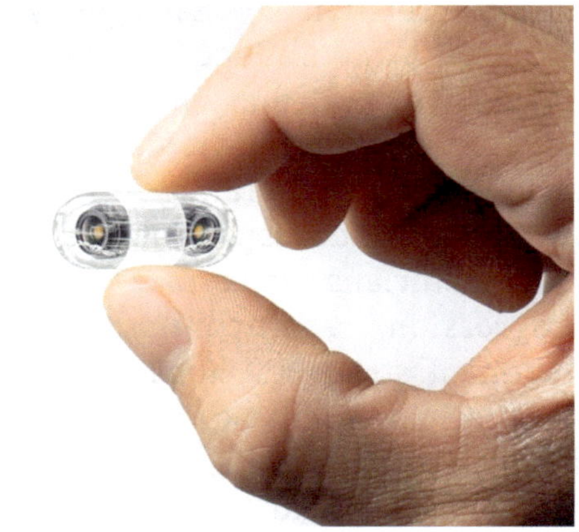

Figure 15.14. Capsule endoscopy.

Source: https://www.carygastro.com/uploads/blog/_1200x720_crop_center-center_100_none/Capsule-Endoscopy.jpg.

15.5.3. Artificial Intelligence (AI) in Endoscopic Procedures

The application of AI in endoscopic procedures is a big step in gastroenterology, particularly in the context of IBD. AI technologies, with computer-aided detection (CADe), have been reported to increase the sensitivity of neoplasia and source bleeding detection during endoscopy. Evidence shows that CADe systems can facilitate the automatic detection of lesions that might be missed by human observers, therefore improving diagnostic outcomes for conditions , such as Crohn's disease and ulcerative colitis. Systematic classification of AI potential brings out its capacity to transform clinical decision-making. As the availability of data increases, AI systems are evolving to identify not only pathology but also decode complex inflammatory patterns, reflecting an overall benefit in the successful management of IBD (Arif et al., 2023). Video capsule endoscopy has emerged as a major technological advancement in the assessment of IBD. The application of AI in VCE raises its diagnostic yield significantly, providing physicians with detailed reports of the small intestine that are difficult to assess with other traditional techniques like colonoscopy. AI can also be used to automate the interpretation of VCE images, with increased sensitivity and reduced analysis time. This is useful in patients with suspected Crohn's disease, whose diagnostic yield can be extremely variable. By incorporating AI technologies like the Capsule Endoscopy Crohn's Disease Activity Index, clinicians can more closely track disease progression, resulting in more customized treatment strategies. Furthermore, the use of AI in lesion identification outside the reach of standard endoscopy highlights its application in both diagnosis and therapy (Pal et al., 2023). The future of AI-assisted endoscopy in IBD care is promising, with ongoing development yet to come on the horizon to shape the direction of clinical practice. The future possibility of novel uses for quality assurance by CADq improves not just efficiency but also procedure quality overall. By constant real-time feedback and maintenance of excellence throughout the entire endoscopy procedure, AI applications have the potential to mitigate risks and enhance patient outcomes. Furthermore, the prospect of multimodal integrated systems represents a revolution in the approach to endoscopy. The visionary technique, with the utilization of AI for therapeutic decision support, supports the technology's role of enhancing the level of care for patients with IBD. With these advancements, AI will be an important driver of endoscopic technique and strategy evolution (Arif et al., 2023) (Figure 15.15).

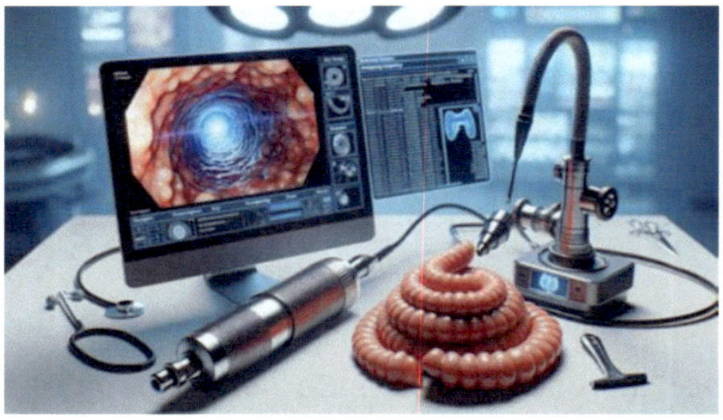

Figure 15.15. Artificial intelligence (AI) in endoscopic procedures.

Source: https://external-content.duckduckgo.com/iu/?u= https%3A%2F%2Ftse2.mm.bing.net%2Fth%2Fid%2FOIP.o_KAe9EOtOBabX8DNPhKFwHaEO%3Fpid%3DApi&f=1&ipt=0e867cacfb261fe0447b25622bd1e7bff1035793ff6d0d9936351302af864b7f.

15.6. Patient Perspectives and Experiences

The intersection of patient experiences with IBD management gives rise to important findings on the application of endoscopy in disease surveillance and treatment response. One qualitative study of 20 patients from various countries noted that the majority of individuals associate remission of disease with the lack of symptoms, demonstrating a symptomatic-centered attitude prevalent among IBD patients. While some were taught the function of endoscopy in defining mucosal healing, others were not made aware of this integral part of their condition. This imbalance shows that healthcare workers should effectively convey the value of endoscopic therapy to bridge the disparity between patient awareness and clinical practice. By encouraging a more educated patient population, clinicians can enhance compliance with treatment and patient satisfaction with their treatment processes, thereby improving the overall management of IBD (Duncan et al., 2024). Even more importantly, patients' compliance in undergoing regular endoscopic assessments proves to be an important attitudinal shift towards invasive therapy when they perceive they are benefiting from its use. The research showed that patients voiced a deep psychological reassurance derived from the awareness of being "healthy inside," which is a form of desire for endorsement that goes beyond symptom control. This reassurance may be one of the driving factors for patients to agree to have frequent endoscopies, with an average willingness score of 5.7 on a scale of 1–7 for annual procedures. But this inclination is offset by caution regarding more frequent invasions, suggesting a cost-benefit assessment patients make of their care. These insights present proof that evidence must be offset with opinions from patients, which will ultimately direct better clinical guidelines in endoscopic IBD treatment (Duncan et al., 2024). Additionally, heterogeneity of IBD diagnostic practice across regions of Asia, as reported in a multinational Asian physicians' survey, reveals profound meaning in patient experiences. While adherence to current European guidelines was common, individualized preferences, such as regional guidelines among Japanese physicians, reveal practice heterogeneity that can affect consistency of patient care. This variation in endoscopic application for assessment of disease activity is international and may lead to variable patient experience based on regional practice. If these differences are recognized, it may be possible to develop more Asia-specific guidelines that respect local clinical needs but find common ground in accommodating the heterogeneous perceptions of patients with IBD. Thus, the integration of physician knowledge with patient recommendations is crucial in the creation of a responsive system of health care that maximizes the treatment of IBD among various populations.

15.6.1. Psychological Impact of Endoscopy

The psychological impact of endoscopy on patients with IBD constitutes a multifaceted problem that has the tendency of complicating disease management. The majority of patients are stressed and worried about the procedure on the basis of fear regarding discomfort, potential complications, and, importantly, uncertain outcomes of their diagnosis. Avoidance of necessary procedures on this basis ultimately renders correct disease management inadequate. Psychological studies have revealed emotional problems, such as fear of pain and vulnerability, which can be a potent factor in persuading patients to undergo endoscopic examination. Thus, identification and management of such psychological hurdles is necessary to enhance patient compliance and optimize care. Pre-procedure counseling and supportive interventions can minimize anxiety levels, thereby enhancing better utilization of endoscopic procedures instrumental in the surveillance and management of IBD. Personality traits and coping styles also have a big impact on the psychological reaction of IBD patients to endoscopy. Literature shows that individuals with certain personality types, for instance, high neuroticism, tend to adjust less after medical interventions, such as endoscopy. Such individuals will cope with their illness and its related treatments using adaptive coping strategies, thereby increasing their distress. For instance, the occurrence of emotion-focused coping strategies has been related to adverse endoscopic evaluation experiences during and after. Thus, intervention of these psychological factors in an individualized fashion can help alter maladaptive coping styles, making a more positive endoscopic experience likely. Personality trait interventions and support for adaptive coping can do much to both improve the psychological well-being of patients and their treatment outcomes. Also, the subjective experience of IBD patients during endoscopy is not only dominated by bodily discomfort but also by psychological state and illness perceptions. The absence of correlation between clinical symptoms and objective disease activity tends to create intensified anxiety and uncertainty about one's state of health.

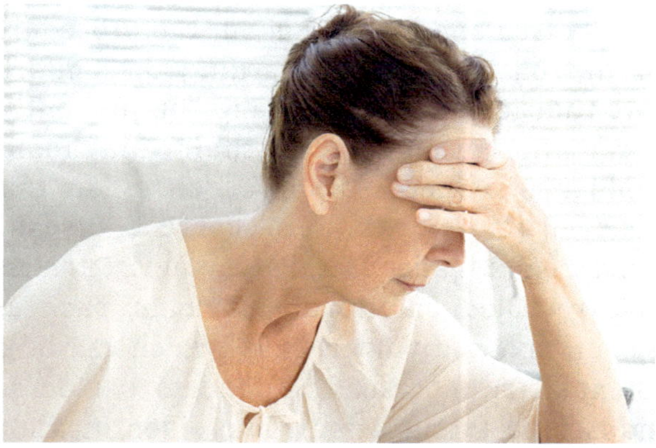

Figure 15.16. Psychological impact of endoscopy.

Source: https://i0.wp.com/intouchwomenshealth.com/wp-content/uploads/2021/10/psychological-effects.png?resize=960%2C640&ssl=1.

This has caused many patients to trust their individual experience to determine their own interpretation of flare-up and disease progression, which does not consistently agree with mucosal inflammation as diagnosed by endoscopic examination. The conflict between symptoms reported by the self and clinically manifest states of disease can cause distress and confusion, as indicated in research that established the poor correlation between patient-reported outcomes and mucosal inflammation (Ford et al., 2018). The psychological implications of these differences emphasize the significance of overall care plans involving psychological counseling as well as medical treatments, urging patients and healthcare professionals alike to adopt a more comprehensive outlook towards IBD (Figure 15.16).

15.6.2. Patient Education and Preparation

Patient education and preparation is vital in optimizing the outcome of endoscopy procedures for IBD patients. Understanding the complexities of IBD and risks of endoscopic procedures has the ability to empower patients, reducing levels of anxiety and ensuring cooperation during the procedure. Education should effectively address matters of the nature of IBD, specific aims of the endoscopic examination, as well as feelings expected during the process. Such information not only eliminates fears but also encourages patients to be proactive in their care processes. Whereas recent findings have shown, patient education is a critical element that can improve the effectiveness of treatment, eventually bringing about a shift in paradigm from symptom control towards mucosal healing in IBD management (Cai et al., 2021). Education programs thus need to be included as an integral part of pre-procedure protocols. Patient preparation for endoscopy in IBD also requires personalized strategies that address the unique issues about their condition. For example, bowel preparation protocols play a key role in preserving visualization quality during endoscopic procedures. Patients with severe colitis, on the other hand, may experience greater distress and discomfort from preparation requirements, which are likely to be underestimated by non-medical professionals (Napolitano et al., 2021). Therefore, it is advisable to individualize bowel preparation guidelines, offer support materials, and provide appropriate instructions to prevent discomfort. The education of patients with regard to preparation procedures enables them to be more compliant with procedures, guaranteeing successful endoscopic procedures and ultimately promoting a greater overall awareness of their management of disease. The role of health professionals in providing patient education and ensuring adequate preparation for endoscopy procedures cannot be overlooked. Furthermore, the involvement of specialist nurses in the management of IBD can greatly enhance the quality of education provided. Existing surveys indicate a concerning lack of awareness among non-IBD healthcare professionals working in endoscopy, which speaks to the need for targeted training programs (Napolitano et al., 2021). These are to focus on raising the awareness of healthcare practitioners regarding IBD patients' psychological and physical concerns regarding the endoscopy procedure. Hence, ongoing education among nurses and other members of the healthcare team becomes essential in equipping them with the necessary competence. This, in turn, leads to a compassionate approach to patient care, ultimately resulting in better prepared patients and better clinical outcomes for the treatment of IBD.

15.6.3. Post-Procedure Care and Follow-Up

Careful post-procedure care and follow-up are critical parameters in the management of patients with IBD following endoscopic procedures. The post-procedure period is typically the time of greatest risk for complications, and thus, it is crucial that caregivers carefully observe patients. After diagnostic or therapeutic endoscopy procedures, the symptoms of abdominal pain, rectal bleeding, or infection should be extensively evaluated. According to ECCO guidelines, healthcare teams must adopt a standard pattern of follow-up post-procedure, especially since a significant proportion of centers lack a protocol for monitoring high-risk patients. In addition, adherence to established guidelines can allow for timely interventions and, therefore, enhance the quality of care provided to IBD-affected individuals (Walsh et al., 2024). Follow-up care is not just limited to direct observation after endoscopy but also involves periodic reviews to evaluate the response to treatment and disease behavior. IBD patients require personalized follow-up intervals according to their individual disease characteristics and therapeutic responses. The use of objective measurements, such as fecal calprotectin and clinical scores, is important in assessing whether management strategies implemented are effective. Furthermore, repeated screening procedures—, such as colorectal cancer through high-definition endoscopy—are in accordance with the appropriateness of care for IBD patients. Regrettably, the majority of centers exhibit remarkable deficiencies in fulfilling these follow-up procedures, emphasizing the need for systemic reform to standardize care protocols for various healthcare facilities (Dipasquale et al., 2021). Furthermore, the discovery of telemedicine has revolutionized the situation of post-procedure follow-up, particularly in the face of ongoing public health concerns. The COVID-19 pandemic has required creative ways to maintain patient care, with telehealth being a viable option for treating IBD safely. Although certain patients would find value in traditional visits to complete their evaluation, telemedicine provides a useful alternative for standard follow-up, particularly for patients in remission or a stable state. Such a shift to remote consultations has the potential to relieve pressure on healthcare facilities while still maintaining the need for psychological support and continued management of the condition. With healthcare systems adapting to integrate such advancements, continuity of care is still vital to improving health outcomes in IBD patients, a paradigm shift in the follow-up care model (Dipasquale et al., 2021) (Figure 15.17).

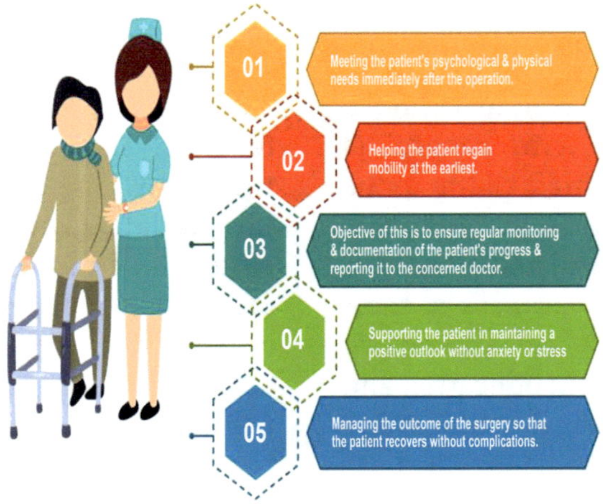

Figure 15.17. Post-procedure care and follow-up.

Source: https://www.collidu.com/media/catalog/product/img/1/0/10ad7e3221f504f1ab75ed370ec24da8605d9a8cb9c60a8702e68ef2cd0fb16a/post-operative-care-slide1.png.

SUMMARY

In considering the role of endoscopy in IBD management, it becomes clear that this procedure serves as a foundation for diagnosis and monitoring of treatment. Endoscopy provides not only direct visualization of the gastrointestinal tract but also targeted biopsies, which play a role in the differentiation between Crohn's disease and ulcerative colitis. Through its ability to assess disease severity and detect complications, endoscopy enables the planning of treatment regimens by clinicians. Greater IBD burden, however, necessitates exploration of other less invasive but no less revealing modalities. New technologies , such as point-of-care intestinal ultrasound (POC IUS), provide promising results in monitoring disease activity and overcoming some of the limitations experienced with traditional endoscopy, according to a recent study indicating its acceptability to both patients and healthcare professionals (Chan et al., 2024). In addition, integration of newer technologies and markers into the clinical practice of IBD depicts the notion of personalized medicine. The advancement in genomic knowledge and biomarkers is transforming the clinical picture, as it provides the possibility of the introduction of precision-based therapeutic approaches that are responsive to the individual patient profile. The existing literature emphasizes the manner in which the innovation can personalize maximum therapeutic effects without undue side effects (Green et al., 2023). The collaboration between endoscopic modalities and novel interventions is a very promising domain for the overall treatment of IBD. With clinicians learning from such ancillary methods, the effectiveness of patient condition monitoring and treatment will more than likely improve, eventually translating to a better quality of life for patients. In conclusion, as much as endoscopy is a vital tool in IBD management, one must be open to adapting practice and technology meant to enhance patient care. The introduction of less invasive technology, such as POC IUS, will minimize the risk and pain associated with conventional endoscopic techniques while still permitting effective surveillance. As ongoing research continues to introduce new information regarding the pathophysiology of IBD, the practice will likely become increasingly integrative blending the advantages of endoscopy with state-of-the-art diagnostic technologies and tailored treatments. The acceptance of such a multidimensional strategy will not only augment disease control but also empower patients with greater knowledge and involvement in their therapy (Chan et al., 2024; Green et al., 2023).

Management of IBD has revolutionized over the last few years, shifting from mere control of symptoms to the objective of mucosal healing. Conventional treatments have long concentrated on pharmacologic treatment, like aminosalicylates, corticosteroids, immunomodulators, and biologics. Despite this, a large number of patients either do not respond or lose the response with time, prompting the need for new therapeutic alternatives. Advanced research in recent times has brought forth innovative possibilities in the form of small molecules, apheresis therapy, and novel treatments to correct intestinal microecology. Also, a key shift in the objectives of treatment highlights the importance of individualized patient education, which has been found to enhance the overall therapeutic effectiveness of IBD therapy. These developments illustrate the evolutionary process of IBD care, emphasizing an overall appreciation of both conventional and contemporary strategies toward achieving the best patient outcomes (Cai et al., 2021). Endoscopic techniques play a crucial role in IBD diagnosis and tracking, particularly in mucosal healing assessment and the diagnosis of disease complications. Bidirectional gastrointestinal endoscopy is the gold standard test for inspecting and biopsying the upper and lower gastrointestinal tracts. The technique is not only important in diagnosis but also in directing treatment and malignancy surveillance. Where traditional endoscopy is lacking, as in the evaluation of occult gastrointestinal bleeding or small bowel illness, wireless capsule endoscopy is priceless. This technology enhances the diagnostic capability by providing a minimally invasive tool to investigate the small intestine, often elusive in standard assessment. Thus, endoscopy is a cornerstone in the treatment of IBD, enabling early intervention and targeted therapeutic intervention that can significantly improve patient quality of life (Snook et al., 2021). Additionally, the integration of endoscopy in the clinical management of IBD has promoted an active approach in addressing complications like iron deficiency anemia (IDA). Chronic intestinal inflammation and damage in patients with IBD usually cause malabsorption and bleeding in the gut, leading to IDA. The realization that a large percentage of one-third of men and postmenopausal women with IDA will have underlying gastrointestinal pathologies has created a need for extensive investigations. Thus, the implementation of rapid referral guidelines for unexplained IDA underlines the extremely critical interface between endoscopy and systemic health problems. Timely and adequate endoscopic evaluation not only aids in the diagnosis of the underlying disease but also directs treatment plans , including intravenous or oral iron supplementation therapy. To sum up, endoscopy is an important tool in the intricate treatment of IBD, impacting both disease understanding and therapy (Cai et al., 2021; Snook et al., 2021).

CLOSER LOOK

PRIMARY SCLEROSING CHOLANGITIS (PSC):

Primary sclerosing cholangitis (PSC) is a chronic, progressive liver disease characterized by inflammation, fibrosis, and stricturing of the bile ducts, both intrahepatic and extrahepatic. This leads to cholestasis, biliary cirrhosis, and, eventually, liver failure in many patients. Although the precise etiology remains unclear, PSC is widely considered an immune-mediated condition with a strong association with inflammatory bowel disease (IBD), particularly ulcerative colitis. Genetic predisposition, environmental triggers, and dysregulated immune responses are thought to contribute to disease development.

PSC can affect individuals of any age but is most commonly diagnosed in middle-aged men. Clinical presentation is variable, ranging from asymptomatic elevations in liver enzymes detected incidentally to symptoms such as fatigue, pruritus, jaundice, right upper quadrant pain, and recurrent cholangitis. Over time, complications including cirrhosis, portal hypertension, and cholangiocarcinoma may arise. Laboratory findings often reveal a cholestatic pattern with elevated alkaline phosphatase and gamma-glutamyl transferase, while bilirubin levels may rise in advanced disease.

Diagnosis relies on a combination of biochemical, imaging, and histological criteria. Magnetic resonance cholangiopancreatography (MRCP) is the imaging modality of choice, revealing characteristic multifocal strictures and segmental dilations of the bile ducts. Endoscopic retrograde cholangiopancreatography (ERCP) may be used for both diagnostic and therapeutic purposes, particularly to relieve dominant strictures. Liver biopsy is reserved for cases where small-duct PSC or overlapping autoimmune hepatitis is suspected.

Management of PSC remains challenging as no medical therapy has been proven to alter disease progression. Ursodeoxycholic acid (UDCA) is often used to improve liver enzyme profiles, though its impact on long-term outcomes is uncertain. Symptomatic management includes treatment of pruritus, fat-soluble vitamin supplementation, and antibiotics for recurrent cholangitis. Endoscopic interventions, such as dilation or stenting of dominant strictures, are commonly employed to manage obstructive symptoms. Liver transplantation is the only definitive treatment for end-stage disease or complications such as cholangiocarcinoma.

Patients with PSC require long-term monitoring due to the risk of disease progression and associated malignancies, particularly cholangiocarcinoma and colorectal cancer in those with IBD. Multidisciplinary care involving hepatologists, gastroenterologists, radiologists, and transplant teams is essential.

In conclusion, PSC is a chronic, progressive cholestatic liver disease with significant morbidity and a high risk of complications. Early recognition, careful monitoring, and timely intervention—particularly for complications and liver transplantation—are critical to improving outcomes and quality of life in affected patients.

REFERENCES

1. Al-Hagawi, Y., Alqahtani, N. I., Alsharif, S. N., Chakik, R. M., Asiri, D. H., Al mani, S. Y., Badawi, A. G., et al. (2024). *Endoscopy of low BMI patients compared to normal BMI patients: A study from the Aseer Region, Saudi Arabia. Cureus, 16.* https://www.semanticscholar.org/paper/9027c50abdb0a1b0eb8252a05b7fc7ab2a6a7f85 (accessed on 15th July 2025).
2. Arif, A. A., Jiang, S., & Byrne, M. F. (2023). Artificial intelligence in endoscopy: Overview, applications, and future directions. *Saudi Journal of Gastroenterology, 29*, 269–277. https://doi.org/10.4103/sjg.sjg_286_23 (accessed on 15th July 2025).
3. Ayala, I., Latorre, R., Soria, F., Carballo, F., López-Albors, O., Buendía, A., & Pérez-Cuadrado, E. (2011). *A case of lymphocytic-plasmacytic jejunitis diagnosed by double-balloon enteroscopy in a dog. Journal of the American Animal Hospital Association, 47*(4), 262–267. https://www.semanticscholar.org/paper/1d9f936db35eb5b2616f24e789f87493e1d86786 (accessed on 15th July 2025).
4. Bakshi, N., Hart, A., Lee, M., Williams, A. C. de C., Lackner, J. M., Norton, C., & Croft, P. (2021). *Chronic pain in patients with inflammatory bowel disease. Pain, 162*, 2466–2471. https://doi.org/10.1097/j.pain.0000000000002304 (accessed on 15th July 2025).
5. Bhattaru, A., Pundyavana, A., Raynor, W. Y., Chinta, S., Werner, T., & Alavi, A. (2024). 18F-FDG-PET and other imaging modalities in the diagnosis and management of inflammatory bowel disease. *American Journal of Nuclear Medicine and Molecular Imaging, 14*(5), 295–305. https://www.semanticscholar.org/paper/69e600ddb7801004b2a0140c52a370cd6cf3bff8 (accessed on 15th July 2025).
6. Cai, Z., Wang, S., & Li, J. (2021). *Treatment of inflammatory bowel disease: A comprehensive review. Frontiers in Medicine, 8.* https://doi.org/10.3389/fmed.2021.765474 (accessed on 15th July 2025).
7. Chalder, T., Fear, N. T., Jordan, C., Sin, F., et al. (2016). *A systematic review of the psychological correlates of adjustment outcomes in adults with inflammatory bowel disease.* https://core.ac.uk/download/46166370.pdf (accessed on 15th July 2025).
8. Chan, R., Stewart, M., & Jones, J. (2024). *A79 Patient and physician perspectives on implementation of bedside intestinal ultrasound for the assessment of inflammatory bowel disease. Journal of the Canadian Association of Gastroenterology, 7*, 54–55. https://www.semanticscholar.org/paper/52671ae636e81ccced6610d388682fe82ac32130 (accessed on 15th July 2025).
9. Chapman, M. H., Thorburn, D., Hirschfield, G. M., Webster, G., Rushbrook, S., Alexander, G., Collier, J., et al. (2019). *British Society of Gastroenterology and UK-PSC guidelines for the diagnosis and management of primary sclerosing cholangitis. Gut, 68*, 1356–1378. https://doi.org/10.1136/gutjnl-2018-317993 (accessed on 15th July 2025).
10. Chen, B. B., Hamilton, Z., Hasosah, M., Zetler, P., Popescu, O., Bush, J., Katz, R., et al. (2024). The role of upper gastrointestinal endoscopy in the diagnosis of pediatric inflammatory bowel disease. *American Journal of Clinical Pathology, 162*, 597–603. https://www.semanticscholar.org/paper/551cb69e838ed39b172480c35d736b7c0fb7343c (accessed on 15th July 2025).
11. Clement, B., & Genere, J. R. (2024). Interventional inflammatory bowel disease: Current and future practice. *Current Opinion in Gastroenterology.* https://www.semanticscholar.org/paper/24356b53809d235018a14e55ac77b76e60d5fca1 (accessed on 15th July 2025).

12. Da Rio, L., Spadaccini, M., Parigi, T., Gabbiadini, R., Dal Buono, A., Busacca, A., Maselli, R., et al. (2023). *Artificial intelligence and inflammatory bowel disease: Where are we going? World Journal of Gastroenterology, 29*, 508–520. https://www.semanticscholar.org/paper/55c517331f2984e1d64fd3ea9a20594448f05777 (accessed on 15th July 2025).

13. Dipasquale, V., Passanisi, S., Cucinotta, U., Cascio, A., & Romano, C. (2021). *Implications of SARS-CoV-2 infection in the diagnosis and management of the pediatric gastrointestinal disease. Italian Journal of Pediatrics, 47.* https://www.semanticscholar.org/paper/fe3d040ee03256dbbe66f2dd45647b889e522ac6 (accessed on 15th July 2025).

14. Duncan, E., Sanon, M., Griffo, C., Amatelli, D., Barthelmes, J., Wirth, D., Kachroo, S., et al. (2024). *Patient perceptions of endoscopic testing in the management of inflammatory bowel disease. Gastroenterology.* https://www.semanticscholar.org/paper/904e41d9351e65fafab74f2a7291aeb6a77582c4 (accessed on 15th July 2025).

15. Fazal, M., Bowron, J., Reeson, M., Zepeda-Gomez, S., & Halloran, B. (2025). *A186 Balloon-assisted endoscopy in the management of small bowel Crohn's disease – An overall experience from a Canadian tertiary care hospital. Journal of the Canadian Association of Gastroenterology, 8*, i77. https://www.semanticscholar.org/paper/c3aa0573df81bb9ad500d79fcb71186a5ef90dad (accessed on 15th July 2025).

16. Ford, A. C., Selinger, C. P., Williams, C. J. M., Gracie, D. J., Bholah, M. H., Hamlin, P. J., Pendse, D. A., et al. (2018). *Factors affecting clinical decision-making in inflammatory bowel disease and the role of point-of-care calprotectin.* https://core.ac.uk/download/153570415.pdf (accessed on 15th July 2025).

17. Foscarini, E., Emoli, V., Petito, V., Di Vincenzo, F., Masi, L., Troisi, S., Pane, C., et al. (2025). *P0167 Circular extrachromosomal DNA (eccDNA): A potential diagnostic and prognostic tool to be introduced into the clinical practice of inflammatory bowel disease. Journal of Crohn's and Colitis.* https://www.semanticscholar.org/paper/59481b0f3955e21977dbcb882ab498e62539a2db (accessed on 15th July 2025).

18. Green, Z., Beattie, R. M., & Ashton, J. (2023). *Recent developments in the assessment and management of inflammatory bowel disease in childhood: A narrative review. Translational Pediatrics, 12*, 1853–1874. https://www.semanticscholar.org/paper/feed7fc7f2c57b0a9a012d985825aac56e7bf331 (accessed on 15th July 2025).

19. Hossain, M. S., Karuniawati, H., Jairoun, A. A., Urbi, Z., Ooi, D. J., John, A., Lim, Y. C., et al. (2022). *Colorectal cancer: A review of carcinogenesis, global epidemiology, current challenges, risk factors, preventive and treatment strategies. Cancers, 14*, 1732. https://doi.org/10.3390/cancers14071732 (accessed on 15th July 2025).

20. Huang, C. W., Yen, H., & Chen, Y. Y. (2025). P0395 Endoscopic approaches for colorectal neoplasia surveillance in inflammatory bowel disease: A systematic review and network meta-analysis. *Journal of Crohn's and Colitis.* https://www.semanticscholar.org/paper/1602c452ccb7bd46870c1aeae871f506ebecd75a (accessed on 15th July 2025).

21. Huang, C. W., Yen, H. H., & Chen, Y. Y. (2025). *Endoscopic techniques for colorectal neoplasia surveillance in inflammatory bowel disease: A systematic review and network meta-analysis. United European Gastroenterology Journal.* https://www.semanticscholar.org/paper/a0fda5a000267ef730d5126dd6d682c1e4fc6761 (accessed on 15th July 2025).

22. Jaison, M., Mahadevan, P., & Menon, R. (2024). *Spectrum of pathological lesions observed in post-transplant gastrointestinal mucosal biopsies. Annals of Pathology and Laboratory Medicine.* https://www.semanticscholar.org/paper/eaa26e451b89a2ac04fcea47b78539b482c1dac5 (accessed on 15th July 2025).

23. Jiang, H., He, S., & Wang, H. (2023). *A rare complication of people with inflammatory bowel disease after ileostomy: A case report. Medicine, 102.* https://www.semanticscholar.org/paper/d1772d9a12e2be05c3a0d409f0794bd02c1772d0 (accessed on 15th July 2025).

24. Kucharzik, T., Allocca, M., Torres, J., & Taylor, S. A. (2025). *Role of non-invasive imaging in the diagnosis and management of patients with suspected and established IBD. Gastroenterology.* https://www.semanticscholar.org/paper/42b585ad1287100de1bddd350ccc7c472f267033 (accessed on 15th July 2025).

25. Kumar, R., Khan, F. U., Sharma, A., Aziz, I. A., & Poddar, N. K. (2021). *Recent applications of artificial intelligence in the detection of gastrointestinal, hepatic and pancreatic diseases. Current Medicinal Chemistry, 29,* 66–85. https://doi.org/10.2174/0929867328666210405114938 (accessed on 15th July 2025).

26. Lamb, C. A., Kennedy, N. A., Raine, T., Hendy, P., Smith, P. J., Limdi, J. K., Hayee, B., et al. (2019). *British Society of Gastroenterology consensus guidelines on the management of inflammatory bowel disease in adults. Gut, 68,* s1–s106. https://doi.org/10.1136/gutjnl-2019-318484 (accessed on 15th July 2025).

27. Lee, H., Park, J. J., Lee, B. I., Hilmi, I., Sollano, J., & Ran, Z. (2023). *Diagnosis of inflammatory bowel disease–Asian perspectives: The results of a multinational web-based survey in the 8th Asian Organization for Crohn's and Colitis meeting. Intestinal Research, 21,* 328–338. https://www.semanticscholar.org/paper/d444d6697ddeb583a0286a80ae06bdbaaac09210 (accessed on 15th July 2025).

28. Li, Z., Zhang, X., Chen, H., Zeng, H., Wu, J., Wang, Y., Ma, N., et al. (2024). *Empagliflozin in children with glycogen storage disease-associated inflammatory bowel disease: A prospective, single-arm, open-label clinical trial. Scientific Reports, 14.* https://www.semanticscholar.org/paper/91a678eb7ec3461361ace44112ba2c304baad2cd (accessed on 15th July 2025).

29. Lightner, A. L., Vogel, J. D., Carmichael, J. C., Keller, D. S., Shah, S. A., Mahadevan, U., Kane, S. V., et al. (2020). The American Society of Colon and Rectal Surgeons clinical practice guidelines for the surgical management of Crohn's disease. *Diseases of the Colon & Rectum, 63,* 1028–1052. https://doi.org/10.1097/dcr.0000000000001716 (accessed on 15th July 2025).

30. Lovén, H., Erichsen, R., Tøttrup, A., & Bisgaard, T. (2025). *Long-term outcomes after elective inguinal hernia mesh-repair in patients with inflammatory bowel disease. Hernia, 29.* https://www.semanticscholar.org/paper/2f8e30d77818408d088e23b423824d9336389e0f (accessed on 15th July 2025).

31. Manchanda, S., Rizvi, Q. U. A., & Singh, R. (2019). *Role of endoscopy in the surveillance and management of colorectal neoplasia in inflammatory bowel disease. World Journal of Clinical Cases, 7,* 1–9. https://www.semanticscholar.org/paper/b05da8442062d16d59085c5e63eab21989315980 (accessed on 15th July 2025).

32. Maselli, R., de Sire, R., Barbaro, F., Cecinato, P., Andrisani, G., Rosa Rizzotto, E., Sferrazza, S., et al. (2024). *P1065 Endoscopic submucosal dissection for high-risk colorectal colitis-associated neoplasia in inflammatory bowel disease: A real-world multicenter study. Journal of Crohn's*

and Colitis. https://www.semanticscholar.org/paper/9bd4aea224b2b67f3d9ec9615f066238 62d628fa (accessed on 15th July 2025).

33. Mureşan, S., Slevin, M., Szász, E., & Loghin, A. (2024). *Monomeric C-reactive protein potential utilization in the histological assessment of inflammatory bowel disease (IBD) patients. Cureus, 16.* https://www.semanticscholar.org/paper/58d3263a55e84283c1638d63970c13a8233ad 2e3 (accessed on 15th July 2025).

34. Napolitano, D., Scaldaferri, F., Fiorino, G., Spagnuolo, R., Leonetti, A., Lopetuso, L. R., & Cocchieri, A. (2021). *Knowledge of diagnostic and therapeutic aspects of IBD among nurses working in digestive endoscopy. Gastroenterology Nursing, 44,* E59–E66. https://doi.org/10.1097/sga.0000000000000593 (accessed on 15th July 2025).

35. Nardone, O., Ghosh, S., & Iacucci, M. (2022). *Endoscopy and histology in inflammatory bowel diseases patients: Complementary or alternatives? – Author's reply. United European Gastroenterology Journal.* https://www.semanticscholar.org/paper/66f69652d1847b60b1ff 52bb5dcb05d548b2ac74 (accessed on 15th July 2025).

36. Núñez, P. F., Krugliak Cleveland, N., Quera, R., & Rubin, D. (2021). *Evolving role of endoscopy in inflammatory bowel disease: Going beyond diagnosis. World Journal of Gastroenterology, 27,* 2521–2530. https://www.semanticscholar.org/paper/c1df788955841d82cc13c6468b7a5f4a2d90c07e (accessed on 15th July 2025).

37. Pal, P., Banerjee, R., Gupta, R., Reddy, P. M., Reddy, D. N., & Tandan, M. (2023). *Capsule endoscopy in inflammatory bowel disease: A systematic review. Journal of Digestive Endoscopy, 14,* 149–174. https://doi.org/10.1055/s-0043-1766122 (accessed on 15th July 2025).

38. Pu, W., Tyler, M. B., Jeremy, R. G. B., Shishira, B., Aymeric, B., Xun, X., Peixi, L., et al. (2019) Real-time automatic detection system increases colono scopic polyp and adenoma detection rates: a prospective randomized controlled study. *Gut., 68,* 1813–1819. doi: https://doi.org/10.1136/gutjnl-2018-317500.

39. Radmard, A., Amouei, M., Torabi, A., Sima, A. R., Saffar, H., Geahchan, A., Davarpanah, A. H., et al. (2024). *MR enterography in ulcerative colitis: Beyond endoscopy. Radiographics: A Review Publication of the Radiological Society of North America, Inc., 44*(1), e230131. https://www.semanticscholar.org/paper/a6da8e95ccbf4f9604e51043ff9d7025b9725f3e (accessed on 15th July 2025).

40. Saitta, D., & Garg, M. (2021). *Letter: Missed opportunities for the diagnosis of colorectal cancer in patients with inflammatory bowel disease—still significant room for improvement. Alimentary Pharmacology & Therapeutics, 54.* https://www.semanticscholar.org/paper/021 4b5601aa3cc37f614213c7ed64ef58885d5b9 (accessed on 15th July 2025).

41. Santacroce, G., Zammarchi, I., Tan, C. K., Coppola, G., Varley, R., Ghosh, S., & Iacucci, M. (2023). *Present and future of endoscopy precision for inflammatory bowel disease. Digestive Endoscopy, 36,* 292–304. https://www.semanticscholar.org/paper/9af7029c550b223c9f74d2affdcc2acb aa9eebc9 (accessed on 15th July 2025).

42. Seyedian, S. S., Nokhostin, F., & Dargahi-Malamir, M. (2019). *A review of the diagnosis, prevention, and treatment methods of inflammatory bowel disease. Journal of Medicine and Life, 12,* 113–122. https://doi.org/10.25122/jml-2018-0075 (accessed on 15th July 2025).

43. Snook, J., Bhala, N., Beales, I., Cannings, D., Kightley, C., Logan, R., Pritchard, D. M., et al. (2021). *British Society of Gastroenterology guidelines for the management of iron deficiency*

anemia in adults. Gut, 70, 2030–2051. https://doi.org/10.1136/gutjnl-2021-325210 (accessed on 15th July 2025).

44. Walsh, A., Fidalgo, C., Adamina, M., Barreiro de Acosta, M., Burisch, J., Drobne, D., Faiz, O., et al. (2024). DOP03 Gaps between ECCO quality standards of care and the real world: The E-QUALITY survey on processes and outcomes. *Journal of Crohn's and Colitis.* https://www.semanticscholar.org/paper/c83d6955e5ed74717869e568c1a6c7ce53b7b999 (accessed on 15th July 2025).

45. Wolf, A. M. D., Fontham, E. T. H., Church, T. R., Flowers, C. R., Guerra, C. E., LaMonte, S. J., Etzioni, R., et al. (2018). Colorectal cancer screening for average-risk adults: 2018 guideline update from the American Cancer Society. *CA: A Cancer Journal for Clinicians, 68*, 250–281. https://doi.org/10.3322/caac.21457 (accessed on 15th July 2025).

46. Yang, Y. J. (2023). *Current status of image-enhanced endoscopy in inflammatory bowel disease. Clinical Endoscopy, 56*, 563–577. https://doi.org/10.5946/ce.2023.070 (accessed on 15th July 2025).

47. Young, J. C., Helsingen, L., Refsum, E., Högdén, A., Perrin, V., Løberg, M., Gantzel, R., et al. (2025). *Temporal trends in characteristics and management of inflammatory bowel disease. Scandinavian Journal of Gastroenterology, 60*, 421–429. https://www.semanticscholar.org/paper/9573f64c4b446a12ada5633d41b6cde57d7139f4 (accessed on 15th July 2025).

48. Younis, M. Y., Khan, M. U., Khan, U., Khan, T. L., Mukarram, H., Jain, K., Ilyas, I., et al. (2024). *The current role of imaging in the diagnosis of inflammatory bowel disease and detection of its complications: A systematic review. Cureus, 16.* https://www.semanticscholar.org/paper/06556885836fe814170c4289205f30cf564e2342 (accessed on 15th July 2025).

49. Zammarchi, I., Santacroce, G., & Iacucci, M. (2023). *Next-generation endoscopy in inflammatory bowel disease. Diagnostics, 13*, 2547. https://doi.org/10.3390/diagnostics13152547 (accessed on 15th July 2025).

INDEX

A

Accordingly 165, 226, 290, 421, 444
Additional precautions 111
Advanced Modular Furnace 58
Aerodigestive clinics 376, 403
Aggressive treatment 362
AI-assisted anesthesia system 21
AI-augmented analysis 357
AI-based algorithms 367
AI-based diagnostics 304
AI-based systems 315
AI-driven advancements 271
AI researchers 327
Although small 7
American Cancer Society 25, 409, 439, 472
American Speech-Language-Hearing Association (ASHA) 427
Anesthesiologists 81, 379, 383, 384, 386, 389, 394, 424, 454
Another great aspect 301
Anticipatory gastrointestinal care 143
Anti-inflammatory drugs 104, 190, 193
Anti-tumor necrosis factor (TNF) 399
Anxiety management 66
Artificial intelligence 1, 4, 11, 25, 30, 32, 33, 46, 52, 55, 96, 116, 117, 143, 208, 209, 210, 218, 228, 239, 270, 278, 287, 304, 316, 330, 331, 338, 344, 349, 351, 353, 359, 364, 371, 372, 373, 379, 423, 443, 450, 451, 452, 454, 458, 460, 468, 469, 470
Atmospheric dispersion correctors (ADCs) 52
Augmented reality (AR) 13, 363
Autism spectrum disorder (ASD) 68
Automated systems 27, 255, 342, 360, 363
Automation and robotics 53

B

Balloon-assisted enteroscopy 252, 258, 259, 265, 274, 287, 289, 292, 293, 297, 299, 300, 301, 313
Bedrest Muscle Stress Apparatus 55, 62
Better-skilled workforce 43
Bleeding and obstruction 323
Blood pressure 79, 80, 81, 82
Body mass index (BMI) 449
Bronchoscopy 11, 12, 383, 384, 411, 412, 413

C

Caecal intubation rate (CIR). 87
Calibration procedures 57
Capsule endoscopy 4, 10, 249, 250, 253, 260, 263, 265, 266, 272, 273, 283, 340, 396, 406, 459, 471
Capsule endoscopy (SBCE) 282, 300
Capsule Ingestion Process 262
Cardiovascular instability 20, 75, 77, 79, 86, 109, 415
Chromatography 43, 44, 63
Chronic inflammation 207, 445, 447, 457
Chronic pain 441, 468

Circulating tumor cells (CTCs) 220
Clavien-Dindo grading 413
Clear liquids 105, 114
Clinical 20, 30, 31, 33, 34, 76, 89, 138, 155, 184, 234, 240, 245, 246, 247, 259, 273, 325, 333, 334, 338, 352, 370, 388, 399, 403, 405, 406, 412, 421, 436, 439, 442, 468, 470, 472
Clinical decision-making 15, 69, 102, 115, 127, 211, 226, 228, 237, 273, 304, 326, 364, 450, 460, 469
Clinical environment 327, 349, 353, 359
Clinical evidence supports 76
Clinical guidelines 11, 25, 112, 120, 128, 163, 195, 237, 367, 428, 461
Clinical indication 177
Clinical management 98, 102, 189, 442, 444, 458, 466
Clinical meaning 230
Clinical practice guidelines 164, 226, 282, 402, 404, 435, 470
Clinical practices 273, 399
Clinical procedures 68, 92, 358, 360
Clinical trials 138, 207, 240, 241, 333, 334, 336, 397
Clinicians excellent tools 281
Co-curricular approach 390
Cognitive-behavioral therapies 75, 87
Cognitive-behavioral therapy 68, 71, 76, 86
Collaborative efforts 44
Colon capsule endoscopy (CCE), 293
Colonoscopy 4, 127, 128, 130, 131, 133, 134, 135, 136, 138, 140, 141, 142, 143, 146, 147, 148, 151
Colonoscopy allows 129
Colonoscopy-done individuals 147
Colonoscopy procedure 133, 139, 144
Colorectal cancer 31, 129, 131, 143, 155, 165, 166, 181, 186, 439, 469, 472
Common bile duct (CBD) 199
Community Health Services 131
Comorbid patients 83
Complicating treatment 387
Complication monitoring 193
Comprehensive assessment 295
Comprehensive patient history 69
Computed tomographic angiography (CTA) 331
Computed tomography (CT) 233, 412, 445
Computer-aided polyp 423
Computer-assisted surgery (CAS) 343, 353
Computer-based data acquisition 42
Consequently 39, 45, 87, 97, 102, 160, 167, 231, 242, 256, 271, 305, 359
Continual learning 82
Continuous education 19
Continuous monitoring 80, 263, 384, 410, 429
Continuous monitoring during 139
Continuous monitoring modalities 80
Continuous wave (CW) 223
Control instrumentation 41
Conversely 177, 179, 223, 417, 444
Convolutional neural networks (CNNs) 271
Corrosive injury treatment 101
Cost-benefit assessment 461
Crohn's disease 6, 132, 133, 252, 258, 264, 265, 286, 289, 291, 295, 297, 307, 308, 323, 349, 395, 442, 444, 448, 452, 459, 460, 465, 469, 470
Crohn's disease (CD) 133, 459
Cross-disciplinary collaboration 375
Cultural perceptions 141
Current systematic reviews 326
Current technical 288
Cutting-edge imaging technology 264, 361

D

Decision-making about healthcare 330
Decision-making tools 143
Deep sedation 72, 75, 296
Determine treatment 446
Device-assisted enteroscopies (DAEs) 302
Diagnosing biliary tract disorders 192
Diagnostic technologies 241, 273, 274, 367, 465
Digital technologies 17, 117
Disruptive technology 266
Doris Sylvanus General Regional Hospital 387, 403
Double-balloon enteroscopy 283, 290

E

Early detection of cancer 141

Effective management 71, 193, 296, 323
Electromagnetic interference (EMI), 58
Emotional support systems 145
Emotion-based fears 146
Endocuff Vision 156, 333, 340
Endoscopic bile duct stone 205
Endoscopic mucosal resection (EMR) 6, 314, 318, 325
Endoscopic procedures 5, 9, 19, 311, 408, 411
Endoscopic retrograde cholangiopancreatography (ERCP) 4, 199, 208, 214, 234, 245, 303, 315, 339, 386, 414, 435
Endoscopic stenting 318
Endoscopic submucosal dissection (ESD) 6, 322, 433
Endoscopic techniques 4, 5, 6, 12, 13, 15, 20, 99, 111, 117, 162, 164, 165, 166, 193, 194, 209, 224, 264, 281, 283, 312, 314, 315, 317, 323, 331, 332, 346, 349, 354, 375, 379, 382, 385, 386, 408, 413, 423, 426, 432, 443, 445, 449, 450, 451, 457, 459, 465
Endoscopic technology 1, 2, 4, 5, 7, 8, 10, 13, 14, 15, 24, 25, 97, 121, 203, 208, 209, 219, 230, 273, 284, 315, 317, 320, 321, 332, 347, 350, 359, 379, 385, 408, 420, 421, 448, 449, 450, 457, 458, 459
Endoscopic tests 21, 159
Endoscopic therapy 331
Endoscopic treatment 285
Endoscopic ultrasonography (EUS) 102, 193, 286
Endoscopic ultrasound (EUS) 4, 10, 224, 225, 228, 230, 232, 234, 238, 246, 409, 420
Endoscopy 1, 2, 3, 4, 5, 7, 10, 12, 13, 16, 20, 23, 30, 31, 32, 34, 92, 95, 96, 99, 105, 116, 118, 123, 124, 125, 154, 185, 214, 216, 242, 245, 247, 249, 250, 251, 253, 257, 263, 270, 271, 277, 279, 285, 296, 299, 307, 308, 309, 311, 312, 315, 317, 318, 320, 321, 331, 332, 338, 341, 342, 345, 346, 348, 349, 352, 353, 375, 376, 379, 381, 382, 385, 388, 394, 395, 397, 404, 405, 407, 408, 409, 411, 412, 413, 414, 422, 427, 432, 435, 436, 438, 439, 441, 442, 443, 444, 445, 446, 447, 450, 451, 453, 454, 455, 456, 458, 459, 460, 461, 465, 468, 471, 472
Enforcing improved recovery after surgery (ERAS) 303
Enteroscopy procedure 294, 295, 297, 298
Enteroscopy techniques 282, 283, 287
Environmental monitoring 35, 38, 39, 41, 43, 44
Eosinophilic esophagitis (EoE) 393
Epstein–Barr virus (EBV) 395
Equipment maintenance 55
Esophagogastroduodenoscopy (EGD) 4, 9, 80, 95, 381, 411, 448
Ethical decision-making 391
Ethical standards 11, 24, 391, 399
EUS-guided fine needle aspiration (EUS-FNA) 217
EUS-guided procedures 228, 231, 237
EUS is in the celiac plexus neurolysis (EUS-CPN) 222
Evidence-based advice 89
Evidence-based recommendations 150, 151

F

Facilitate early treatment 171
Faecal occult blood test (FOBT) 163
False-negative diagnosis 135
Fecal Immunochemical Test (FIT) 147
Fiber-optic instruments 163
Fiber-optic technology 6, 321, 346, 347
Fine-needle aspiration 116, 219, 220, 221, 225, 226, 231, 245, 300, 327
Fine needle aspiration (FNA) 224
First-line treatment 175
Follow-up appointments 84, 113, 115, 174
Follow-up care 19, 23, 85, 111, 113, 176, 330, 429, 430, 464
Four-dimensional imaging 220

G

Game-changing technology 396
Gastric cancer 95, 402, 435
Gastric premalignant conditions (GPCs) 97
Gastroenterology history 284
Gastroesophageal reflux disease (GERD) 10, 101, 393, 411
Gastrointestinal 10, 23, 31, 32, 34, 92, 95, 96, 100, 105, 118, 123, 124, 132, 143, 156, 164, 214, 225, 245, 252, 257, 258, 268, 273, 277, 282, 283, 292, 296, 307, 308, 309, 318, 319, 321, 338, 339, 381, 382, 383, 404,

405, 409, 411, 412, 422, 427, 432, 435, 438, 439, 448, 455
Gastrointestinal bleeding 10, 13, 26, 95, 96, 97, 99, 100, 102, 106, 118, 125, 185, 220, 247, 250, 251, 257, 258, 259, 262, 264, 269, 271, 273, 277, 282, 283, 285, 286, 289, 290, 291, 292, 293, 297, 299, 302, 305, 308, 309, 315, 317, 321, 322, 331, 332, 340, 377, 379, 454, 456, 466
Gastrointestinal cancers 23, 217, 227, 230, 325
Gastrointestinal disease (GID) 395
Gastrointestinal disorders 14, 95, 97, 100, 105, 106, 116, 132, 133, 165, 177, 181, 205, 223, 224, 225, 239, 252, 257, 265, 291, 313, 318, 321, 322, 340, 377, 388, 399, 405, 419
Gastrointestinal endoscopy 4, 5, 9, 10, 11, 13, 21, 22, 30, 32, 68, 87, 95, 96, 97, 98, 100, 101, 102, 104, 105, 107, 108, 109, 111, 112, 113, 117, 119, 120, 123, 124, 185, 214, 215, 226, 245, 246, 277, 307, 318, 319, 322, 335, 338, 339, 340, 350, 355, 356, 381, 382, 383, 406, 411, 412, 416, 436, 439, 465, 468
Gastrointestinal health 115, 117, 120, 139, 145, 159, 181, 273, 282, 286, 300, 399
Gastrointestinal illness 13, 14, 97, 115, 117, 120, 144, 165, 219, 231, 242, 252, 274, 290, 318, 351, 376, 387, 391, 419
Gastrointestinal intervention 107, 192, 299, 415
Gastrointestinal neoplasia 100, 110, 124
Gastrointestinal symptoms 96, 100, 101, 102, 124, 164, 169, 178, 281, 290, 298, 389
Gastrointestinal tract 2, 4, 6, 7, 10, 15, 16, 17, 18, 21, 24, 96, 102, 104, 106, 107, 110, 111, 112, 114, 118, 120, 124, 132, 135, 147, 159, 160, 161, 163, 165, 171, 189, 196, 198, 220, 221, 222, 223, 224, 225, 227, 229, 230, 231, 234, 235, 238, 239, 250, 251, 252, 253, 254, 255, 256, 258, 260, 261, 262, 263, 264, 266, 268, 269, 270, 272, 274, 275, 279, 283, 285, 286, 287, 291, 292, 294, 296, 299, 305, 309, 312, 313, 314, 318, 319, 321, 323, 324, 325, 332, 339, 344, 346, 349, 352, 354, 363, 378, 379, 385, 386, 396, 399, 408, 411, 414, 426, 442, 443, 444, 445, 448, 449, 450, 452, 454, 455, 456, 459, 465
Gastrointestinal Ultrasound (GIUS) 282
Gavriel Iddan 286, 300, 304
General equipment 42
GI bleeding 98, 117, 166, 199, 270, 277, 291, 319, 332, 338
GI endoscopy 9, 79, 99, 103, 109, 125, 411
GI health 129, 270
Global diagnostic accuracy 275
Global health emergencies 397
Good discharge planning 84
GPT-capable chatbot 17

H

Harmonious equilibrium 204
Health-care coverage 157
Health care management 98
Healthcare practice 66, 174, 342
Healthcare professionals 11, 19, 23, 67, 68, 69, 77, 78, 79, 80, 81, 84, 85, 90, 104, 114, 117, 147, 171, 179, 231, 251, 271, 282, 324, 335, 367, 388, 394, 420, 421, 429, 444, 459, 462, 463, 465
Healthcare systems 10, 83, 120, 128, 132, 135, 142, 144, 150, 152, 174, 178, 182, 218, 252, 253, 313, 335, 362, 364, 387, 410, 424, 463
Healthcare workers 72, 168
Health disparities among 129
Health professionals 83, 90
Heat treatment 236
High-deductible health plans (HDHPs) 144
High-definition and optical 342
High-definition imaging 24, 116, 128, 143, 173, 317, 330, 331, 354, 355, 356, 375, 380, 449, 450
High-definition visualization 25, 107, 341, 378
High-efficiency operations 53
High-end imaging technology 354
Higher-risk patients 424, 429
High-quality images 148, 251, 255, 263, 282, 305
High-resolution images 147, 217, 218, 222, 224, 234, 235, 236, 254, 265, 279, 322
High-resolution imaging 10, 45, 201, 220, 227, 229, 230, 236, 242, 351, 367
High-resolution imaging capability 229
High-risk environments 58
High-risk populations 107, 130, 137, 198, 328
High-risk regions 120

High-tech imaging techniques 6
High-technology 38, 304, 446, 451
High-technology measuring 38
Hoped-for benefit 392

I

Image-enhanced endoscopy (IEE) 457
Immunomodulators 465
Increasingly patient-centered 259
Inflammatory bowel disease (IBD) 2, 121, 388, 441, 442, 445, 446, 471
Internal body structures 45
Intraperitoneal onlay mesh (IPOM) 393
Invasive surgical techniques 3, 5, 8, 165, 172, 387

L

Laboratory tests 389
Langley Research Center 54
Life-threatening gastrointestinal 26
Liver transplantation (LT) 426
Longer depending 109
Long-term outcomes 144, 176, 205, 322, 398, 399, 449, 452, 454
Long-term patient management outcomes 291

M

Machine learning 8, 23, 25, 26, 51, 54, 96, 117, 134, 143, 239, 271, 272, 287, 304, 315, 344, 348, 351, 353, 356, 363, 366, 378, 396, 443
Magnet-controlled capsule 107, 123
Magnetic Resonance CholangioPancreatography (MRCP) 234
Magnetic resonance enterography (MRE) 295, 446
Magnetic resonance imaging (MRI) 233, 258, 360, 445
Maintaining measurement integrity 56
Maternal pregnancy-associated 327
Medical clinicians 149
Medical equipment 37
Medical intervention 3, 110, 143, 248, 329, 376
Medical procedures 71
Medicare coverage 140
Medication classes 420
Minimally invasive transforaminal lumbar interbody fusion (MI-TLIF). 8
Minimal sedation 73, 74
Moderate sedation 74, 105
Monitoring devices 47
Monitoring post-procedure 111
Mother-baby 408
Multi-functional ultrasound modalities 223
Multi-view pose estimation 344

N

Narrow-band imaging 6, 25, 163, 208, 270, 317, 330, 331, 332, 345, 357, 358, 426
Narrowband imaging (NBI) 348
Natural Language Processing (NLP) 192
Necessitates vigilant monitoring 171
Nevertheless 50, 147, 201, 289, 390, 423
New EUS techniques 116
Nishtar Hospital Multan 18, 33
Non-invasive methods of monitoring 239
Non-invasive monitoring 380
Non-invasive nature 147, 149, 265
Non-invasive technologies 297, 380
Non-invasive way 250, 260, 300
Non-screened individuals 142
Non-surgical intervention 320
Non-surgical method 148

O

Office of Aeronautics and Space Technology (OAST) 53
On-board equipment 57
Operator skill 302
Optical coherence tomography (OCT) 45, 224, 348
Oral squamous cell carcinoma (OSCC) 351
Organizational guidelines 360
Over-the-scope clips (OTSC) 325

P

Pain control techniques 391
Pain management 175
Pancreatic assessment 226

Pancreatitis-related disease 195
Parental involvement 390, 404
Patient care practices 48
Patient-centered areas 251
Patient-centered treatment 331
Patient-centric 317, 432
Patient demographics 115
Patient-driven comprehensive 67
Patient education 16, 18, 21, 22, 66, 76, 103, 104, 134, 142, 144, 151, 173, 175, 198, 294, 295, 296, 297, 329, 412, 415, 418, 430, 431, 432, 438, 462, 463, 465
Patient experience 144
Patient-focused tools 72
Patient history 69, 180, 196, 298
Patient-oriented medicine 48
Patient preparation 66, 67, 77, 89, 462
Patient-related factors 233, 421
Patient-reported outcomes 442, 462
Patient safety 3, 5, 10, 11, 16, 17, 19, 20, 21, 24, 67, 68, 70, 71, 75, 76, 77, 78, 79, 80, 81, 82, 83, 87, 89, 97, 100, 102, 103, 104, 105, 111, 112, 113, 118, 135, 136, 139, 172, 175, 190, 196, 197, 198, 199, 200, 201, 202, 204, 208, 211, 212, 229, 233, 234, 237, 239, 241, 252, 263, 273, 296, 297, 301, 302, 314, 321, 328, 329, 330, 334, 346, 352, 356, 362, 363, 378, 379, 385, 389, 394, 395, 407, 409, 410, 417, 419, 420, 421, 423, 425, 426, 427, 428, 429, 432, 433, 457
Patient sedation and preparation 65
Patients need 168, 261, 265
Patient-specific recommendations 149
Patients typically report 260
Patients undergoing sigmoidoscopy 174
Patient teaching regarding 113
Percutaneous endoscopic gastrostomy (PEG) 382
Percutaneous nephrolithotomy (PCN) 12
Personalized approaches 332, 385
Personalized medicine's 367
Personalized scheduling 143
Personalized treatment 285, 316, 331, 335, 356, 357, 445
Pharmacological strategy 77
Photodynamic diagnosis (PDD) 316
Photodynamic therapy (PDT) 316
Physiological variations 377
Pill-sized camera 10, 249, 250
Point-of-care intestinal ultrasound (POC IUS) 465
Post-anesthesia care 197
Post-anesthesia care unit (PACU) 105
Post-EGDEX 99
Post-ERCP complications 200, 202, 206
Post-polypectomy bleeding 139
Postprocedural complications 384
Post-procedure after colonoscopy 136
Post-procedure bleeding 171, 457
Post-procedure cannot 85
Post-procedure care 22, 67, 85, 99, 108, 112, 113, 119, 136, 137, 145, 174, 176, 188, 197, 207, 295, 430, 463, 464
post-procedure instructions 75
Post-procedure monitoring 22, 263, 299
Post-procedure recovery needs 15
Post-procedure surveillance 456
Post-sedation care 82
Power sources 254
Pre-emptive measures 145
Pre-exam bowel preparation 158
Pre-existing cardiac 196
Pre-existing gastrointestinal 105, 110, 137, 138, 269
Pre-procedural dietary 196
Pre-procedure anxiety 10, 18, 67, 81, 146
Pre-procedure counseling 18, 139, 168, 172, 393
Pre-procedure discussion 174
Pre-sedation physical assessment 70
Pre-sedation protocols 76
Preventive maintenance measures 56
Probe-based confocal laser endomicroscopy (pCLE) 222, 354
Proper monitoring 85, 201
Proper preparation 134
Public health goals 160
Pulmonary artery sling (PAS) 383

Q

Qualitative assessment 89
Quality improvement 71

R

Radio frequency (RF) 267
Real-time feedback during 25, 366, 380
Real-time images 163, 218, 221
Real-time imaging 6, 191, 200, 208, 226, 229, 233, 235, 257, 264, 345, 351, 363, 365, 368, 451
Real-time imaging and assessment 208
Real-time navigation 237
Real-time video 1
Real-time visualization 9, 13, 170, 229, 230, 238, 343
Real-world ice protection 40
Registered nurses (RNs) 118
Research and clinical trials 240, 241
Research-technologists 52
Rigid bronchoscopy 382
Risk-increasing factors 140
Robot-assisted techniques 15
Robotic-assisted systems 8
Rudolf Schindler 5, 7

S

Safer environment 396
Saturn IB rocket systems 59
Scanning electron microscopy (SEM) 45
Screening for colorectal cancer 165
Screening tests 154, 163
Second major shortcoming 270
Self-expanding metal stents (SEMS) 312, 426
Sigmoidoscopy 157, 158, 159, 160, 161, 165, 167, 168, 169, 172, 175, 177, 178, 179
Sigmoidoscopy and proctoscopy 157, 160, 165, 167, 168, 172, 178
Since biliary disease 202
Single-operator cholangioscopy 357
Small body anatomical dimensions 392
Small bowel disease 257, 291
Social networking sites (SNSs) 390
Soft-tissue structures 365, 367
Space-like environments 46
Space Station Freedom (SSF) 54
Specific interventions 106
Statistical process control (SPC) 50
Stent-related infections 207
Successful troubleshooting 58
Super minimally invasive surgery (SMIS) 15
Surgery-sparing approach 454
Surgical Data Science (SDS) 378
Surgical decision-making 8
Sustained learning 12

T

Targeted biopsies 166
T-cell lymphoma patient 322
Techniques and technology 143, 160
Technologies 25, 56, 128, 271, 360, 379, 395, 448
Technology and pharmacologic 378
Thick Gas Electron Multipliers (THGEM) 37
Total Quality Management (TQM) 50
Traditional biopsy procedures 354
Traditional endoscopy 4, 116, 219, 251, 256, 264, 290, 332, 365, 445, 465, 466
Traditionally 14, 286, 328
Transanal endoscopic microsurgery (TEM) 161
Transanal minimal invasive surgery (TAMIS) 167
Transient bowel habit disturbances 172

U

Ultrasound capsule endoscopy (USCE) 218, 250
Unilateral Biportal Endoscopy (UBE) 408
United States increases 181
United States Preventive Services Task Force (USPSTF) 131

V

Variations demonstrate 165
Various age groups 100
Various clinical circumstances 178
Various clinical settings 3
Various cystic neoplasms 237
Various fields 35
Various medical fields 355, 356
Various multidisciplinary techniques 210
Various physical properties 38
Varying external environment 49
Vascular architecture 350

Virtual reality (VR) 361
Vision during endoscopy 16
Volatile organic compounds (VOCs) 14
Vulnerable populations 77, 79, 89, 105, 200, 324, 329, 380

W

Water-assisted colonoscopy (WAC) 15
Well-prepared bowel 261
Well-rounded appreciation 36
White light endoscopy (WLE), 354
Wireless capsule endoscopy (WCE) 132, 252, 253, 308, 317, 364

X

X-ray fluorescence spectrometry 39
X-ray phase-contrast imaging (XPCI) 49

Z

Zollinger-Ellison syndrome 323